W9-BME-187

TRANSCULTURAL

ASSESSMENT AND
INTERVENTION **NURSING**

Joyce Newman Giger, Ed.D., R.N., C.S.
Professor and Chair, Department of Nursing,
Columbus College,
Columbus, Georgia;
Formerly Associate Professor and Chair,
Health Professions/Nursing,
Bethel College,
Mishawaka, Indiana

Ruth Elaine Davidhizar, D.N.S., R.N., C.S.
Director of Nursing,
Logansport State Hospital,
Logansport, Indiana;
Associate Professor,
Health Professions/Nursing,
Bethel College,
Mishawaka, Indiana

Illustrated

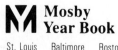 **Mosby
Year Book**

St. Louis   Baltimore   Boston   Chicago   London   Philadelphia   Sydney   Toronto

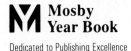

Mosby
Year Book

Dedicated to Publishing Excellence

Editor: Linda L. Duncan
Editorial assistant: Rebecca Sweeney
Project manager: Patricia Gayle May
Production editor: Judith Bange
Designer: Susan Lane

Copyright © 1991 by Mosby—Year Book, Inc.
A Mosby imprint of Mosby—Year Book, Inc.

All rights reserved. No part of this publication may be reproduced, stored
in a retrieval system, or transmitted, in any form or by any means,
electronic, mechanical, photocopying, recording, or otherwise, without prior
permission from the publisher.

Printed in the United States of America

Mosby—Year Book, Inc.
11830 Westline Industrial Drive, St. Louis, Missouri 63146

Library of Congress Cataloging-in-Publication Data

Transcultural nursing: assessment and intervention/[edited by]
  Joyce Newman Giger, Ruth Elaine Davidhizar.
        p.   cm.
    Includes bibliographical references.
    Includes index.
    ISBN 0-8016-1928-9
    1. Transcultural nursing.   I. Giger, Joyce Newman.
  II. Davidhizar, Ruth Elaine.
    [DNLM: 1. Cross Cultural Comparison.   2. Ethnic Groups.
  3. Nursing Assessment.   4. Nursing Care.   WY 87 T7715]
  RT86.54.T73   1991
  610.73—dc20
  DNLM/DLC
  for Library of Congress   90-6173
                                                    CIP

C/C/D   9 8 7 6 5 4 3 2 1

······ Contributors

Margaret Bowen, B.S.N., R.N.
Assistant Director of Nursing Service,
Logansport State Hospital,
Logansport, Indiana

Karen Chang, M.S.N., R.N.
Assistant Professor,
Purdue University School of Nursing,
West Lafayette, Indiana

Brenda Cherry, B.S.N., R.N., C.C.R.N.
Staff Nurse, CCU,
Emory University Hospital,
Decatur, Georgia

Robert E. Cosgray, M.A., B.S.N., R.N.C.
Nursing Supervisor,
Logansport State Hospital,
Logansport, Indiana

Ruth Elaine Davidhizar, D.N.S., R.N.,
C.S.
Director of Nursing,
Logansport State Hospital,
Logansport, Indiana;
Associate Professor,
Health Professions/Nursing,
Bethel College,
Mishawaka, Indiana

Joyce Newman Giger, Ed.D., R.N., C.S.
Professor and Chair, Department of Nursing,
Columbus College,
Columbus, Georgia;
Formerly Associate Professor and Chair,
Health Professions/Nursing,
Bethel College,
Mishawaka, Indiana

Catherine E. Hanley, M.S.N., R.N.,
F.A.C.H.E.
Health Systems Administrator,
Deputy Service Unit Director,
USPHS Indian Hospital,
Tuba City, Arizona

Joan Kuipers, M.S.N., R.N.
Assistant Professor,
Purdue University School of Nursing,
Lafayette, Indiana

Dolly Lefever, M.S., R.N., A.N.P.,
C.N.M.
Nurse Practitioner,
Palmer, Alaska

Cheryl Martin, M.S.N., R.N.C.
Associate Professor of Nursing,
Bethel College,
Mishawaka, Indiana

Scott Wilson Miller, M.S., R.N., C.P.A.N.
Nursing Information Systems Manager,
Saint Agnes Medical Center,
Fresno, California

Enid A. Schwartz, M.S., R.N.C.
Instructor of Nursing,
Cochise College,
Douglas, Arizona

Cynthia C. Small, M.S.N., R.N.
Instructor, Medical-Surgical Nursing,
Lake Michigan College,
Benton Harbor, Michigan

Linda S. Smith, M.S.N., R.N.
Editorial Director, ADvancing CLINICAL
    CARE;
Nurse Educator,
Gateway Technical College,
Nursing Division,
Kenosha, Wisconsin

Ruth Yoder Stauffer, M.S.N., R.N.
Staff Nurse,
Hospice Care,
Honolulu, Hawaii

Jill Nerala Supersad, B.S.N., R.N.
Staff Nurse—Coronary Care Unit,
Pacific Presbyterian Medical Center,
San Francisco, California

Anna Rambharose Vance, Ph.D. candidate,
M.A., R.N.
Assistant Professor of Nursing,
Bethel College,
Mishawaka, Indiana

TO

OUR PARENTS
Ionia Holmes Newman and Lucille and Ralph Holderman
and the late Naomi Holderman

OUR HUSBANDS
Argusta Giger, Jr., and Ronald Davidhizar

OUR MENTORS
Frances P. Dixon, B.S., and Angela Barron McBride, Ph.D., R.N., F.A.A.N.

AND
the students of Bethel College, past and present

Foreword

Caring has long been regarded as the foundation of nursing practice (Benner & Wrubel, 1988; Leininger, 1988; Watson, 1985). The American Nurses' Association has gone on record as describing the profession as "committed to the care and nurturing of sick and well people, individually and in groups" (1980, p. 9). Fry (1989) has argued that the central value of nursing ethics is caring that protects and enhances the human dignity of patients. A 1989 Wingspread Conference on *Knowledge about Care and Caring: State of the Art and Future Development*, cosponsored by the American Academy of Nursing and Sigma Theta Tau International in collaboration with the Johnson Foundation and select nursing schools, discussed care and caring as core representations of nursing and set an agenda for the future that called for elaborating on the characteristics of the need for care, agents of care, recipients of care, context of care, methods of care, and goals of care in a range of specific clinical situations (McBride, 1989).

This volume on transcultural nursing, edited by Giger and Davidhizar, addresses aspects of that agenda by elaborating in great detail on what constitutes culturally appropriate care. In proposing a framework for assessment that focuses on six key cultural phenomena thought to shape care—communication, space, social organization, time, environmental control, and biological variations—the authors provide students and practitioners with a template for systematically exploring how caregivers' responses, recipients of care, contexts of care, and goals of care may vary, given the cultural diversity in the United States. Not only do the many chapters specifying how a particular cultural group (for example, Black, Appalachian, Navajo, Eskimo, or Mexican American) may vary in these six areas provide rich information that heightens awareness of the special perspectives that must be taken into account in planning care, but these chapters also provide a model for looking at the experience of other populations not included in this book.

It has become commonplace for nurse educators to advocate culturally appropriate care, but what that really means other than some general admonition to be aware that not all patients with the same medical diagnosis are likely to have the same experience is not clear. Indeed, the notion that patients make choices based on the unique meaning of their illness experience is often discounted on a day-to-day basis when the emphasis seems to be more on the importance of routine, procedures, and covering the unit than it is on providing individualized attention. Yet this volume forces the reader to confront the many ways in which an individual's experience is likely to vary in ways that go well beyond the patternings of medical diagnosis: Is this man or who responds well to high touch? Does this woman need considerable personal space? Will an effective intervention necessarily have to involve the client's extended family? Does this patient have little future orientation? What are this person's beliefs about the nature of illness? What does well-oxygenated skin color look like when the infant being rated on the Apgar Scale is not White?

This volume, which draws on the clinical experience of many individuals, speaks to the needs of our pluralistic society by providing a wealth of insights about how cultural assessment is that part of the nursing process that considers the meaning of behaviors that might, if not understood within the context of ethnic values, be regarded as puzzling or even negative. The details make us sensitive to the concerns of various population groups; the framework provides a general approach to cultural assessment; the case studies and study questions encourage further creative thinking on this broad topic. In the final analysis, this volume is a part of the growing health care revolution that is critical of the professional who paternalistically sets out to do what is best for the patient, and that emphasizes, instead, the importance of the patient's concept of his or her own good for directing the professional's caregiving.

Angela Barron McBride, Ph.D., R.N., F.A.A.N.
Professor and Associate Dean for Research,
Indiana University School of Nursing

REFERENCES

American Nurses' Association. (1980). *Nursing—A social policy statement*. Kansas City, Mo.: Author.

Benner, P., & Wrubel, J. (1988). *The primacy of caring*. Reading, Mass.: Addison-Wesley.

Fry, S.T. (1989). The role of caring in a theory of nursing ethics. *Hypatia, 4*(2), 88-103.

Leininger, M. (Ed.). (1988). *Care: The essence of nursing and health*. Thorofare, N.J.: Slack.

McBride, A.B. (1989). Knowledge about care and caring: State of the art and future development. *Reflections, 15*(2), 5-7.

Watson, J. (1985). *Nursing: The philosophy and science of caring*. Boulder: Colorado Associated University Press.

Preface

This book was written for all nurses and nursing students who are interested in developing a knowledge of transcultural concepts to apply to patient care. A good foundation in transcultural nursing is essential for the nurse, since it can provide a conceptual framework for holistic patient care in a variety of clinical settings and assist the nurse throughout a nursing career.

The concept of transcultural nursing is relatively new to the nursing literature. In fact, it has only been in the last two decades that nurses have begun to develop an appreciation for the need to incorporate culturally appropriate clinical approaches into the daily routines of patient care. Although nurses have begun to recognize the need for culturally appropriate clinical approaches, the literature on this subject is either scanty or does not provide a systematic method for comprehensive assessment.

Several years ago we were challenged by the nursing students at Bethel College to develop a systematic approach to patient assessment for use with patients from diverse transcultural backgrounds. The nursing students reported difficulties in finding adequate literature to assist in planning care for patients from transcultural backgrounds. We also had identified this need by virtue of our own diverse cultural backgrounds; one of us is African American and was raised in the South, and the other is White and was raised in an Eskimo setting in Alaska. Thus in response to both personal interest and the need identified by the students, we set about synthesizing a body of literature that would assist students and nurses in developing the theoretical knowledge necessary to provide culturally appropriate care.

We selected contributing authors with expertise and clinical backgrounds in the care of selected cultural groups. The uniqueness of this book is that many of the chapters were written by contributing authors who actually represent by ethnic heritage the cultural group described. Not only are unique and diverse cultures represented, but the contributing authors span the continent with representation literally from coast to coast, for example, from California to Alaska and Hawaii.

We believe this book has applicability across other disciplines, such as psychology, sociology, medicine, and anthropology, since it provides not only a nursing perspective but also a historical and bioethnological approach to transcultural nursing care.

In our commitment to transcultural nursing we have made every effort, through extensive research, to be as culturally sensitive as possible and not offend our readers or specific cultural groups.

The text is divided into two parts. The first part, which focuses on theory, includes an introduction and six chapters describing the six cultural phenomena that make up our transcultural conceptual theory of assessment. The six cultural phenomena that we have identified as being evidenced in all cultural groups include (1) communication, (2) space, (3) social organization, (4) time, (5) environmental control, and (6) biological variations. The chapters describe how these phenomena vary with application and utilization across cultures.

The second part contains chapters by contributing authors in which the six cultural phenomena are systematically applied to the assessment and care of individuals in specific cultures. Thus the assessment model is applied to persons in diverse cultural settings by nurses who have expertise and sensitivity in the cultural group and in the unique care strategies that a nurse should use in providing culturally appropriate care.

ACKNOWLEDGMENTS

We would first like to acknowledge and thank our editor, Linda Duncan, whose belief in this project allowed it to come to fruition. Special recognition is given to Margaret Bowen, B.S.N., R.N., for emotional support and for critiquing and reviewing the manuscript; to Robert Cosgray, M.A., B.S.N., R.N.C., and Jeanne Larson, M.L.S., for computer searches; and to Melba Nunemaker for assistance in typing the final manuscript. In addition, we would like to acknowledge Curtis Stump and Gail Reichart, student research assistants, Bethel College, for the countless hours spent assisting us in locating the materials to complete this project. We would also like to acknowledge and thank Joan Tapp, M.L.S., reference librarian, Bethel College, for her valuable assistance. In addition, we would like to thank the many cultural experts involved in individual review of each chapter for ethnic authenticity.

Recognition is also given to Dotty Kauffmann, B.S.N., R.N., for excellent photographic work, as well as to the many individuals who submitted willingly to being photographed and included in this text.

Finally, we would like to thank each other for the unselfish sacrifice of more than 3 years of our time to this project and acknowledge the friendship and respect that have grown over the years.

Joyce Newman Giger
Ruth Elaine Davidhizar

······· Contents

PART ONE

FRAMEWORK FOR CULTURAL ASSESSMENT AND INTERVENTION TECHNIQUES

··

CHAPTER 1

Introduction to Transcultural Nursing

Theories of transcultural nursing with established clinical approaches to patients from varying cultures are relatively new. According to Madeline Leininger (1987), the education of nursing students in the area of transcultural nursing, which began in the mid-1960s, is only now beginning to yield significant results.

Today, nurses with different cultural insights and a deeper appreciation of human life and values are developing a sensitivity for culturally appropriate, individualized clinical approaches as a result of the introduction of transcultural concepts into nursing curricula and movements such as the development of the Transcultural Nursing Society, founded in 1974, to promote interest and preparation of nurses in transcultural nursing (Giger & Davidhizar, 1990; Wenger, 1989).

Since its inception the Transcultural Nursing Society has promoted such efforts as an annual transcultural nursing conference in different, worldwide locations. In addition, the Transcultural Nursing Society publishes the *Transcultural Nursing Society Newsletter* and implemented the first certification plan in transcultural nursing. Through the efforts of the Transcultural Nursing Society, 28 nurses received certification in 1988. Since July 1989 the Transcultural Nursing Society has also published the *Journal of Transcultural Nursing,* which has joined the already existing international nursing journals, the *International Journal of Nursing Studies* and the *International Nursing Review*. Other international conferences such as that supported by the Rockefeller Foundation in October 1988 in Bellagio, Italy, have sought to promote international health care management. Although the literature on patient approaches in culturally diverse situations is mushrooming and nurses are beginning to do transcultural research studies, relatively few theories on transcultural nursing to date have provided a systematic method for comprehensive nursing assessment (Leininger, 1985a; Tripp-Reimer, 1983, 1984; Tripp-Reimer & Dougherty, 1985; Tripp-Reimer & Friedl, 1977).

TRANSCULTURAL NURSING DEFINED

To understand transcultural nursing and implications for nursing practice, one must have a basic understanding of culture, cultural values, and culturally diverse nursing care. *Culture* may be defined as the values, beliefs, norms, and practices of a particular group that are learned and shared and that guide thinking, decisions, and actions in a patterned way (Leininger, 1985a). Leininger (1985a) goes on to define *cultural values* as a desirable or preferred way of acting or knowing something that over time is reinforced and sustained by the culture and ultimately governs one's actions or decisions. *Culturally diverse nursing care* refers to the variability in nursing approaches needed to provide culturally appropriate patient care. Culturally diverse nursing care must take into account six cultural phenomena that vary with application and use, yet are evidenced among all cultural groups: (1) communication, (2) space, (3) social organization, (4) time, (5) environmental control, and (6) biological variations.

CULTURAL ASSESSMENT

In a pluralistic society nurse practitioners need to be prepared to work with all patients regardless of cultural background and to provide culturally appropriate nursing care for each patient. To provide culturally appropriate nursing care, nurses must understand specific factors that influence individual health and illness behaviors (Tripp-Reimer, Brink, & Saunders, 1984). According to Affonso (1979), cultural assessment can give meaning to behaviors that might otherwise be judged negatively. If cultural behaviors are not appropriately identified, their significance will be confusing to the nurse.

In recent years transcultural nursing theories have appeared in the literature (Affonso, 1979; Leininger, 1985a, 1985b); however, adequate nursing assessment methods to accompany these theories have not been consistently provided. One of the most comprehensive tools used for nursing cultural assessment is the *Outline of Cultural Material* by Murdock et al. (1971); however, this tool was primarily developed for anthropologists who were concerned with ethnographic descriptions of cultural groups. While the tool is well developed and contains 88 major categories, it was not designed for nurse practitioners; thus it does not provide for systematic use of the nursing process. Another assessment tool is found in Brownlee's (1978) *Community, Culture and Care: A Cross-Cultural Guide for Health Care Workers*. Brownlee's work is devoted to the process of practical assessment of a community, with specific attention given to health areas. It deals with three aspects of assessment: what to find out, why it is important, and how to do it. Brownlee's assessment tool has been criticized as being too comprehensive, too difficult, and too detailed for use with individual patients. While this tool was developed for use by health care practitioners, it is not exclusively a nursing assessment tool.

In response to the apparent lack of practical assessment tools available in nursing for evaluating cultural variables and their effects on health and illness behaviors, this text provides a systematic approach to evaluating the six essential cultural phenomena to assist the nurse in providing culturally appropriate nursing care.

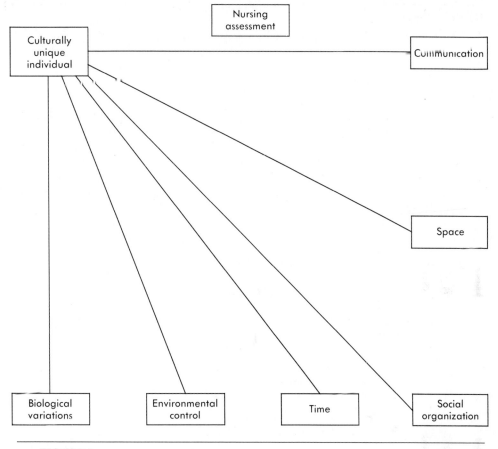

FIGURE 1

Application of cultural phenomena to nursing care and nursing practice.

TRANSCULTURAL ASSESSMENT MODEL

Although the six cultural phenomena mentioned previously—(1) communication, (2) space, (3) social organization, (4) time, (5) environmental control, and (6) biological variations—are evidenced among all cultural groups, they vary with application and use across cultures. Thus an individualized assessment approach of these six areas is indicated when working with patients from diverse cultural groups (Figure 1).

In this book the six cultural phenomena are presented in individual chapters with areas that need to be assessed when working with patients from multicultural populations. In addition, these six phenomena are applied to the care and management of patients in 14 subcultural groups found in the United States and throughout the world. A comprehensive nursing assessment is necessary for both the nurse practitioner and the researcher in order to provide culturally appropriate nursing care.

REFERENCES

Affonso, D. (1979). Framework for cultural assessment. In A.L. Clark (Ed.), *Childbearing: A nursing perspective* (2nd ed.), (pp. 107-119). Philadelphia: F.A. Davis.

Brownlee, A.T. (1978). *Community, culture, and care: A cross-cultural guide for health workers.* St. Louis: C.V. Mosby.

Giger, J., & Davidhizar, R. (1990). Transcultural nursing assessment: A method of advancing nursing practice. *International Nursing Review, 37*(1), 199-202.

Leininger, M. (1985a). *Qualitative Research Methods in Nursing.* Orlando, Fla.: Grune & Stratton.

Leininger, M. (1985b). Transcultural care diversity and universality: a theory of nursing. *Nursing and Health Care, 6*(4), 209-212.

Leininger, M. (1987). A new generation of nurses discover transcultural nursing (editorial). *Nursing and Health Care, 8,* 5.

Murdock, G., et al. (1971). *Outline of cultural materials* (4th ed.). New Haven, Conn.: Human Relations Area Files.

Tripp-Reimer, T. (1983). Retention of a folk-healing practice (matiasma) among four generations of urban Greek immigrants. *Nursing Research 32*(2), 97-101.

Tripp-Reimer, T. (1984). Research in cultural diversity. *Western Journal of Nursing Research, 6*(3), 353-355.

Tripp-Reimer, T., Brink, P., & Saunders, J. (1984). Cultural assessment: Content and process, *Nursing Outlook, 32*(2), 78-82.

Tripp-Reimer, T., & Dougherty, M.C. (1985). Cross-cultural nursing research. *Annual Review of Nursing Research, 3,* 77-104.

Tripp-Reimer, T., & Friedl, M. (1977). Appalachians: A neglected minority. *Nursing Clinics of North America, 12*(1), 41-54.

Wenger, F. (1989). President's address. *Transcultural Nursing Society Newsletter, 9*(1), 3.

CHAPTER 2

. . . .

Communication

BEHAVIORAL OBJECTIVES
After reading this chapter, the nurse will be able to:

1 Describe the importance of communication as it relates to transcultural nursing assessment.

2 Delineate barriers to communication that hinder the development of a nurse-patient relationship in transcultural settings.

3 Understand the importance of dialect, style, volume, use of touch, context of speech, and kinesics, and their relationship to transcultural nursing assessment and care.

4 Describe appropriate nursing intervention techniques used by the nurse to develop positive communication in the nurse-patient relationship.

5 Understand the significance of nonverbal communication and the use of silence, and their relationship to transcultural nursing assessment and care.

6 Explain the significance of the structure and format of names in various cultural groups.

7 Explain the significance of variations in word meanings across and within various cultural and ethnic groups.

The word *communication* comes from the Latin verb *communicare:* "to make common, share, participate, or impart" (Guralnik, 1972). Communication, however, goes further than this definition implies and embraces the entire realm of human interaction and behavior. All behavior, whether verbal or nonverbal, in the presence of another individual is communication (Potter & Perry, 1989; Watzlawich, Beavin, & Jackson, 1967).

As the matrix of all thought and relationships between people, communication provides the means by which people connect. It establishes a sense of commonness with another and permits the sharing of information, signals, or messages in the form of ideas and feelings. Communication is a continuous process by which one person may affect another through written or oral language, gestures, facial expressions, body language, space, or other symbols.

Nurses have long recognized the importance of communication in the healing process. Communication is the core of most nursing curricula. In spite of this, communication frequently presents barriers between nurses and patients, especially when the patients are from diverse cultural backgrounds. If the nurse and the patient do not speak the same language, or if communication styles and patterns differ, both the nurse and the patient may feel alienated and helpless. A patient who does not understand what is happening or who feels misunderstood may appear angry, noncompliant, or withdrawn. The physical healing process may be impaired. Nurses may also feel angry and helpless if their communication is not understood or if the patient cannot be understood. Without the ability to communicate, care will be inadequate. Nurses need to have not only a working knowledge of communication with patients of the same culture, but also a thorough awareness of racial, cultural, and social factors that may affect communication with persons from other cultures. Fielding and Llewelyn (1987) recently related that while communication skills are needed in nursing curricula, the more important issue is the broader understanding of the patient from a cultural perspective.

Nurses need to have an awareness of how an individual, although speaking the same language, may differ in communication patterns and understandings as a result of cultural orientation. Nurses must also have communication skills in relating to individuals who do not speak a familiar language (Kasch, 1984; Knowles, 1983). Most nurses generally assume that their perceptions and assessment of the patient's health status are accurate and congruent with those of the patient. Despite the patient education process, however, there is evidence that discrepancies in perceptions persist. These discrepancies should be of particular concern to the nurse when providing transcultural nursing care because they may interfere with the provision of that care. Many factors obstruct quality patient care, including poor communication, noncompliance with the treatment regimen, inadequate or unnecessary treatment, and ethical problems. All of these factors combine to create discrepancies in perceptions between nurse and patient (Molzahn & Northcott, 1989).

COMMUNICATION AND CULTURE

Communication and culture are closely intertwined. Communication is the means by which culture is transmitted and preserved (Delgado, 1983). On the other hand, culture influences how feelings are expressed and what verbal and nonverbal expressions are appropriate. Americans may be more likely to conceal feelings, and the United States is considered a low-touch culture, whereas a member of an Eastern culture may be open and loud with expressions of grief, anger, or joy, and may use touch more (Hall, 1966; Thayer, 1988). Other cultural variables, such as the perception of time, bodily contact, and territorial rights, also influence communication. The cultural differences in contact can be quite dramatic. Sidney Jourard (1971) reported that when touch between pairs of people in coffee shops around the world was studied, there was more touch in certain cities. For example, it was reported that touch occurred as frequently as 180 times an hour between couples in San Juan, Puerto Rico, and 110 times an hour in Paris, France. In other cities there was less touch; specifically, touch occurred two times an hour between couples in Gainesville, Florida, and zero times an hour in London, England.

Cultural patterns of communication are embedded early and are found in child-rearing practices. Gibson (1984) studied the playgrounds and beaches of Greece, the Soviet Union, and the United States and compared the frequency and nature of touch between caregivers and children ranging in age from 2 to 5 years. The analysis of data suggests that while rates of touching for retrieving or punishing the children were similar, rates of touching for soothing, holding, and play were dissimilar. American children were less likely to be touched than children from other cultures.

The communication practices of persons in individual cultural groups affect the expression of ideas and feelings, decision making, and communication strategies. The communication of an individual reflects, determines, and consequently molds the culture (Hedlund, 1988; Kretch, Crutchfield, & Ballachey, 1962). In other words, a culture may be limited and molded by its communication practices. Sapir (1929) proposed that individuals are at the mercy of the particular language that has become the medium of expression of their society. Experiences are determined by language habits that predispose the individual to certain conceptions of the world and choices of interpretation.

Variations in communication may be limited to specific meanings for a few individuals in a small group, for example, a family group. On the other hand, some communication patterns appear to be found in persons from a certain culture. In any case, the nurse must be cautious about assuming that a certain communication pattern can be generalized to all persons in a designated cultural group, since communication patterns are often unique. While the nurse assessing the patient should keep in mind common cultural patterns, it is essential to approach the patient as an individual who should not be categorized because of cultural heritage.

LINGUISTICS

Since communication is a broad concept and encompasses all of human behavior, it has been conceptualized in many ways. One way is to consider the structure of communication, as in linguistics. The major focus on the structure of communication has been developed within the fields of ethnomethodology in sociology and linguistics in anthropology. Structure may be perceived as a form of language and the use of words and behaviors to construct messages. The role of ethnomethodologists is to consider the structure and effects of communication and to look at rules of communication and the consequences of breaking these rules. Ethnomethodologists not only have emphasized the study of the structure and rules of language, but also have studied the structure and rules of nonverbal communication (Sudnow, 1967). Linguistics is the area within anthropology concerned with the study of the structure of language. Linguistic patterns represent more than the use of grammatically nonequivalent words; these patterns can create real disparity in social treatment.

FUNCTIONS OF COMMUNICATION

Another way to think about communication is to consider what it achieves or accomplishes in human interaction. Consideration of the functions of communication refers to examining what the communication accomplishes rather than how the communication is structured. A relationship exists between communication structure and communication function in the sense that structure does affect function.

As a part of human interaction, communication discloses information or provides a specific message. Messages can be sent with no expectation of a response. Included in the disclosure of information may be an element of self-disclosure. Communication may or may not be intended as a method of self-disclosure or a means to provide information about the self or the individual's perception of self (Luft & Ingham, 1963; Hedlund, 1988). Perceptions of self include acts that describe the self and estimations of self-worth. In some situations self-awareness may be achieved through communication. This function of communication involves interaction with people. Through communication with others an individual may become more aware of personal feelings.

PROCESS OF COMMUNICATION

Communication may be conceptualized as a process that includes a sender, a transmitting device, signals, a receiver, and feedback (Murray & Zentner, 1985). A sender attempts to relay a message, an idea, or information to another person or group through the use of signals or symbols. Many factors influence how the message is given and how it will be received. For example, physical health, emotional well-being, the situation being discussed and the meaning it has, other distractions, knowledge of the matter being discussed, skill at communicating, and attitudes toward the other person and the subject being discussed may all affect the communication that takes place (see box). In addition, personal needs and interests; background, including cultural, social, and philosophical values; the senses and their functional ability;

FACTORS INFLUENCING COMMUNICATION

1. Physical health and emotional well-being
2. The situation being discussed and the meaning it has
3. Distractions to the communication process
4. Knowledge of the matter being discussed
5. Skill at communicating
6. Attitudes toward the other person and toward the subject being discussed
7. Personal needs and interests
8. Background, including cultural, social, and philosophical values
9. The senses involved and their functional ability
10. Personal tendency to make judgments and be judgmental of others
11. The environment in which the communication takes place
12. Past experiences that relate or are related to the present situation

personal tendency to make judgments and be judgmental of others; the environment in which the communication takes place; and past experiences that relate or are related to the present situation can all affect the message that is received. The receiver then interprets the message. Feedback is given to the sender about the message, and more communication may occur. In the event that no feedback is given, there may be no reciprocal interaction.

While the process of communication is universal, nurses should be aware that styles and types of feedback may be unique to certain cultural groups. For example, before the assimilation of the Eskimo into the American culture, the Eskimo would indicate a message was received by blinking rather than making a verbal response (Davidhizar, 1988c). This is also found in the Vietnamese. A Vietnamese person may smile, and yet the smile may not indicate understanding. A Vietnamese person may say yes simply to avoid confrontation or out of a desire to please. A smile may cover up disturbed feelings. Nodding, which nurses commonly interpret as understanding and compliance, may not have the same connotation for a Vietnamese individual, who may simply be smiling to indicate respect for the person talking (Rocereto, 1981; Hoang & Erickson, 1982; Stauffer, 1989). The nurse may be surprised later when the Vietnamese patient who smiled and nodded does not follow through with the instructions given.

VERBAL AND NONVERBAL COMMUNICATION

Another way to conceptualize communication is in terms of verbal and nonverbal behavior (see box). Communication first of all involves language or verbal communication, including vocabulary or repertoire of words and grammatical structure. Along

---

Language or verbal communication

1. Vocabulary
2. Grammatical structure
3. Voice qualities
4. Intonation
5. Rhythm
6. Speed
7. Pronunciation
8. Silence

Nonverbal communication

1. Touch
2. Facial expressions
3. Eye movement
4. Body posture

Communications that combine verbal and nonverbal elements

1. Warmth
2. Humor

with vocabulary and grammatical structure, significant communication cues are received from voice quality, intonation, rhythm, and speed, as well as from the pronunciation used. Dialect may differ significantly among persons both across and within cultures. Silence during communication may itself be a significant part of the message. Communication secondly involves nonverbal messages, which include touch, facial expressions, eye behavior, body posture, and the use of space. Spatial behavior also affects communication and encompasses a variety of behaviors, including proximity to others, objects in the environment, and movement (see Chapter 3). While nonverbal communication is powerful and honest, its importance and meaning vary among and within cultures; therefore it is essential that the nurse have an awareness and appreciation of the role that body language may have in the communication process. In addition, some communications combine nonverbal and verbal components in the message that is sent. Two examples of combination messages are warmth and humor.

Language or Verbal Communication

Language is basic to communication. Without language the higher-order cognitive processes of thinking, reasoning, and generalizing cannot be attained. Words are tools or symbols used to express ideas and feelings or to identify or describe objects. Words shape experiences and influence cultural perceptions. Words convey interpretations and influence relationships (Murray & Zentner, 1985; Pirandello, 1970). Although words provide a special way of looking at the world, the same words often have different meaning for different individuals within cultural groups. In addition, word meanings change over time and in different situations. It is important to ascertain that the message is received and understood as the sender intended it. As early as 1954, Sullivan emphasized the importance of ongoing validation in a therapeutic relationship to verify interpretations made on the behavior and words of another. Even today this remains valid in a nurse-patient relationship where many experiential, educational, and cultural differences are present. Smith and Cantrell (1988) have reported a study comparing the effect of personal questions and physical distance on anxiety rates. Pulse rates were found to be higher when the investigator asked personal questions regardless of the physical distance from subjects. While the data from this study suggest that the most important part of a message is verbal, the opposite has also been found to be true. Thus both verbal and nonverbal communication must be considered before a conclusion about the true meaning of a message can be determined.

To provide culturally appropriate nursing care, it is essential that nurses separate values based on their own cultural background from the values of the patients to whom care is given. Transcultural communication and understanding break down when caregivers project their own culturally specific values and behaviors onto the patient. Thiederman (1986) has suggested that projection of values, as well as hindering care, may actually contribute to noncompliance.

Vocabulary

Even though people may speak the same language, establishing communication is often difficult, since word meanings for both the sender and the receiver vary based on past experiences and learning. Words have both denotative and connotative meanings. A denotative meaning is one that is in general use by most persons who share a common language. A connotative meaning usually arises from a person's personal experience. For example, while all Americans are likely to share the same general denotative meaning for the word *pig,* depending on the occupation and cultural perception of the person, the connotation may be entirely different and may precipitate completely different reactions. The word *pig* will invoke negative or positive reactions from certain people based on occupation and culture. For example, an Orthodox Jew's reactions will differ from those of a pig farmer. For an Orthodox Jew the word *pig* is synonymous with the word *unclean* or *unholy* and thus should be avoided. On the other hand, for a pig farmer the word *pig* implies a clean, wholesome means of making a living. Numerous conflicts resulting from differences in word meaning among various ethnic and racial groups are reported in the literature. Among her many famous cultural studies, Margaret Mead (1947) reported on the different meanings that the word *compromise* carries for an Englishman and an American:

In Britain, the word "compromise" is a good word, and one may speak approvingly of any arrangement which has been a compromise, including, very often one in which the other side has gained more than fifty per cent of the points at issue. . . . Where, in Britain, to compromise means to work out a good solution, in America it usually means to work out a bad one, a solution in which all the points of importance are lost.

Often people who have learned a language have only learned the meaning for the word in one context. For example, Diaz-Duque (1982) reported that a Hispanic person who was told he was going "to be discharged tomorrow" somehow interpreted this to mean he was going to develop "a discharge from below." Diaz-Duque also indicated that for Hispanics problems arise with cognates such as *constipation,* since for Hispanics this term generally refers to nasal congestion rather than intestinal constipation.

While barriers exist when people speak the same language, more profound barriers are present when different languages are spoken. Each language has a whole set of unconscious assumptions about the world and life. Understanding differences in the meaning of words can provide insight into people of different cultures. For example, many English-speaking Americans are puzzled by what seems to be a different time orientation among Spanish people. An understanding of the meaning of the word *time* helps provide insight into this different orientation. In Spanish, *time* is defined as "passing"—a clock "passes time" or "moves"—whereas in English a clock "runs." If time is moving rapidly, as Anglo usage declares, we must hurry. On the other hand, the Spanish definition allows for a more leisurely attitude (Saunders, 1954). Such cultural understandings can provide insight into the reasons why Spanish individuals are often late for health care appointments.

Language reflects the dominant concerns and interests of a people. This can be noted in the number of words for certain things. Some classic studies have reported that certain cultures use many words to describe a particular object of importance. For example, Thomas (1937) explained that in the Arabic language there are about six thousand names for camels. Boas (1938) pointed out that Eskimos have many words for snow. The language of a people is a key that unlocks their culture. A nurse who is familiar with the language of patients will have the best chance of gaining insight into their culture.

Names. Names have a special psychological and cultural significance. All people have names, and in every culture naming a newborn is considered important. The considerations that go into the naming process vary greatly from culture to culture. For example, in Roman tradition there is a given name for boys; a family name, which is second; and a third name that specifies an extended family unit. The name Caius Julius Caesar illustrates the importance of tribal connections, as well as male chauvinism (Clemmens, 1988). In Roman times girls had only one name, the female version of the family name; for example, Caesar's sister was Julia, as was his aunt, father's sister, etc. During the early Roman times women lacked individuality and thus in Roman society were not worth being named.

The Hebrew tradition has a patrilineal way of looking at names, that is, a given name plus "son of." Mothers' names were not included. A spiritual and traditional continuity is evidenced in this system of naming. The Hebrew tradition can be seen today in Iceland, where all males have their given names, followed by their father's given name, ending in "son." In contemporary Western society, as well, there are systems of naming. The most common one in the dominant culture in the United States is a patrilineal succession plus one or more given names. In the United States the middle name is often one that relates to the family, for example, the mother's maiden name.

The Russian system of naming provides a clue to the significance placed on relating son and father, as well as daughter and father. The mother is left out, with Russians habitually addressing each other by the individual's given name together with the patronymic. The family name is omitted. Spaniards and Latin Americans include women more than other cultures, with children carrying their father's name first and their mother's name second. The mother's name usually appears only on documents and for formal occasions, since the addition of the mother's name makes the name quite long. Another variation is seen in the Dutch, who have the option of using both the husband's and the wife's family names jointly.

Among the various cultures the most common theme of naming is pride in lineage (Clemmens, 1985, 1988).

Grammatical structure

Cultural differences are reflected in grammatical structure and the use and meaning of phrases. For example, "That's all right" is a phrase frequently used by Blacks when it actually means, "I have some plans but I am not telling you what they are" (Mitchell, 1978). However, it is important for the nurse to keep in mind that there is little validity in generalizations about the meaning of phrases by persons in varying cultures. Calnek (1970) has stated that Black therapists who work with Black patients have an unusual burden. The problem is not only the possible projection of personal self-image onto other Blacks, but also the adoption of White stereotypes of how Blacks think, act, and feel.

Length of sentence and speech forms may vary not only with culture, but also with social class. For example, Argyle (1967) noted that persons from the lower class commonly use short, simple sentences and are more direct than are persons with more education. Word choice, grammatical structure, speech fluency, and articulation provide cues to social status and class. Jargon is also a speech variation that may prove to be a barrier to communication. Nurses frequently have difficulty expressing things in simple jargon-free language (without medical terms) that patients can understand. On the other hand, a nurse who does not know the jargon used by the patients served may have a difficult time relating to them.

For some cultures patterns of social amenities can create communication problems. Small talk, social chitchat, and discussion of mundane topics that may appear to "kill time" are necessary as preliminaries for more purposeful discussion. Yet the busy nurse seeking short, succinct answers to questions may be annoyed by the amount of anecdotal information that the Hispanic patient, for example, gives. Many patients tend to add irrelevant material because it lessens embarrassment. They may be more comfortable if attention is not focused on their medical problem, so they may intersperse actual symptoms with other biographical data. Cultural factors may also play a role in what seems to be verbal ramblings. Patients who are used to folk healers believe that information on the weather, the environment, and eating habits are really important pieces of information for the health professional.

Voice qualities

Paralinguistics, or paralanguage, refers to something beyond the words themselves. Voice quality, which includes pitch and range, can add an important element to communication. The commonly used phrase, "Don't speak to me in that tone of voice," provides an indication of the significance of this aspect of the communication message.

The softer volume of Asian or Native American speech may be interpreted by the nurse as shyness. On the other hand, the nurse's behavior may be viewed as loud and boisterous if the volume is loud and if there is a deliberate attempt to accent particular words. Sometimes people who speak softly and slowly and without emphasis on particular words are viewed as "wishy-washy." It is important for the nurse to remember that paralinguistic behavior is an important cultural consideration when assessing the patient. This behavior can be recognized by the nurse by listening to nonword vocalizations such as sobbing, laughing, and grunting, the tone of the voice, and, finally, the quality of the voice.

Intonation

Intonation is an important aspect of the communication message. When people says they feel "fine," this may mean they genuinely do, or they do not feel fine but do not wish to discuss it. If said sarcastically, it may also mean they feel just the opposite of fine. There is often a latent or hidden meaning in what a person is saying, and intonation frequently provides the clue that is needed to interpret the true message.

Techniques of intonation vary among cultures. For example, Americans put commands in the form of suggestions and often as questions, whereas Arabic speech contains much emphasis and exaggeration (Argyle, 1967). Some cultures value indirectness and subtlety in speech and may be alienated by the frankness of American health care professionals. Asian patients, for example, may interpret this method of communication as rude, immature, and lacking finesse. On the other hand, health care professionals may label Asian patients as evasive, fearful, and unable to confront problems (Sue, 1981).

Rhythm

Rhythm also varies from culture to culture; some people have a melodic rhythm to their verbal communication, whereas others appear to lack rhythm. Rhythm may also vary among persons within a culture. For example, some Black American ministers use a singsong rhythm to deliver fiery sermons.

Speed

Rate and volume of speech frequently provide a clue to an individual's mood. A depressed person will tend to talk slowly and quietly, whereas an aggressive, dominating person is more apt to talk rapidly and loudly .

Pronunciation

Persons from some cultural groups may be identified by their dialect, for example, Black dialect or Black English, an Irish brogue, or a Brooklyn accent. Black dialect includes words and expressions not commonly found in Standard English and is spoken by Blacks, or African Americans. It ranges on a continuum from being more to less Africanized, with the mild end of the continuum being much like Standard English (Taylor, 1976). However, even persons with dialects at the mild end of the continuum may have a "Black sound" that identifies them as African American. A person may hear a boil called a "risin" or difficulty breathing called "athe smothers" (Snow, 1976); dentures may be called "racks" (Dillard, 1973). Some Blacks speak in dialect when they do not want others to understand what is being said. One function of the Black language may be to enhance the in-group solidarity of Black Americans (Taylor, 1976).

"Ahs," "ers," and grunts also provide important dimensions to communication. While hesitations may indicate a person who is unsure of self and slow to make a commitment, for some cultures this can have the opposite meaning.

Silence

The meaning of silence varies among various cultural groups. Silences may be thoughtful, or they may be blank and empty when the individual has nothing to say. A silence in a conversation may also indicate stubbornness and resistiveness, or apprehension or discomfort. Silence may be viewed by some cultural groups as extremely uncomfortable; therefore attempts may be made to fill every gap with conversation. Persons in other cultural groups value silence and view it as essential to understanding a person's needs. Many Native Americans have this latter view of silence, as do some traditional Chinese and Japanese persons. Therefore when one of these persons is speaking and suddenly stops, what may be implied is that the person wants the nurse to consider the content of what has been said before continuing. Other cultures may use silence in yet other ways. For example, English and Arabic persons use silence for privacy, whereas Russian, French, and Spanish persons may use silence to indicate agreement between parties. Some persons in Asian cultures may view silence as a sign of respect, particularly to an elder.

Nurses need awareness of possible meanings of a silence so that personal anxiety does not prompt the silence to be interrupted prematurely or untherapeutically. A nurse who understands the therapeutic value of science can use this understanding to enhance care of patients from other cultures.

Nonverbal Communication

In his early and classic work Hall (1966) suggested that 65% of the message received in communication is nonverbal. Through body language or motions (kinetic behavior), the person conveys what cannot or may not be said in words. For a message to be accurately interpreted, not only must words be translated, but also the meaning held by nuances, intonation patterns, and facial expressions. Just as verbal behavior may undo nonverbal behavior, nonverbal behavior may repeat, clarify, contradict, modify, emphasize, or regulate the flow of communication. Nonverbal behavior is less significant as an isolated behavior, but it does add to the whole communication message. To understand the patient, the nurse may wish to validate impressions with other health team members, since nonverbal behavior is often interpreted differently by different people. It is important for the nurse to be aware not only of the patient's nonverbal behavior, but also of personal nonverbal behavior that may add to, undo, or contradict verbal communication (Reusch, 1961).

Touch

Touch, or tactile sensation, is a powerful form of communication that can be used to bridge distances between nurse and patient (Davidhizar & Giger, 1988). Touch has many meanings (see box). It can connect people, provide affirmation, be reassuring, decrease loneliness, share warmth, provide stimulation, and increase self-concept. Being touched can be highly valued and sought after. On the other hand, touch can also communicate frustration, anger, aggression, and punishment; invade personal space and privacy; and convey a negative (for example, subservient) type of relationship with another. In certain situations touch can be disconcerting because it signals power. In a study reported by Thayer (1988), higher-status individuals were found to

---

MEANINGS OF TOUCH

Touch may:
1. Connect one individual with another both literally and figuratively by indicating availability
2. Provide affirmation and approval
3. Be reassuring by providing empathy, interest, encouragement, nurturance, caring, trust, concern, gentleness, and protection
4. Decrease loneliness by indicating a relationship with another
5. Share warmth, rapport, love, intimacy, excitement, and happiness
6. Provide stimulation by being a mode of sensation, perception, and experience
7. Increase self-concept
8. Communicate frustration, anger, aggression, or punishment
9. Invade personal space and privacy by physical and psychological assault or intrusion
10. Convey a negative type of relationship with another
11. Cause sexual arousal
12. Allow a person to perform a functional or professional role, such as a physician, barber, or tailor, and be devoid of personal message
13. Reflect cordiality, such as a handshake by business associates and among strangers and acquaintances

enjoy more liberties concerning touch than their lower-status associates. It is generally considered improper for individuals to put their hands on superiors.

Politicians have long known the value of touch. Ignoring security precautions, politicians find that handshakes and touching people in a crowd can pay off later at election time with positive reactions from those touched.

Touching or lack of touch has cultural significance and symbolism and is a learned behavior. Cultural uses of touch vary. Each culture trains its children to develop different kinds of thresholds to tactile contacts and stimulation so that their organic, constitutional, and temperamental characteristics are accentuated or reduced. Some cultures are characterized by a "do not touch me" way of life. These persons may view fondling and kissing as embarrassing. Some cultures include every possible variation on the theme of tactility. In America the mainstream culture generally tolerates hugs and embraces among intimates and a pat on the shoulder as a gesture of camaraderie. The firm, hearty handshake is symbolic of good character and a sign of strength. In some American Indian groups, however, the hand is offered in some interpersonal interactions but the expectation is different. Rather than a firm handshake, there is a light touch or grasp or even just a passing of hands. Some American Indians interpret vigorous handshaking as an aggressive action and are offended by a firm, lengthy handshake (Montagu, 1971). Americans often give a lingering touch a sexual connotation. For some Americans, even casual touching is considered taboo and may be a result of residual Victorian sexual prudence (DeThomaso, 1971). Other cultures also consider touching taboo; the English and Germans carry untouchability further than Americans do. On the other hand, highly tactile cultures do exist, such as the Spanish, Italians, French, Jews, and South Americans (Montagu, 1971). However, generalizations about different national or ethnic groups in the area of touch can be problematic. For example, Shuter (1976) reported on studies of touch in Costa Rica, Columbia, and Panama. While Latin Americans are commonly considered highly contact oriented, Thayer (1988) compared couples in Costa Rica, Columbia, and Panama and found that partners in Costa Rica were touched and held more often than partners in the other two countries.

Most cultures give touch different rules and meanings depending on the sex of the persons involved. Whitcher and Fisher (1979) reported that women in a hospital study had a strikingly positive reaction to being touched, with subsequent lowering of blood pressure and anxiety before surgery, whereas men found the same experience upsetting, with a subsequent increase in blood pressure and anxiety. Thayer (1988) reported on a study at the Kansas City International Airport in which it was found that women greeted women and men more physically, with lip kisses, embraces, and more kinds of touch and holding and for longer periods, than did men. For men a more common greeting was to shake hands. Regardless of sex, some research has been reported showing that people who are most uncomfortable with touch are also uncomfortable with communicating through other means and have lower self-esteem (Thayer, 1988). Other studies have shown that people who touch more are less afraid and suspicious of other people's motives and intentions and have less anxiety and tension in their everyday lives. In some cultures leaning back, showing the palm of the hand, and fussing with the other person's collar may be perceived as possible courting behaviors because they may convey an invitation for closeness or affiliation. Touching behaviors such as reaching out during conversation to poke the other person in the chest may be viewed as domineering behavior. However, laughing while being poked may be a way to submit and at the same time trivialize or eliminate the other person's aggressive intent (Scheflen, 1972).

In some cultures touch is considered magical and healing. For example, Mexicans and some American Indians view touch as symbolic of "undoing" an evil spell, as a means for prevention of harm, or as a means for healing (Montagu, 1971). On the other hand, the Vietnamese may find touching shoulders with another to be anxiety producing, since it is believed that the soul can leave the body on physical contact, and health problems may result (Rocereto, 1981). The human head is regarded by the Vietnamese as the seat of life and is therefore highly personal. Procedures that invade the surface or any orifice of the head can frighten the Vietnamese, who fear that this could provide an exit for the essence of life (Muencke, 1983).

It is important that the nurse be alert to the rules of touch for individuals encountered in the work role. Lane (1989) found that nurses appeared to perceive male patients as being less receptive to touch and closeness than their female counterparts. This was possibly attributed to the fact that males, overall, have a larger personal space than females. Thus it is thought that people generally maintain a greater distance from males (Insel, 1978; Sommer, 1959). Lane concluded that there may be a double standard concerning touch because of societal norms and expectations: male patients may be more receptive to touch, but female nurses are perhaps more comfortable with the closeness and touch of female patients.

While the rules of touch may be unspoken and unwritten, they are usually visible to the observer. A nurse should stay within the rules of touch that are culturally prescribed. It is essential that the nurse use touch judiciously and avoid forcing touch on anyone. The nurse must keep in mind that the message conveyed through touch depends on the attitude of the persons involved and the meaning of touch both to the person touching and to the person being touched. In general, the need for intimacy and touch is so strong that the satisfaction of that need is a greater influence on behavior than the fears about its inappropriateness (Johnson, 1965). A momentary and seemingly incidental touch can establish a positive, temporary bond between strangers, making them more compliant, helpful, positive, and giving. In all cases touch needs to be applied deliberatively, with empathy, and with close attention given to the person's unique and particular needs. All cultural groups have rules, often unspoken, about who touches whom, when, and where. The astute nurse must be mindful of the patient's reaction to touch in order to avoid being perceived as intrusive.

Facial expression

Facial expression is commonly used as a guide to a person's feelings. Research shows that generally in Americans, facial expression is noted and used as a part of the communication message. A constant stare with immobile facial muscles indicates coldness. During fear, the eyes open wide, the eyebrows raise, and the mouth becomes tense with the lips drawn back. When a person is angry, the eyes become fixed in a hard stare with the upper lids lowered and the eyebrows drawn down. An angry person's lips are often tightly compressed. Eyes rolled upward may be related to tiredness or may show disapproval. Narrowed eyes, upper lip curled up, and a moving nose commonly signal disgust. A person who is embarrassed or self-conscious may turn the eyes away or down; have a flushed face; pretend to smile; rub the eyes, nose, or face; or twitch the hair or beard/mustache. A direct gaze with raised eyebrows shows surprise (Ekiman & Friesen, 1975; Polhemus, 1978).

Facial expression also varies with culture. Italian, Jewish, Black, and Spanish-speaking persons smile readily and use a lot of facial expression, along with gestures and words, to communicate feelings—happiness, pain, or displeasure. Irish, English, and Northern European persons tend to have less facial expression and are generally less responsive, especially to strangers. Facial expression can also be used to convey an opposite meaning of the one that is felt; for example, in the Orient negative emotions may be concealed with a smile (Sue, 1981).

Eye movement

Eye movement is an important aspect of interpersonal communication. Generally during social interaction, most people look each other in the eye repeatedly but for short periods of time (Argyle and Dean, 1965; Davidhizar, 1988a). People use more eye contact while they are listening and may use glances of about 3 to 10 seconds in length. When glances are longer than this, anxiety is aroused.

Eye contact is an important tool in transcultural nursing assessment and is used both for observation and to initiate interaction. The dominant American culture values eye contact as symbolic of a positive self-concept, openness, interest in others, attentiveness, and honesty. Eye contact can communicate warmth and bridge interpersonal gaps between people. A nurse who wears glasses and wants to make a point may increase the intensity of eye contact by taking the glasses off. The removal of glasses has also been cited as a technique that can humanize the manager's face, since barriers to eye contact are removed (Davidhizar & Giger, 1989; *Personal Report*, 1987). Lack of eye contact may be interpreted as a sign of shyness, lack of interest, subordination, humility, guilt, embarrassment, low self-esteem, rudeness, thoughtfulness, or dishonesty. In social interaction the speaker glances away from the listener to indicate collecting thoughts or planning what is to be said. If contact is not resumed, disinterest may be interpreted. Pupil dilation and constriction can also be assessed as a clue to anxiety level and positive response (Hess, 1965, 1975).

Most African American and Mexican American patients are comfortable with eye contact (Murray & Huelskoetter, 1987). In fact, in the United States avoidance of eye contact is sometimes considered rude, an indication of lack of attention, or a sign of mental illness (Bigham, 1964; Giger & Davidhizar, 1990; Paynich, 1964). On the other hand, McKenzie and Chrisman (1977) reported that for some Filipino Americans eye contact that turns away is associated with the possibility of being a witch. Other groups that find eye contact difficult include some Oriental people and some American Indians who relate eye contact to impoliteness and an invasion of privacy. Persons in certain Indian cultures avoid eye contact with persons of a higher or lower socioeconomic class. The Vietnamese generally practice less eye contact (Giger & Davidhizar, 1990; Rocereto, 1981), and prolonged eye contact is also avoided by some African Americans (Giger & Davidhizar, 1990). In some Indian cultures eye contact is given a special sexual significance. Some Orthodox Jews also attribute a sexual significance to eye contact by an elderly man for a woman other than his wife (Sue, 1981). Still another group that might consider direct eye contact impolite is the Appalachians. Some Appalachian people tend to avert their eyes because eye contact is related to hostility and aggressiveness (Tripp-Reimer & Friedl, 1977). Certain cultures place more focus on the eyes than others; for example, in India and Greece the use of the eyes is all important (Eibl-Eibesfelt, 1972).

Body posture

Communication is also affected by body posture. A nurse can bridge distance in an interaction by placing the forearms on the table, palms up. In the United States palms up can send a message of acquiescence even while disagreeing. However, the nurse should also recognize that palms up in other cultures may have a sexual implication. Therefore the decision to use this gesture should be weighed carefully.

Body posture can provide important messages about receptivity. In the United States the closer a listener's overall posturing matches the posture of the speaker, the higher the likelihood of receptivity. If the individuals' unconscious gestures are different, probably their perspective on the matter at hand is also different. Matching body movements to those of another person can communicate a sense of solidarity even if solidarity is not present. Body posture can also communicate attitude toward a person. For example, in the United States an attentive posture is indicated by leaning toward a person. Attentive posture is used toward people of higher stature and toward people who are liked (Mehrabian, 1968, 1981). An American man may indicate sexual attraction by having the arms in front of the body with the legs closed. An American woman, on the other hand, indicates attraction by a more open posture, that is, arms down at the side (Hall, 1966). Physical pain is communicated by rigid muscles, flexed body, and cautious movements. Argyle et al. (1970) reported that in England dominance is communicated when the dominant person stands or sits more erect than the compliant or submissive person. Knowledge of sociocultural heritage is essential in interpreting body language, since various body parts are used differently in different cultures.

Communications That Combine Verbal and Nonverbal Elements

A number of interpersonal communications combine both verbal and nonverbal elements. The communications of warmth and humor are two of these.

Warmth

Warmth is a quality or state that promotes feelings of friendship, well-being, or pleasure. Warmth can be communicated verbally ("You really lay still during the procedure, and that surely helped us to do it as quickly as possible") and may also be communicated nonverbally, as by a pat on the shoulder or a gentle smile.

Although warmth is also a matter of perception, communication that focuses on human needs is more likely to be related to warmth in the speaker. Statements that show respect, address the human need to be needed, and promote self-acceptance will usually be interpreted positively and can increase motivation, morale, and cooperation. Personal recognition and concern also communicate warmth. Verbal recognition (for example, a "hello" on meeting) or a statement of genuine concern (for example, "How are you feeling?") can convey interest and may facilitate a positive relationship between patient and family and the nurse (Davidhizar, 1989).

The nurse's communication of warmth is an important and dynamic aspect of a therapeutic nurse-patient relationship. If the patient is from another culture and is having difficulty with understanding communication, the nurse's warmth may be vital to promoting a positive relationship.

Humor

Humor is a powerful component of verbal and nonverbal communication. Humor can create a bond of shared pleasure between people, can decrease anxiety and tension, can build relationships, can promote problem solving and learning, can provide motivation, and can enable personal survival. As a healthy and constructive coping mechanism, humor can provide a discharge for aggressive feelings in a more or less acceptable way and can enable stressful situations to be managed (Davidhizar, 1988b). Humor that is therapeutic does not ridicule and rarely uses cynicism (Huckaby, 1987). Personality, culture, background, and levels of stress and pain may influence reactions to humor. When people are from a different culture, humor must be used in limited and well-thought-out situations, since humor can be an obstacle to a relationship if it is misunderstood. The nurse must carefully assess the individual patient and the situation to evaluate if humor is appropriate. Humor not only can improve communication when used appropriately, but may also affect the immune system by promoting the body's ability to combat such problems as cancer and diseases of the connective tissue such as arthritis and lupus (Simonton & Matthews-Simonton, 1978).

When the individual spoken with does not have a full grasp of the language and the nuances and puns that are often involved in humor, jokes and statements meant as humorous may not be understood or may be misinterpreted. It is also important for an individual who tries to speak in another language to be prepared to precipitate laughter. A statement meant to be serious may be perceived as comical. The ability to laugh at oneself and with others can ease the anxiety that may be present in an intercultural situation.

IMPLICATIONS FOR NURSING CARE
Guidelines for Relating to Patients from Different Cultures

Nurses commonly relate to patients in an interview setting. The nurse may also relate during the process of patient care or at a more informal level on the hospital unit or in the clinic. While cultural issues may cause the patient to interpret the nurse's behavior from a unique perspective, adherence to the following guidelines will increase the likelihood that the nurse-patient relationship will be positive.

1. *Assess personal beliefs surrounding persons from different cultures.* Awareness of the nurse's personal beliefs is vital in relating to patients from diverse cultural backgrounds. A nurse working with a patient from another background should carefully review personal beliefs and past experiences to determine conscious and unconscious attitudes. It is important for the nurse to set aside personal values, biases, ideas, and attitudes that are judgmental and may negatively affect care.

2. *Assess communication variables from a cultural perspective.* To communicate with a patient from another culture, it is important to assess each patient receiving care from a cultural perspective. Each individual has a dominant culture and also belongs to a subculture. The cultural phenomena of communication cannot be minimized when

providing culturally appropriate nursing care. The nurse who understands differences in communication variables can attempt to transcend communication barriers to provide quality patient care.

It is important to realize that cultural assessment does not require information on every aspect of a specific culture. However, data should elicit ethnic identity, including generation in America (that is, first or second generation); the beliefs of a first-generation immigrant, regardless of ethnic heritage, who is a Roman Catholic, Orthodox Greek, Baptist, or Jehovah's Witness in the United States may differ from those of a second-generation person. Whenever possible, the patient should be used as the primary informant, since others, even though close to the patient, may have different ideas and beliefs.

After a careful assessment of cultural factors that may enter into a relationship, it is necessary to respond appropriately. For example, for African Americans and Mexican Americans, who tend to value eye contact, it is important for the nurse to use eye contact. On the other hand, when relating to Filipino Americans, who are afraid of eye contact, the nurse should avoid eye contact.

3. *Plan care based on the communicated needs and cultural background.* When planning care for persons from other cultures, it is important that the care be consistent with the life-style and unique needs of the patient that have been communicated by the patient to the nurse and mutually agreed on. To establish an appropriate plan, it is essential that the nurse improve personal knowledge about the customs and beliefs of the culture of the patients cared for. The nurse should encourage the patient to communicate cultural interpretations of health, illness, and health care. A patient's perception of illness will affect not only communication, but also the care that is planned. Sensitivity to the uniqueness of each patient is required if the nurse is to work effectively, particularly with patients from different cultures. This sensitivity can be gained only through appropriate communication techniques.

The best teacher in learning about culture is people themselves. Individuals must be communicated with at their own personal level of functioning. Values and beliefs of persons from different cultures may affect the way care is delivered. For example, Tripp-Reimer (1982) found that when relating to Appalachian people, questions about income, how often children go to school, other persons in the household, and neighbors should be avoided, since such questions can be given a negative connotation. Many cultures have similar idiosyncrasies that must be considered. Finally, it is important to evaluate the effectiveness of nursing actions with patients from diverse cultural groups. It may be necessary to modify the plan in order to provide an effective intervention based on communicated needs.

The nurse may need to identify sources of discrepancy between the patient's and the health provider's conceptions of health and illness. While it may be stoic to ignore pain, if the pain results from cancer that could be cured by surgery, education may be preferable to tolerance of this cultural difference.

4. *Modify communication approaches to meet cultural needs.* A factor that commonly interferes with care delivery to a person from another culture is confusion and fear about the treatment process. The fact that a non-English patient is ill and receiving treatment can interfere with the patient's ability to communicate. The nurse must be attentive to signs of anxiety and respond in a reassuring manner in keeping with the person's cultural orientation.

When working with persons from diverse cultural backgrounds, the astute nurse must recognize that the communication process may be impeded by encompassing people other than the individual involved. For example, many Navajo Indians feel it is ethically wrong to speak for another individual. This ethical belief makes it difficult to obtain a history from a relative or person other than the patient. While some cooperation may be given in an emergency, the nurse must creatively use methods to get around this cultural practice.

5. *Understand that respect for the patient and communicated needs is central to the therapeutic relationship.* The need to communicate respect for the patient is a nursing concept that crosses all cultural boundaries. Regardless of the language spoken or the cultural orientation, communication is increased and interpersonal distance is reduced by the nurse whose approach focuses on individuals and their human as well as physical needs. Communication of respect is central to a focus on human needs. Respect for patients is communicated by a kind and attentive approach where the patient is heard. Active listening techniques are used, such as encouraging patients to share thoughts and feelings by reflecting back what has been heard. The nurse should be attentive to how listening is communicated in the culture that the patient represents. For example, for some persons listening may be indicated by eye contact, whereas for others listening may mean having the listener turn a listening "ear." Predictions about what the patient is trying to express may be made to encourage elaboration. Listening communicates genuine interest and caring. The feeling of being heard is powerful, and reduces distance and draws people together into positive interpersonal interactions. An attitude of flexibility, respect, and interest can bridge artificial barriers of distance imposed by culture and role.

6. *Communicate in a nonthreatening manner.* The interview should be started in an unhurried manner with adherence to acceptable social and cultural amenities. It is usually wise to start with general social topics. During the information-gathering stage, general rather than specific questions should be asked. The interviewer should allow time for the respondent to give what appears to be unrelated information. For many persons a direct approach appears rude and uncaring. For example, persons of European background and Spanish-speaking individuals often value "small talk" and will not relate optimally to the nurse who talks only about illness-related matters. Many persons, specifically Oriental and Spanish-speaking persons, respond better to a nondirective approach with open-ended questions than to direct questions and answers (Giger & Davidhizar, 1990).

When personal matters are discussed, it is important to allow time for the development of a relationship. For example, American Indians tend to be hesitant to discuss personal affairs quickly. For such individuals it is important to first develop trust. This may be difficult in an emergency where answers to questions are needed quickly. Because of this hesitancy on the part of American Indians to speak, it is especially important for the nurse to listen carefully and give the patient full attention.

The appearances of being too busy, of not having time to listen, of not giving sufficient time for an answer, and of not really wanting to hear are equally effective in "cutting off" the patient. Patients will be encouraged to talk by a nurse who "wants" to hear.

7. *Use validating techniques in communication.* While validating techniques are always important, they are especially important when the patient is from a different cul-

ture. The nurse should be alert for feedback that the patient is not understanding and should use restating and validating techniques such as "Did I hear and understand you correctly?"

Even if an interpreter is used, the nurse should not assume the meaning has been transmitted without some distortion. It is difficult to transmit exact meaning when both persons speak the same language and even more so when both persons do not.

8. *Be considerate of reluctance to talk when the subject involves sexual matters*. Spanish-speaking patients and American Indians, who tend to be hesitant to talk about sexually related matters, may talk more freely to a nurse of the same sex. When talking about sexual matters with a male child from certain cultures (for example, Spanish-speaking, Pakistani, or Arabic), it is important to have the father rather than the mother present.

9. *Adopt special approaches when the patient speaks a different language*. A patient who enters the health care system without being able to speak to the caregiver enters a frightening and frustrating world. Without the availability of words, the nurse must relate to the patient at an affective level. A tone and facial expression of caring can be vital to alleviating the patient's fear.

The nurse should guard against the common assumption that the patient will understand better if the nurse talks loudly. If an interpreter is not available and the patient seems to have some understanding of the language, speaking slowly and distinctly, using a lot of gestures, acting out, using pictures, and repeating the message several times in different ways may enable the patient to understand what is being said. The nurse should be alert for words that the patient seems to understand so that these words can be used more frequently. Messages should be kept simple and stated sentence by sentence, not paragraph by paragraph.

It is especially necessary to avoid using medical terms and jargon when speaking to a patient with only partial understanding of the language. Abbreviations such as *TPR* and *BP* should be avoided. An individual usually first understands standard words and picks up slang expressions and professional terms at a much later stage of language acquisition.

The nurse should select a dictionary that has both the language the nurse speaks and the language the patient speaks, for example, a Spanish/English dictionary. In addition, standard nursing references such as *Taber's Cyclopedic Medical Dictionary* have sections that give common medical statements and questions in several languages.

10. *Use interpreters to improve communication*. When a patient does not speak the nurse's language, an interpreter should be obtained. This person may be either a family member or a person from an agency or the community. It is important to obtain an interpreter who can translate not only the literal meaning of the words, but also the nonverbal messages that accompany the communication. Interpreters who "act out" their message through intonation, facial expression, or gestures are more likely to be effective in getting the message across. Even when every effort is made to ensure effective translations, neither the nurse nor the interpreter can be completely sure that accurate communication has been accomplished; therefore obtaining feedback remains essential. Communication through a third party compounds the problem of sending a message clearly. Interpreters often face the difficulty of interpreting versus translating. While a message may be translated into another language, helping another understand is much more complex and involves interpreting the message into

understandable terms. An interpreter must have transcultural sensitivity, understand how to impart knowledge, and understand how to be a patient advocate to represent the patient's needs to the nurse. Interpreting with cultural sensitivity is much more complex than simply putting the words in another language (Diaz-Duque, 1982; Muencke, 1970; Putsch, 1985).

CASE STUDY

A 35- to 37-year-old Black woman who has been recently diagnosed as having hypertension is admitted for a medical workup. Her history reveals that she has just recently moved from New Orleans to Chicago. The nurse is having difficulty communicating with the patient because she not only speaks in Black English but has a heavy southern drawl and tends to speak in Pidgin English. Another factor complicating the development of the nurse-patient relationship is that not only does the patient not understand the hospital jargon and medical terms, but word meanings for the nurse and the patient vary. For example, when the nurse asks if the patient likes her physician, she responds, "He's bad." Only later does the nurse discover that the patient was speaking in an argot that is a special linguistic code for some Black Americans. The patient appears very fearful and anxious about being in the hospital. When the nurse questions the patient, the nurse finds that the fear and anxiety are related to the connotative and denotative meanings of the word *hospital*. In this case the patient believes that hospitals are associated with death and that she may not leave the hospital alive. When the nurse communicates with the patient, she speaks very loudly and repeats the same words again and again.

STUDY QUESTIONS

1. Describe at least two problems encountered by the nurse when giving nursing care to persons who use Black English as opposed to Standard English.
2. List at least three words commonly used in Black English that have varying connotative and denotative meanings.
3. Describe four communication approaches that the nurse can use to give culturally appropriate care.
4. Describe approaches the nurse can use when relating to a patient whose primary language is not Standard English.
5. Describe at least two nonverbal indicators of anxiety the nurse may encounter when dealing with a patient who does not speak Standard English.
6. List at least two problems encountered by the nurse who assumes that speaking louder will improve communication.

REFERENCES

Argyle, M. (1967). *The psychology of interpersonal behavior*. Baltimore: Penguin Books.

Argyle, M., & Dean, J. (1965). Eye-contact, distance, and affiliation. *Sociometry, 28*, 289-304.

Argyle, M., Salter, H., Nicholson, N., Williams, M., & Burgess, P. (1970). The communication of inferior and superior attitudes by verbal and nonverbal signals. *British Journal of Social and Clinical Psychology, 9*, 221-231.

Bigham, C. (1964). To communicate with Negro patients. *American Journal of Nursing, 64*(9), 113-115.

Boas, F. (Ed.). (1938). *General anthropology*. Boston: D.C. Heath.

Calnek, M. (1970). Racial factors in the countertransference: The Black therapist and the Black client. *American Journal of Orthopsychiatry, 40*(1), 39-46.

Clemmens, E. (1985). An analyst looks at languages, cultures, and translations. *American Journal of Psychoanalysis, 45*(4), 310-321.

Clemmens, E. (1988). Some psychological functions of language. *American Journal of Psychoanalysis, 43*(4), 294-304.

Davidhizar, R. (1988a). Distance in managerial encounters. *Today's OR Nurse, 10*(10), 23-29.

Davidhizar, R. (1988b). Humor—No nurse should be without it. *Today's OR Nurse 10*(1), 18-20.

Davidhizar, R. (1988c). Personal communication.

Davidhizar, R. (1989). Developing managerial warmth. *Dimensions of Critical care, 8*(1), 28-34.

Davidhizar, R., & Giger, J. (1988). Managerial touch. *Today's OR Nurse, 10*(7), 18-23.

Davidhizar, R., & Giger, J. (1989). Personal space and the patient from another culture. Unpublished manuscript.

Delgado, M. (1983). Hispanics and psychotherapeutic groups. *International Journal of Group Psychotherapy, 33*(4), 507-520.

DeThomaso, M. (1971). Touch power and the screen of loneliness. *Perspectives in Psychiatric Care, 9*(3), 112-117.

Diaz-Duque, O. (1982). Advice from an interpreter. *American Journal of Nursing, 82*(9), 1380-1381.

Dillard, J.L. (1973). *Black English.* New York: Vintage Books.

Eibl-Eibesfelt, I. (1972). Similarities and differences between cultures in expressive movements. In R.A. Hinde (Ed.), *Nonverbal communication* (pp. 297-312). Cambridge, U.K.: Cambridge University Press.

Ekiman, P., & Friesen, W. (1975). *Unmasking the face.* Englewood Cliffs, N.J.: Prentice Hall.

Fielding, R., & Llewelyn, S. (1987). Communication training in nursing may damage your health and enthusiasm: Some warnings. *Journal of Advanced Nursing, 12*(3), 281-290.

Gibson, J. (1984, Jan.). As they grow: 1 year olds. *Parents,* p. 128.

Giger, J., & Davidhizar, R. (1990). Crosscultural nursing and implications for nursing care. *International Nursing Review 37*(1), 199-202.

Guralnik, D. (Ed.). (1972). *Webster's new world dictionary* (2nd college ed.). New York: William Collins & World Publishing.

Hall, E.T. (1966). *The silent language.* New York: Doubleday.

Hedlund, N. (1988). Communication. In C.K. Beck, R.P. Rawlins, & S. Williams (Eds.), *Mental health–psychiatric nursing: A holistic life-cycle approach* (2nd ed.). St. Louis: C.V. Mosby.

Hess, E.H. (1965). Attitude and pupil size. *Scientific American, 212,* 46-54.

Hess, E.H. (1975). The role of pupil size in communication. *Scientific American, 233*(5), 110-119.

Hoang, G., & Erickson, R. (1982). Guidelines for providing medical care to Southeast Asian refugees. *JAMA 248*(6), 710-714.

Huckaby, D. (1987). Take time to laugh. *Nursing '87, 17,* 81.

Insel, P.M. (1978). *Too close for comfort: The psychology of crowding.* Englewood Cliffs, N.J.: Prentice Hall.

Johnson, B. (1965). The meaning of touch in nursing. *Nursing Outlook, 13*(2), 59-60.

Jourard, S. (1971). *The transparent self.* New York: D. Van Nostrand.

Kasch, C. (1984). Interpersonal competence and communication in the delivery of nursing care. *Advances in Nursing Science, 62,* 71-88.

Knowles, R. (1983). Building rapport through neuro-linguistic programming. *American Journal of Nursing, 83,* 1011-1014.

Kretch, D., Crutchfield, R., & Ballachey, E. (1962). *Individual in society.* New York: McGraw-Hill.

Lane, P. (1989). Nurse-client perceptions: The double standard of touch. *Issues in Mental Health Nursing, 10,* 1-13.

Luft, J., & Ingham, H. (1963). The Johari window: A graphic model of awareness in interpersonal relations. In J. Luft (Ed.), *Group processes: An introduction to group dynamics.* Palo Alto, Calif.: National Press Books.

McKenzie, J., & Chrisman, N. (1977). Healing herbs, gods, and magic: Folk health beliefs among Filipino-Americans. *Nursing Outlook, 25*(5), 326.

Mead, M. (1947). The application of anthropological technique to cross-national communication. *Transcultural New York Academy of Science, Series II, 9,* 4.

Mehrabian, A. (1968). The influence of attitudes from the posture, orientation, and distance of a communicator. *Journal of Consulting Clinical Psychology, 32,* 296-308.

Mehrabian, A. (1981). *Silent messages: Implicit communication of emotion and attitude.* Belmont, Calif.: Wadsworth.

Mitchell, A. (1978). Barriers to therapeutic communication with Black clients. *Nursing Outlook, 26,* 109-112.

Molzahn, A., & Northcott, H. (1989). The social bases of discrepancies in health/illness perceptions. *Journal of Advanced Nursing, 14*(2), 132-140.

Montagu, A. (1971). *Touching: The significance of the human skin.* New York: Columbia University Press.

Muencke, M. (1970). Overcoming the language barrier, *Nursing Outlook, 18*(4), 53-54.

Muencke, M. (1983). Caring for Southeast Asian refugee patient in the USA. *American Journal of Public Health, 74*(4), 431-438.

Murray, R., & Huelskoetter, N. (1987). *Psychiatric/mental health nursing: Giving emotional care* (2nd ed.). Norwalk, Conn.: Appleton & Lange.

Murray, R., & Zentner, J. (1985). *Nursing concepts for health promotion* (3rd ed.). Englewood Cliffs, N.J.: Prentice Hall.

Paynich, M. (1964). Cultural barriers to nurse communication. *American Journal of Nursing, 64*(2), 87-90.

Personal Report for the Executive. (1987). New York: National Institute of Business Management.

Pirandello, L. (1970). Language and thought. *Perspectives in Psychiatric Care, 8*(5), 230.

Polhemus, T. (Ed.). (1978). *The body reader: Social aspects of the human body.* New York: Pantheon Books.

Potter, R., & Perry, A. (1989). *Fundamentals of Nursing: Concepts, Process, and Practice* (2nd ed.). St. Louis: C.V. Mosby.

Putsch, R. (1985). Crosscultural communication. *JAMA, 254,* 3347-3348.

Reusch, J. (1961). *Therapeutic communication.* New York: W.W. Norton.

Rocereto, L. (1981). Selected health beliefs of Vietnamese refugees, *Journal of School Health, 51*(1), 63-64.

Sapir, E. (1929). The status of linguistics as a science. *Language, 5,* 207-214.

Saunders, J. (1954). *Cultural differences and medical care.* New York: Russell Sage Foundation.

Scheflen, A. (1972). *Body language and social order.* Englewood Cliffs, N.J.: Prentice Hall.

Shuter, R. (1976). Proxemics and tactility in Latin America. *Journal of Communication, 26*(3), 46-52.

Simonton, O.C., & Matthews-Simonton, S. (1978). *Getting well again.* Los Angeles: Jeremy P. Tarcher.

Smith, B., & Cantrell, P. (1988). Distance in nurse-patient encounters. *Journal of Psychosocial Nursing, 26*(2), 22-26.

Snow, L. (1976, June). " High blood" is not "high blood pressure." *Urban Health,* pp. 54-56.

Sommer, R. (1959). Studies in personal space. *Sociometry, 22,* 247-260.

Stauffer, R. (1989). Personal communication.

Sudnow, D. (1967). *Passing on.* Englewood Cliffs, N.J.: Prentice Hall.

Sue, D. (1981). *Counseling the culturally different: Theory and Practice.* New York: John Wiley & Sons.

Sullivan H. (1954). *The interpersonal theory of psychiatry.* New York: W.W. Norton.

Taylor, C. (1976). Soul talk: A key to Black cultural attitudes. In D. Luckroft (Ed.), *Black awareness: Implications for Black patient care.* New York: American Journal of Nursing Company.

Thayer, S. (1988, March). Close encounters. *Psychology Today,* pp. 31-36.

Thiederman, S. (1986). Ethnocentrism: A barrier to effective health care. *Nurse Practitioner, 11*(8), 52-59.

Thomas, W.I. (1937). *Primitive behavior: An introduction to the social sciences.* New York: McGraw-Hill.

Tripp-Reimer, T. (1982). Barriers to health care: Variations in interpretation of Appalachian clients' behavior by Appalachian and non-Appalachian health professionals. *Western Journal of Nursing Research, 4*(2), 179-191.

Tripp-Reimer, T., & Friedl, M. (1977). Appalachaians: A neglected minority. *Nursing Outlook, 32*(2), 41-45.

Watzlawich, P., Beavin, J., & Jackson, D. (1967). *Pragmatics of human communication.* New York: W.W. Norton.

Whitcher, S.J., & Fisher, J.D. (1979). Multidimensional reaction to therapeutic touch in hospital setting. *Journal of Personality, Sociology, and Psychology, 37*(1), 87-96.

....

CHAPTER 3

Space

BEHAVIORAL OBJECTIVES

After reading this chapter, the nurse will be able to:

1 Discuss factors related to distance and immediate receptors that influence spatial behavior.

2 Define the term *personal space* and relate its significance to care plan development for patients from varying cultures.

3 Explain how actions of the nurse may contribute to feelings of anxiety and loss of control for patients from transcultural backgrounds.

4 List actions the nurse can take to promote feelings of autonomy and self-worth when caring for patients from transcultural backgrounds.

5 Delineate the difference between tactile space and visual space and the relationship to transcultural nursing care.

Personal space is the area that surrounds a person's body; it includes the space and the objects within the space (Sommer, 1969). Personal space is an extension of the body and is also referred to as outer space; inner space refers to the personal state of consciousness or awareness (Haber et al., 1987). An individual's comfort level is related to personal space, and discomfort is experienced when personal space is invaded. While personal space is an individual matter and varies with the situation, dimensions of the personal space comfort zone also vary from culture to culture.

Spatial behavior is an important consideration in measuring distance in relationships. Since spatial behavior is usually judged to be spontaneous and unintentional, individuals are typically more likely to trust the accuracy of actions rather than words as a reflection of true feelings. Although a large percentage of spatial behaviors are spontaneous and unintentional, communication in this domain can be managed to promote favorable and desired impressions. For example, a nurse may choose to stand when greeting a patient in order to show respect.

To understand human behavior, one must understand something of the nature of our receptor systems and how the information received by these systems is modified by culture. Since spatial behavior is a response to sensory stimulation in the internal and external environment, the phenomenon of space can only be understood as an integral part of the sensory systems, that is, sight, sound, touch, and smell. Spatial behavior encompasses a variety of behaviors, including proximity to others, objects in the environment, and movement.

PERCEPTION OF SPACE

Sensory apparatuses fall into two categories:

1. *Distance receptors:* Those apparatuses that are concerned with the examination of distant objects. The sensory receptors for distance include the eyes, ears, and nose.
2. *Immediate receptors:* Those apparatuses that are used to examine the world up close. Sensory receptors that are used to examine the world up close include touch, which is the sensation received from the skin membranes (Hall, 1966a).

These two classifications can be broken down even further to facilitate the nurse's understanding of the phenomenon of space. For example, the skin is the chief organ of touch, and it is also sensitive to heat gain and heat loss—both radiant and conducted heat are detected by the skin. Therefore the skin must be perceived as both an immediate and a distance receptor. In general, there is a relationship between the evolutionary age of the receptor system and the amount and quality of information it can convey to the central nervous system. Many psychologists estimate that the touch system is as old as life itself (Hall, 1966b); because the ability to respond to stimuli is based on touch, the response to touch is one of the basic criteria for the maintenance of life. In comparison, sight is thought to be the last and most specialized sense to be developed in humans. Vision, from an anthropological view, became more important than olfactory response when our ancestors left the ground and took to trees in search of food and safety. Stereoscopic vision became essential for primitive man because without it jumping from branch to branch was difficult and dangerous.

Distance Receptors

Distance receptors include sensory apparatuses for visual, auditory, and olfactory perception. It is essential that the nurse understand the relationship between sight, touch, and smell and how the reaction to these stimuli can be modified by culture.

Visual and auditory perception

As indicated earlier, vision was the last of the senses to evolve. However, it is by far the most complex. Seemingly, more data are fed to the nervous system through the eyes at a much greater rate than through the senses of touch or hearing. For example, the information that can be gathered by a blind person outdoors is limited to a circle of 20 to 100 feet—a blind person can perceive by way of auditory or olfactory stimuli only what is immediately surrounding him or her. However, with sight a person can see the stars if they are out. Even the very talented blind are limited to an average speed of perception of 2 to 3 miles an hour over familiar territory. In contrast, with sight, a person has to fly faster than sound before additional visual aids are needed to avoid bumping into things. The amount of information that can be gathered by the eyes as contrasted to the ears cannot be precisely calculated. If such a calculation were possible, it would require not only a translation process but the ability on the part of scientists to know precisely what to count. A general notion held by most scientists is that the relative complexities of the two systems, visual and auditory, can be obtained by comparing the size of the nerves connecting the eyes and the ears to the centers of the brain (Brown, Leavitt, & Graham, 1977).

The optic nerve contains roughly 18 times as many neurons as the cochlear nerve; therefore one might assume that it transmits at least that much more information. The eyes may act as a defense mechanism, because they normally alert us to danger; the eyes may be as much as a thousand times as effective as the ears in gathering information to protect us from harmful stimuli. The area that the unaided ear can effectively cover in the course of daily living is quite limited. The ear is very efficient, but only up to a distance of 20 feet. At about 100 feet one-way vocal communication is possible, but at a somewhat slower rate than at a conversational distance. While two-way conversation is also possible at this distance, it is considerably altered, and beyond this distance the auditory cues begin to break down rapidly. The unaided eye, on the other hand, can gather an extraordinary amount of information within a 100-yard radius and is efficient for human interaction at up to a mile (Hall, 1966a).

The impulses that activate the eyes and the ears differ in speed and quality. For example, at a temperature of 0° C (32° F) at sea level, sound waves can travel 1100 feet per second and be heard in frequencies of 50 to 1500 cycles per second (c/s). On the other hand, light rays can travel 186,000 miles per second and thus are visible at a frequency of 10 zillion c/s (Hall, 1966a).

A number of complex and remarkable instruments have been invented to extend the eyes and ears. Radio and television have revolutionized the perception of space and shortened distances between people worldwide. During World War II radio was relied on quite extensively to bring news from the occupied countries to parts of the free world. Perhaps one of the most famous broadcasts of this time period was done by Tokyo Rose, whose broadcasts, while reported to be untrue, influenced many people in the listening audience about the nature and direction of World War II. However, radio lacked the visual stimuli offered later by television, which filled in perception gaps left by radio. Television came of age in the 1960s, when for the first time, brighter, clearer, bolder, and color pictures were offered to viewers. The addition of color filled another perception gap and enhanced our receptor fields. President Kennedy was the first U.S. president to be seen frequently on television. For the first time in history, from their living rooms, the American people could view their president doing the ordinary, the extraordinary, and the unusual. For example, the American people were informed about the Cuban missile crisis by Kennedy on television. They were also able to see this president playing with his children in the Oval Office. In 1963, when President Kennedy was assassinated, nothing was left to the imagination of the American people, who were mesmerized by complete television coverage from assassination to burial. Because of television the nation and the world at large experienced grief still present today and mourned collectively.

In summary, visual space has an entirely different character than auditory space. The overriding quality that differentiates visual space from auditory space is that visual information tends to be less ambiguous and more focused than auditory information. Therefore visual information is less subject to external manipulation than is auditory information. One major exception to this rule is the blind person who has learned to understand selectively the higher audio frequencies that assist him or her in locating objects within a familiar or unfamiliar room. For example, a blind person may know where the door is in a room by the relationship of the sound that comes from that direction.

Even today it is not known what effects the incongruencies between auditory and visual space have on individuals. Some data suggest that auditory space is a factor in performance. J.W. Black, a phonetician, demonstrated that the size and reverberation (vibrations of external sounds) of a room can affect an individual's reading rate. In a classic 1950 study, Black found that people read more slowly in larger rooms, where the reverberation time, or circulation of sound, is slower than in smaller rooms. Hall (1966a) interviewed subjects in regard to the slowing of reverberation time in a larger room. Among the interviewees was a gifted English architect who improved the performance of a malfunctioning committee by simply blending the auditory and visual worlds of the conference chamber where the committee met. The complaint the architect had received was that the chairman was inadequate and was about to be replaced. However, the architect had reason to believe that the difficulties encountered by this committee were caused by more in the environment than just the chairman. In this situation the meeting room was next to a busy street where traffic noises were intensified by reverberations from the hard walls and rugless floors inside the building and particularly in the meeting room. The architect was able to readjust the room by adding an acoustic ceiling, carpet, and soundproof walls. Once interferences were reduced, the chairman was able to conduct the meeting without undue strain, and complaints about the chairman ceased.

People who are brought up in different cultures learn unknowingly to screen out various information and to sort information into relevant or irrelevant categories, and, once set, these perceptual patterns remain stable throughout life. For example, Japanese people screen visually in a variety of ways and are more perceptive to visual stimuli. Japanese people are therefore perfectly content with paper walls as acoustic screens. A Westerner who finds himself in a Japanese inn where a party is going on next door may be in for a new sensory experience, since only paper thin walls separate each room. In contrast, German and Dutch people depend on double doors and thick walls to screen out sound and may have difficulty if they must rely on their own powers of concentration to screen out sound. If two rooms are the same size and one screens out sound and the other one does not, a sensitive German or Dutch person who is trying to concentrate will feel less intruded on in the former and thus less crowded (Hall, 1966a).

Olfactory perception

Some cultures place more importance on olfactory perceptions than do others. For example, Hall (1966a) found Americans culturally underdeveloped in the use of the olfactory apparatus. Hall (1966a) contended that the deprivations of the olfactory stimulus are a result of the extensive use of deodorants and the suppression of odors in public places, which has resulted in a land of olfactory blandness and sameness that is difficult to duplicate anywhere else in the world.

People in the United States are continuously bombarded with commercials for room deodorizers, antiperspirants, mouthwashes, carpet deodorizers, etc. All of these factors result in bland, undifferentiated spaces and deprive many Americans of the richness and variety of life. For example, if one is cooking with garlic, a room deodorizer may be used during the cooking process, causing the garlic smell to be eliminated. It is this type of behavior on the part of American people that obscures memories. It is thought that smells evoke much deeper memories than either vision or sound; when the sound or the sight of what has happened has passed, the memory of the smell lingers on. Even today many Americans equate certain holidays, such as Christmas, with certain smells. For example, since Christmas traditionally has been equated with the smell of baked goods, holly, pine, and fruit, today many Americans try to reproduce these smells at Christmas. An individual who has an artificial Christmas tree may buy a pine-scented spray to create the effects of a fresh tree. Another old-fashioned scent for many Americans is country potpourri, which has now been simulated in aerosol cans for easy dispensing. A new car can be simulated by a car spray that smells like new leather. Soap may be purchased to recreate a desired feeling; for example, the soap mother used at home may create a feeling of hominess. Smells may also create a negative reaction. For example, an individual who washes with lye soap may be thought to have body odor, since the smell is unusually strong and medicinal. A medicinal smell is perceived by most individuals in the United States to be appropriate for a hospital room but not in a non-health-care setting.

Odor is perhaps one of the most basic methods of communication. It is primarily chemical in nature and is therefore referred to in a chemical sense. The olfactory sense has diverse functions and not only differentiates individuals, but also makes it possible to identify the emotional state of others. Even an infant can learn to identify his or her parents through the sense of smell. Although the young infant has not learned to see and discriminate patterns well, the infant can distinguish identity through the olfactory sense.

In a hospital setting an employee who has an unpleasant odor creates a real management dilemma. The supervisor may counsel and even reprimand the employee for poor hygiene. Employees who present themselves with the smell of alcohol may be sent home. It is important that the nurse appreciate that odors may be pathological, such as with certain diabetic states, or the result of certain mouthwashes or soaps. If a patient has an unpleasant odor, the nurse's first response should be to assess whether some pathological condition is ensuing, such as an inflammatory process. In a psychiatric hospital a patient's odor could be associated with a condition such as schizophrenia; while there is some thought that such an odor may be pathological, it is more likely to be related to a lack of motivation for self-care skills.

Immediate Receptors

Immediate receptors are those that examine the world up close and include tactile stimuli received by way of the skin membranes. It is important that the nurse appreciate the effect culture may have on an individual's reaction to these stimuli and how these stimuli can be modified by cultural influences.

Skin membranes

Human beings receive a tremendous amount of information from the distance receptors, which include the eyes, ears, and nose. Because of the vast amount of information that is received from the distance receptors, few people think of the skin as a major sense organ. However, if we humans lacked the ability to perceive heat and cold, we would soon perish. Without the ability to perceive heat and cold, or to react appropriately to these stimuli, we would freeze in the winter and become overheated in the summer. The skin, as a major sense organ, is so grossly overlooked that even some of its subtle sensing and communicating qualities are overlooked. Nerves called proprioceptors keep us informed as to exactly what is happening as we work our muscles. These nerves provide the feedback that enables us to move our bodies smoothly; thus they occupy a key position in kinesthetic space perception. The body also has another set of nerves called exterioceptors, which are located in the skin and convey the sensations of heat, cold, touch, and pain to the central nervous system. In light of the fact that two different systems of nerves are employed in the perception of space, kinesthetic space is viewed as being qualitatively different from thermal space. However, it must be kept in mind that these two systems work together and that they are mutually reinforcing most of the time.

It has only been in modern scientific times that some remarkable thermal characteristics of the skin have been discovered. The capacity of the skin for emitting and detecting radiant or infrared heat is extraordinarily high. One might assume that since the capacity of the skin to both emit and detect radiant or infrared heat is so highly developed, it was important to survival in the past and most certainly had a significant function in early man. Although the discovery of the thermal characteristics of the skin has only been within recent times, the importance of the skin as an immediate receptor should not be overlooked by the nurse.

Humans are well equipped to send and receive messages concerning emotional states according to changes in skin temperature. Skin temperatures can give very important clues to the emotional state of an individual. A common indicator of embarrassment or anger in fair-skinned individuals is the blush. However, dark-skinned people also blush. Therefore blushing cannot be perceived as simply a matter of change in skin coloration. The nurse must carefully observe dark-skinned persons when looking for changes in emotional state such as embarrassment or anger by noting a swelling of the regions of the forehead. The additional blood to these areas will raise the temperature, and these areas will appear flushed. Therefore even if there is no significant change in color to these areas in dark-skinned individuals, these areas will appear warm to the touch.

Many novel instruments have been developed that make it possible to study heat emission. These instruments should make it possible to study the thermal details of interpersonal communication, an area not previously accessible to direct observation. Thermographic devices (infrared detaching devices and cameras) that were originally developed for satellites and homing missiles have been developed for recording subvisual phenomena. Photographs taken in the dark using radiant heat of the human body have shown that an inflamed area of the body actually emits more heat than the surrounding areas. Diagnosis of cancer is also possible with thermographic devices that measure blocked circulation of blood. Thermographic devices have been useful in health care delivery because skin color does not affect the amount of heat delivered;

dark skin does not emit more or less heat than light skin. Thus the observable phenomenon in all individuals in regard to heat emission is the blood supply in a given area of the body.

Increased heat on the surface is detected in three ways:

1. Thermal detectors in the skin, particularly if two individuals are close enough to each other.
2. Intensified olfactory interactions, which are augmented when skin temperature rises. Perfumes or body or face lotions may be smelled at a greater distance when the body temperature is increased.
3. Visual examination, which can give clues to an increase or decrease in body temperature. For example, an individual who is pale may have a decrease in body temperature, whereas a person who appears flushed may have an increase in body temperature.

Certain individuals and/or racial groups are more aware of subtle changes in skin temperature. In addition, some persons accentuate or take advantage of this medium of communication. For example, an individual knowledgeable about variations in skin temperature according to location may apply perfume to certain parts of the body. The phenomenon of crowding is a chain reaction set in motion when there is not enough space to dissipate the heat within a crowd and the heat becomes more intense. A hot crowd will require more room than a cool crowd if they are to maintain the same degree of comfort and lack of involvement. It is important for the nurse to remember that when thermal spaces overlap and people can smell each other, they become more involved and may even be under the chemical influences of each other's emotions. Some individuals by virtue of cultural heritage have trouble with the phenomenon of crowding. These individuals are more likely to be unable to sit in a chair soon after someone else has vacated it. An example of this phenomenon is often given by sailors on submarines who are forced to participate in "hot bunking," the practice of sharing a bunk as soon as someone gets out of it. It is not understood why one's own heat is not objectionable whereas a stranger's may be. It may be due in part to the fact that humans have a great sensitivity to small differences; therefore individuals respond negatively to a heat pattern that is not familiar (Hall, 1966a).

Body heat regulation lies deep in the brain and is controlled by the hypothalamus. Culture affects attitudes in regard to the perception of skin temperature changes. Human beings exert little or no conscious control over the heat system of the body. Many cultural groups tend to stress phenomena that can be controlled and deny those that cannot. In other words, because some individuals by virtue of their cultural heritage have been taught to ignore certain uncontrollable stimuli, these individuals experience body heat as a highly personal stimulus. Body heat is therefore linked to intimacy, as well as to the experiences of childhood. An adult who as a child was used to close personal contact with parents and other loved ones may have a pleasant association when in a crowded environment where heat and warmth are radiated. On the other hand, an adult who was subjected to discomfort in close relationships or who was not exposed to closeness as a child may experience a great deal of difficulty and anxiety when in a close environment, for example, an overcrowded bus.

A person born in a heavily populated country where closeness was necessitated by overcrowding may experience conscious discomfort in moving to another locality where closeness is not the norm. On the other hand, persons born in thinly populated countries may have a conscious feeling of overcrowding in a country where closeness is the norm. For example, a tourist from the United States visiting a country such as Hong Kong, Jamaica, or China, all of which are extremely overpopulated, may quickly react to the experience of closeness and associate the country with unpleasantness. This experience is not limited to different cultures but may also be noted when a rural person visits an urban setting, such as a person from rural Mississippi visiting New York.

The English language is full of expressions that relate to skin sensation and body temperature changes. For example, it is not uncommon in the United States to hear individuals say that another made them hot under the collar, gave them a cold stare, involved them in a heated argument, or warmed them up. These expressions may be more than just a figure of speech; they may be a way of recognizing the changes in body temperature that occur both personally and in other people. Thus these common experiences have been incorporated into language in the United States.

Relationship between Tactile Space and Visual Space

Touch and visual spatial experiences are so interwoven with one another that the two cannot be easily separated. Young children and infants learn to reach, grasp, fondle, and mouth everything in the environment. Teaching children the relationship between tactile and visual space is a difficult task that requires many years of training in order for children to subordinate the world of touch to the visual world. Visual and tactile space can be distinguished by the fact that tactile space separates the viewer from the object, whereas visual space separates objects from each other. As early as 1945 Michael Baliant described two different perceptual worlds: one was described as sight oriented and the other as touch oriented. According to Baliant, the touch-oriented world is both immediate and friendlier than the sight-oriented world, in which space is friendly but filled with dangerous and unpredictable objects, namely people. Using Baliant's definition of tactile space, it is difficult to conceive that designers and engineers have failed to grasp in all of their scientific research the deep significance of touch, particularly active touch (actually contacting others or objects). Individuals incorporate both tactile and visual stimuli in relating to the world. For example, although automakers tend to rely heavily on visual perception when designing a particular automobile for marketing purposes, they are also concerned with tactile perception, as evidenced by their giving attention to such things as luxury upholstery, automatic windows, doors, gas cap locks, ornate trimmings, and carpeting. In response to this stimuli, prospective buyers stroke and fondle both the car's interior and exterior before making a purchase.

Some objects in the environment are appraised and appreciated almost entirely by touch, even when these objects are visually presented, such as objects made from wood, cloth, or ceramics. The Japanese are very conscious of the significance of texture. Emphasis is placed on the smoothness of the item being crafted. It may be perceived that it requires more time to make a smoothly crafted item than a roughly textured item and that the time spent on the crafted item is related to the care and concern of the craftsman. The objects that are produced by Japanese people may be perceived as being made by caring craftsman.

Touch is the most personal of all of the sensations. It is described by some as the most important sense, because it confirms the reality perceived through the other senses (Montagu, 1971). Touch is central to the human communication process and is often used to communicate messages. Beyond general communication, touch is associated with breaking down the distance between individuals. Most people associate life's most intimate moments with touch. For example, during lovemaking or in a loving relationship, touch takes on a private and special meaning. Nurses have long appreciated touch as an important component of the nurse-patient interaction (Clement, 1987). Nurses face the challenge of developing trust, creating a humanistic and responsive atmosphere, and effectively exchanging information in a system energized by high technology and concern for cost-effectiveness. Most nursing literature focuses on touch as a communication behavior and describes using touch to communicate caring (Geldard, 1960; Leininger, 1977; Mintz, 1969; Montagu, 1971), the physiological and psychological dynamics of touch (Davidhizar & Giger, 1989; Goodykoontz, 1980; Hedlund, 1988; Heidt, 1981; Kreiger, 1975; Lynch, 1978; West, 1981), and the components of touch behavior. Research also supports the belief that using touch appropriately with patients can bring about positive physiological and psychological responses (Day, 1973; Seaman, 1982; Ujhely, 1979). Nurses need to be aware of the characteristics of touch and how they can affect the entire communication process.

In contrast to tactile space is the phenomenon of visual space. To understand visual space, the nurse must understand that no persons see exactly the same thing when actively using their eyes in a natural situation; people do not relate to the world around them in exactly the same way. For example, different persons will visually notice different objects because of perceptual differences. It is important for the nurse to recognize these differences and at the same time be able to translate from one perceptual world to another. The distance between the perceptual worlds of two persons of the same culture may be considerably less than the distance between the perceptual worlds of two persons of different cultures. There is significant evidence that people brought up in different cultures live in different perceptual worlds. Americans tend to have a more linear perceptual field, whereas Chinese and Japanese persons tend to have a more depth-oriented perceptual field. This difference is demonstrated in art and architectural design. Designs that have a linear perspective are preferred by Americans. On the other hand, Chinese and Japanese artists symbolize depth and yet at the same time maintain constancy in the design.

SPATIAL BEHAVIOR

Spatial behavior is often described in the nursing literature in relation to the universal need for territoriality (Allekian, 1973; Davidhizar, 1988; Hayter, 1981; Hedland, 1988; Oland, 1978). People by nature are territorial. Territoriality refers to a state characterized by possessiveness, control, and authority over an area of physical space. If the need for territoriality is to be met, the person must be in control of some space and be able to establish rules for that space. The need for territoriality cannot be fully met unless individuals can defend their space against invasion or misuse by others (Roberts, 1978). Hayter (1981) has suggested three important aspects of territoriality to consider when planning nursing care: a physical space of one's own, a personal space, and the territory of expertise or role. One can also relate territoriality needs to spatial behaviors of or proximity to others, to objects in the environment, and to body movement or position. Territoriality serves to achieve diverse functions for individuals, including meeting needs for security, privacy, autonomy, and self-identity. A variety of factors may influence needs for territoriality, including culture, age, sex, and health status. It is important for the nurse to understand the effect such variables may have on spatial behavior.

Proximity to Others

Generally, in Western culture there are three primary dimensions of space: the intimate zone (0 to 18 inches), the personal zone (18 inches to 3 feet), and the social or public zone (3 to 6 feet) (Hall, 1966b). The intimate zone may be used for comforting, protection, and counseling and is reserved for people who feel close. The personal zone usually is maintained with friends or in some counseling interactions. Touch can occur in the intimate and personal zones. The social zone is usually used when impersonal business is conducted or with people who are working together. Sensory involvement and communication are often less intense in the social zone. Wide variations to these general dimensions do occur and are often influenced by cultural background. Montagu (1971) has suggested that child-rearing practices affecting sleep behavior may have an effect on the use of space, especially as it determines acceptable interaction distance. He reported on varying cultural approaches apparently related to family group sleeping arrangements and the Western middle-class practice of separating the child from parents for sleep. According to Oland (1978), the Western practice of putting small children in a room of their own, which separates them from other family members, may enculturate children to desire isolation and separation, and cause or facilitate a desire for more extensive territory.

Spatial needs and the desire for a certain proximity to certain people continue through life and have been studied in the elderly. In nursing homes the elderly patients may have certain chairs identified as theirs and become upset when a stranger sits in their chair or in the seat nearby that is reserved for a special friend. Moving from household to household to stay with children on a rotating basis, rather than being viewed as a pleasant variation, is also likely to be upsetting. Since the elderly are more likely to experience separation from others through the death of a spouse and the moving away of offspring, their spatial needs may appear to change; that is, they way withdraw or may reach out more for others (Ittelson et al., 1974).

Interpersonal messages are communicated not only by body proximity, but also by the location and availability of the nurse during the day. A patient who knows that the nurse will answer when the call bell is pressed feels differently than the patient who does not understand how the call bell works or feels it is an imposition to ask for help and waits for the nurse to ask what can be done (Schuster & Ashburn, 1986).

Individuals have different requirements for sensory stimulation. Either overstimulation, such as by crowding, or understimulation, such as may be present when a person cannot communicate with others, may cause an untoward reaction. For example, in times of disaster overstimulation induced by crowding can be so extreme it can result in insanity or death. In this example, a person is perceived as being in a little black box and unable to move about freely, which causes the person to jostle, push, and shove. How the individual responds to jostling and therefore to the enclosed space depends on how he or she feels about being touched by total strangers. It is this constant touching and being touched that may result in widespread panic and "freezing" in disaster situations (Hall, 1966b).

An enclosed space requirement can also be overstimulating. For example, a patient who must remain in a hospital room in bed and in isolation for a lengthy period can be overstimulated because of the spatial limits presented by the boundaries, including bed rest and the four walls of the room. Nursing interventions for this patient include opening window curtains, calling by intercom frequently to check on the patient, and stopping by to see the patient as often as possible. A patient in isolation can also suffer from understimulation in regard to tactile stimulation. The few people who do enter the room may hesitate to touch the patient out of fear of contracting the illness. One of the greatest problems expressed by patients with acquired immunodeficiency syndrome (AIDS) today is the isolation they experience because of physical distances from others. Family members afraid of catching AIDS may hesitate to touch, hug, or kiss the AIDS victim. Caregivers also may show their fear by standing a greater distance from the patient, wearing gloves, and having less frequent encounters with the patient (Zook & Davidhizar, in press).

The strong link between curing, the major focus of health care, and caring by health care practitioners has been emphasized by Leininger (1977), who cites touch as one of the special constructs of the caring process. As a therapeutic element of human interaction, touch can help the nurse to show caring.

Cultural implications

Watson (1980) noted that while there are variations in spatial requirements from individual to individual, persons in the same cultural group tend to act similarly. For example, nomads do not seem to desire a permanent territory but are content with establishing a very temporary territory and then moving on. Since individuals are usually not consciously aware of their personal space requirements, they frequently have difficulty understanding a different cultural pattern. What may be considered an act of friendliness by one person (for example, standing close to another person) may be perceived by the other as a threatening invasion of personal space. A person who wishes to maintain distance will indicate this by body language. Individuals who step back, do not face the nurse directly, or pull their chair back from the nurse are sending messages indicating additional space requirements. The nurse's responsiveness to the patient's spatial requirements is an important factor in the patient's emotional comfort. It is important that the nurse be cognizant of the effects of culture on the patient's spatial needs and use sensitivity in responding to the patient's need for personal territory. Subtle cultural variations in the use of nonverbal signals often lead to misunderstanding; thus to meet patient needs, it is essential that the nurse have knowledge of cultural variations in spatial requirements.

Watson (1980) studied cultural differences in the use of personal space. He compiled a range of space by nationality and found that Americans, Canadians, and the British require the most personal space, whereas Latin American, Japanese, and Arabic persons need the least. Japanese, Arabic, and Latin American persons seemingly have a much higher tolerance for crowding in public spaces than do some other cultural groups, such as Americans and Northern Europeans, but they also appear to be more concerned about their own requirements for the space they live in. In particular, the Japanese tend to devote more time and attention to the proper organization of their living space for perception by all the senses (Hall, 1966b). A South American male patient may stand in the intimate zone while describing symptoms to the nurse.

Touching between persons of the same sex, including men, is more common among Arabs or South Vietnamese persons than it is among Americans. In America this kind of familiarity may be considered a homosexual pass (Hall, 1966b). Argyle and Dean (1965) reported that members of primitive societies in Africa and Indonesia came closer still and maintained bodily contact during conversation.

In America a person who stands at a slight angle to another indicates a body position of readiness to communicate. A desire to exclude a third person can be shown by two persons who face each other directly and have ongoing eye contact. Rejection is also communicated by a person who stands at right angles to another (Scheflen, 1972). The position of the toes can create distance by communicating rank. A person who feels subordinate will usually stand with the toes inward, whereas a person who feels superior will stand with the toes facing out (*Personal Report,* 1987). A comparison of the recent American movie *Three Men and a Baby* and the French comedy it was based on *(Three Men and a Cradle)* illustrates the differences in responses in the two cultures. In the French version when the natural father returns to the two bachelors who have been inconvenienced by the care of the baby, icy silence occurs, with the men sitting stiffly in their chairs and refusing to answer their friend's questions or even acknowledge his presence. In the American version when the natural father returns, he is pummeled and a loud scene occurs (Grosvenor, 1989).

Territoriality influences relationships between people. Some German people tend to need a larger space and are less flexible in their spatial behavior than some American, French, and Arab people. Differences in spatial patterns between persons in different cultures apply not only to their body proximity, but also to such behavior as changing geographic location. For example, whereas Germans often live in the same house their entire lives, Americans tend to change houses approximately every 5 years. Differences in patterns of permanance are also noted in nomads, who for the most part are content with establishing temporary territories rather than permanent ones. According to Evans and Howard (1973), some Puerto Ricans and Blacks may have different perspectives about space. Some Blacks have more eye contact when they speak, have greater body activity, and have a closer personal space (Sue, 1981).

Objects in the Environment

Objects in the environment offer additional dimensions to communication and can provide both positive and negative qualifiers to verbal communication. Easily movable chairs in a waiting room or office can be pulled together to provide physical closeness or, if the patient prefers it, separated to provide distance. Positioning chairs at a 90-degree angle can communicate a cooperative stance, whereas a side-by-side arrangement of chairs can decrease communication.

Cleanliness in the environment may also be a significant factor in creating a healthy and comfortable milieu. Comfortable air conditioning in a patient waiting room on a hot day can facilitate a patient's ease and decrease anxiety. On the other hand, when the air conditioning is absent or malfunctioning on a hospital ward on a hot day, patient and staff anxiety can escalate. Discomfort and consequently emotional distance can be created by uncomfortable furniture. The nurse's position during the conversation (for example, behind a desk or leaning against the corner of the desk looking down on the patient seated at a lower level) can also promote the perception of psychological distance. In any case, the nurse needs to be aware of the effect culture may play on the patient's reaction to objects in the environment and should respond in a way that patient comfort will be increased (Pearlin, 1982).

The nurse's clothes, hair, and jewelry also affect the message that the patient receives. For example, a child may be fearful of white, relating it to being hurt. A male patient may perceive any female nurse with red hair as "sexy." Medical symbols such as a stethoscope around the nurse's neck or a name pin may indicate to the patient that the nurse is a knowledgeable professional. On the other hand, lack of a cap or uniform, if the patient expects nurses to have caps or uniforms, may cause the patient to doubt the competency or professionalism of the nurse.

Structural boundaries

The term *personal boundaries* is sometimes used to describe the use of structural boundaries in the environment. A boundary separates a person from others and also helps define a person's space. Fences, doors, curtains, and walls, as well as desks, chairs, and certain objects, may create a boundary between the individual and others (Scott, 1988). The purpose of a boundary is to facilitate individuation or separation from the environment. Developmentally, this concept begins at approximately 6 months of age. Mahler, Pine, and Bergman (1975) have described an infant's first attempts at separation/individuation as consisting of behaviors such as pulling at the parent's hair, ears, or nose and straining the body away from the parent to get a better look at him or her. At 7 to 8 months the infant begins to differentiate self from the parent. The child may examine the parent's jewelry or glasses and is anxious around others. These crucial developmental steps are indicative of the child's beginning formation of boundary. The process of boundary formation continues through the toddler stage. By age 3 the toddler has a fairly stable sense of identity and self-boundaries.

Doors, walls, glass panels, and waist-high partitions serve as structural boundaries for nurses' territories in health care settings. Doors, curtains, and furniture arrangements may define patient territories. Structural boundaries can help the individual adapt to both internal and external stresses. On the other hand, when structural boundaries are violated, anxiety may increase. The nurse needs to assess whether the patient has rigid or flexible boundaries. If a patient has open boundaries, less anxiety will be encountered in interactions with health professionals that may violate personal boundaries. If the patient has rigid boundaries, the nurse should guard against approaches that may be perceived as threatening.

The use of restraints with agitated patients involves physical invasion of both intimate space and body boundaries. Patients who resist restraints and become aggressive and combative may be viewed as resisting this personal invasion.

Just as individuals can be described by personal boundaries that determine comfort levels in relation to others, territoriality can also be used to describe an interpersonal phenomenon in the environment. As indicated earlier, territoriality is a state characterized by possessiveness, control, and authority over an area of physical space (Hayter, 1981). For the need for territoriality to be fully met, the person must be in control of some space, be able to establish rules for that space, and be able to defend it against invasion or misuse by others. In addition, the person's right to do things in the space must be acknowledged by others (Roberts, 1978). For example, a psychiatric patient needs not only a personal sleeping area, but also a place to put and arrange personal belongings without fear that they will be bothered by others. There should also be freedom to do things in the personal space, such as take a nap.

Nursing staff also have professional territorial imperatives. Nurses' stations and lounges may be designated as staff territory. When a psychiatric unit is renovated and staff are asked by administration to move from a locked nursing station concept to an open nursing station concept wherein patients may come to an open half wall to interact openly with staff who may be inside, staff may find this very intrusive of "their" territory and object to this invasion of their space. Staff needs for territory must also be considered when unit staff and patients' areas are designed. When certain staff are restricted from certain hospital areas (for example, the mailroom or the copy machine room), this may be seen as punitive and dehumanizing. Thus it is essential that explanations given for this restriction be clearly understood to avoid paranoid interpretations of this action.

Cultural implications

In American culture warm colors such as yellow, red, and orange stimulate creative, happy responses. Cool colors such as blue, green, and gray tend to encourage meditation and deliberation and have a dampening effect on communication. The nurse should plan color in the environment to be therapeutic and to enhance communication (Bartholet, 1968).

Many immigrants to America not only decorate their houses to remind them of their cultural heritage, such as with pictures, curtains, or furniture from their homeland, but their houses may resemble those of their native land on the outside as well. For example, a German American may have a garden in Pennsylvania that resembles the garden of the parental home in Germany. Cultural artifacts may be worn by the patient or nurse and provide a nonverbal message. Artifacts that act as nonverbal stimuli when interactions occur include clothes, cosmetics, perfume, jewelry, wigs or hairpieces, and beards and mustaches. A full-length mink coat, hair that has been dyed purple, earrings on a man, a nose ring, two earrings in one ear, a military uniform, a sorority pin, a wedding band—all provide nonverbal information to others.

Body Movement or Position

Body movement or position can also communicate a message to others. This concept has been well documented by the pioneering work of Birdwhitstell (1970), Efron (1941), Scheflen (1972), Ekman and Friesen (1975), and Ekman (1985) and by recent reviews of the state of the art in this field (Bull, 1983; Davis, 1975; Davis & Skupien, 1982; Hickman & Stacks, 1985; Leathers, 1986; Wolfgang, 1984). This information has been further applied to counseling and psychotherapeutic techniques through the work of Moreno (1946); Perls, Hefferline and Goodman (1951); Gendlin (1969); Marcus (1985); and Steere (1982), who have made body movement and awareness central aspects of their therapeutic approach. Thus a broad body of knowledge supports the premise that through body movement a person may convey what is not verbalized.

It is well known that body movements may be of particular importance during periods of stress. Expressions of self through movement are learned before speech; therefore when stress is experienced, a person may revert to a form of expression used at an earlier level. Attention to body movement can facilitate understanding of a person experiencing stress. There are endless expressions of body movement, such as finger pointing, head nodding, smiles, slaps on the back, head and general body movements, and even body sounds, including belching, knuckle cracking, and laughing. A seemingly insignificant act such as how a door bell is rung may bear the stamp of an individual's personality, as well as emotional state. For example, the door bell may be rung loudly, impatiently, repetitively, tentatively, feebly, or aggressively (Bendich, 1988).

The nurse must also consider the effect of slow versus fast movements (Newman, 1976). In an emergency rapid movements are essential. On the other hand, a young child in the hospital for the first time may be frightened by a health professional who enters the room quickly, approaches the child rapidly, and picks the child up. In another situation an agitated psychiatric patient who is approached slowly and with a quiet voice may be calmed by the slow movements of the nurse, which are seen as reassuring.

Nurses are also exploring movement as a therapeutic medium, for example, movement therapy for the aged (Goldberg & Fitzpatrick, 1980; Stevenson, 1989), movement therapy following inactivity or infection (Folta, 1989; Kasper, 1989), dance and movement therapy, and exercise to music. It has been thought that movement therapy can provide a way to communicate when the ability to communicate feelings is limited. Movement therapy has also been used for relaxation and to provide relief of blocked emotion.

Body motions, or kinetic behaviors, can be categorized as follows (Knapp, 1980):

1. *Emblems:* Nonverbal actions that have a verbal translation into a word, phrase, or symbol. This includes sign language used in the operating room or the gesture of thumb and forefinger to form a circle to say "A-OK" in America or to indicate an obscenity in Brazil.
2. *Affect displays:* Facial expressions such as a frown, smile, or lips pulled down at the corners.
3. *Illustrations:* Nonverbal acts accompanying speech. Examples of this include an up-turned thumb to indicate a ride is desired or pointing a finger to indicate a direction.
4. *Adapters:* Nonverbal behavior that modifies or adds to what is being said. For example, folded arms may indicate disgust or that a person is feeling closed to others; a wave may be used as a friendly greeting; leg swinging and finger tapping may indicate anxiety.
5. *Regulators:* Movements that maintain interaction and provide feedback. Head nods or changing gaze can indicate that it is the other person's turn to talk. A head nod can also indicate listening.

Cultural implications

Body movement is also related to culture. For example, in America head nodding is common, whereas in Africa the torso is frequently moved (Eibl-Eibesfeldt, 1972). Gestures are used by Americans and the English to denote activity and by Italian or Jewish persons to emphasize words (Bigham, 1964). In the United States certain actions are not considered proper with strangers, for example, touching, standing close to, or looking directly at the individual. Some cultures give certain body movements a sexual interpretation. In the United States stroking the hair, adjusting the clothes, or changing position to accent maleness or femaleness may have or be given a sexual connotation (Scheflen, 1972). While a kiss is often given a sexual connotation in the United States, the Japanese kiss to show deference to superiors (Sue, 1981).

IMPLICATIONS FOR NURSING CARE

It is important for the nurse to remember that territoriality, or the need for space, serves four functions: security, privacy, autonomy, and self-identity (Oland, 1978). Security includes actual safety from harm and gives the person a feeling of being safe. It is important for the nurse to remember that if a patient is in a place where a feeling of control is experienced, the patient will feel safer, less threatened, and less anxious. People generally tend to feel safer in their own territory because it is arranged and equipped in a familiar manner. In addition, most people believe there is a degree of predictability associated with being in one's own personal space and that this degree of predictability is hard to achieve elsewhere. Nurses must also keep in mind that the anxiety level of a patient is increased when the patient is hospitalized. However, the same patient may experience a decrease in anxiety if the patient is allowed to return home, even if still sick. Some terminally ill patients request to go home because of the feeling of security experienced in one's own personal space.

In addition to security, personal space provides privacy and at the same time protected communication. Most people feel it is not necessary to be on guard or to keep up pretenses in the security of one's own personal space. In other words, most people have a need to be themselves. The fulfillment of the desire to be oneself contributes to feelings of decreased anxiety and promotes relaxation. Many people may complain of feeling tense and tired after a long day at work but may experience relaxation and ease of tension as soon as they get home. Two factors that contribute to these feelings are the fact that activities at home are different from those at work and the fact that people experience more relaxation in their own personal space (Hayter, 1981). If it becomes necessary to transfer a patient from one room to another or from one floor to another, the nurse should keep in mind that the patient may experience increased anxiety because of a sense of loss of security and privacy (Smith, 1976). This feeling of loss of security and privacy can also be related to nursing practice. For example, a nurse manager who returns from vacation to find office furniture rearranged may feel dissettled until the furniture is returned to a familiar arrangement. The nurse should keep in mind that patients may already be experiencing feelings of anxiety that are related to the reasons for seeking health care. Additional anxiety invoked by issues involving territoriality can be minimized by the nurse who develops an understanding of culture and its implications for territoriality or interpersonal space.

Another important aspect of territoriality for nursing is the function of autonomy. Autonomy is the means by which a person controls what happens. In personal territory a person may feel free to ask questions, resist suggested actions, hold out for those things that are most important personally, and share personal feelings. A patient, on the other hand, is out of personal territory and lacks control. Therefore it is important for the nurse to ascertain whether the patient has an adequate understanding of the treatment regimen and is not submitting to treatment merely because of a lack of control of territory. Statements to the patient that maximize feelings of control, such as "How do you want to arrange the room?" or "Are you concerned about your treatment? We can walk down the hall to the visiting room, where it is private, to discuss your feelings" should promote feelings of security and autonomy for the patient. Feelings of autonomy are also evidenced in nursing practice. For example, when a nurse manager needs to counsel an employee, the manager's control will be maximized if the counseling occurs in the manager's office. On the other hand, if the manager is viewed as too controlling, the manager may intentionally select a more neutral territory for the conference, such as a conference room.

It is important for the nurse to keep in mind that having personal space promotes self-identity by affording opportunities for self-expression. Another way to define self-identity in relation to personal space is to view self-identity as a mode of individuality. The personal space over which a person has jurisdiction often becomes a personal extension of self and a reflection of characteristics, personality, and interest. People have a need to organize and arrange personal space so that it maximizes functioning and at the same time meets needs. An excellent example of this is that when a person purchases a new home, it becomes essential for that home to take on the person's identity. This is evidenced by the desire of the new occupants to change such items as the wallpaper, colors of the walls, the carpet, lighting fixtures, and draperies. Regardless of whether or not these items are new, each person has a need for self-expression or individuality. When patients set out personal pictures of their family and other personal items from home and wear their own sleepwear, self-identity is enhanced. Therefore changing items to reflect this individuality becomes an essential aspect of personal security and autonomy.

SUMMARY

To give culturally appropriate nursing care, the nurse must have an understanding of interpersonal space. Understanding the way in which a patient may use space requires open-mindedness, an observing attitude, and an attitude in which inferences and hypotheses are made from repeated observations and checked against further observations until a reasonably comprehensive understanding develops. This understanding is then continually reconciled with any new discrepant verbal or nonverbal data that may appear (Bendich, 1988). The nurse must guard against an interpretation that just because a patient is from a certain cultural group, the patient's use of space is similar to that of others in that culture. While a person's cultural heritage may have some bearing on certain aspects of that person's use of space, use of space also varies with the individual.

CASE STUDY   Mr. Bernhard Wolfgang, a 56-year-old German immigrant who works as an engineer, is admitted with chest pain and shortness of breath. Mr. Wolfgang is admitted to the coronary care unit to rule out myocardial infarction. Immediately after admission Mr. Wolfgang's wife comes to the coronary care unit with personal items such as family portraits, some roses from the patient's garden, and some personal clothing. However, since the coronary care unit is restricted in space, personal items are not allowed, and the wife is instructed to take the items home. On admission, Mr. Wolfgang's vital signs are stable and his color is good. He reports that the chest pain is not debilitating and is more or less an occasional dull ache. After 2 days the diagnosis of myocardial infarction is confirmed, and Mr. Wolfgang remains restricted to bed but is transferred to a semiprivate room in the coronary care step-down unit . After admission to the coronary care step-down unit, the nurse notes that Mr. Wolfgang is anxious, somewhat withdrawn, and unable to express his needs and feelings.

STUDY
QUESTIONS

1. When assessing Mr. Wolfgang, the nurse should realize that some German people have specific needs that are related to territoriality and space. Name at least two factors that affect some Germans and their spatial behavior.
2. List ways the nurse could enable Mr. Wolfgang to meet his needs for privacy and autonomy while in a semiprivate room.
3. Identify markers that would indicate Mr. Wolfgang's need for the establishment of a temporary territorial space.
4. Identify ways in which illness and hospitalization could threaten Mr. Wolfgang's personal sense of territoriality.
5. Identify factors present in a coronary care unit that could negatively affect spatial behavior.
6. List two factors related to perceptual and visual stimuli that adversely affect some German patients.
7. List ways the nurse could control perceptual and verbal stimuli that may affect Mr. Wolfgang.

REFERENCES

Allekian, C.E. (1973). Intrusions of territory and personal space. *Nursing Research, 22,* 236-241.

Argyle, M., & Dean, J. (1965). Eye-contact, distance, and affiliation. *Sociometry, 28,* 289-304.

Baliant, M. (1945). Friendly expanses—hard empty spaces. *International Journal of Psychoanalysis, 4,* 38-46.

Bartholet M. (1968). Effects of color on dynamics of patient care. *Nursing Outlook, 6*(10), 51-53.

Bendich, S. (1988). Appreciating bodily phenomena in verbally oriented psychotherapy sessions. *Issues in Mental Health Nursing, 9,* 1-7.

Bigham, C. (1964). To communicate with Negro patients. *American Journal of Nursing, 64*(9), 113-115.

Birdwhitstell, R. (1970). *Kinesics and context.* Philadelphia: University of Pennsylvania Press.

Black, J.W. (1950). The effect of room characteristics on vocalizations and rate. *Journal of Accoustical Society in America, 22,* 174-76.

Brown, J.W., Leavitt, L., & Graham, F. (1977). Response to auditory stimuli in six and nine-week-old infants. *Developmental Psychobiology, 10,* 255-266.

Bull, P. (1983). *Body movement and interpersonal communication.* New York: John Wiley & Sons.

Clement, J. (1987). Touch. *Association of operation room nurses, 45*(6), 1429-1439.

Davidhizar, R. (1988). Distance in managerial encounters. *Today's OR Nurse, 10*(10), 23-30.

Davidhizar, R., & Giger, J. (1989). Managerial touch. *Today's OR Nurse, 10*(7), 18-25.

Day, F. (1973). The patient's perception of touch. In E.H. Anderson, B.S. Bergerson, M. Duffey, M. Lohr, & M.H. Rose (Eds.), *Current concepts in clinical nursing* (Vol. 4, pp. 266-275). St. Louis: C.V. Mosby.

Davis, M. (1975). *Towards understanding the intrinsic body movement.* New York: Ayer.

Davis, M., & Skupien, J. (1982). *Body movement and nonverbal communication: An annotated bibliography, 1971-1981.* Bloomington: Indiana University Press.

Efron, D. (1941). *Gesture and environment.* New York: King's Crown Press.

Eibl-Eibesfeldt, I. (1972). Similarities and differences between cultures in expressive movements. In R.A. Hinde (Ed.), *Nonverbal communication* (pp. 297-312). Cambridge, U.K.: Cambridge University Press.

Ekman, P. (1985). *Telling lies.* New York: W.W. Norton.

Ekman, P., & Friesen, W.V. (1975). *Unmasking the face.* Englewood Cliffs, N.J.: Prentice Hall.

Evans, G.W., & Howard, R.B. (1973). Personal space. *Psychological Bulletin, 80,* 335-344.

Folta, A. (1989, April 3). *Exercise and functional capacity after myocardial infarction.* Paper presented at the 13th Annual Midwest Nursing Research Society Conference, Cincinnati.

Geldard, F. (1960). Some neglected possibilities of communication. *Science 131,* 1583-1588.

Gendlin, E.T. (1969). Focussing. *American Journal of Psychotherapy, 1,* 1-18.

Goldberg, W., & Fitzpatrick, J. (1980). Movement therapy with the aged. *Nursing Research, 29,* 339-346.

Goodykoontz, L. (1980). Touch: dynamic aspect of nursing care. *Journal of Nursing Care, 13,* 16-18.

Grosvenor, G.M. (1989, July). Viva la difference (President's editorial). *National Geographic,* p. 15.

Haber, J., Hoskins, P., Leach, A., & Sideleau, B. (1987). *Comprehensive psychiatric nursing.* New York: Mc-Graw-Hill.

Hall, E.T. (1966a). *The hidden dimension.* New York: Doubleday.

Hall, E.T. (1966b). *The silent language.* Westport, Conn.: Greenwood Press.

Hayter, J. (1981). Territoriality as a universal need. *Journal of Advanced Nursing, 6,* 79-85.

Hedlund, N. (1988). Therapeutic communication. In C.K. Beck, R.P. Rawlins, & S. Williams (Eds.), *Mental health–psychiatric nursing* (2nd ed., pp. 65-91). St. Louis: C.V. Mosby.

Heidt, P. (1981). Effect of therapeutic touch on anxiety level of hospitalized patients. *Nursing Research, 30,* 32-37.

Hickson, M.L., & Stacks, D.W. (1985). *Nonverbal communication studies and applications.* Dubuque, Iowa: Wm. C. Brown.

Ittelson, W., Proshansky, H., Rivlin, I., & Winkel, H. (1974). *An introduction to environmental psychology.* New York: Holt, Rinehart, & Winston.

Kasper, C. (1989, April 3). *Exercise-induced degeneration of skeletal muscle following inactivity.* Paper presented at the 13th Annual Midwest Nursing Research Society Conference, Cincinnati.

Knapp, M. (1980). *Nonverbal communication in human interaction* (2nd ed.). New York: Holt, Rinehart, & Winston.

Kreiger, D. (1975). Therapeutic touch: The imprimatur of nursing. *American Journal of Nursing, 75,* 785-787.

Leathers, D.B. (1986). *Successful nonverbal communication principles and applications.* New York: Macmillan.

Leininger, M. (1977, Dec.). Caring: The essence of central focus of nursing. *Nursing Research, Report I,* p. 2.

Lynch, J. (1978). The simple act of touching. *Nursing '78, 8,* 32-36.

Mahler, M., Pine, F., & Bergman, A. (1975). *The psychological birth of the human infant.* New York: Basic Books.

Marcus, N. (1985). Utilization of nonverbal expressive behavior in cognitive therapy. *American Journal of Psychotherapy, 39*(4), 467-478.

Mintz, E. (1969). On the rationale of touch in psychotherapy. *Psychotherapy: Theory, Research, and Practice, 6*(4), 232-234.

Montagu, A. (1971). *The significance of the human skin.* New York: Columbia University Press.

Moreno, J.L. (1946). *Psychodrama* (Vol. 1). New York: Beacon House.

Newman, M. (1976). Movement therapy and the experience of time. *Nursing Research, 25,* 273-279.

Oland, L. (1978). The need for territoriality. In H. Yura & M.B. Walsh (Eds.), *Human needs and the nursing process* (pp. 97-140). New York: Appleton-Century-Crofts.

Pearlin, L. (1982). The social context of stress. In L. Goldberger & S. Breznitz (Eds.), *Handbook of stress* (pp. 367-379). New York: Free Press.

Perls, F.S., Hefferline, R., & Goodman, P. (1951). *Gestalt therapy.* New York: Dell.

Personal Report for the Executive. (1987, July 15). New York: National Institute of Business Management.

Roberts, S.L. (1978). *Behavioral concepts and nursing throughout the life span.* Englewood Cliffs, N.J.: Prentice Hall.

Scheflen, A. (1972). *Body language and social order.* Englewood Cliffs, N.J.: Prentice Hall.

Schuster, C., & Ashburn, S. (1986). *The process of human development: A holistic approach* (2nd ed.). Boston: Little, Brown.

Scott, A. (1988). Human interaction and personal boundaries. *Journal of Psychosocial Nursing, 26*(8), 23-28.

Seaman, L. (1982). Affective nursing touch. *Geriatric Nursing, 3,* 162-164.

Smith, M. (1976). Patient responses to being transferred during hospitalization. *Nursing Research, 25,* 192-196.

Sommer, R. (1969). *Personal space: The behavioral basis of design.* Englewood Cliffs, N.J.: Prentice Hall.

Steere, D.A. (1982). *Bodily expressions in psychotherapy.* New York: Brunner/Mazel.

Stevenson, J. (1989, April 3). *Exercise in frail elders: Findings and methodological issues.* Paper presented at the 13th Annual Midwest Nursing Research Society Conference, Cincinnati.

Sue, D. (1981). *Counseling the culturally different: Theory and practice.* New York: John Wiley & Sons.

Ujhely, G. (1979). Touch: Reflections and perceptions. *Nursing Forum, 18*(1), 18-32.

Watson, O.M. (1980). *Proxemic behavior: A cross-cultural study.* The Hague, Netherlands: Mouton.

West, B. (1981). Understanding endorphins: Our natural pain relief system. *Nursing 81, 11,* 50-53.

Wolfgang, A. (Ed.) (1984). *Nonverbal behavior: Perspectives, applications, and intercultural insights.* Lewiston, N.Y.: C.J. Hogrete.

Zook, R., & Davidhizar, R. (in press). Caring for the psychiatric inpatient with AIDS. *Perspectives in Psychiatric Care.*

■ ■

CHAPTER 4

Social Organization

BEHAVIORAL OBJECTIVES

After reading this chapter, the nurse will be able to:

1 Describe how cultural behavior is acquired in a social setting.

2 Define selected terms unique to the concept of social organization, such as *culture-bound, ethnocentrism, homogeneity, bicultural, ethnicity,* and *race.*

3 Describe significant social organization groups.

4 Define family groups, including nuclear, nuclear dyad, extended, alternative, blended, single-parent, and special forms of family groups.

5 List at least two primary goals inherent to the American culture in regard to the family as a unit.

6 Describe the significant impact that religion may have on the way individuals relate to health care practitioners.

Cultural behavior, or how one acts in certain situations, is socially acquired, not genetically inherited. Patterns of cultural behaviors are learned through a process called enculturation (also referred to as socialization), which involves acquiring knowledge and internalizing values. Most people achieve competence in their own culture through enculturation. Children learn to behave culturally by watching adults and making inferences about the rules for behavior. Patterns of cultural behavior are important to the nurse because they provide explanations for behavior related to life events. Life events that are significant transculturally include birth, death, puberty, childbearing, child rearing, illness, and disease. Children learn certain beliefs, values, and attitudes about these life events, and the learned behavior that results persists throughout the entire life span unless necessity or forced adaptation compels the learning of different ways. It is important for the nurse to recognize the value of so-cial organizations and their relationship to physiological and psychological growth and maturation.

CULTURE AS A TOTALITY

Most anthropologists believe that to understand culture and the meaning assigned to culture-specific behavior, one must view culture in the total social context. The concept of holism requires that human behavior not be isolated from the context in which it occurs. Therefore culture must be viewed and analyzed as a totality—a functional, integrated whole whose parts are interrelated and yet interdependent. The components of culture, such as political, economic, religion, kinship, and health systems, perform separate functions but nevertheless mesh to form an operating whole. Culture is more than the sum of its parts (Goldsby, 1971; Henderson & Primeaux, 1981).

Culture-Bound

As children grow and learn a specific culture, they are to some extent imprisoned without knowing it. Some anthropologists have referred to this existence as culture-bound. In this context the term *culture-bound* describes a person living within a certain reality that is considered "the reality." Most people have learned ways to interpret their world based on enculturation. Thus although certain interpretations are understandable and persuasive to persons brought up to share the same frame of reference, other people may not share these interpretations and therefore may make little sense out of the context. Nurses are also culturally bound within the profession, because they are likely to bring a unique scientific approach—the nursing process—to determining and resolving health problems. Many nurses are likely to consider the nursing process the best and only means of meeting the needs of all patients regardless of their cultural heritage. However, patients may view this modern scientific approach differently, thinking that the nursing process meets their needs in some ways, but not in others. The nursing process may not take into consideration alternative health services, such as folk remedies, holistic health care, and spiritual interventions. In contrast to the nursing process, medicine is often practiced in unscientific ways according to the Western viewpoint. Therefore desirable outcomes for treatment may occur independently of medical and health care interventions.

Ethnocentrism

For the most part, people look at the world from their own particular cultural viewpoint. Ethnocentrism is the perception that one's own way is best. Even in the nursing profession, there is a tendency to lean toward ethnocentrism. Nurses must remain cognizant of the fact that their ways are not necessarily the best and that other people's ideas are not "ignorant" or "inferior." Nurses must remember that the ideas of lay individuals may be valid for them and, more important, will influence their health care behavior and consequently their health status. In contrast to the term *ethnocentrism* is the word *ethnic*, which relates to races or to large groups of people classed according to common traits or customs. In populations throughout the world, people are bound by common ties, elements, life patterns, and basic beliefs germane to their particular country. Because people in the United States have differing cultural traditions and today's population is more mobile, the result has been a heterogeneous cultural population. Therefore it is difficult to find a homogeneous culture in the United States.

Homogeneity

If a homogeneous culture did exist in the United States, all individuals would share the same attitudes, interests, and goals. When homogeneity does occur, the phenomenon is referred to as ethnic collectivity. People who are reared in ethnic collectivity share a bond that includes common origins, a sense of identity, and a shared standard for behavior. These values are often acquired from experiences that are perceived to be cultural norms and that determine the thoughts and behaviors of individual members (Harwood, 1981; Saunders, 1954). The ultimate consequences of enculturation are carried over to health care and become an important influence on activities relative to health and illness behaviors. In the American culture there is a tendency to speak of culture as if it included a set of values shared by everyone. However, even within an ethnic collectivity, intraethnic variations occur and are obvious in health behaviors. For example, intraethnic variations are seen in the concept of mental illness (Guttmacher & Elinson, 1972), in cultural definitions of health and illness, in skepticism about medical care and consequently the use or lack of use of health care services (Potter & Perry, 1989; Berkanovic & Reeder, 1973), and finally in the willingness of the individual to assume a dependent role when ill (Suchman, 1964).

Bicultural/Ethnicity

The term *bicultural* is used to describe a person who crosses two cultures, lifestyles, and sets of values. To understand biculturalism, the nurse must understand the differences in meaning for the terms *ethnicity, race,* and *minority. Ethnicity* is frequently and perhaps erroneously used to mean *race,* but the term *ethnicity* includes more than the biological identification. Ethnicity in its broadest sense refers to groups whose members share a common social and cultural heritage passed on to each successive generation. The most important characteristic of ethnicity is that members of an ethnic group feel a sense of identity.

Race

In contrast to the term *ethnicity* is the term *race,* which is related to biology. Members of a particular group share distinguishing physical features such as skin color, bone structure, or blood group. Ethnic and racial groups can and do overlap, because in many cases the biological and cultural similarities reinforce one another (Bullough & Bullough, 1982).

Minority

In contrast to the definitions of *ethnicity, ethnic group, biculturalism,* and *race* is the definition of *minority.* A minority can consist of a particular racial, religious, or occupational group that constitutes less than a numerical majority of the population. Using this definition for the term *minority,* it is obvious that all kinds of people can belong to various kinds of minorities (Bullough & Bullough, 1982). Often a minority group is designated because of its lack of power, assumed inferior traits, and/or supposedly undesirable characteristics. Persons who belong to a bicultural group may share ethnic and racial characteristics of the larger group of which they are a part but at the same time have common cultural differences from the larger group.

SOCIAL ORGANIZATION GROUPS AS SYSTEMS

Social organizations are structured into a variety of groups, including family, religious, ethnic, racial, tribal, kinship, clan, and other special interest groups. Groups are dependent on particular persons and are more affected by changes in members than are other systems. In most groups, with the exception of racial and ethnic groups, members may come and go. Thus the formation and the disintegration of groups are more likely to occur during the members' lifetime than are the formation and the disintegration of other systems.

According to the general systems theory, social organization groups are characterized by a steady state and a sense of balance or equilibrium that is maintained even as the group changes. Most groups form, grow, and reach a state of maturity. Social organization groups begin with a variety of elements that include individuals with unique personalities, needs, ideas, potentials, and limits. In the course of development of the group, a pattern of behavior and a set of norms, beliefs, and values evolve. As the group strives toward maturity, parts become differentiated and each member assumes special functions.

Family Groups

One group of paramount concern for the nurse when working with persons transculturally is the family. Regardless of cultural background, the family is a basic unit of society. From a sociological perspective the family may be defined as a social unit that interacts with a larger society. The discipline of economics may define the family in terms of how it works together to meet material needs. From a psychological perspective the family may be defined as a basic unit for personality development and the development of subgroup relationships, such as parent-child relationships. Still another definition is offered from a biological perspective, which conceptualizes the family as a unit with the biological function of perpetuating the species.

The most predominant family system in the United States is the nuclear family, which is defined as a small group consisting of parents (or a parent) and their non-adult children living in a single household (Farber, 1973; Robischon & Scott, 1969). A similar definition to that of the nuclear family views the family as a cluster of people whose relationship is stipulated by law in terms of marriage and descent and whose precise membership varies according to the circumstances. A broader conceptualization of the term *family* views the family as a relationship community of two or more persons in which individuals may come from the same or different kinship groups. Mauksch (1974) views the family as a basic human unit with generic properties. According to Mauksch, these generic properties include the coexistence of more than one human being involved in continuous, presumably permanent, sharing of living facilities; a perception of reciprocal obligations; a sense of commonness; and a perception of certain obligations toward others. These varying definitions of the family range from viewing the family as having one structure exclusively to perceiving the family as a household unit representative of various types of family structures.

Types of family structures

Traditional nuclear family. According to Virginia Satir (1972), the traditional nuclear family consists of one man and one woman of the same race, religion, and age; who are of sound mind and body; and who marry during their early or middle 20s, are faithful to the other for life, have and raise their own children, retire, and finally die. This definition appears narrow; however, it has maintained popularity over the years and is still seen by many persons as the most desirable family form. Today a more current definition of the nuclear family allows for more variation. This newer definition defines the nuclear family as a family of two generations formed by a married woman and man with their children by birth or adoption (Govaets, 1987). Within this particular family form, as within all identified family forms, the assigned roles and functions performed by each member vary. One example is a common family structure that has the father working outside the home and the mother working at home taking care of the children and household tasks. However, today the traditional nuclear family often finds both mother and father working outside the home. Thus child rearing and child care may be shared by both parents, as well as by others outside the family, such as a day care center.

Nuclear dyad family. The nuclear dyad family consists of one generation and is made up of a married couple without children. There are numerous reasons why this particular family remains childless: the family may have chosen not to have children; they may not be able to have children or to adopt them; or the children may have died. In some cultures this family form is frequently thought of as a beginning point for the formation of the family. However, in other cultures the nuclear dyad family is considered a part of the mainstream of the social organization of the family. The number of nuclear dyad families continues to grow and survive as a functioning unit throughout the world.

Extended family. The extended family is multigenerational and includes all relatives by birth, marriage, or adoption. The family group is made up of grandparents, aunts, uncles, nieces, nephews, cousins, brothers, sisters, and in-laws. In today's society there is a tendency for children to leave the homes and communities of their parents, which has resulted in a separation of the nuclear family from the extended family.

Alternative family. The alternative family consists of adults of a single generation or a combination of adults and children who live together without social sanction of marriage. The alternative family is often either a communal arrangement—composed of roommates who might be either homosexual or heterosexual—or a love relationship between a man and a woman.

Single-parent family. The single-parent family consists of two generations and is made up of a mother or father and children by birth or adoption. The reasons for a single-parent family include electing to be a single parent, divorce, death, separation, or abandonment. The prevalence for the single-parent family is increasing because of a number of factors such as divorce and the acceptability of being a single parent (Zinn & Eitzen, 1987).

Reconstituted or blended family. The reconstituted or blended family is a family that is formed by "put-together parts" of previously existing families with the intention of forming a new nuclear family (Satir, 1972). The blended family, like the traditional nuclear family, is two-generational. However, the blended family differs in form and may be made up of a single person who marries a person with children, or a man and a woman, both of whom have children, who marry. This family form may also yield biological children; thus there may be a composition of "yours," "mine," and "ours" in the family. The blended family can become very complicated because of the composition and blending of family members, which may include stepbrothers, stepsisters, stepparents, and stepgrandparents. With the rate of divorce and remarriage increasing in the United States, one of every five children belong to a blended family (Romanzuk, 1987).

Special forms of families: gay families and communal families. The typical American family has become a rarity. In 1983 approximately 6.2% of American families included a breadwinning husband, a full-time housewife, and two children (Skolnick, 1987). In some cultures an even wider array of family forms than the ones mentioned above is observed, particularly if ideas about marriage and the requirement that the nuclear family is essential to family definition are put aside. These groups do function as families and therefore must be recognized. These special forms of families may be either one-generational or multigenerational. Two or more adults constitute these special family forms, and both adults may or may not be of the same sex.

A commune is a group of people that intertwines husband-wife, parent-child, and brother-sister types of relationships of individuals who have elected to live together in one household or in closely adjoining structures. Family members in a commune must express a feeling of commitment to others in the group. Assigned family roles, as well as responsibilities, are divided among the members of the group. Generally, there are specific rules and expectations for each member of the group. A commune may be formed when people have a common goal, such as a religious, philosophical, or political goal, or a common need, such as an economic, social, or physical need. Examples of communes include Israeli kibbutzim, religious cults, retirement homes for the elderly, and households where couples share resources.

Some gay households consist of two persons and generally function as a nuclear dyad. Other gay households may consist of more members, for example, a commune. Today, perhaps as a result of the gay rights movement, homosexual couples have openly taken up residence together. Nevertheless, many members of society continue to be nonaccepting of this particular family form. Thus it remains difficult for the gay couple to either adopt children or be given custody of children when a gay partner is divorced.

Characteristics of a family system

According to the general systems theory, a system is a group of interrelated parts or units that form a whole. When the general systems theory is applied to the family, the individual family members are those units that make up the identifiable family system. These parts or units act as one or more subsystems within the larger system. Within the family system the subsystems are meant to refer to the way in which the members align themselves with one another. For example, in the family system the parents may be one subsystem whereas the children may be another subsystem. At the same time, males and females of the family system may be two other subsystems. A subsystem may consist of any number of members who are linked by some common factor. Within the family system membership to a particular subsystem may be determined by generational considerations, sexual identity, areas of interest, or a specifically designated function. Individual family members may belong to several different subsystems. At the same time, family members also belong to external systems, such as the community system, the school system, and career systems. Subsystems may be constructed to ensure that important functions within the family system are carried out to maintain the overall family structure.

Family systems theory as applied to nursing is referenced in the nursing literature. Fawcett (1975) studied the family as a living open system and thus viewed family nursing as an emerging conceptual framework for nursing care. Nurses have cared for families for years; however, it is only recently that nurse researchers have begun to study the family as a whole (Murphy, 1986). Nursing studies in family health are increasing. For example, qualitative studies in family health include those by Campbell (1989), Phipps (1989), and Breitmayer et al. (1989).

The family as a behavioral system. The family is conceptualized as a behavioral system with unique properties inherent to the system. There is a close interrelationship between the psychosocial functioning of the family as a group and the emotional adaptation of individual family members. There is a distinguishable link between disorders of family living and disorders of family members. This link can best be understood in the context of systems theory. Systems theory is an orientation whereby people are recognized and defined by who they are within the context of their relationship with family, friends, and the society within which they live. Family systems theories were developed in the 1950s on both the East and West Coasts of the United States. On the West Coast a group of people that included Jackson, Haley, and their associates in Palo Alto explored the notions of communication theory and homeostasis applied to the family with a schizophrenic member (Bateson et al., 1968; Satir, 1967). On the East Coast, in Washington, D.C., Bowen (1978) conceptualized a family systems theory based on a biological systems model. In Philadelphia Minuchin (1974) used a systems model in his research with families with psychosomatic disorders.

More recently Lewis et al. (1976) and Caplan (1975) explored not only disturbed families but also healthy families from a systems perspective. A system is a whole that consists of more than the sum of its parts; a system can be divided into subsystems, but the subsystems are not representative pieces of the whole. To study the family from a cultural perspective, one must understand the basic characteristics of a family system and of a living system. Today in nursing the family nursing process is the same whether the focus is on the family as the patient or the family as the environment. Therefore the nursing process used in family nursing is the same as that used with individuals, that is, assessment, nursing diagnosis, planning, intervention, and evaluation. According to Friedman (1986), the only distinguishable difference is that both the individual and the family receive care simultaneously. There are some inherent underlying assumptions germane to the family approach to the nursing process, including the beliefs that all individuals must be viewed within their family context, that families impact on individuals, and that individuals impact on families.

Independent units. All systems have basic units that make functioning possible. Within the structure of the family system, the basic interdependent units are the individual family members. As with any open system, change within one family member affects the entire family system. For example, when one family member becomes physically or emotionally ill, the entire family system is changed in some way. Additional alterations in the family system occur because of the changing composition of family membership. Family membership changes as a result of events such as a birth, divorce, death, hospitalization, leaving home for college, or marriage. All of these variables can result in disequilibrium within the family system. All changes, regardless of whether positive or negative, may bring about disruption and disequilibrium in the system. All family systems have dynamic characteristics that must be used when disruption or disequilibrium occurs if the family system is to be permitted to return to equilibrium as matter, energy, and information are exchanged (Lewis, 1979).

Environment.   As with all open systems there is an internal and external environment that controls the direction of growth of the family system. The internal environment involves the social and physical factors within the family boundaries, the quality of which is reflected by such factors as (1) marital relationship, (2) location of power, (3) closeness of the family members, (4) communication, (5) problem-solving abilities, (6) free expression of feelings, (7) ability to deal with loss, (8) family values, (9) degree of intimacy, and (10) autonomy of family members. Within the family system the external environment involves the social and physical world outside of the family, such as church, neighbors, extended family, school, friends, work, health care system, political systems, and recreation.

Boundaries.   Within the family system the "boundary" is the imaginary line or area of demarcation that helps keep the family system separate and unique from its external environment. As with all open systems, energy, in the form of information, material goods, and feeling states, passes between family members and the external environment. Openness and closeness in a family system is governed by the degree of information or energy that is exchanged and the nature of the boundaries. Information coming into the family system provides the family with information about the environment and about family functioning. If the family accepts the information, it may be used to formulate and respond to the environment, to assist the family in coping with disequilibrium, or to rejuvenate the family. Energy coming into the family can also be stored until needed. Finally, energy or information coming into the family can be rejected or ignored (Satir, 1972).

As with all open systems, the amount of energy or information that enters and leaves the system must be balanced within certain limits to maintain a steady state of functioning or homeostasis if proper adaptation of the system is to occur. Any system can become dysfunctional if the system is allowed to become too open or too closed. No truly closed systems exist, except in a theoretical sense. On the other hand, if a family system were totally open, the family system would probably lose its identity as a system separate from other systems to which family members belong. Therefore the family members might suffer from alienation, rootlessness, and a lack of belonging. The opposite extreme, or a theoretically closed family system, would be composed of boundaries that were very rigid, and thus family members would become enmeshed, fixed, and unable to move out, grow, or change.

Communication within the family system

The verbal and nonverbal interaction between family members is called communication. Factors that contribute to the family member's pattern of communication include (1) the pattern of members acknowledging each other's verbal and nonverbal messages; (2) the degree of responsibility taken by each member for expressing individual feelings, thoughts, and reactions in a constructive way; (3) the extent to which the family encourages a clear exchange of words; (4) whether family members are allowed to talk for themselves; and (5) patterns of spontaneous talking. Bonding between family members occurs as a result of the form of communication patterns that are present.

Roles in the family

Family member roles are patterns of wants, goals, beliefs, feelings, attitudes, and actions that family members have for themselves and others in the family. Roles are both assigned and acquired, and they specify what individuals do in the family. Although they are usually dependent on social class and cultural norms, roles are dynamic and change in response to factors both within the family and without. Roles are reciprocal and complement roles taken by other family members. Family equilibrium is dependent on how well roles in the family are balanced and reciprocated (Duvall, 1977; Friedman, 1986; Robischon & Scott, 1969).

The way in which a family member takes on a particular role is influenced by various factors. Such variables as temperament, height, weight, gender, birth order, age, and health status all play a part in the role(s) a family member takes on. For example, a female member of a family can be sister, daughter, wife, mother, or girlfriend. Other roles, such as breadwinner, homemaker, cook, handyman, or gardener, are performance roles and are dependent on the person's ability to perform a certain task. In contrast to performance roles are emotional roles, such as leader, nurturer, scapegoat, caretaker, jester, arbitrator, or martyr, which may be adopted at certain times as a means of adjusting to the demands of a family system, to an extended family crises such as a long-term family illness, or to long-term family conflict. The functions of emotional roles are to reduce conflict between family members and to promote temporarily adaptation among family members. However, consistent use of emotional roles may serve to impair adaptation, thus hindering the growth of the family. An example of this is when one family member, perhaps the oldest child, assumes the role of family caretaker, supporting other members and arbitrating disputes. The role may take on negative characteristics in this instance because the family caretaker may appear outwardly strong and capable but inwardly have unrealistic feelings, such as "I can't fail," or "I can't be weak." In this emotional role this person may function under pressure to be perfect but at the same time have feelings of self-doubt and fear. It is important for the nurse to remember that roles have a significant impact on individual adjustment.

Family organization

To understand family organization, it is important for the nurse to remember that structuring of both functions and goals must be addressed. It is also important for the nurse to remember that most families are not static but dynamic, endlessly adaptable, and continuously evolving in both structure and function. The functional ability of a family is dependent in part on the individual needs and wants of the members. If the nurse is unable to assist family members in meeting needs within the family structure, pain may be felt and confusion may exist. The nurse must keep in mind that in the American culture families are expected to be self-perpetuating and at the same time be the primary system for the transfer of social values and norms.

In the American culture two primary goals that are inherent to the family include (1) the encouragement and nuturance of each individual and (2) the production of autonomous, healthy children. In the American culture marital partners are expected to be supportive and at the same time protective of each other. Both the husband and the wife are expected to share a sense of meaning and emotional closeness within the boundaries of their relationship, thus fostering the goal of personality development. In families where supportive relationships do not exist, the achievement of the first goal (the encouragement and nuturance of each individual) is not attainable. The second goal of the family includes encouraging children to develop their own identity and individuality by allowing them to develop ideals, feelings, and life directions. At the same time, children are encouraged to sense both similarities to and differences from others and to be able to initiate activities based on this information (Lewis, 1979). Factors that must be addressed in order to determine the degree to which the family will accomplish these two primary goals include the patterns of relationship and adaptive mechanisms present.

There are many reasons why some families fail to accomplish these two primary goals, including psychiatric disturbance among family members, incomplete maturation of children, and disintegration of the family system. When adaptive mechanisms are used by the family, internal equilibrium may result. These adaptive mechanisms are dependent on (1) the level of communication skills within the family; (2) the individual contributions of each family member to the family welfare; (3) mutual respect and love within the family; (4) the type, kind, and amount of stressors encountered; (5) the response pattern to stressors encountered in the internal and external environment; and (6) the support or resources available and the opportunity to participate in support systems (Ackerman, 1984; Black, 1981). For example, a family that has an alcoholic father may not be able to accomplish goals, because this problem may result in psychiatric disturbances in the wife and children, and, ultimately, the family system may disintegrate. The reasons for the disintegration of this family include not only the individual psychiatric disturbances, but also accompanying difficulties such as incomplete maturation of children and adult members, financial instability, inability to adapt successfully to stressors, and, more important, the inability of each family member to perceive the family unit as caring and loving (Brown, 1986).

Levels of functioning.   Four levels of family functioning that have been identified form a continuum in increasingly abstract levels (see box on p. 59): (I) family functions and activities, (II) intrafamilial interactions, (III) interpersonal relationships, and (IV) the family system (Averaswald, 1973).

To understand the family from a cultural perspective, it is essential that the nurse recognize that family relationships are stronger among some ethnic or cultural groups than among others. However, the importance of socioeconomic class cannot be overlooked. According to Casavantes (1976), a pattern of strong family relationships exists particularly among poor people, who have few resources and must rely on the support of the family kinship network to meet physical and emotional needs. Middle- or upper- class people often have resources that extend beyond the extended family

LEVELS OF FAMILY FUNCTIONING

Least abstract: Level I—Family functions and activities
Level II—Intrafamilial interactions
Level III—Interpersonal relationships
Most abstract: Level IV—The family system

Level I deals with family affairs and functions. Included in this level are tangible, pragmatic activities that are either observable or easily identified; more important, these are things that family members are most comfortable in discussing. Four categories of family functioning have been identified in Level I:

1. *Activities of family living.* Families are expected to provide physical safety and economic resources. Included in this category is the ability of family members to obtain such necessities as food, clothing, shelter, and health care.
2. *Ability of the family members to assist one another.* Included in this category is the family's ability to assist one another in developing emotionally and intellectually and at the same time attaining a personal as well as family identity.
3. *Reproduction, socialization, and release of children.* Included in this category are functioning goals that would allow the family to become closely aligned, thereby allowing the transmission of subcultural roles and values.
4. *Integration between the family, its culture, and society.* Included in this category is the ability of the family to use external environmental resources for support and feedback.

Level II basically deals with communication and various interactions between family members, including what is said, how it is said, patterns of communication over time, the ability of each family member to communicate, and the quality of communication skills. Also included in this level is the transfer of information from family member to family member.

Level III deals with the way family members interact in relationships that occur within the family constellation. The dimensions of closeness and power, and the degree of empathy, support, and commitment that exist among family members are important. How the family functions in regard to decision making and problem solving is included in this level.

Level IV deals with the concepts of the family system, as well as how the family functions as a system. Level IV is the most abstract level of family functioning. It encompasses the concepts of wholeness, openness or closedness, homeostasis, and rules.

Data from Schneider, R. (1980, June). *Conceptual scheme of family organization and function.* Paper presented at St. Louis University Medical Center conference, St. Louis.

and are therefore able to avail themselves of physical and emotional support within the community. It is often thought that when people do not have money or other available resources for recreation and social activities in the community, they tend to spend more time together and depend on the family group for recreational and social outlets.

Regardless of socioeconomic class, families must organize and structure themselves. Structure refers to the organization of the family and includes the type of family, such as nuclear or extended. The value system of the family dictates the roles assigned in the family, communication patterns within the family, and power distribution within the family (Friedman, 1986; Schneflen, 1972). The basic beliefs about humankind, nature, the supernatural (fate), time, and family relationships constitute a family's value system. Value systems are often clustered by socioeconomic status or ethnic groups. For example, families from lower socioeconomic groups tend to have a present-time orientation and view themselves as being subjugated to the environment or the supernatural (fate). Often the family relationships are disrupted by desertion of a spouse or by the early emancipation of the children because of severe economic difficulties. These families have been able to survive and adapt by taking in other extended family members' children; for example, a grandmother may provide direct assistance by raising her son's or daughter's children. In these families power is usually authoritarian or not exerted at all.

Middle- and upper-class families in the United States for the most part espouse the Protestant work ethnic values prevalent in this country today, which dictate the importance of working and planning for the future. These values encompass the belief that although man is somewhat evil, his behavior is changeable by hard work. In the middle- and upper-class family structure, financial stability and success are viewed as rewards for hard work. Within these classes family relationships center around the nuclear family, socialization takes place with work-related or neighborhood friends, and power may be more egalitarian than in the lower-class family. Power tends to become more male dominated as the economic level of a family rises. Middle- and upper-class families often see themselves as able to control or have mastery over their environment.

The nurse must keep in mind that these statements on structure and organization of a family by class are broad generalizations of social class values and in themselves cannot account for cultural differences. For example, many ethnic groups, such as the Black American family, regardless of socioeconomic status, place great importance on extended family relationships rather than the individualism valued by White, Protestant, middle-class Americans. A family with a good income but with a time orientation in the present, such as that commonly found among persons in the lower-socioeconomic class, may fail to recognize the importance of saving money and thus may always struggle financially. To understand whether a family system organizes itself around a family unit, such as the extended family, or tends to be a more individualistic system, such as the nuclear family, the nurse must assess the family as a group.

The structure and function of the American family must be perceived somewhat differently from the structure and function of families from other countries. It is also important to remember that the United States is virtually a cultural melting pot; therefore it is essential to understand family functioning from a transcultural perspective. Thus although the persons that make up an American family are often viewed as a homogeneous group, this is not necessarily the case. The American family is composed of diverse multicultural populations and is defined by three criteria: kinship, function, and location.

Kinship In the first criterion, kinship, there are three dyads that imply the existence of or location for the individual within the family structure: husband-father, wife-mother, or child-sibling. There are several conventional forms of family structures that are composed of these positions, including the nuclear family and the stem family. The nuclear family, which is discussed earlier, may consist of a husband, a wife, and their nonadult children and is based on all three dyads, with their marital, parental, and sibling elements. Whereas the nuclear family is restricted to a depth of two generations, the stem family encompasses three generations: grandparents, parents, and children.

Function   The second criterion, function, describes the purpose, goals, and philosophy of the family organization. Family function is defined as the expected action of an individual in a given role. In a description of family organization, the term *function* is used to depict family roles and the assigned tasks for those roles. Every family has unit functions that must be performed to maintain the integrity of the family unit and to meet the needs of the family. If individual family members' needs and societal expectations are to be met, the functioning role of the family must be clearly delineated. In family systems with two or more individuals, the family members have unit functional responsibilities related to their social positions. Depending on the position within the family structure, an individual may function in a variety of roles such as breadwinner, homemaker, companion, health motivator, or sexual partner. It is important for the nurse to remember that the maintenance of the family system is dependent on these various roles. Some cultural groups function in traditional ways in which the family is viewed as a holistic functioning unit. Other cultural groups may function as a disaggregate unit, meaning that the family does not function as a unit but members function independently.

Murray, Meili, and Zentner (1975) have described one approach to examining family functions in relation to the family's physical, affectional, and social properties. Physical functions include the provision of food, clothing, and shelter; protection against danger; and the provision for health and illness care. Affectional functions include the meeting of emotional needs, and social functions include the provision for social togetherness, the fostering of self-esteem, and the support of creativity and initiative. Another approach to examining family functions views the family from a task-oriented perspective (Sussman, 1971). Tasks include socialization of children, strengthening competency of family members in relation to their adjustments within organizations, appropriate use of social organizations, providing an environment that fosters the development of identities and affectional behavior, and creating a satisfying, emotionally healthy environment essential to the family's well-being. Adaptation is essential to the family's ability to carry out functions and tasks and to meet the changing needs of society and other social systems, for example, political and health-illness systems.

Location   Family location is also a significant criterion for understanding the family. Martin and Martin (1978) and Leininger (1985) discussed the variations that occurred among values of Black families when families were evaluated in urban versus rural settings. Martin and Martin found that when families moved from rural to urban settings there was an erosion of values emphasing "mutual aid," and a contrasting increase in individualism, materialism, and secularism. When urban Blacks are compared with their rural counterparts, it appears that urban Blacks may view their counterparts as lacking the toughness and sophistication needed to make headway in a dominant urban culture. Despite the variations that occur with location changes, geographic separation does not mean a severing of kinship ties, according to Martin and Martin; rather, geographic separation may serve to strengthen the emotional bonds between relatives. Today there is a tendency among American Blacks, whether urban or rural, toward a migration back home and getting back to their people. For some Black Americans there has been an increasing awareness that the urban centers have not met their hopes and aspirations. From the 1940s to the 1970s there was a migration by some Black Americans away from the rural South. In the 1980s there was a trend toward the migration of some Black Americans away from the urban North back to the South. For example, the migration of urban northern Blacks has occurred in significant numbers to such cities as Atlanta, Dallas, and Houston (Bernard, 1966; Billingsley, 1968; Blasingame, 1972; Blaxton, 1976; Frazier, 1964).

Religious Groups

According to many sociologists, religion is a social phenomenon (Carroll, Johnson, & Marty, 1979), which implies an interactive relationship with the other social units that constitute a society. However, many persons, particularly those with religious convictions, tend to think of religion in an entirely different way. For some people religion is seen in the context of a person's communion with the supernatural, and religious experiences fall outside ordinary experiences, whereas other people view religion as an expression of an instinctual reaction to cosmic forces (Johnstone, 1988). Another world view of religion depicts religion as an explicit set of messages from a deity. For the most part, all of these beliefs tend to deemphasize, ignore, and perhaps even reject the sociological dimensions of religion. Nevertheless, whether it is being considered in general, in regard to a particular religious family such as Christianity or Buddism, or in regard to a very specific religious group such as Baptists, religion is thought to interact with other social institutions and forces in society and to follow and illustrate sociological principles and laws. In other words, regardless of what religion is or is not, it is a social phenomenon and as such is in a continual reciprocal, interactive relationship with other social phenomena.

Regardless of its definition, be it theological or sociological, many different kinds of groups are based on religion. Generally, religious structures fall into two basic types: the church type and the withdrawal-group type. The church-type structure is broadly based and represents the normative spiritual values of a society that most people adhere to by virtue of their membership in the society, such as Hinduism in India or Catholicism in Spain. For the most part, membership in certain societies dictates the faith that the person should belong to if that person has not made a conscious, deliberate choice to adhere to something else. The church-type structure is generally a comprehensive system that allows for individual variations and in practice does not make extremely rigorous demands on its members. In America the church-type structure is encompassed within a number of major denominations. This denominational structure is in sharp contrast with the church-type structure in other countries, such as India or Spain, where most of the people belong to one faith and one church. In some countries, particularly the United States, individual churches are often closely identified with an ethnic group rather than with a social class, and churches thrive, more or less, as a means of asserting ethnic identity. For example, the Black church, regardless of denominational faith, has become synonymous with the Black life experience. The Amish people, on the other hand, subscribe to one denominational belief; however the belief is synonymous with the Amish life experience.

The second type of religious structure is the withdrawal group, which expresses the beliefs of those for whom personal commitment and experience are more important than the family and the community functions of religion (Ellwood, 1987). Withdrawal groups meet the needs of those who feel that the faith or lack of faith by the majority is not for them. Persons involved in withdrawal groups define themselves by making a separate choice. These groups include such religions groups as the Amish or

Jehovah's Witnesses, which tend to represent a more intense or unbending commit-ment than that held by the average person adhering to a religion. These groups may be called sects. Groups that combine separation with syncretism and new ideas and that place emphasis on mystical experience are often referred to as cults. However, the word *cult* is often used in Western society with caution, since it has acquired a nega-tive connotation. In some religious groups such as the Mormons, Muslims, Jehovah's Witnesses, Seventh-Day Adventists, Buddhists, or Hindus, as well as that of the gypsy culture, the extended social organization of the religion is considered more important than membership in the individual family. Two groups that may have particular sig-nificance for the nurse are Jehovah's Witnesses and Seventh-Day Adventists.

Jehovah's Witnesses

The founder of the religious group now referred to as Jehovah's Witnesses was Charles Taze Russell. The name "Jehovah's Witness" was taken in Columbus, Ohio, in 1931 in an attempt to differentiate between the Watchtower Tract Society and the true followers of Russell, who were represented by the Dawn Bible Students and the Layman's Home Missionary Movement. During the period 1876 to 1879 Russell served as pastor of the Bible class that he organized in Pittsburgh, Pennsylvania, and was also the assistant editor of a small monthly magazine in Rochester, New York. However, he resigned from the editorial position in 1879 when controversy arose over his counterarguments on the "Atonement of Christ." In 1879 he founded the magazine, *Herald of the Morning,* which developed into the magazine that is distrib-uted today entitled *The Watchtower Announcing Jehovah's Kingdom.* This magazine has grown from a circulation of 6000 to 17.8 million per month. Today there is another Watchtower periodical entitled *Awake,* which has a circulation of 15.6 million per month and is published in 34 languages.

In 1884 Russell incorporated Zion's Watchtower Tract Society in Pittsburgh. This group published a series of seven books. Russell, himself, actually wrote six of these books. The seventh volume, *The Finished Mystery,* caused a split in the group that culminated in a clean division. The larger portion of the group followed Joseph Franklin Rutherford, while the smaller portion remained by itself and subsequently became known as the Dawn Bible Students Association. Under Rutherford's leader-ship the Watchtower Bible Society began to attack the doctrines of organized reli-gion. This group eventually became known as the present-day Jehovah's Witnesses and today has branches in 100 countries, with members doing missionary work in over 250 countries. Watchtower literature is distributed in 110 languages (Martin, 1985).

Modern-day Jehovah's Witnesses still await the Millennium. They regard Christ as a creature who will come to destroy the forces of evil, at Armageddon, and they teach that sinners who are not saved will perish, whereas the faithful will enter into the Kingdom of Joy and Happiness. Because they believe in the Second Coming of the Kingdom, they undertake no military services. They also hold the belief that the institutions of government are under the control of Satan. It is this belief that has been the basis for some of the persecution they have undergone over the years. One view of this group is that Jehovah's Witnesses are peaceful but somewhat fanatical and that they know their Bible backward and forward (Smart, 1984). Some theologians believe that this religion appeals to persons of very modest education (Smart, 1984). The Jehovah's Witness faith is based on the doctrines presented in the box on p. 64.

BELIEFS OF JEHOVAH'S WITNESSES

1. Jehovah's Witnesses believe that there is one solitary Being from all eternity and that that Being is Jehovah God, the creator and preserver of the universe in all things that are visible and invisible.

2. Jehovah's Witnesses do not believe in the Holy Trinity of three Gods in one—God the Father, God the Son, and God the Holy Ghost—who are equal in power, substance, and eternity (Watchtower Bible and Tract Society, 1953). Rather, they believe that Satan is the originator of the Trinity doctrine and that this doctrine is just another of Satan's attempts to keep people from learning the truth about Jehovah and his Son, Christ Jesus, which is that there is no Trinity (Watchtower Bible and Tract Society, 1953).

3. Jehovah's witnesses believe there is only one God and that he is greater than his Son. They believe that the Son, the firstborn and only begotten, was sent by God but is not God, himself, and is not equal with God.

4. On the subject of the Virgin Birth, Jehovah's witnesses believe that Jehovah God took the perfect life of his only begotten Son and transferred it from heaven to the womb of the unmarried virgin, Mary. They believe that Jesus' birth was not an incarnation, but that he was emptied of all things heavenly and spiritual. This was a miracle in the sense that Jesus was born a man (and was flesh) instead of a spirit-human hybrid (Martin, 1985).

5. Jehovah's Witnesses believe that the human life that Jesus Christ laid down in sacrifice must be viewed as exactly equal to the life that Adam forfeited for all of his offspring. Thus Jesus' life must be viewed as a perfect human life, no more and no less (Watchtower Bible and Tract Society, 1955).

6. Jehovah's Witnesses believe that immortality is a reward for faithfulness and that it does not come automatically to a human at birth (Watchtower Bible and Tract Society, 1953).

7. On the subject of the Resurrection of Christ, Jehovah's Witnesses believe that Christ was raised from the dead, not as a human creature, but as a Spirit (Watchtower Bible and Tract Society, 1953).

8. Jehovah's Witnesses believe that Christ Jesus will return again, not as a human, but as a glorious spirit. National flags or symbols of the sovereign power of a nation are forbidden by Exodus 20:2-6. Thus those who believe and ascribe salvation only to God may not salute a national emblem without violating Jehovah's commandments against idolatry (Watchtower Bible and Tract Society, 1953).

9. Jehovah's Witnesses believe that the hell mentioned in the Bible is mankind's common grave and that even an honest child can understand it. Thus the doctrine of a burning hell where the wicked are tortured after death cannot be true.

10. Jehovah's Witnesses believe that man is a combination of two things: dust of the ground and breath of life. The combining of these two things produces a living soul, or a creature called man.

11. Jehovah's Witnesses believe that the undefeatable purpose of Jehovah God is to establish a righteous kingdom in these last days and that this purpose has already been fulfilled.

12. Jehovah's Witnesses believe that the Levitical commandments given by God to Moses included the commandment that no one in the House of David should eat blood or he would be cut off from people.

Implications for nursing care. There are many implications for nursing care for the nurse who provides culturally appropriate nursing care to a Jehovah's Witness. The paramount concern for the nurse is the fact that Jehovah's Witnesses are opposed to blood transfusions. Pesons who subscribe to this belief are likely to refuse to have any surgical or medical interventions that will require a blood transfusion. Even in the face of ominous danger and with the impending threat of loss of life, a Jehovah's Witness will refuse treatment for self and family members. There have been many legal battles waged in the courts in regard to minor children and the parents' refusal to allow surgical or medical interventions. The consensus of the Supreme Court of the United States has been that a person of adult majority age has the right to refuse treatment but not to withhold treatment from a minor child.

A second concern for the nurse is in regard to the refusal of Jehovah's Witnesses to eat certain foods wherein blood has been added, such as certain sausages and lunch meats. The nurse must take extra care to ensure that blood has not been added to foods that are served to Jehovah's Witnesses. Because Jehovah's Witnesses are pacifists and are conscientious objectors in wartime, the nurse must take extra care to avoid raising such issues during interaction. In general, topics related to politics, government rule, or the like, should be avoided. Since Jehovah's Witnesses do not observe any national holidays or ceremonies, including Christmas, the nurse should avoid any attempts to involve the patient in preparations for such celebrations.

Seventh-Day Adventists

The Seventh-Day Adventist religion sprang from the "Great Second Advent Awakening" that shocked the religious world just prior to the middle of the nineteenth century. During this period reemphasis on the second advent of Jesus Christ was rampant in England and on the continent of Europe. It was not long before many of the Old World views and prophetic interpretations crossed the Atlantic and began to penetrate American theological circles (Martin, 1985). The American Seventh-Day Adventist group began in upper New York.

The first leader of the Seventh-Day Adventist group was William Miller, a Baptist minister who was a resident of Lower Hampton, New York. The Seventh-Day Adventist religion is based largely on the apocalyptic books of Daniel and Revelation. Many of the early students of the Seventh-Day Adventist religion, following the chronology of Archbishop Ussher, interpreted the 2300 days of Daniel as 2300 years, and thus they concluded that Christ would come back in about the year 1843. In 1818 Miller taught many of his followers that in about 25 years (1843) Jesus Christ would come again. Miller and his associates were able to pinpoint a specific final date that Jesus Christ would return for his saints, visit judgment on sin, and establish the Kingdom of God on earth. They concluded that this specific final date would be October 22, 1843. Many theologians disagreed with Miller's contentions because it was believed that Miller was teaching in contradiction to the Word of God. According to biblical scripture, "the day and hour knoweth no man, no, not the angels of heaven but God alone" (Matthew 24:36). Because of Miller's early teaching, the first group of Seventh-Day Adventists were called Millerites. However, the mistake of setting an exact date for Christ's Second Coming led to failure for the first Seventh-Day Adventist movement in the United States.

The modern Seventh-Day Adventist movement is based on the prophecy of Ellen

G. White. White made an early assertion about Miller's prophecy that supported the prophecy and gave a date that she considered to be correct: October 22, 1844. In spite of this failure in prediction, the group has grown and been active in evangelism. Today Seventh-Day Adventists believe Christ will return again very soon and that Christians have an obligation to keep some of the laws of Moses, which includes worship on Saturday, the old Sabbath. Thirteen issues on doctrine that give direction for living and that are upheld by the Seventh-Day Adventist church are presented in the box on p. 67.

In America the Seventh-Day Adventist church has a membership of approximately 606,000 persons (Ellwood, 1987). The historic center of the Seventh-Day Adventist church is Calhoun County, Michigan. Other Adventist strongholds include Takoma, Maryland; Los Angeles County, California, particularly around Loma Linda; and Battle Creek, Michigan.

Implications for nursing care. The religious doctrines of Seventh-Day Adventists teach that the body is a temple of God and thus should be kept healthy. Persons who prescribe to this faith may avoid such items as seafood, meat, caffeine, alcohol, drugs, and tobacco in all forms. To provide culturally appropriate nursing care to a Seventh-Day Adventist, the nurse requires a knowledge and understanding of the religious doctrines of the Seventh-Day Adventist church. A Seventh-Day Adventist may refuse surgical intervention on a Friday evening or Saturday morning or afternoon because the patient may interpret such an intervention as being in direct conflict with religious doctrines. This same patient may also refuse other medical interventions that might normally take place at these times, such as respiratory or physical therapy.

The religious doctrine in regard to unclean foods may cause some patients to refuse to eat certain foods with shells, such as lobster or crab; scavenger fish, such as catfish; or certain meats. This refusal to eat certain foods that are high in iodine or protein may cause these patients to have iodine and protein deficiencies; thus it is important for the nurse to teach these patients that iodine and protein substitutes are necessary in the diet. In some specialty shops that have Seventh-Day Adventist clientele, many protein substitutes for meats are found. These substitutes are often made from vegetables such as soybeans and may take the place of meats such as ground beef. These substitutes should be encouraged, particularly when they appear to be free of preservatives.

The nurse and the nurse manager should also be aware that a colleague who is a Seventh-Day Adventist may refuse to accept assignments on Friday evenings or Saturday during the day, since the Sabbath begins on Friday at dusk and extends to Saturday at dusk. It is important for the nurse who is a Seventh-Day Adventist to ascertain at the time of employment whether working on Friday evenings or Saturday during the day is a requirement of the job. On the other hand, it is also important for the nurse manager to include staff in making nondiscriminatory policies in this regard. Inclusion of staff in policy making may serve to minimize implementation difficulties.

Ethnic Groups in Relation to Family
Arab Americans

According to the 1980 census, there are 3 million Arabs in the United States (U.S. Department of Commerce, Bureau of the Census, 1981). Arab Americans include people from Egypt, Palestine, Lebanon, Iraq, Jordan, Syria, and other Arabic

BELIEFS OF SEVENTH-DAY ADVENTISTS

1. *Inspiration and authority of the scriptures.* Seventh-Day Adventists believe that the scriptures of both the Old Testament and the New Testament were inspired by God and constitute the very word of God. They hold the Protestant position that the Bible is the sole root of the faith and practice of Christians.
2. *The nature of Christ.* Christ, called the Second Adam, is pure and holy, and connected with God and beloved by God. Seventh-Day Adventists believe that Christ is God and that he has existed with God for all eternity (Martin, 1985).
3. *The Atonement.* Seventh-Day Adventists do not believe that Christ made partial or incomplete sacrificial atonement on the cross. The all-sufficient sacrifice of Jesus was completed on the cross at Calvary.
4. *The Resurrection.* Seventh-Day Adventists believe that Jesus rose from the grave, ascended literally and bodily into heaven, and serves before God. They believe there will be a resurrection of both the just and the unjust. For the just, this resurrection will take place at the Second Coming of Christ, whereas the resurrection of the unjust will take place 1000 years later, at the close of the Millennium (Revelation 20:5-10).
5. *The Second Coming.* Seventh-Day Adventists believe Jesus Christ will assuredly come the second time and that his second advent will be visible, audible, and personal.
6. *The plan of salvation.* Seventh-Day Adventists believe that one must be born again and fully accepted by the Lord. They believe there is nothing an individual can ever do that will merit the salvation of God. Salvation is by grace (Roman 3:20).
7. *The spiritual nature of man.* Seventh-Day Adventists believe man rests in the tomb until the resurrection of the just, when the righteous will be called forth by Christ (Revelation 20:4-5). It is at this point that the just will enter into everlasting life in their eternal home in the Kingdom of Glory.
8. *Punishment of the wicked.* Seventh-Day Adventists reject the doctrine of eternal torment, because everlasting life is a gift from God (Romans 6:23). The wicked do not possess this and therefore shall not have eternal life (John 3:36).
9. *Sanctuary and investigative judgment.* Seventh-Day Adventists believe that the acceptance of Christ at conversion does not seal a person's destiny; rather, it determines his life's work after conversion. Man's record is closed when he comes to the end of his days; he is responsible for his influences during life and is likewise responsible for his evil influences after he is dead.
10. *Scapegoat teaching.* Seventh-Day Adventists repudiate the idea that Satan is the sin bearer.
11. *The Sabbath and the Mark of the Beast.* This doctrine is based on the Bible as interpreted by Seventh-Day Adventists and not according to Ellen White's writings. Seventh-Day Adventists do not believe that keeping the Sabbath is a means of keeping salvation or willing merit before God. They believe that man is saved only by grace.
12. *The question of unclean food.* Seventh-Day Adventists refrain from eating certain foods, not because of the laws of Moses, but because it is a Christian duty to preserve the body in the best of health for the service and glory of God (I Corinthians 3:16).
13. *The "remnant church."* Seventh-Day Adventists believe God has a precious remnant, a multitude of earnest and sincere individuals, in every church. The majority of God's children are scattered throughout the world and may practice their religion on Sunday.

countries. About 1 million Arab Americans have permanent resident visas in America, and another 2 million Arabs are in the United States to study or work (Meleis & LaFever, 1984).

For some Arab Americans an affiliation with family is needed if the individual is to cope satisfactorily with stressful events or life crises (Meleis & Sorrell, 1981). On the other hand, family members may be hesitant to seek help actively within the family, waiting instead until help is offered. Visiting between family members is viewed as a social obligation during illness and a variety of other significant events and consequently assumes great importance to the hospitalized patient.

Families are expected to be supportive. Particularly in psychiatric care, the family of an Arab American patient is often disapointed at the family's failure to take care of its kin, and the patient is angry at being sent to the hospital (Meleis & LaFever, 1984). Family members may present themselves as overbearing, and the patient may seem docile. A family member's overprotectiveness may be better understood when considered in this cultural context. The nurse should understand that family members are often overindulging and may appear to interfere in the patient's care.

Meleis and Sorrell (1981) have emphasized that topics of sex and reproduction may have special cultural significance when the patient is Arabic. Topics of sex and reproduction are traditionally discussed with female relatives and friends but not with men or strangers. When the nurse wishes to involve the husband in a discussion dealing with sex or reproduction, extreme tact is necessary.

Some Arab American families are oriented to the present and may believe that planning ahead may be defying God's will. The "efficient, time-conscious" manner in which Americans conduct business varies considerably from what may be construed as a casual Arabic style (Meleis & LaFever, 1984). With Arab American patients, as with patients from any other cultural group, however, it is important to individualize care and not provide care based on cultural stereotyping.

Japanese Americans

According to the 1980 census, there are 716,331 Japanese persons in the United States (U.S. Department of Commerce, Bureau of the Census, 1981), with 37.5% residing in California (268,814). Today the ability of Japanese Americans to identify with Japanese culture depends largely on when they arrived or whether they were born in the United States, where they live, and how much acculturation and assimilation have taken place. Before the 1890s a few Japanese scholars and businessmen came to the United States and settled along the East Coast. Because of the small numbers and the desire of these early Japanese settlers to be acculturated and assimilated into the mainstream society in the United States, these early immigrants were more readily accepted than later ones.

There was a large influx of Japanese immigrants between 1890 and 1924. These new Japanese immigrants settled primarily along the West Coast and in Hawaii. Because of the prejudice they experienced, their lack of knowledge about the new country, and the language barrier, these immigrants kept to themselves and formed relatively self-sufficient communities where they were able to retain familiar cultural values. Second-generation Japanese Americans who were born and educated in the United States remained largely influenced by the values and norms of their parents. However, third- and fourth-generation Japanese Americans may be unfamiliar with the Japanese language and customs. In addition, 50% of the Japanese people in the United States have married outside of the Japanese ethnic group, promoting further assimilation into the mainstream of American culture (Kikumura & Kitano, 1973).

The Japanese American people are the only immigrant group to identify themselves by the generation in which they were born, and these generational groups are distinguishable by the individual's age, experience, language, and values. The generational groups are the Issei, the first generation to live in the United States; the Nisei, the second generation; the Sansei, the third generation; and the Yonsei, the fourth generation (Hashizume & Takano, 1983)

These generational categories provide a framework for understanding family-related cultural values. For the Issei generation it was the family that provided an anchor for the values and traditions of Japan. Today the family remains one of the most important factors in the lives of the Japanese people. The Issei generation withstood extreme hardships and made personal sacrifices for the benefit of their children.

Before the 1890s the majority of Japanese persons who immigrated to the United States were men. Generally speaking, it often took many years before a Japanese man was able to afford a wife or family. These men might have been 30 or 40 years of age before they looked back to Japan to find their brides through the exchange of photographs and letters. Thus these Japanese women were often 10 to 20 years younger than their husbands, and even today it is not unusual to find elderly Japanese men with much younger wives. For the Issei descendants there was a strong, stable family support system. The exclusion law of 1924 prevented some of the early Japanese male immigrants from finding a spouse. This is a significant fact because it resulted in a group of single elderly men who continue to reside in the United States without the support of a family.

It was not until 1965, with the lifting of the immigration restrictions based on race, creed, and nationality, that Japanese immigrants were able to reestablish the continuity of family life (Kobata, 1979). The general pattern of the Japanese family is the vertical family structure, with the father and other male members in the topmost position. Many of the activities in the Japanese family take place in the nuclear family, as well as in the extended family. Problems are handled within the structure, and the achievement or accomplishment of the individual member is a reflection on the entire family (Kitano, 1976).

Today intergenerational relations are close among most Japanese Americans. There continues to be a flow of goods, money, and services between the generations. The younger generation continues to be willing to assist and give more than what is requested and expected by the older generation (Osako, 1979). The Issei descendants continue to emphasize the importance of caring for their elderly parents; however, it is important to remember that the Issei generation never experienced caring for their own parents, since they left them in Japan. Today the tradition of caring for aged parents is seen in the Issei descendants wherein aged parents continue to maintain separate but close residences, receive contributions from all of their children, and spend blocks of time with each child. Generally one child, often the oldest son or an unmarried child, assumes full responsibility for the care of elderly parents (Kobata, 1979). As indicated, family contacts are frequent among the elderly.

In a 1979 study (Osako, 1979) done in Chicago, researchers found that 65% of the elderly Japanese Americans surveyed indicated that they had at least daily contact with at least one child, 30% had contact once a week, and the remaining 3% lived with their children. Similar studies have been conducted that support these findings (Kiefer, 1974; Modell, 1968). Seemingly, reliance on the family structure has resulted in less dependence on outside individual agencies and organizations.

For both the Issei and the Nisei generations, parent-child relationships tended to be intense with open expressions of emotion displayed. For these generational groups there was much tolerance and permissiveness for the child until the age of 5 or 6, at which time parents began to place emphasis on the child's learning emotional reserve and control. On the other hand, the Sansei group tended to adopt the child-rearing practices and attitudes of contemporary and middle-class Americans and showed much less traditionalism than the earlier generations (Kiefer, 1974).

Native Americans

According to the 1980 census, there are 1,366,676 Native Americans living in United States. This figure is increased to 1,423,043 if Eskimo and Aleut Indians are included (U.S. Department of Commerce, Bureau of the Census, 1981). Because there are more than 400 different tribes of Native American Indians, it is difficult to predict patterns of residency unless one is dealing with specific tribes. The 1980 census reported large Indian populations in Arizona, Oklahoma, New Mexico, Alaska, California, North Carolina, South Dakota, New York, Montana, Washington, and Minnesota. Providing culturally appropriate nursing care is complicated by the fact that each nation or tribe of Native Americans has its own language and religion, and belief-system practices differ significantly among groups, as well as among members of the same tribe (Vogel, 1970).

The Native American family is composed frequently of extended family members who may encompass several households. Through various religious ceremonies other individuals can become the same as a parent in the family network. In some Native American tribes grandparents are viewed as the family leaders, and respect for individuals increases with age. Also, in some tribes the family is viewed as important, particularly in periods of crises, when family members are expected to serve as sources of support and security. It is important for the nurse to remember that since some Native American tribes tend to place great emphasis on the extended family as a unit, the opinions and ideas of the family members should be solicited when one is giving culturally appropriate nursing care. Even though physicians and hospitals may be available to Native Americans, traditional healing ceremonies may still be held in high regard by some families, and it may be important to incorporate old ways to treat illnesses in order for a treatment plan to be effective.

IMPLICATIONS FOR NURSING CARE

When nurses provide care to patients from a sociocultural background other than their own, they must have an awareness of and a sensitivity to the patient's sociocultural background, including knowledge of family structure and organization, religious values and beliefs, and how ethnicity and culture relate to role and role assignment within group settings. Any social organization or group can be viewed as the environment in which the patient strives for health. The approach to nursing care depends on the situation. It is important for the nurse to remember that if even one family member (other than the patient), regardless of culture and ethnic heritage, is receptive to nursing care, it is realistic and practical to view the family as an environment. Fried-man (1986) contends that nursing care must be directed to the family as a whole, as well as to the individual family member. The nurse must therefore view the family as having two separate entities, the first being the family as an environment and the sec-ond being the family as the patient. Both approaches to patient care can be useful when the nurse attempts to provide culturally appropriate nursing care.

If the family is viewed as an environment, the primary focus of nursing care is the health and development of individual family members within a very specified environ-ment. In this context it is important for the nurse to assess the extent to which the family provides the individual basic needs of each person. It is also essential to re-member that individual needs vary depending on developmental level and the situa-tion present. The nurse should be cognizant of the fact that families provide more than just the physical necessities; the ability of the family to help the patient meet psychosociological needs is paramount.

When families are viewed as an environment, it is extremely important for the nurse to recognize that other family members may need intervention, as well as the patient. For example, when a child is hospitalized, the parents may feel anxiety and stress; therefore intervention with them is just as important as intervention with the hospitalized child.

When families are viewed as patients, it is important to assess crucial factors that are germane to family structure and organization. For example, if a hypertensive pa-tient is admitted to a hospital unit, it is crucial that the nurse assess several factors related to the family, including the following:

1. The family's current dietary patterns
2. The family's desire, as well as resources, for changing the dietary patterns
3. The family's knowledge about hypertension and its effects on the body
4. The family's capabilities to support a hypertensive family member
5. The family's ability to cope with and manage stress and anxiety

Whether the family is viewed as an environment or as the patient, it is essential to incorporate cultural concepts when developing the nursing plan of care. The nursing process is used regardless of whether the family is viewed as an environment or as the patient. The delineations or differences that occur in the nursing process are the result of cultural variables and beliefs that are germane to a particular ethnic or cultural group. Therefore it is essential that the nurse incorporate cultural beliefs and concerns shared by family members into the plan of care.

CASE
STUDY

Susie Chung, a 24-year-old Chinese American, is admitted with right lower quandrant ab-dominal pain. Within a few hours Miss Chung is taken to surgery for an appendectomy. When she returns to the floor, her vital signs remain stable. The nurse notes that even though she is rapidly recovering, her immediate and extended family appear to hover about her. The nurse also notes that it is very difficult to administer nursing care because of the number of family members who are keeping a constant vigil.

STUDY
QUESTIONS

1. List at least three social organization factors that influence the interactions between members of the same ethnic group or members of varying ethnic groups.
2. List at least two social organization factors that contribute to the development of cul-tural behavior.

3. Explain the role that religion may play for Susie Chung in regard to sociopsychological adaptation to her illness.

4. List at least three nursing interventions that may serve to minimize the confusion caused by the large number of family members who are keeping constant vigil in Susie Chung's room.

5. List at least two reasons why the family members of Susie Chung have congregated in the hospital room.

6. List at least three factors that would support Susie Chung's family being defined as a behavioral system.

7. List at least two imaginary and two real boundaries that would be found within Susie Chung's family structure.

8. List at least two roles that Susie Chung may take on in a social context within her family structure.

REFERENCES

Ackerman, N. (1984). *The theory of family systems*. New York: Gardner Press.

Averaswald, E. (1973). Families, change and the ecological perspective. In A. Ferber (Ed.), *The book of family therapy*. Boston: Houghton Mifflin.

Bateson, G., Jackson, D., Haley, J., & Weakland, J. (1968). Toward a theory of schizophrenia. In D.D. Jackson (Ed.), *Communication, family and marriage*. Palo Alto, Calif.: Science & Behavior Books.

Berkanovic, E., & Reeder, L.G. (1973). Ethnic, economic and social psychological factors in the source of medical care. *Social Problems, 21,* 246-259.

Bernard, J. (1966). *Marriage and family among Negros*. Englewood Cliffs, N.J.: Prentice Hall.

Billingsley, A. (1968). *Black families in White America*. Englewood Cliffs, N.J.: Prentice Hall.

Black, C. (1981). *It will never happen to me*. Denver: MAC.

Blasingame, J. (1972). *The slave community*. New York: Oxford University Press.

Blaxton, E. (1976). Structuring the Black family for survival and growth. *Perspectives in Psychiatric Care, 4*(14), 165-173.

Bowen, M. (1978). *Family therapy in clinical practice*. Northvale, N.J.: Jason Aronson.

Breitmayer, B., Gallo, A., Knafl, K., & Zoeller, L. (1989, April 3). *Correlates of social competence among children with a chronic illness*. Paper presented at the 13th Annual Midwest Nursing Research Society Conference, Cincinnati.

Brown, S. (1986). Children with an alcoholic parent. In N. Estes & M. Heinemann (Eds.), *Alcoholism: Development, consequences, and interventions* (3rd ed., pp. 207-220). St. Louis: C.V. Mosby.

Bullough, V.L., & Bullough, B. (1982). *Health care for the other Americans*. East Norwalk, Conn.: Appleton-Century-Crofts.

Campbell, J. (1989, April 3). *Self-care agency in battered women*. Paper presented at the 13th Annual Midwest Nursing Research Society Conference, Cincinnati.

Caplan, G. (1975). The family as a support system. In G. Caplan & M. Killilea (Eds.), *Support systems and mutual help: Multidisciplinary exploration*. New York: Grune & Stratton.

Carroll, J., Johnson, D., & Marty, M. (1979). *Religion in America: 1950 to present*. New York: Harper & Row.

Casavantes, E. (1976). Pride and prejudice: A Mexican American dilemma. In C.A. Hernandez, M.J. Haug, & N.N. Wagner (Eds.), *Chicanos: Social and psychological perspectives* (2nd ed., pp. 9-14). St. Louis: C.V. Mosby.

Duvall, E. (1977). *Marriage and family development* (ed. 2). East Norwalk, Conn.: Appleton-Century-Crofts.

Ellwood, R. (1987). *Many peoples, many faiths* (3rd ed.). Englewood Cliffs, N.J.: Prentice Hall.

Farber, B. (1973). *Family and kinship in modern society*. Glenview, Ill.: Scott, Foresman.

Fawcett, J. (1975). The family as a living open system: An emerging conceptual framework for nursing. *International Nursing Review, 22,* 113.

Frazier, I. (1964). *The Negro in the United States*. New York: Macmillan.

Friedman, M.M. (1986). *Family nursing: Theory and assessment*. East Norwalk, Conn.: Appleton-Century-Crofts.

Goldsby, R. (1971). *Race and races*. New York: Macmillan.

Govaets, K. (1987). Cultural and socioeconomic dimensions in mental health nursing. In J. Norris, M. Kunes-Connell, S. Stockhard, P.M. Ehrhart, & G.R. Newton (Eds.), *Mental health – psychiatric nursing: A continuum of care*. New York: John Wiley & Sons.

Guttmacher, S., & Elinson, J. (1972). Ethno-religious variation in perception of illness: The use of illness as an explanation for deviant behavior. *Social Science Medicine, 5,* 117-125.

Harwood, A. (Ed.). (1981). *Ethnicity and medical care*. Cambridge, Mass.: Harvard University Press.

Hashizume, S., & Takano, J. (1983). Nursing care of Japanese American patients. In M.S. Orque, B. Bloch, & L.S.A. Monrroy (Eds.), *Ethnic nursing care: A multicultural approach* (pp. 219-243). St. Louis: C.V. Mosby.

Henderson, G., & Primeaux, M. (1981). *Transcultural health care*. Reading, Mass.: Addison-Wesley.

Johnstone, R. (1988). *Religion in society* (3rd ed.). Englewood Cliffs, N.J.: Prentice Hall.

Kiefer, C.W. (1974). *Changing cultures, changing lives*. San Francisco: Jossey-Bass.

Kikumura, A., & Kitano, H. (1973). *Changing lives*. San Francisco: Jossey-Bass.

Kitano, H.L. (1976). Japanese Americans: The development of a middleman minority. In N. Hundley, Jr. (Ed.), *The Asian American* (pp. 81-100). Santa Barbara, Calif.: ABC-CLIO.

Kobata, F. (1979). The influence of culture on family relations: The Asian American experience. In P.K. Ragan (Ed.), *Aging parents*. Los Angeles: Ethel Percy Andrus Gerontology Foundation, University of Southern California.

Leininger, M. (1985). Southern rural Black and White American lifeways with focus on care and health phenomena. In M. Leininger (Ed.), *Qualitative research methods in nursing*. Orlando, Fla.: Grune & Stratton.

Lewis, H. (1979). *How's your family?* New York: Brunner/Mazel.

Lewis, J.M., Beavers, W.R., Gossett, J.T., & Phillips, V.A. (1976). *No single thread: Psychological health in family systems*. New York: Brunner/Mazel.

Martin, E.P., & Martin, J.M. (1978). *The Black-extended family*. Chicago: University of Chicago Press.

Martin, W. (1985). *The kingdom of the cults*. Minneapolis, Minn.: Bethany House.

Mauksch, H. (1974). A cosial science basis for conceptualizing family health. *Social Science Medicine, 8,* 521.

Meleis, A.L., & La Fever, C. (1984). The Arab American and psychiatric care. *Perspectives in Psychiatric Care, 22*(2), 42-85.

Meleis, A.L., & Sorrell, L. (1981). Arab American women and their birth experiences. *American Journal of Maternal Child Nursing, 6,* 171-176.

Minuchin, S. (1974). *Families and family therapy*. Cambridge, Mass: Harvard University Press.

Modell, J. (1968). The Japanese American family: A perspective for future investigations. *Pacific Historical Review, 37,* 67-81.

Murphy, S. (1986). Family study and nursing research. *Image: Journal of Nursing Scholarship, 18*(4), 170.

Murray, R., Meili, P., & Zentner, J. (1975). The family—Basic unit for the developing person. In R. Murray & J. Zentner (Eds.), *Nursing concepts for health promotion*. Englewood Cliffs, N.J.: Prentice Hall.

Osako, M.N. (1979). Aging and family among Japanese Americana: The role of ethnic tradition in the adjustment to old age. *Gerontologist, 19,* 448-455.

Phipps, S. (1989, April 3). *A phenomenological study of males' experience with infertility*. Paper presented at the 13th Annual Midwest Nursing Research Society Conference, Cincinnati.

Potter, P., & Perry, A. (1989). *Fundamentals in nursing: Concepts, process and practice*. St. Louis: C.V. Mosby.

Robischon, P., & Scott, D. (1969). Role theory and its application in family nursing. *Nursing Outlook, 17*(7), 52-57.

Romanzuk, A. (1987). Helping the stepparent parent. *Maternal Child Nursing, 12,* 106.

Satir, V. (1967). *Conjoint family therapy*. Palo Alto, Calif.: Science & Behavior Books.

Satir, V. (1972). *Conjoint family therapy* (2nd ed.). Palo Alto, Calif.: Science & Behavior Books.

Saunders, L. (1954). *Cultural differences and medical care*. New York: Russell Sage Foundation.

Schneflen, A. (1972). *Body language in social order*. Englewood Cliffs, N.J.: Prentice Hall.

Schneider, R. (1980, June). *Conceptual scheme of family organization and function*. Paper presented at St. Louis University Medical Center conference, St. Louis.

Smart, N. (1984). *The religious experience of mankind* (3rd ed.). New York: Charles Scribner's Sons.

Suchman, E.A. (1964). Sociomedical variations among ethnic groups. *American Journal of Sociology, 70,* 319-331.

Sussman, M.B. (1971, July). Family systems in the 1970's: Analysis, politics, and programs. *Annuals of American Academy of Political Social Science, 396,* 40-56.

U.S. Department of Commerce, Bureau of the Census. (1981). 1980 provisional race and Spanish-origin counts announced. *Data User News, 16,* 1-3.

Vogel, V.J. (1970). *American Indian medicine.* Norman: University of Oklahoma Press.

Watchtower Bible & Tract Society. (1953). *Let God be true* (rev. ed.). Brooklyn, N.Y.: Author.

Watchtower Bible & Tract Society. (1955). *You may survive Armageddon into God's new world.* Brooklyn, N.Y.: Author.

Zinn, M., & Eitzen, D. (1987). *Diversity in American families.* New York: Harper & Row.

■ ▪ ■

CHAPTER 5

Time

BEHAVIORAL OBJECTIVES

After reading this chapter, the nurse will be able to:

1 Postulate an adequate definition for the term *time* in relation to transcultural nursing care.

2 Understand the significant role that culture plays in the understanding and perception of time.

3 Understand the significant role that the developmental process plays in the understanding and perception of time.

4 Understand the significance of the measurement of time and the relationship to transcultural nursing care.

5 Differentiate the terms *social time* and *clock time*.

6 Describe the world view of clock time and social time.

7 Define the following three broad areas of the structure of social time: temporal patterns, temporal orientation, and temporal perspectives.

Since the beginning of life on earth, time has been the greatest mystery of all. The mystery of time becomes evident as soon as thought is given to the concept. Our experience with time continuously leads us into puzzles and paradoxes. According to Wessman and Gorman (1977), it is through an awareness and conception of time that the products of the human mind, that is, time itself, seem to possess an existence apart from time's passage, which is perceived as personal and inexorable. We measure time, and time measures us. It is this intimate and personal, yet aloof and detached, character that constitutes the paradox of human time.

CONCEPT OF TIME

The concept of the passage of time is very familiar to most people regardless of cultural heritage. The days and nights come and go, and with each passing day and night humankind grows older. In the highly mechanized world of today there are numerous clocks and watches that ceaselessly tick away time and determine the schedules by which hundreds of millions of people live. Thus it would seem that the concept of the passage of time should be second nature to humankind and thoroughly understood by all people.

However, developing an awareness of the concept of time is not a simple phenomenon but a gradual process (Hymovich & Chamberlin, 1980). Most people, regardless of cultural heritage, remember a time when their perception of the passage of time was altered. Such occasions might have been during times of boredom, or highly emotional and stressful events. During these events time might have seemed to have passed very slowly, or it might have seemed to have passed all too quickly. It must be remembered that a sense of time is not innate but is developed early as a result of everyday experiences that are common to all people. Thus a sense of time results from learning. It becomes a part of human nature before one is conscious of its presence. Even infants perceive the essence of time. Infants are fed on demand or according to a strict timetable and experience the sucession of day by night. Thus infants are exposed to regular rhythmic changes that are reflected in rhythmic changes in bodily conditions, including the conditions of being sated, awake, or asleep. Thus one phenomenon about time is that it is associated with rhythm and change.

Infants grow and develop, and begin to move through crawling. The speed with which crawling occurs determines the time it takes to get from one place to another. Thus even this simple task makes individuals aware that time is associated with speed and velocity, which is the second phenomenon about time. As individuals grow older, speech is learned by listening to stories that begin with "once upon a time." It is through these story-telling sessions that children learn that things did happen before they were born; thus time is associated with history and goes backward as well as forward with the succession of events. As the growth and development of the child continues, an awareness of punctuality is developed. Children may be punished for being slow or late, and regardless of their reaction to it, the punishment contributes to the formation of character and the development of understanding of time. Thus the third phenomenon about time is that it is associated with social behavior (Haber et al., 1987).

The child begins to become conscious of time and to ask questions such as "Where was I before I was born?" "What did God do before He created the world?" "What will happen to me after I die?" Such questions lead to an understanding that time is associated with philosophy and religion. Children are taught to read time on a clock, and as they grow to adulthood they learn that the clock is ubiquitous and that life is governed by the clock. Thus there is an erroneous identification of time with the clock. Through questioning, individuals begin to contemplate existence on earth and to develop an understanding that time is associated with something external over which there is no control and that appears absolute (Elton & Messel, 1978; Haber et al., 1987).

Developing an understanding of the definition of time by looking at the developmental process is clearly too simple. The development of the awareness of time is directly influenced by earlier ideas and prejudices that are mostly unconscious. However, because it is the nature of humankind to have a questioning frame of mind, ideas and prejudices may become conscious.

Other considerations concerning time include the question of whether time is concrete or abstract. Time is perceived as real in the sense of being concrete and having direct effects, or it is regarded as not real in the sense of being abstract. The mathematical and physical sciences adopt the view that time is an abstract dimension with only a locational or reference function (McGrath & Kelly, 1986). On the other hand, the biological sciences adopt the view that time is an essential ingredient in many life and behavioral processes such as gestation, healing, and metamorphosis. This difference in conceptualization of time may be related to an obvious difference between the physical and biological sciences and how each treat the concept of *entropy*. For the physical sciences entropy, or randomness, continuously increases over time, whereas the biological sciences see organization, structure, and information residing within the organism and in the organism's relation to its environment as increasing over time.

MEASUREMENT OF TIME

Time has two distinct, although related, meanings. The first meaning is that of duration, which is an interval of time. The second meaning is that of specified instances, or points in time. These two meanings are related because a point in time is identified as being the end of a time interval that starts at an arbitrary or fixed reference point, such as the founding of Rome or the birth of Christ. Thus if one asks the question, "What is the time?" and the answer given is "It is 10:00 AM," this answer refers to a point in time. At the same time, the answer refers to a time interval, since it indicates the time from a certain reference point, which in this case is midnight the previous night (Elton & Messel, 1978; Haber et al., 1987). The two meanings are quite different and must not be confused with each other. Measuring devices are meant to determine intervals of time, and clocks and watches are designed to read direct points in time. Clocks and watches therefore have to be standardized against a standard clock. The purpose of a standard clock is to measure accurately the time interval up to the present time. This phenomenon goes back to one universal standard clock against which all standard clocks are calibrated.

The purpose of a universal standard clock is to define operational time in terms of both time interval and point in time (Landes, 1983). The purpose of measuring devices is to define time; however, people need to have intuitive ideas about time in order to specify the properties of the instrument. Measuring devices of a phenomenon such as time are more accurate than measuring devices of some other phenomena. For example, if an individual wanted to measure the weight of a person, this weight could be defined operationally as a point or reading on a scale. Thus a good scale would give accurate weight, just as any good clock would give accurate time. On the other hand, if an individual wanted to define a person's intelligent quotient (IQ) as the score obtained on an intelligence test but there was no general agreement about what constituted intelligence and what constituted a good intelligence test, the scores would not be as relevant or as meaningful as the weight or time measures.

Throughout the entire history of humankind there have been two obvious standards of time: the day and the year. The day is a remarkably easy period of time to recognize because of the experience of daylight and darkness, which result from the earth's spinning on its axis. The year is also easy to recognize because of the passage of the seasons, which are caused by the tilting of the earth's axis. Thus a day is the period of time for one complete revolution of the earth about its axis, whereas a year is the time taken for the earth to make one complete revolution around the sun, which takes just under 365¼ days. Therefore it is completely natural that we choose to mark the passage of time by first marking the days and then marking the years. Time measurement during the day has been divided into hours, and the hours in turn have been divided by 60 to give minutes. The minutes have been divided by 60 to give seconds.

Very early in the history of civilization the middle of each day was determined as the point when the sun was at its highest point during the day. This point was defined as noon, and clocks were made to read 12 when it occurred. Thus if it is noon in one place, it is midnight at the opposite side of the earth, and different times at other places on the earth. To understand how time varies, the earth must be viewed as a circle that passes through both the North and South Poles.

Traditionally in science, Greenwich, the observatory in London, has been taken to have 0 degrees of longitude; all other places on earth are given as so many degrees east or west of Greenwich. Therefore, one half of the earth's surface has a longitude of up to 180 degrees east of Greenwich, whereas the other half has a longitude of up to 180 degrees west of Greenwich. The times of all places east of Greenwich are ahead of that of Greenwich, and the times of all places west of Greenwich lag behind that of Greenwich. For example, if an individual started from Greenwich and traveled eastward to a longitude of 45 degrees, the time would be 3 hours ahead of Greenwich time. The converse is that if an individual started at Greenwich and traveled westward to a longitude of 180 degrees, the time would be 12 hours behind that of Greenwich. In simpler terms, if it were 2 AM on Sunday morning at Greenwich, it would be 2 PM on Sunday at a longitude 180 degrees east of Greenwich and 2 PM on Saturday at a longitude 180 degrees west of Greenwich (Elton & Messel, 1978).

This phenomenon of time presents some interesting effects on persons who travel great distances. For example, it is possible for an international traveler to have two birthdays; that is, if an individual crosses the international date line traveling eastward at 2 AM Sunday morning, at which point it suddenly becomes 2 AM Saturday, the individual has Saturday all over again and thus is able to celebrate the birthday again. If this same international traveler who is about to celebrate a birthday on Saturday leaves from the point of origin at 2 AM on Saturday but crosses the international date line westward, the traveler suddenly finds that it is 2 AM Sunday morning and apparently has missed almost the entire day of Saturday and the birthday as well (Elton & Messel, 1978).

Time-Measuring Devices
Clocks

According to historians and philosophers the earliest clocks were undoubtedly sundials of various kinds, which were probably followed by devices that used the regular flow of a substance such as water, oil, or sand, or the steady combustion of oil or candles. The earliest clocks have been dated back to 1600 BC in Egypt and were used throughout classical times and the Middle Ages.

The thirteenth century saw the invention of a rhythmic motion clock, which was a sawtoothed crown wheel. However, the most important development in clock construction occurred with the introduction of the pendulum, which was first discovered by Galileo in 1581. Galileo discovered that a swinging pendulum would readily tick away a unit of time by a specific number of swings, and that even if the swings gradually died, the unit of time would remain relatively unaffected. Thus for the first time in history, time was measured more accurately.

Tropical years

An important distinction that has been made by scientists is the difference between a calendar year and a tropical year. According to scientists, a calendar year consists of 365 days, whereas a tropical year consists of 365.242199 solar days (the word *tropical* in this instance has nothing to do with a hot climate). The difference between these two numbers (tropical year and calendar year) is the reason for the necessity of leap years. Time that is based on the length of a tropical year is called ephemeris time. One tropical year is defined in terms of seconds as having 31,556,925.9747 seconds. Today atomic clocks have replaced the old, outdated pendulum and weight and gravity–driven clocks. These clocks are so accurate that in due course scientists speculate that the difference between atomic time and ephemeris time will become very apparent. In fact, atomic clocks are said to be 10 million times more accurate than any other clock on earth and are never more than 1 billionth of a second off. Atomic clocks are considered to be so accurate that the exact second of an event can be obtained at the time of the event.

Solar time

Solar time is perhaps the earliest way that time was measured (Dossey, 1982). Solar time takes into consideration a focal point, 12:00 noon, which is precisely the point at which the sun passes directly overhead (vertically above the meridian). The time period between successive crossings of the sun directly over the same meridian is called a solar day. However, this measurement of time is not without its problems. When days are measured in this way, they turn out to be not exactly constant. A solar day varies slightly in length throughout the year because of the orbiting of the earth around the sun. The concept of solar time has many implications for nurses who work at extreme southern or northern points of the earth, for example, at the North or South Pole. A nurse working in northern Alaska may find Eskimos operating on "Eskimo time," since the sun remains up during most of the summer and down during much of the winter (see Chapter 12 on American Eskimos).

Calendar

Inventing a simple yet efficient calendar has presented difficulties since the invention of the first calendar. It is thought by scientists that these difficulties lie in the fact that the three obvious periodicities are due to the rotation of the earth, the revolution of the moon about the earth, and the revolution of the earth about the sun. These three revolutional periods are not simply related one to the other. In fact, they have obvious differences. For example, 1 tropical year equals 365.224 solar days and 1 month, which is considered to be the observed time between one full moon and the next, is 29.5306 solar days.

Throughout history we have measured time by counting the months and the calendar years, and combining the two. However, this combination of months and years has proved to be most confusing. Even if we ignored the moon, there would still be the problem of the solar year not being a whole number of days, although this problem has conceivably been dealt with by the system of leap years. With so many different civilizations contributing to the development of the calendar it is no wonder that we are left with a complicated system that children and even adults, regardless of ethnic or cultural heritage, find difficult to remember or understand. Many of the significant events that are linked with the calendar can also be traced to specific persons in history such as Julius Caesar.

It was Julius Caesar who decreed that months should alternately have 30 and 31 days with the exception of February (which at that time was the last month of the Roman calendar). Historians believe that all would have been well with the calendar if Julius Caesar had not decided to call the fifth month Julius in his honor. The problem began when Augustus followed Julius Caesar and also wanted a month. He promptly chose the month that followed Julius and named it Augustus. However, he very soon realized that his month was shorter than Caesar's month and promptly took a day from February, added it to his month, and readjusted the rest of the year. The result was that there were three long months in succession, that is, June, July, and August. Even today, because of the vanity of Emperor Augustus, children continue to chant "Thirty days has September."

According to the earlier decree by Julius Caesar, September would have been an alternate month with 31 days if August had been given 30 days as originally planned (Elton & Messel, 1978). While there have been attempts over the last 50 years to standardize the calendar by international agreement through the League of Nations and the United Nations, these attempts have uniformly failed. For example, the day that is considered the beginning of the New Year in the United States is January 1, but the beginning of the New Year differs in many countries.

SOCIAL TIME VERSUS CLOCK TIME

The word *time* immediately presents an image of a clock or calendar. However, the term *social time* is not equivalent with *clock time*. Social time refers to patterns and orientations that relate to social processes and to the conceptualization and ordering of social life. For centuries, many of the great thinkers of the universe have recognized and argued that social time must be distinguished from clock time. As early as 1910, Henri Bergson insisted that the homogeneous time of newtonian physics was not the time that revealed the essence of humankind. On the other hand, Phillip Bock (1964), an anthropologist, showed that an Indian wake could be meaningfully analyzed in terms of "gathering time," "prayer time," "singing time," "intermission time," and "meal time." None of these times has a particular relationship to clock time. They all simply imply the passage of the mourner from one time to another by consensual feelings rather than by the clock.

According to some sociologists, certain kinds of psychological disorders may be viewed in terms of the individual living wholly in the present, the implication being that both the past and the future are completely severed from the consciousness. The difference therefore between social time and clock time is that the former is a more inclusive concept whereas the latter may or may not be. Hoppe and Heller (1974) conducted a study on Mexican Americans and proposed that Mexican Americans have a present time orientation that may possibly account for the tendency to be late for appointments. It is thought that present time orientation, particularly in high-risk settings such as mental health facilities, may result in a crisis approach rather than a preventive one. For example, a patient who has an immediate need at home may be late for appointments at the clinic or hospital, or may miss them altogether. The nurse should also keep in mind that patients with a present time orientation may be reluctant to leave an appointment simply because the time is up.

This same lack of correlation between social time and clock time can be seen in mystical beliefs. According to mystical thought, magic can be employed to negate the temporal order that infers causality. For example, an Indian warrior who is wounded by an arrow may attend to his pain by hanging the arrow up where it is cool or by applying ointment to the arrow. What the Indian warrior is attempting to do is to reverse the clock time, that is, wrench the present back into the past to alter the course of events. For people who have mystical beliefs, temporal intervals are not simple, homogeneous series; rather, they contain an inherent quality and meaning or an essence and efficacy of their own (Cassirer, 1955). Therefore the objectivity represented by clock time is unknown to a person with mystical beliefs.

Many sociologists believe that people who lack or minimize clock time also lack regularity or temporal measurement. It is the natural and social phenomena that may dictate regularity and measurement. Ariotti (1975) has given a number of examples of natural events that have been used to time human activities:

> The arrival of the cranes in ancient Greece marked the time for planting.
> The return of the swallow marked the time for the end of pruning.
> The South African bush men note the rising of Sirius and Canopus and are able to depict the progress of winter across the night sky by the movement of these celestial bodies across the night sky.

In modern times certain natural events continue to be linked with certain activities. In the United States folklore has it that if the groundhog sees his shadow on February 2, there will be 6 more weeks of winter. However, if the groundhog does not see his shadow, an early spring is imminent. The return of the robin is also considered an early indicator of spring. If spring and summer birds fly south very early in the fall, it is considered a sign of a very hard and early winter. If flowers are to be planted in the spring, they should not be planted until after Mother's Day. The passage of Mother's Day should assure the planter that all possible chances of frost have passed.

Archeologists have been able to piece together the history of humankind by measuring the passage of time, using the method of geologists. This measure of time is based on rates of deposits to and erosion of natural early elements. An example of this kind of measurement is tree ring chronology (Weyer, 1973).

World View of Social Time versus Clock Time

People throughout the world view social time and clock time differently. For example, Sorokin (1964) noted that the division of time by weeks reflects social conditions rather than mechanical newtonian divisions. Most societies have some kind of week, but the weeks vary in length of days from 3 to 16 or more days. In most cases weeks are a reflection of the cycle of market activities. The Khasi people have an 8-day week because they hold market every eighth day. The Khasi people have named the days of the week after the places where the principal markets occur (Sorokin, 1964).

Some cultural groups exhibit a social time that not only is different from clock time, but is actually scornful of clock time. For example, there are peasants in Algeria who live with a total indifference to the passage of clock time, and who despise haste in human affairs. These peasants have no notion of exact appointment times; they lack exact times for eating meals; and they have labeled the clock as "the devil's mill" (Thompson, 1967).

Despite the way people in various cultures view clock time as opposed to social time, it is important for the nurse to remember that clock time should not be regarded as unimportant or irrelevant. Although for some people in some cultural groups there is no necessary correlation of clock time with social time, clock time does take on paramount importance in a social context such as the modern Western world, where the watch or the clock can become something of a tyrant. In Jonathan Swift's *Gulliver's Travels,* Gulliver never did anything without looking at his watch, which he called his oracle. He said that his watch pointed out the time for every action of his life. Because of Gulliver's obsession with his watch, the Lilliputians concluded that the watch was Gulliver's God.

Aside from literature, many actual examples of human obsessive behavior in regard to clock time can be found. Lebhar (1958) wrote that he was exactly 43 years old and had probably only 227,760 hours to live, and he proceeded to detail how he would maximize the use of those remaining hours of his life. He concluded that if he reduced his sleep time from 8 hours to 6 hours, the 2 hours a day saved from sleeping would amount to 18,980 hours over a period of 26 years. If this savings were converted into 18-hour days, which is the equivalent of about 2 years and 11 months, he could virtually lengthen his remaining years by 2 years and 11 months. This example illustrates how human life can be turned into a lengthy succession of minutes and hours, with the individual's existence reduced to a compulsive and frantic effort to avoid waste.

Gilles and Faulkner (1978) conducted a study of the role of time in television news work. They found that time is a major factor in the production of unscheduled "hard" news. The definition for "hard" news refers to events such as fires, homicides, and accidents, which have a certain urgency to them. They summarized the findings of their research in three propositions. In the first proposition they concluded that the news value of an event is directly proportional to the time invested in covering it. An event may turn out to be relatively minor in the sense of not involving the trauma or shock value that was anticipated, but this factor was not considered when a film crew invested time in the event, and the story is likely to be used in the evening news program, anyway. They found in the second proposition that what is considered news by the news crew depends on when it happens and how long it lasts. Although viewers tend to believe that what they see on the evening news is a compilation of the universal news events for that particular day, what is telecast each evening is actually a compilation of news events that the news crew were able to learn about, get a story line on, capture the film of, and then process and edit the film. The researchers found in the third proposition that bias in the news reflects occupational assumptions and temporal constraints more than it does the political or social views of the news crew; more important than political and social biases are the assumptions that the news crew make about what will make good news on television and the severe time constraints on those persons assigned to locate film and write about events in time for the evening news program. The researchers concluded that because of deadline pressures, it is inevitable that events are reduced to surface actions and that the visuals seen each evening are of only the most dramatic events.

In today's modern technological society clock time is of paramount importance. However, we need to keep in mind that even in a modern society the clock may be a relatively peripheral part of social life. Not all people in a modern technological society function under the ineluctable tyranny of the clock.

In a survey of a representative sample of the French population, approximately 21% of the respondents indicated a belief that there was no urgency about being punctual and also stated they had not experienced the feeling of wasting time (Stoetzel, 1953). It is the perception of some people in some cultural groups that there is little correlation between being punctual and wasting time (Hein, 1980). Hein further postulated that assumptions and definitions in regard to time are determined by culture and cultural variables and are reflected in interactions with others, personal views concerning punctuality, the use or waste of time, and, finally, value and respect for time or a lack thereof. Waiting is a cultural counterpart to time because a particular behavior, person, or event is anticipated within a particular time frame. Waiting may have a meaning similar to that of time for some Black patients. The nurse may schedule an appointment for a Black patient and wait for the Black patient to arrive for the appointment. However, the patient may not arrive for several hours, or perhaps even a few days, because of other important issues that took precedence over the appointment. While this was experienced by the nurse as waiting and therefore wasting time, time for the patient waiting for the appointment was not being wasted.

In the American nursing profession, many nurses have related professionalism and success in their career to a sense of precision about clock time. For example, in many health care facilities, a medication error is considered to occur when a medication is not given within 30 minutes of the prescribed time, even when the medication is given daily and is not a time-released medication. Thus the nurse must complete a medication error form for not giving a routine daily medication such as a vitamin or laxative, which is neither time released nor urgent.

Most agencies relate medication errors to disciplinary action and dismissal. In some facilities the nurse is expected to complete all morning or evening care in a precise time frame even though many patients may not operate in the same time sphere as the agency schedule for patient care. For example, a patient may become upset when the night nurse refuses to help the patient to shower at 3 AM because showering is a stated day shift activity. In this case the patient may be used to starting the day at 3 AM and unwilling to wait until 7 AM to do so. Another example is early morning vital signs, which may be taken by the night nurse to facilitate a timely assessment of the patient's condition for the physician who makes early morning rounds. The patient may be annoyed at being awakened for such a brief procedure and then instructed by the nurse to return to sleep.

According to Zerubavel's (1979) analysis of the temporal order of the hospital, any unit of clock time is equal to any other unit whether one is talking about minutes, hours, days, or weeks. However, Zerubavel concluded that different days mean quite different things to different people. Because people perceive days differently, it is important to remember that some days are more or less desirable for some people. For example, some personnel may perceive the fact of working two weekends in succession as unfair. Similarly, evening or night duty is usually considered more undesirable than day duty. Thus it is important for hospital administrators to understand the necessity for fairness in scheduling. In some hospitals it is the policy that all personnel are expected to work their share of the less desirable times. In other hospitals staff are paid differentials for working what is perceived as the less desirable times, that is, evenings, nights, weekends, and holidays.

STRUCTURE OF SOCIAL TIME

The structure of social time is a complex phenomenon. To understand the structure of social time, three broad areas of social time must be analyzed: temporal pattern, temporal orientation, and temporal perspective.

Temporal Pattern

Hawley (1950) identified the temporal pattern of social time as one of the most important aspects of ecological organization. He concluded that there are five basic elements in the temporal pattern of any social phenomenon: periodicity, tempo, timing, duration, and sequence.

Periodicity

Periodicity refers to the various rhythms of social life and is characterized by activities related to both the needs and the activity or people. For example, every community has a functional routine that is supposedly peculiar to that community, such as the search for food, shelter, and mates, which occurs more or less with regular periodicity. People also have transcendental needs that are pursued with regular periodicity. For example, people may attend church weekly in pursuit of satisfying transcendental needs. Even physical functions of the body occur in a periodic manner. There are cyclic variations in physiological functions of the body such as body temperature, blood pressure, and pulse.

Nelkin (1970) studied the behavior patterns of migrant workers and found a number of daily, weekly, and seasonal rhythms that were germane to their existence. Nelkin concluded that these migrant workers seemed to alternate between compact and diffuse time. "Migrant time" was seen to be very present oriented, irrational, and highly personal. Nelkin concluded that migrant time was in sharp contrast to the typical time perception, which was future oriented, rational, and impersonal. Findings from the study suggest that social time for the migrants differed because it was a series of disconnected periods rather than a continuous and predictable process, which in part accounted for maladaptive behaviors such as excessive drinking, gambling, volatile social relationships, and apathy.

Periodicity is also considered important at the managerial level. An important aspect of managerial life concerns the periodicity of meetings. For example, it is inappropriate for managers of a volunteer organization to plan frequent meetings for the membership. It is thought that a volunteer organization can engage in systematic self-destruction and ensure itself of a high turnover of membership if the body seeks to gather its members too often. These organizations must justify their demands on the members' time and at the same time create the novelty necessary to maintain the interest of the membership. In contrast to this are nonvoluntary groups, such as those that are part of a job assignment. For example, in nursing administration regular meetings are necessary as part of the required management structure and are not usually planned with the intent of being novel and interesting. Because the management structure requires regular meetings to take place, the meetings are planned regardless of specific agenda items.

Periodicities are also noted at the individual level. It is thought that when people are able to control their own work patterns (periodicity), satisfaction and productivity are maximized (Strauss, 1963). Some individuals spontaneously choose to alternate bouts of intense work with bouts of idleness.

It is important for managers to realize that productivity is cyclic and that equal periods of productivity cannot always be maintained. For example, after a period in which a nursing care unit experiences high patient acuity necessitating an extremely heavy work load for staff, employees will need to recover with a period of less intense pressure. It is unwise to follow a period of high acuity with another assignment that requires major time on the task. However, some work environments by their very nature cannot and do not provide for individual periodicity. For example, industrial worker often must work at a continuous rhythmic pace, such as that seen on an automobile assembly line.

To understand periodicity, the nurse must remember that it is an important aspect of human life and the first aspect of the temporal pattern. Periodicity therefore refers to the recurrence of a social phenomenon with some kind of regularity that can be measured by clock time or by comparing the social phenomenon with other social phenomena.

Tempo

Tempo is the second aspect of the temporal pattern and refers to rate (Morgenstern, 1960). Tempo may refer to the frequency of activities in some unit of social time or to the rate of change of some phenomenon. An example of this is the industrialization of the United States, which differs from that of the Soviet Union and China because of different rates (Gioscia, 1970). In a study done by the Southern Illinois University Foundation (Veterans World Project, 1972), it was suggested that one major problem among Vietnam veterans resulted from the rapidity with which they were brought home. The study concluded that the sudden transition from combat back to the United States by way of jet flights required a psychological adjustment that was often quite traumatic for these veterans.

Tempo also includes perceived rapidity of time and experience and the rapidity of various modes of social life, such as urban versus rural and work versus leisure. For example, the tempo of life in a large urban city such as Chicago or New York is much different from the tempo of life in a small rural midwestern town. Thus a person who relocates may have difficulty adjusting to the different tempo.

Tempo has a number of important consequences at the individual level because control of the tempo of one's work seems to be important for a healthy self-concept (Kohn, 1969). The tempo of change in social order appears to be related to emotional health; thus the more rapid the change, the greater the stress on the individual. This thought became the theme of Alvin Toffler (1970), who coined the phrase "future shock."

The term *future shock* is used to describe the psychological disruptions that result from experiencing too much change in too short a time. An example of this is noted with Japanese people, who traditionally have had to change their culture and society at a very rapid pace. The very rapid tempo of the deliberative transformation of the Meiji era in Japan produced considerable stress for the Japanese people. Some historians have concluded that the 1878 revolution of Japan did save Japan from Western domination, but the generations that followed experienced the brunt of the hectic rate of change and suffered extraordinary mental agonies as a result of these forced changes (Pyle, 1969).

Timing

Timing is the third element in the temporal pattern and is referred to as synchronization. Timing involves the adjustment of various social units and processes with each other. It is the necessity for synchronization that has led to the emphasis on clock time in modern society. Timing can be a crucial factor in the initiation of planned social changes and is of obvious importance in numerous social contexts, such as industrial processes, military campaigns, and political campaigns. A presidential candidate who supports a particular view that is not popular or timely may lose an election but win at a later time when the view becomes popular or another view emerges. An example of this is the case of Richard Nixon, who ran for president in 1960 and lost. Eight years later Nixon ran for president again at the height of the Vietnam War, and since the issue of the war was a timely one, he campaigned on this issue and won. Success is related to being at the right place at the right time with popular ideas.

Another example of the importance of timing is provided by research data on institutionalized disturbed children. These children, because of their psychological limitations, can be permitted to engage in activities such as competitive sports for only limited amounts of time. The restrictions on time must be placed because the process of the game and psychological processes can mesh for only limited periods of time before the two processes begin to conflict and lead to destructive behavior (Doob, 1970).

Some researchers have concluded that one of the most serious problems of the modern American family is the difficulty of synchronizing family life because of the diverse activities in which each member is engaged. Another difficulty that has emerged over the years lies in the efforts of rural immigrants to adjust to the stringent demands of industrial life. It has been suggested by some researchers that habitual functioning of these rural immigrants must be synchronized with the industrial process and that such synchronization disallows the individual's self-actualization.

Duration

Duration is the fourth element of the tempo pattern and has been the concern of psychologists more than it has been the concern of sociologists. The psychological concern of duration is related to the duration of which the individual is conscious, or to what has been referred to as the "spacious present." According to the classic early work of James (1890), one of the early writers in the field of social psychology, longer or shorter periods are conceived symbolically by adding to or dividing the vaguely bound unit that is the spacious present.

Duration has significance beyond the psychological level, however. Some noted sociologists have set forth a number of laws that relate to duration and behavior in organizations (Parkinson, 1970). Parkinson developed the laws of triviality and delay. The law of triviality states that the amount of time spent on any item in the agenda of an organizational meeting is inversely proportional to the money involved with that item. People may quibble far more about an item costing $50 than about an item costing $10,000. For example, in professional staff meetings at a state psychiatric hospital, an inordinate amount of time was spent discussing the purchase of a 75-cent plastic receptacle for holding patients' personal items such as toothbrushes and soap. A year later, when some plastic lids were missing, several meetings were devoted to developing a strategic nursing procedure for safeguarding these "valuable plastic receptacles." The policy developed to safeguard these receptacles mandated that the staff send a written requisition to the director of nursing, who in turn was required to write a written justification for replacement of the receptacle or the lid. The law of delay asserts that delay is the deadliest form of denial. In addition, duration is perceived as a useful variable.

Researchers continue to investigate the effects of various phenomena such as perceived importance of time, anxiety, and boredom on the perception of time. For example, researchers have concluded that morale may be improved among workers if time is subjectively made to pass more quickly and if there are a number of methods whereby the apparent length of a period of time can be manipulated (Meade, 1960).

Sequence

Sequence is the final element of temporal pattern and is derived from the fact that there are activities requiring the ordering of actions. An obvious evidence of the utility of sequence is the measuring of values. For example, work before play is an ordering of activity that reflects a valuing hierarchy. In a classic 1946 study, Friedman measured values relating to physical activities, theoretic-scientific interests, and esthetic interests and found that subjects made similar choices on both time and money scales. Friedman concluded that when cost and time are equalized, similar preferential orderings are made for various activities.

In modern American society time is indeed money. It is conceivable, however, that the sequential ordering of activities may reflect necessity rather than values as an industrial process. It is also possible that conflict may arise over whether the sequence actually does represent necessity rather than values. Generally, this kind of conflict is more common in organizational settings where disputes arise over the necessity of sequential orderings that are demanded by bureaucratic rules.

Finally, sequential ordering may reflect habit. Rituals of primitive societies are ordered in accordance with custom. Modern rituals also fall in this category, even though some are more appropriately viewed as reflections of values. For example, the ritual of a man removing his hat before entering a room or elevator is a habitual sequence. However, the ritual of the same man removing his hat before the national anthem is played is a sequence demanded by values.

Temporal Orientation

Temporal orientation refers to the ordering of past, present, and future and to the fact that both individuals and groups may be differentiated according to whether behavior is primarily related to the past, present, or future. Psychologists and sociologists, however, have raised objections to this particular ordering. One objection is that past, present, and future are perceived to make up an organic whole that cannot be separated (Cassirer, 1955; Haber et al., 1987).

A second objection is in respect to variations in the ordering of past, present, and future among various groups. For example, the argument is made that an actor's orientation to a situation always contains "an expectancy aspect," which implies that all orientations are to a future state of a situation, as well as to the present. However, this may be true only in a limited sense, because actors generally do not anticipate their demise in the situation. It is also not true that orientation to the future is a universal and inherent aspect of all social action.

Future orientation refers to the fact that the future is a dominant factor in present behavior, and as such this kind of orientation is by no means universal. For example, the Navajo Indians' view of time does not include the expectancy aspect. In years past, efforts to get the Navajo Indians to engage in range control and soil conservation programs were extremely frustrating for government employees because the Navajos simply do not have a view of temporality that would lead them to act on the basis of an expected future (Hall & William, 1960). For the Navajo people the only real time, like the only real space, is that which is here and now. For some Navajo Indians there is little reality of the future; thus the promise of future benefits is not worth thinking about (Hall & William, 1960). It is important for the nurse to remember that the way in which a society, group, or individual orders past, present, and future will be consequential for behavior.

Kluckhohn and Strodtbeck (1961) have argued that the knowledge of rank ordering of these three modes can tell much about a social unit and the direction of change for that unit. Some Americans have typically placed a dominant emphasis on the future, which does not imply that they ignore either the past or the present. Although there are some undesirable connotations for the label "old fashioned," few Americans express total contentment with the present state of affairs. According to Kluckhohn and Strodtbeck, American values change easily as long as the change does not contradict what is perceived as the American way of life. There is a direct relationship between the extended future orientation and the amount of change. However, the change perceived is not expected to be the kind that threatens the existing order.

Generally speaking, resistance to change should be expected where there is a past orientation. Thus it should be expected that serious problems would arise in efforts to industrialize a society where a future orientation was lacking. For example, in a classic 1953 study, Ritzenthaler found that among the Chippewa Indians, who traditionally lack any concern for the future, there were serious problems when attempts were made to industrialize their work. In the study it was found that the Chippewa Indians quit work as soon as they had sufficient money for immediate needs.

Temporal orientations are not immutable; they can change, and along with change come various behavioral changes. Therefore a shift of orientation to the present may have significant consequences in a number of contexts (Ketchum, 1951). For example, in a crowd situation the orientation may be drawn to the present, wherein some of the typical behaviors of crowds may manifest themselves as overre-acting behaviors, such as struggling at a department store sale, racing to the exit doors in a fire, or panic in an airplane during turbulence. Similarly, in a marriage or rela-tionship where the partners perceive the relationship to be of uncertain duration, they may begin to act in accordance with feelings rather than stable values. For example, one of the partners may transfer joint banking accounts and charge card accounts to individual status. In other words, when situations are structured so that people func-tion in a present orientation that lacks future and past orientations, a variety of self-destructive and self-limiting behaviors may result.

Whenever a change is anticipated, orientation to the change may be resisted by individuals or groups, and serious consequences generally follow. The intermingling of traditional orientation, which is somewhat past oriented, with the pressures mani-fested by modernization, which may be somewhat present or future oriented, may cause societal agony. For example, many problems arose in a factory in Cantal, Gua-temala, because the management refused to be sensitive to market variations or to the problem of obsolete equipment (Nash, 1967). Worse situations occurred in Iran, which is a past-oriented society. In past-oriented societies the past is of primary im-portance and the future of minimal significance. In Iran businessmen invested consid-erable sums of money in factories without any real plan on how to use these factories (Hall & William, 1960).

Temporal orientation is an important variable in societal behavior and is also sig-nificant at the societal level. Some psychological studies suggest that temporal orien-tation is directly related to various kinds of emotional disorders, such as alcoholism, and to certain kinds of deviant behaviors, such as juvenile delinquency.

Temporal Perspective

Temporal perspective refers to the image of past, present, and future that prevails in a society, a social group, or individuals. The rank ordering of past, present, and future is of significance, yet it is insignificant in gaining an adequate understanding of social time. For example, if a particular group is future oriented, that is, it ranks the future highest in its hierarchy of values, this group's behavior will depend largely on the way they perceive the future. If people in a society perceive that they may be ex-tinct in the future, efforts may be made to ensure survival. The converse of this is that if people in a society perceive that they do not have a future (for example, they will be eradicated in a nuclear holocaust), they may adopt a present orientation, desiring to live life now at its fullest. An excellent example of this is found with the dying pa-tient's perception of time. For the dying patient, living in the present is very impor-tant; however, the nurse should recognize other realms of time perception. The nurse should ascertain precisely how the patient views the past, present, and future, because these views may assist the nurse in helping the patient cope with death and the chal-lenges faced in the process (Maguire, 1975). An image of the future functions to di-rect present behavior in accordance with specific values, and some sociologists view a society as being magnetically pulled toward a future fulfillment of their own image of the future, as well as being pushed from behind by their actual past (Polick, 1961).

A future orientation to illness, disease, and health care is essential to preventive medicine. Actions are taken in the present to safeguard the future, particularly in re-gard to certain disease conditions, for example, using condoms to prevent AIDS, practicing safe sex, adhering to a diet to prevent elevated cholesterol or blood glucose levels, not driving while under the influence of alcohol, and using seat belts.

TIME AND HUMAN INTERACTION

Up to this point an effort has been made to create an awareness that social time arises out of interaction. Regardless of the cultural heritage of an individual or group, there is no kind of time that is natural to humans. Instead, time is a result of the structuring and functioning of social order. When a particular temporality emerges, it tends to persist and to influence subsequent interaction. Various cultural groups construct systems of time that have diverse meanings and therefore diverse consequences on social interactions. The most fundamental differences in the meaning of time occur when cultural groups measure time predominantly by either social events or the clock.

Cultural groups that measure time predominantly by social events construct time according to the activities of the group. Conversely, cultural groups that measure time by the clock schedule activities according to the clock. In this regard, time is perceived basically as qualitative for those who measure time by social life and activities and as quantitative for those who measure time by the clock. When time is measured by social activities, it has significance only in terms of the activities that are taking place. When time is measured by the clock, it often has significance primarily in terms of money, which is perceived to be a scarce commodity, and all activities that take place do so in the shadow of the clock.

There are few cultural groups or societies that could be characterized as bound exclusively by the clock or as wholly independent of any constraints of temporality. How a group perceives time, nevertheless, has implications for interactions. For example, the Balinese people have a detemporalizing conception of time (Geeretz, 1973). For these people social time includes a calendar with a complex system of periodicities. According to Geeretz, this is called a premutational calendar because it contains 10 different cycles of days ranging in length from 1 to 10 days. While this is a complex system, it nevertheless serves various religious and practical purposes; it identifies nearly all the holidays and temple celebrations and at the same time guides the individual in daily activities. According to Geeretz, the structure of this complex system allows and disallows certain activities on certain days. For example, there are certain days that are good or bad for building a house, starting a business enterprise, moving from one location to another, going on a trip, harvesting and planting crops, etc.

In contrast to the Balinese people is the belief held by some Americans that time is money and therefore a scarce commodity. Thus human interactions are controlled in accordance with some notion of the appropriate amount of time for a particular situation. For example, some Americans distinguish the amount of time that can rightfully be consumed by strangers from that which can be given to friends and relatives. Weigert (1981) concluded that interaction time is a measure of the meaning of the relationship between two persons. In the event that two casual acquaintances meet somewhere, it is unlikely that they will take more than a few minutes to express recognition or perhaps exchange a pleasantry or two; therefore the interaction time for such a meeting is limited. The converse of this is that if two good friends meet and one of the friends attempts to limit the interaction, the other friend may feel rejected. Therefore the violator is expected to account for the behavior, and if this accounting is not forthcoming, the friendship may be severely strained. A single logical conclusion is that interaction can be evaluated in terms of time consumption.

In the United States methods to save time or to use time more effectively are in high demand. Numerous books, articles, workshops, tapes, and seminars imply that most Americans value time but at the same time do not think they use it wisely. Many busy professionals feel torn between wise use of time and taking time for interpersonal relationships with fellow workers or friends. For example, a dilemma may arise when a person is busy and a co-worker drops in and asks, "Do you have a minute?" If time is considered money, then a minute is costly. Since this worker values time, a reply of "yes," may be viewed as costly and thus unjustifiable. On the other hand, "no" may be perceived by the other person as a lack of sensitivity, coldness, and a lack of interest. Therefore much of the advice given by time efficiency experts can do much to depersonalize human interactions. An individual who follows the advice of these experts to the letter may have far more hours in which to accomplish tasks but at the same time may have fewer friends and fewer intimate relationships.

Drucker (1966) called the executive a captive, because everyone can move in on an executive's time, and, generally speaking, everybody does. An executive's time is often preempted by matters that are important to other people; therefore the executive has little or no time for self. A nurse manager who is responsive to others may find there is little time to do paperwork in the office and thus may take a lot of paperwork home. A nurse manager's personal priorities are often adapted when employees present "more urgent" problems.

CULTURAL PERCEPTIONS OF TIME

Appreciating cultural differences regarding time is important for the nurse in relating to both peers and patients. When people of different cultures interact, as is frequently the case in health care settings, there is a great potential for misunderstanding. If nurses are to avoid misreading issues that involve time perceptions, they must have an understanding of how other persons in different cultures view time.

Tripp-Reimer (1984) compared time orientation among certain groups in relation to future and present time orientation:

Dominant American	Future over present
Southern Black	Present over future
Puerto Rican	Present over future
Southern Appalachian	Present
Mexican American	Present
Traditional Chinese American	Present

Individuals with Future-Oriented Perceptions

Most middle-class Americans, regardless of ethnic or cultural heritage, tend to be future oriented (Tripp-Reimer & Lively, 1988). For example, some middle-class Americans tend to defer gratification of personal pleasure until some future objective has been met, such as advanced education. Thus they will delay starting families, purchasing homes, buying an expensive car, or investing money until they have prepared for a profession through advanced education, etc. Another noted difference among members of the dominant American culture is that these individuals tend to structure time rigidly. For these people adhering to a time-structured schedule is a way of life, regardless of whether the schedule involves work or leisure. For the nurse who works with future-oriented individuals, it is important to talk about events in relation to the future and to adhere to the schedule for planned events in a timely and precise manner.

Individuals with Present-Oriented Perceptions

Present-oriented individuals do not necessarily adhere strictly to a time-structured schedule. The present takes precedence over the future and the past with these individuals. More specifically, whatever is occurring at a precise moment may be more important than a future appointment, etc. It is important for the nurse to avoid labeling such individuals as lazy, disrespectful, or lacking interest. Hoppe and Heller (1974) concluded that present time orientation may be a reason why some Hispanic clients are late for appointments. Carter (1979) noted that it is important to gain an awareness of differences in values for Black Americans from low socioeconomic groups and proposed that instead of labeling tardiness as a blatant disregard for time, problems related to health, economics, and transportation should be considered with these individuals. Another explanation of individuals with present time orientation is that they tend to react to time in a linear fashion. Because they perceive time as being on a straight plane, they believe that a present moment spent on a particular task or with a particular individual cannot be regained: "We will never have this moment again," or "We must do it now, because you'll only pass this way once." This idea is in contrast to the thoughts held by persons with circular time orientation, who say, "I'll get back with you," or "We can do it later." The implication of these latter statements is that both persons will be around and the essence of the moment can be relived.

A common belief shared by some Black Americans and Mexican Americans is that time is flexible and events will begin when they arrive. For Black Americans this belief has been translated down through the years as a perception of time wherein lateness of 30 minutes to an hour is acceptable. Mbiti (1970) traced this perception of time back to West Africa, where the concept of time was elastic and encompassed events that had already taken place, as well as those that would occur immediately.

It is important for the nurse to remember that time perception may also be related to socioeconomic status. For example, while some Black Americans and Mexican Americans can be characterized as present-oriented individuals, others have been assimilated into the dominant culture, and are very time conscious and take pride in punctuality. These Black Americans and Mexican Americans are more likely to be future oriented and therefore are more likely to save and plan for important events. They are also likely to be well educated and to hold professional positions. This may not always be the case, since some individuals may not be well educated or hold professional positions, yet may value time and have future hopes for themselves and their children. According to Pouissant and Atkinson (1970), these individuals are more apt to encourage their children to seek higher education and to begin saving for the future.

Time perception may also be related to religious orientation. Some Native Americans, Mexican Americans, and Black Americans hold strong religious beliefs, and their concept of time is therefore very future oriented. These individuals, who may come from all socioeconomic and educational levels, have in common the belief that life on earth, with all of its pain and suffering, is only bearable because of the chance for future happiness after death. Such individuals, according to Smith (1976), may plan future activities related to their death; for example, they may plan their funeral, including their eulogy; purchase a grave plot; make a will; and otherwise prepare to die. Such individuals may also threaten heirs with disinheritance and talk about what the heirs will do with their hard-earned money.

Levine and Wolff (1985), with the assistance of colleagues Laurie West and Harry Reis, compared the time sense of male and female students in Niteroi, Brazil, with similar students at California State University at Fresno. A total of 91 Brazilian students and 107 students from California were surveyed. The universities selected in Brazil and California were similar in academic quality and size, and the cities in which they were located were secondary metropolitan centers with a population of approximately 350,000. The researchers asked students about their perception of time in several situations, including what they considered late or early for a hypothetical lunch appointment with a friend. According to the data, the average Brazilian student defined lateness for the hypothetical lunch as 33½ minutes after the scheduled lunchtime, whereas the Fresno students defined lateness for the hypothetical lunch as 19 minutes after the scheduled lunchtime. The Brazilian students allowed an average of 54 minutes before they considered someone early for an appointment, whereas the Fresno students drew the line for earliness at 24 minutes. When the Brazilian students were asked to give typical reasons for lateness, they were less likely to attribute it to a lack of caring than their North American counterparts were. Instead, the Brazilian students pointed to unforeseen circumstances that an individual could not control without prior knowledge. In addition, the Brazilian students appeared less inclined to feel personally responsible for their own lateness. The question that comes to mind for the nurse is, "Are Brazilians more flexible in their concepts of time and punctuality?" Another question for the nurse to consider is, "If Brazilians are more flexible in their concepts of time and punctuality, how does this relate to the stereotypical picture of the fatalistic and irresponsible temperament associated with Latins?" This example illustrates the need for nurses to guard against formulating stereotyped images of persons from other cultures. Instead, the nurse must have an understanding of cultural variables that differ among cultures, such as the variations in viewing time.

Levine and Wolff (1985) found similar differences in how students from North America and Brazil characterize people who are late for appointments. In the survey, the Brazilian students indicated that a person who is consistently late is probably a person who is more successful than one who is consistently on time. These students seemed to accept the premise that someone of great stature is expected to arrive late; therefore a lack of punctuality is a badge of success. In contrast, according to the North American students, persons who arrive late for scheduled appointments, rush in late to meetings, turn in assignments late, or fail to notify others when they find they are going to be late are generally unorganized, have trouble with priorities, are inconsiderate, and thus will fail to advance professionally and will be less successful.

Popular literature in the United States on creating a successful business and professional image espouses the need for continued punctuality.

PHYSIOCHEMICAL INFLUENCES IN RELATION TO TIME

Research on biological rhythms has found that internal body rhythms fluctuate within a 24-hour period. Biological capacities for some individuals are on a low ebb in the daytime, whereas for others, they are at a high level during the day (*Biological Rhythms,* 1970; Yogman, Lester, & Hoffman, 1983; Ziac, 1984). Research has shown that the time of day in which medication is given influences its effectiveness and its side effects; drugs may be more potent when biological capacities are on a low ebb. However, it is important for the nurse to remember that while drugs might be more potent with low biological capacities, the treatment may be less therapeutic. Health care professionals often fail to take into account the patient's biological rhythms when scheduling surgical procedures and diagnostic tests. For example, surgical interventions should be avoided when a patient's biological capacities are low. Persons who are on a low ebb of biological functioning may be at greater risk for an exaggerated response to anesthesia or may be less able to respond to blood loss (Bremmer, Vitiello, & Prinz, 1983; Haber et al., 1987). There is also evidence that diagnostic tests and treatments may be tolerated better by certain patients when they are timed according to biological rhythms. Hormones and other homeostatic physiological mechanisms fluctuate in the body in a rhythmic way. Finally, the timing of the collection of blood and urine samples is important and influences the interpretation of the information obtained.

Physiochemical levels also are related to age. Children have a higher metabolic rate, which tends to make time appear to move more slowly for children. On the other hand, older individuals have a slower metabolic rate, which results in time appearing to move more quickly.

Body rhythms may influence waking at a preselected time. Waking, however, is also a conditioned response. Body systems, including the nervous and endocrine systems, are the result not only of internal biological rhythms, but also of psychological phenonema, such as the time or date of previous traumatic events.

IMPLICATIONS FOR NURSING CARE

The nurse who gains an understanding of time as a cultural variable with a significant impact on patients and ultimately on patient care must also gain an understanding of how time is managed in order to give quality patient care. A general attitude shared by health care professionals is that time is irreplaceable and irreversible, and that to waste time is to waste life. Moreover, there is no such thing as a lack of time; regardless of the way individuals spend time, it goes at the same pace (Salmond, 1986). That is, each individual has 168 hours to live per week—no more and no less. As health care needs have changed over the years, so have the demands that are placed on nurses. Nurses are constantly being challenged to work in a more time-efficient manner, and these demands have placed a high level of stress on them. Some nurses maintain that they are losing control and lack personal satisfaction, and thus are becoming burned out. However, it is important for the nurse to remember that one way to remain in control and to have personal satisfaction as opposed to burnout is to adopt an efficient system of time management. Getting organized and precisely articulating priorities is related to job satisfaction (MacStavic, 1978; McNiff, 1984; Feldman, Monicken, & Crowley, 1983). Nurses have long known the importance of working smarter rather than longer or harder (Barros, 1983).

Conflicts between nurses and physicians are sometimes complicated by differences in time perception. Nurses tend to operate on an hourly time sense with adherence to rigid schedules in order to complete patient care assignments. Physicians tend to measure time with the patient not in actual time spent with the patient, which often is quite brief, but in the duration of the illness or its treatment. Physicians are less likely to schedule time strictly and often appear not to appreciate the nurse's sense of time (Sheard, 1980; Young & Hayne, 1988).

For the nurse, time management issues involve how to manage personal time as well as time at work in order to meet professional goals. In addition, as cost-containment issues are gaining increased attention in nursing, time management concerns also necessitate precise assessment of patient care needs in order to plan the hours of nursing time required to meet these needs and to manage the time of staff who are supervised in the delivery of care (Vestal, 1987). In the 1970s the concern with cost-effectiveness of patient care and the realization that census may not be an adequate determinant of the demand for care prompted the development of patient classification systems. These classification systems were used initially in general hospitals to determine needs for nursing resources by grouping patients into categories that reflected the magnitude of nursing care time. By 1979 over 1000 hospitals reported using some method of classifying levels of care and the time required (Schroder et al., 1986). In 1983 the development of patient classification systems received a significant impetus when the Joint Commission on Accreditation for Hospitals and American Hospital Association Standards recommended patient classification systems in all hospitals. As psychiatric hospitals began to seek accreditation under the American Hospital Association Standards, increasing attention was given to patient classification systems in psychiatric hospital settings.

Appropriate grouping of patients in a hospital (for example, having a unit for colostomy patients) can contribute to effective use of staff time. In addition, grouping patient activities into a logical sequence (for example, changing the patient's bed after the colostomy irrigation is finished) can save the nurse time.

Organization of supplies and tasks is important when activities are grouped together. Organizing items prevents multiple interruptions during a procedure in order to collect things that were forgotten. A nurse who must leave a procedure to get items that are needed but were forgotten not only wastes time but appears incompetent.

Nursing efforts to reduce hospitalization time is a serious concern today as health care costs spiral (Midgley & Osterhage, 1973). Yet another dimension of time management for nurses in the 1990s involves appropriately timed data collection to determine patient needs and to collect data about the nursing process (Polit & Hungler, 1983; Felton, 1970). If assessment of patient and nursing needs is not adequately timed, inaccurate solutions may be planned. The nurse who is aware of the importance of time must also consider the time constraints of data collection. While a 24-page nursing assessment may provide optimal patient data, if the time taken to collect this data would result in other patient care being neglected, time constraints will by necessity influence the length of the assessment. Time constraints also influence data collection for research purposes in a health care setting. If financial restraints prohibit additional staff for research purposes, a decision must be made about the priority of the research versus the priority of other nursing staff duties (Monette, Sullivan, & Dejong, 1986).

As change agents, nurses are also concerned with time in relation to change. According to organizational change theory, if change merely involves knowledge, change can be achieved in a short time with little difficulty. If attitudes are involved, somewhat longer periods of time are needed. If the behavior of an individual is involved, a moderate amount of time is required, and moderate difficulty may be encountered. If the behavior of a group is involved, a large amount of time may be required and a high level of difficulty may be encountered (Hersey & Blanchard, 1982).

Nurses are also concerned with time in other areas. The optimal time for medication procedures (Dittman & Pulski, 1977), the effect of shift rotation (Tooraen, 1972), and the effect of changing shift assignments are all issues related to time that are being investigated by nursing research. As nurses struggle to manage nursing time more effectively, the complexity of the problem becomes more apparent. One way to develop a time management system that allows for increased productivity is for the nurse to understand how time perception and time orientation differ among and across cultural groups.

Lest the nurse stereotype all persons in the United States as valuing timeliness, it must be emphasized that time and punctuality vary considerably from place to place or region to region even in the United States. Each region and even each city has its own rhythm and rules. Words such as *now* and *later* can convey vastly different meanings to a New Yorker and a Californian. *Now* and *later* may also be interpreted differently by persons from different ethnic or cultural groups. For some Black Americans *now* may not really imply immediately; rather, *now* may mean "soon," so that it could be hours before an action is taken. For the same Black American *later* may not really imply within a few hours but "when you get around to it" (Mbiti, 1970). In contrast, for some White Americans *now* means immediately and thus action is expected at once. For these same White Americans *later* means within a few hours.

For Americans who travel abroad, major differences encountered, surpassed only by language problems, are the contrasting paces of life and the punctuality differences of people from other countries. These differences can also be noted in the United States when one travels from region to region. For example, in the South, regardless of whether the area is rural or urban, the general pace of life is slow and laid back, and punctuality is not of paramount importance; thus people from this region may be given the stereotyped label of being "country." In contrast, in a large metropolitan area such as New York, the pace of life is associated with more rapid activity, such as walking fast, talking fast, and making decisions quickly. Time differences are not only indigenous to different localities of the country, but are also sometimes seen in various agencies and among various health professionals. For example, the nurse may find that a more rapid pace is required in a particular hospital setting, and the pace may vary from clinical discipline to clinical discipline. Duties may differ and the pace may be more accelerated in high-risk areas such as the intensive care unit, coronary care unit, emergency room, operating room, and psychiatric unit. On the other hand, these areas also experience "slow time" or "down time" when the census is low.

When caring for patients who may have present-oriented time perceptions, such as some Black Americans, some Puerto Rican Americans, some Appalachians, some American Indians, some Mexican Americans, and some traditional Chinese Americans, it is important for the nurse to remember that it is necessary to avoid adhering to time as a fixed resource (an example would be rigid schedules for nursing care procedures such as baths, medications, and meals). In this case the nurse may find that the standards of the institution regarding time and the time orientation of the patient may be in conflict with each other. Again, it is important for the nurse to remember that such individuals may perceive time as flexible and that what is happening now is more important than what is going to happen in the future. Therefore the nurse must be able to adapt patient care within a range in time rather than fixed hours.

CASE STUDY

Miss Susie Jones is a 37-year-old Black patient who has been coming to the hospital's outpatient clinic because she is a brittle diabetic. Miss Jones' diabetes was diagnosed 6 months previously; however, the diabetes remains uncontrolled by insulin. The patient was put on a regimen of 40 units of lente insulin with 5 units of regular insulin at 7 AM and at 4 PM. When Miss Jones comes to the clinic today, she relates to the nurse that she had an episode of "blacking out," or an "insulin reaction," because she forgot to eat after taking her morning insulin. This morning, as frequently in the past, Miss Jones is at least 1 hour late for her scheduled appointment. The following questions relate to variable time and its significance in relation to Susie Jones.

STUDY QUESTIONS

1. List at least two things in relation to the perception of time and culture that may be contributing factors in Susie Jones' tardiness for appointments.
2. List at least two things that the nurse could suggest to Susie Jones that would assist her in being on time for future clinic appointments.
3. List at least two factors about time that contribute to Susie Jones' noncompliance to the medical regimen.
4. Identify ways that the nurse could assist Susie Jones in developing an understanding about time and its relationship to important medications such as insulin.
5. Identify a contributing factor to the insulin reaction that was described to the nurse by Susie Jones.

REFERENCES

Ariotti, P.E. (1975). The concept of time in Western antiquity. In J.T. Fraser & N. Lawrence (Eds.), *The study of time* (Vol. 3, pp. 69-80). New York: Springer-Verlag.

Barros, A. (1983, Aug.). Time management: Learn to work smarter, not longer. *Medical Laboratory Observer,* pp. 107-111.

Biological rhythms in psychiatry and medicine. (1970). Chevy Chase, Md.: U.S. Department of Health, Education, and Welfare, National Institute of Mental Health.

Bock, P. (1964). Social structure and language structure. *Southwestern Journal of Anthropology, 20,* 393-403.

Bremmer, W.J., Vitiello, M.V., & Prinz, P.N. (1983). Loss of circadian rhythmicity in blood testosterone levels with aging in normal man. *Journal of Clinical Endocrinology and Metabolism, 56*(6), 1278-1281.

Carter, J. (1979). Frequent mistakes made with Black clients in psychotherapy. *Journal of the National Medical Association, 71*(10), 56-64.

Cassirer, E. (1955). *An essay on man.* New York: Bantam Books.

Dittman, S.S., & Pulski, T. (1977). Early evening administration of sleep medication to the hospitalized aged: A consideration in rehabilitation. *Nursing Research, 26,* 299-303.

Doob, L. (1970). *Patterning of time.* New Haven: Yale University Press.

Dossey, L. (1982). *Space, time, and medicine.* Boulder, Colo.: Shambhala Publications.

Drucker, P. (1966). *The effective executive.* New York: Harper & Row.

Elton, L., & Messel, H. (1978). *Time and man.* New York: Pergamon Press.

Feldman, E., Monicken, L., & Crowley, M. (1983). The systems approach to prioritizing. *Nursing Administration Quarterly, 7*(2), 57-62.

Felton, G. (1970). Effect of time change on blood pressure and temperature in young women. *Nursing Research, 19,* 48-58.

Friedman, B. (1946). *Foundations of the measurement of values.* New York: Columbia University Press.

Gilles, R., & Faulkner, R. (1978). Time and television news work: Task temporalization in the assembly of unscheduled events. *Sociological Quarterly, 19,* 89-102.

Geeretz, C. (1973). *The interpretation of culture.* New York: Basic Books.

Gioscia, V. (1970). On social time. In H. Yaker, H. Osmond, & F. Cheek (Eds.), *The future of time* (pp. 73-141). New York: Doubleday.

Haber, J., Hoskins, P., Leach, A., & Sideleau, B. (1987). *Comprehensive psychiatric nursing.* New York: McGraw-Hill.

Hall, E., & William, F. (1960). Intercultural communication: A guide to men of action. *Human Organization, 19,* 7-9.

Hawley, A. (1950). *Human ecology.* New York: Ronald Press.

Hein, E.C. (1980). *Communication in nursing practice* (2nd ed.). Boston: Little, Brown.

Hersey, P., & Blanchard, K.H. (1982). *Management of organizational behavior.* Englewood Cliffs, N.J.: Prentice Hall.

Hoppe, S., & Heller, P. (1974). Alienation, familism, and the utilization of health services by Mexican-Americans. *Journal of Health and Social Behavior, 15,* 304.

Hymovich, D.P., & Chamberlin, R.W. (1980). *Child and family development.* New York: McGraw-Hill.

James, W. (1890). *Principles of psychology* (Vol. 1). New York: Dover Publications.

Ketchum, J.D. (1951). Time, values, and social organization. *Canadian Journal of Psychology, 5,* 97-109.

Kluckhohn, F., & Strodtbeck, F. (1961). *Variations in value orientation.* Evanston, Ill.: Row, Peterson.

Kohn, M. (1969). *Class and conformity.* Chicago: Dorsey Press.

Landes, D. (1983). *Revolution in time.* Cambridge, Mass.: Belknap Press of Harvard University Press.

Lebhar, G. (1958). *The use of time* (3rd ed.). New York: Chain Store.

Levine, R., & Wolff, E. (1985, March). Social time: The heartbeat of culture. *Psychology Today,* pp. 29-35.

MacStavic, R.E. (1978). Setting priorities in health planning: What does it mean? *Inquiry, 45*(1), 20-24.

Maguire, D.C. (1975). *Death by choice.* New York: Schocken Books.

Mbiti, S.S. (1970). *African religions and philosophies.* New York: Anchor Press.

McGrath, J., & Kelly, J. (1986). *Time and human interaction.* New York: Guilford Press.

McNiff, M. (1984, June). Getting organized—at last. *RN, 47,* 23-24.

Meade, R. (1960). Time on their hands. *Personnel Journal, 39,* 130-132.

Midgley, J.W., & Osterhage, R.A., Sr. (1973). Effect of nursing instruction and length of hospitalization on postoperative complications in cholecystectomy patients. *Nursing Research, 22,* 69-72.

Monette, D., Sullivan, T., & Dejong, C. (1986). *Applied social research.* New York: Holt, Rinehart, & Winston.

Morgenstern, I. (1960). *The dimensional structure of time.* New York: Philosophical Library.

Nash, M. (1967). *Machine age Maya.* Chicago: University of Chicago Press.

Nelkin, D. (1970). Unpredictability and life style in a migrant camp. *Social Problems, 17,* 472-87.

Parkinson, C. (1970). *The law of delay.* London: John Murray.

Polick, F. (1961). *The image of the future* (Vols. 1-2). New York: Oceana Publications.

Polit, D., & Hungler, B. (1983). *Nursing research: Principles and methods.* Philadelphia: J.B. Lippincott.

Pouissant, A., & Atkinson, C. (1970). Black youth and motivation. *Black Scholar, 1,* 43-51.

Pyle, K. (1969). *The new generation of Meiji Japan.* Stanford, Calif.: Stanford University Press.

Ritzenthaler, R. (1953). The impact of small industry on an Indian community. *American Anthropologist, 55,* 143-48.

Salmond, S. (1986). Time management: The time is now. *Orthopedic Nursing 5*(3), 25-32.

Schroder, P., Washington, P., Deering, C., & Coyne, L. (1986). Testing validity and reliability in a psychiatric patient classification system. *Nursing Management, 17(1),* 49-54.

Sheard, T. (1980). The structure of conflict in nurse-physician relations. *Supervisor Nurse, 11*(8), 14-16.

Smith, J.A. (1976). The role of the Black clergy as allied health care professionals in working with Black patients. In J.D. Luckraft (Ed.), *Black awareness: Implications for Black care* (pp. 12-15). New York: American Journal of Nursing Company.

Sorokin, P. (1964). *Sociocultural causality, space, time.* New York: Russell & Russell.

Stoetzel, J. (1953). The contribution of public opinion research techniques to social anthropology. *International Social Science Bulletin, 5,* 494-503.

Strauss, G. (1963). Group dynamics and intergroup relations. In A.O. Lewis, Jr. (Ed.), *Of men and machines* (pp. 321-327). New York: E.P. Dutton.

Thompson, E. (1967). Time, work-discipline, and industrial capitalism. *Past and Present, 38,* 58-59.

Toffler, A. (1970). *Future shock.* New York: Random House.

Tooraen, L.A., Sr. (1972). Physiological effects of shift rotation on ICU nurses, *Nursing Research, 21,* 398-405.

Tripp-Reimer, T. (1984). Cultural assessment. In J. Bellack & P. Bamford (Eds.), *Nursing assessment: A multidimensional approach.* Monterey, Calif.: Wadsworth.

Tripp-Reimer, T., & Lively, S. (1988). Cultural considerations in therapy. In C.K. Beck, R.P. Rawlins, & S. Williams (Eds.), *Mental health–psychiatric nursing* (pp. 185-199). St. Louis: C.V. Mosby.

Vestal, K. (1987). *Management concepts for the new nurse.* Philadelphia: J.B. Lippincott.

Veterans World Project. (1972). *Wasted men: The reality of the Vietnam veteran.* Edwardsville, Ill.: Southern Illinois University Foundation.

Weigert, A. (1981). *Sociology of everyday life.* New York: Longman.

Wessman, A., & Gorman, B. (1977). The emergence of human awareness and concepts of time. In B.S. Gorman & A.E. Wessman (Eds.), *Personal experience of time* (p. 3). New York: Plenum Press.

Weyer, E. (1973). *Primitive peoples today.* New York: Doubleday.

Yogman, M.W., Lester, B.M., & Hoffman, J. (1983). Behavioral rhythmicity and circadian rhythmicity during mother, father, stranger, infant social interaction. *Pediatric Research, 17*(11), 872-876.

Young, L., & Hayne, A. (1988). *Nursing administration: From concepts to practice.* Philadelphia: W.B. Saunders.

Zerubavel, E. (1979). *Patterns of time in hospital life.* Chicago: University of Chicago Press.

Ziac, D.C. (1984). Menstrual synchrony in university women. *American Journal of Physical Anthropology, 63*(2), 237.

. . . . .

CHAPTER 6

Environmental Control

BEHAVIORAL OBJECTIVES
After reading this chapter, the nurse will be able to:

1 Recognize relevant cultural factors that affect health-seeking behaviors related to environmental control.

2 Recognize relevant cultural factors that affect illness behaviors related to environmental control.

3 Identify factors affecting external locus of control for persons in selected cultural groups.

4 Recognize the relationship between external locus of control and fatalistic and/or health-seeking behaviors.

5 Recognize various types of cultural folk health practices and the impact on health-seeking behaviors.

Environmental control refers to the ability of an individual or persons from a particular cultural group to plan activities that control nature. Environmental control also refers to the individual's perception of ability to direct factors in the environment. This definition in itself implies that the concept of environment is broader than just the place where an individual resides or where treatment occurs. In the most practical sense, the term *environment* encompasses relevant systems and processes that affect individuals. (Haber et al., 1987).

Systems are organized structures that may influence and be influenced by individuals. Processes may be viewed as organized, purposeful patterns of operations. Processes generally include the dynamics and interactions between families, groups, and the community at large. On the basis of these definitions, it becomes evident that the environment and humans have a reciprocal relationship in the sense that humans and the environment are constantly exchanging matter and energy. When this exchange has purpose and is goal directed, the interaction and exchange processes are considered functional and useful. However, when the exchange has no purpose and lacks goal direction, a dysynchronous relationship occurs (Giuffra, 1987).

In the broadest sense, health may be viewed as a balance between the individual and the environment. Health practices such as eating nutritiously, subscribing to preventive health services available in the community, and installing hazard- and pollution- control devices are all believed to have a positive effect on the individual, who in turn can positively affect the environment.

Complex systems of health beliefs and practices exist across and within cultural groups. In addition, variations, whether extreme or modest, to cultural beliefs and practices are found across ethnic and social class boundaries and even within family groups. Today, the most widely accepted approach to health care views is the biomedical model. The biomedical model emphasizes biological concerns, which are considered by those who support this model as more "real" and significant (in contrast to psychological and sociological issues) (Kleinman, Eisenberg, & Good, 1978).

Today, in modern Western society health care practitioners remain primarily interested in abnormalities in the structure and function of body systems and in the treatment of disease. According to Kleinman, Eisenberg, and Good (1978), the biomedical approach is culture specific, culture bound, and value laden. The biomedical model represents only one end of a continuum. At the opposite end of the continuum is the traditional model, which espouses popular beliefs and practices that diverge from medical science (Chrisman, 1977). Persons who subscribe to beliefs encompassed in the traditional model have varying health beliefs and practices, including folk beliefs and traditional beliefs that are also shaped by culture.

DISTINCTION BETWEEN ILLNESS AND DISEASE

During the last decade, scientists and anthropologists began to make a distinction between the terms *illness* and *disease*. The individual experiences that relate to illness do not necessarily correlate with the biomedical interpretation of disease. *Illness* can be defined as an individual's perception of being sick. On the other hand, *disease* is diagnosed when the condition is a deviation from clearly established norms based on Western biomedical science (Fabrega, 1971). Illness can and does occur in the absence of disease; approximately 50% of visits made by individuals to physicians are for complaints without a definite basis. According to Kleinman, Eisenberg, and Good (1978), illness is culturally shaped in the sense that it is individually perceived. In other words, how one experiences and copes with disease is based on the individual's explanation of sickness. Disease is described in detail in medical-surgical nursing textbooks. However, nurses need to remember to incorporate both personal and cultural reactions of the patient to illness, disease, and discomfort in order to give culturally appropriate nursing care.

Just as culture influences health-related behavior, it also has a profound effect on expectations and perceptions of sickness that shape the labeling of sickness, as well as how, when, and to whom communication of health problems occurs. The astute nurse must keep in mind the fact that perceptions of health and illness are shaped by cultural factors. As a direct result of cultural shaping, individuals vary in health care behaviors, health status, and health-seeking attitudes.

The term *health care behavior* is inclusive and is defined as the social and biological activities of an individual that are based on maintaining an acceptable health status or manipulating and altering an unacceptable condition (Bauwens & Anderson, 1988). The term *health status,* on the other hand, is defined as the success with which an individual adapts to the internal and external environment (Bauwens & Anderson, 1988). Thus health care behavior influences health status, which in turn influences health care behavior. Because health care behavior and health care status are reciprocal in nature, they both can be affected by sociocultural forces such as economics, politics, environmental influences, and the health care delivery system itself (Elling, 1977).

CULTURAL HEALTH PRACTICES VERSUS MEDICAL HEALTH PRACTICES

Cultural health practices are categorized as efficacious, neutral, dysfunctional (Pillsbury, 1982), or uncertain.

Efficacious Cultural Health Practices

According to Western medical standards, efficacious cultural health practices are those practices that are viewed as beneficial to health status, although they can differ vastly from modern scientific practices. Since efficacious health practices can facilitate effective nursing care, nurses need to actively encourage the use of these practices among and across cultural groups. Nurses must keep in mind that a treatment strategy that is consistent with the patient's beliefs may have a better chance of being successful. For example, persons from cultural groups who subscribe to the theory of hot and cold, such as some Mexican Americans, may actually benefit from this particular belief. Individuals who subscribe to this theory may avoid hot foods in the presence of stomach ailments such as ulcers, and this practice is consistent with the bland diet used in a medical regimen for the treatment of ulcers. Thus scientific health care practices may be blended with efficacious cultural health practices.

Neutral Cultural Health Practices

Neutral cultural health practices have no effect on the health status of an individual. Although some health care practitioners may consider neutral health practices irrelevant, the nurse must keep in mind that such practices may be extremely important because they may be linked to beliefs that are closely integrated into an individual's behavior (Pillsbury, 1982). Greene and Johnston (1980) have cited several examples of neutral practices, including "the ritual disposal of the placenta and cord," interpretation of signs in the cord, avoidance of sexual activity during various stages of pregnancy, certain hygiene practices, and avoidance of exposure to illuminous rays of the moon during a lunar eclipse. While these practices require no planned nursing interventions, the astute nurse must recognize their significance and respect the patient's right to subscribe to and practice such beliefs.

Dysfunctional Cultural Health Practices

Dysfunctional cultural health practices are harmful. An example of a dysfunctional health practice found in the United States is the excessive use of such items as overrefined flour and sugar. The nurse must be cognizant of practices that are dysfunctional and should work to establish educational training programs that will help individuals identify dysfunctional health practices and develop beneficial practices.

Uncertain Health Practices

In 1972 Williams and Jelliffe developed a cultural assessment system that included a category of cultural health practices with unknown effects. Classified as uncertain, these practices included such things as swaddling an newborn infant to maintain body temperature and the use of an abdominal binder for mother and infant to prevent umbilical hernias.

The nurse must keep in mind that in most instances health practices do not fit perfectly into one category or another. According to Greene and Johnston (1980), health practices are subjectively evaluated as more or less beneficial or harmful when they are compared with the alternative practices available to the user.

VALUES AND THEIR RELATIONSHIP TO HEALTH CARE PRACTICES

Values may be viewed as individualized sets of rules by which people live and are governed. They serve as the cornerstone for beliefs, attitudes, and behaviors. Cultural values are often acquired unconsciously as an individual assimilates the culture throughout the process of growth and maturation. It is important for the nurse to recognize that because cultural values are believed to exist almost solely on an unconscious level, they are the most difficult to alter. Cultural values therefore have a pervasive and profound influence on the individual.

Value Orientations

Kluckhohn and Strodtbeck (1961) defined value orientations as "complex but definitely patterned principles . . . which give order and direction to the ever-flowing stream of human acts and thoughts as they relate to the solution of common human problems." Kluckhohn and Strodtbeck also proposed that it is entirely possible for an individual to hold a different value orientation from the rest of the same cultural group. However, they concluded that despite differences in value orientation within a cultural group, dominant value orientations can be identified for most persons of a particular cultural group.

Kluckhohn and Strodtbeck (1961) compared the way people in different cultural groups organize their thinking about such things as time, personal activity, interpersonal relationships, and the relationship to nature and the supernatural, and they developed an orientation framework that includes temporal, activity, relational, people-to-nature, and innate human nature orientations.

Temporal orientation

Temporal orientation refers to the method by which persons from particular cultural groups divide time. Time is generally divided into three frames of reference: past, present, and future. According to Kluckhohn and Strodtbeck (1961) and Haber et al. (1987), most cultures combine all three orientations but one is more likely to dominate than another.

Activity orientation

Activity orientation refers to whether a cultural group is perceived as a "doing"-oriented culture, which is oriented toward achievement, or as a"being"-oriented culture, which values "being" and views people as an important link between generations. In other words, the "doing"-oriented culture values accomplishments, whereas the "being"-oriented culture values inherent existence.

Relational orientation

Relational orientation from a cultural perspective distinguishes among interpersonal patterns. More specifically, relational orientation refers to the way in which persons in a culture set goals for individual members. Relational orientations are found in three modes: lineal, individualistic, and collateral.

Lineal mode. When the lineal mode is dominant within a particular cultural group, the goals and welfare of the group are viewed as major concerns. Another major concern is the continuity of the group, as well as orderly succession of the group over time. Cultures that are perceived as subscribing to the lineal mode view kinship bonds as the basis for maintaining lineage.

Individualistic mode. Cultures wherein the dominant mode is individualistic value individual goals over group goals. Thus each individual is responsible for personal behaviors and ultimately is held accountable for personal accomplishments.

Collateral mode. When the collateral mode is dominant in a cultural group, the goals and welfare of lateral groups such as siblings or peers are of paramount importance. Examples are found in the Soviet Union and in Israel, where the goals of individuals are subordinate to those that affect the entire lateral group.

People-to-nature orientation

People-to-nature orientation implies that people either dominate nature, live in harmony with nature, or are subjugated to nature. The conceptual framework of people dominating nature is based on the view that humans can and do dominate nature and further suggests that humankind can master or control natural events. When people live in harmony with nature, there is an integration among them, nature, and the universe. When the view that humans are subjugated to nature is held, a philosophy of fatalism is adopted; that is, fate is considered inevitable and individuals perceive themselves as having no control over nature or their future—they consider themselves powerless to guide personal destiny. An example is the belief held by some Appalachians that "If I'm going to get cancer, I'm going to get it," so that taking preventive measures to avoid cancer would be of no benefit. This fatalistic attitude, however, is not completely consistent, because most Appalachian people will go to a physician or hospital if they believe they are extremely ill.

Innate human nature orientation

The final orientation perspective is the innate human nature orientation, which distinguishes an individual's human nature as being good, evil, or neutral. Some cultural groups view human beings as having a basic nature that is either changeable or unchangeable. For example, an individual may be viewed as evil and unchangeable, evil but changeable, or neutral (subject to both good and negative influences).

Locus-of-Control Construct as a Health Care Value

The locus-of-control construct, which originated in social learning theory, is defined as follows:

> When a reinforcement is perceived as following some action but not being entirely contingent upon (personal) action then in our culture it is typically perceived as a result of luck, chance, and fate, as under the control of powerful others, or unpredictable because of the great complexity of the forces surrounding [the individual]. When the event is interpreted in this way by an individual, we have labeled this belief in external control. If a person perceives that the event is contingent upon his own behavior or his own permanent characteristics, we have termed this a belief in internal control. (Rotter, 1966)

The above definition presupposes that individuals who believe that a contingent relationship exists between actions and outcomes have internal feelings of control and thus act to influence future behaviors and situations. Individuals who believe that efforts and rewards are uncorrelated, and who thus have external feelings of control, view the future as the result of luck, chance, or fate and are less likely to take action to change the future. The locus-of-control construct can be applied to a variety of phenomena, including the weather, preventive health, curative health actions, and feelings of well-being. For example, individuals who believe that a contingent relationship exists between compliance to preventive and treatment regimens and health have an internal locus of control and are likely to respond positively to affect the future and thus promote good health. On the other hand, individuals who believe that compliance behaviors and health are unrelated have an external locus of control and have little motivation to develop behaviors that could affect the future and enhance good health. Rotter (1975) concluded that the locus-of-control construct does not in itself represent a behavior trait and can be modified by interaction with others.

The astute nurse should recognize that persons who subscribe to an external locus of control tend to be more fatalistic about nature, health, illness, death, and disease. For example, some Mexican Americans, Appalachians, and Puerto Ricans are reported to have an external locus of control. Some American Indians, Chinese Americans, and Japanese Americans are said to be more or less in harmony with nature; therefore their cultural beliefs fall outside of the locus-of-control construct. However, Northern European Americans and Black Americans are reported to fall within both the internal and the external locus-of-control constructs (Kluckhohn & Strodtbeck, 1961). The nurse can help the patient modify behaviors that fall within the realm of the external locus-of-control construct by showing the effects of certain behaviors on illness, health, and disease, and thus promote the development of an internal locus of control.

FOLK MEDICINE

Folk medicine, or what is commonly referred to as Third World beliefs and practices, is often called "strange or weird" by nurses and other health professionals who are unfamiliar with folk medicine beliefs (Snow, 1981). In reality, whether or not something is considered "strange or weird" depends on familiarity with the beliefs. In most instances folk medicine practices will not be considered "strange or weird" once health care providers become familiar with them.

The astute nurse must distinguish between practices that are familiar and practices that are desirable, since becoming familiar with something does not imply acceptance. In this situation tolerance becomes a two-way process: people who subscribe to folk medicine practices need not feel compelled to abandon these beliefs and practices when they become familiar with modern medicine, and health care practitioners should not feel compelled to abandon modern medical practices when they become familiar with folk medicine practices.

An individual's world view largely determines beliefs about disease and the appropriate treatment interventions. For example, if one holds a belief in magic, this belief may lead to the assumption that a disease is a result of human behavior and that a cure can be achieved by magical techniques. If one holds a religious belief, this belief may lead to the assumption that the disease is a result of supernatural forces and that a cure can be achieved by appealing to supernatural forces. The scientific view may lead to the assumption that the disease is a result of the cause-effect relationship of natural phenomena and that a cure is achieved by scientific medicine (Henderson & Primeaux, 1981).

Folk Medicine Beliefs as a System

The folk medicine system classifies illnesses or diseases as natural or unnatural. This division of illnesses or diseases into natural and unnatural phenomena is common among Haitians, persons from Trinidad, Mexicans and Mexican Americans, American Blacks, and some southern American Whites (Snow, 1981).

Distinction between natural and unnatural events

The simplest way to distinguish between natural and unnatural illnesses is to state that according to this belief system, natural events have to do with the world as God made it and as God intended it to be. Thus natural laws allow a measure of predictability for daily life. Unnatural events, on the other hand, imply the exact opposite, because they upset the harmony of nature. Unnatural events can therefore be viewed as events that interrupt the plan intended by God and at their very worst represent the forces of evil and the machinations of the devil. Unnatural events are frightening because they have no predictability. They are outside the world of nature, so that when they do occur, they are beyond the control of ordinary mortals.

Germane to the tendency to view phenomena in terms of opposition, such as good versus evil and natural versus unnatural, is the belief held by some folk medicine systems that everything has an exact opposite. For example, some Black Americans who subscribe to a folk medicine system believe that for every birth there must be a death, for every marriage there must be a divorce, and for every person with good health there must be someone with bad health. This belief is so encompassing that such individuals believe that every illness has a cure, every poison has an antidote, every herb has a healing purpose, etc. (Snow, 1981). This belief contributes to the lack of acceptance by persons in some cultural groups to the chronicity of such diseases as AIDS, herpes, or syphilis.

Distinction between natural and unnatural illnesses

Illnesses are generally classified as natural or unnatural, and this classification affects the type of cure or practitioner sought. All illnesses can be viewed as representing disharmony and conflict in some particular area of life and thus tend to fall into two general categories: natural illness/environmental hazards and unnatural illness/divine punishment.

Natural illness/environmental hazards. Natural illnesses in the folk medicine belief system are those that occur because of dangerous agents, such as cold air, impurities in the air, impurities in food, and impurities in water. Natural illnesses are based on the fact that everything in nature is connected and that events can be both interpreted and directed by an understanding of these relationships. Sympathetic magic, the basis for popular folk medicine beliefs and practices, can be divided into two categories: contagious and imitative magic. At the root of contagious magic is the premise that the parts do represent the whole. Many witchcraft practices are based on contagious magic, including such practices as an evildoer obtaining a lock of the victim's hair or shavings from the victim's skin to do harm. Imitative magic, on the other hand, is based on the premise that like will follow like. An example of imitative magic is the belief that a knife under the bed will cut labor pains. For the nurse to assist the patient in preventing natural illnesses, it becomes imperative for the nurse to comprehend the direct connections between the body and natural phenomena such as the phases of the moon, the positions of the planets, and the changing of the seasons. Because in this belief system good health is contingent on these phenomena, it is imperative that one be able to read these signs if the body is to remain in harmony with nature.

Unnatural illnesses/divine punishment. Unnatural illnesses are thought to occur because an individual may become so grave a sinner that the Lord withdraws his favor. In fact, illnesses may be attributed to punishment for failure to abide by the proper behavior rules given to man by God. The etiology of unnatural illnesses, for those who subscribe to these beliefs, is based on the continual battle between the forces of good and evil as personified in God and the devil. Evil influences may be blamed for any unnatural illness, which may range from nightmares to tuberculosis. An example of a person subscribing to this belief would be a diabetic Black woman who consistently refuses to inject herself with insulin because she believes her illness is the direct result of punishment by the devil for her sinful youth. However, unnatural illnesses are also thought to occur as a result of witchcraft. Witchcraft is based on the belief that there are individuals who have the ability to mobilize unusual powers for good and evil.

Comparison of the folk medicine system and other medical systems

To develop an understanding of folk medicine as a system, the system itself must be examined along with the ecological model, the Western medical system, and religious systems. Every medical system is based on the philosophy of survival of the human organism. According to the classic work of Thomas Weaver (1970), both folk practices and Western medical practices are social systems with interdependent parts or variables that include beliefs, attitudes, practices, and roles associated with the concepts of health and disease and with the patterns of diagnoses and treatment.

All medical systems have an adaptive nature. As such, the term *medical system* can be defined as the pattern of cultural tradition and social institutions that evolves from deliberative behavior to improve health status regardless of the outcome of a particular behavior (Dunn, 1975).

If an individual is to achieve good health, then this individual must develop an idea of what constitutes disease, with its counterpart conditions of pain and suffering. Once a philosophy of health is adopted by an individual, various health roles are delineated. These health roles require specific health care practitioners who are duly initiated into the rights of practice. Practitioner status may be granted by medical societies or, in the case of folk medicine practices, by supernatural forces. The body is an integral part of each individual; therefore all medical systems use body parts or excreta for diagnostic purposes. In addition, folk medicine practices, in most cases, prescribe medicines to rub into the skin, to irrigate the body, or to anoint the sick.

Ecological model. The ecological model is closely related to the folk medicine system. Kay (1978) defined ecology as having three foci: (1) biological, or the branch of biology that deals with the relationship between organisms and the environment; (2) social, or the relationship between people and institutions, and the interdependence between the two; and (3) cultural, or the relationship between culture and the environment, which also includes culture and societies in the environment. Ecological dimensions of health care can assist the nurse in providing plausible explanations as to why certain individuals contract specific diseases and why other individuals do not. Over the past decade, health care practitioners have become increasingly concerned with the ecological dimensions of race and ethnic minority group health problems such as AIDS, sickle cell anemia, and other such diseases.

Western medical system. In contrast to the folk medicine system, which attempts to explain illness in terms of balances between an individual and the physical, social, and spiritual worlds, is the Western medical system of diagnoses and scientific explanations for illness. Western medical practices focus on preventive and curative medicine, whereas folk medicine practices focus on personal rather than scientific behavior. In the folk medicine system, it may make all the sense in the world to burn incense and to avoid certain individuals, cold air, and the "evil eye." According to Kay (1978), one person's religion is another person's magic, witchcraft, or superstition. However, it is very difficult for health care professionals to see these entities as directly relevant to medical practice, or to recognize that for some cultural groups religion is the equivalent of a science.

Although many differences in focus can be seen when a comparison between Western and folk medicine health practices is made, some of these differences may not be that significant. For example, Western medical relationships are generally dyads, such as physician-patient, physician-nurse, and nurse-patient relationships, whereas folk medicine networks are generally multiperson health care networks that may consist of parents, other relatives, and nonrelatives as health care givers. However, today multiperson health care networks are no longer dismissed by Western health care practitioners as being irrelevant and thus dysfunctional. In fact, multiperson networks are slowly being incorporated into the Western medical system of health care.

Ethnic diets are an important aspect of human ecology because health care providers are beginning to incorporate into practice the use of ethnic diets and to understand their significance. An individual, regardless of ethnic group, must consume enough food to meet nutritional requirements for energy, fat, protein, vitamins, and minerals in order to keep the body functioning. Rittenbaugh (1978) noted that very little is known in regard to the range of human variability both among and within human populations, particularly in regard to common parameters such as nutritional requirements, physiological response to malnutrition, and digestive capabilities. It is perhaps this lack of knowledge that has in the past resulted in Western-oriented health care providers prescribing diets unacceptable to persons from diverse and multicultural backgrounds. In fact, some individuals from diverse cultural backgrounds may be physically incompatible with certain Western foods. Therefore factors regarding ethnic diets and other such folk practices need to be considered by the nurse when developing plans of care in order to give culturally specific nursing care.

Religious systems. Some religious groups have elaborate rules concerning health care behaviors, including such things as the giving and receiving of health care. Religious experiences are based on cultural beliefs and may include such things as blessings from spiritual leaders, aberrations of dead relatives, and even miracle cures. Healing power based on religion may also be found in animate as well as inanimate objects. Religion can and does dictate social, moral, and dietary practices that are designed to assist an individual in maintaining a healthy balance and in addition plays a vital role in illness prevention. Examples of religious health care practices include illness prevention through such acts as the burning of candles, rituals of redemption, and prayer. Religious practices such as "the blessing of the throats" on St. Blise Day are performed to prevent illnesses such as sore throats and choking. Baptism may be seen as a ritual of cleansing and dedication, as well as a prevention against evil. As well as being related to dedication to God's will and a preparation for death, annointing the sick is related by some religious and cultural groups to recovery and may be performed in the hope of a miracle. Circumcision is also a religious practice in that it may be viewed as having redemptive values that may prevent illness and harm (Morganstern, 1966; Spector, 1989).

It is important for the nurse to distinguish between a shaman and a priest. A shaman derives power from the supernatural, whereas a priest learns a codified body of rituals from other priests and from Biblical laws. In traditional folk medicine systems, some of the most significant religious rituals are those that mediate between events in the "here and now" and events in the hereafter or "out there" in the "nether" world (Morley & Wallis, 1978).

IMPLICATIONS FOR NURSING CARE

The nurse must keep in mind that regardless of whether a patient believes in internal or external locus of control, or whether the patient uses a folk medicine system, religious system, or ecological system, there is still safety in harmony and balance and there may be danger in anything that is done to the extreme. In other words, it is bad for the body to eat too much, drink too much, stay out too late, etc. In a classic 1972 study in Harlem, it was reported that 90% of Black adolescents surveyed believed that good health was largely a matter of looking after oneself. These adolescents concluded that the results of excess may not be immediately visible but sooner or later will affect the individual because the body has become weakened (Brunswick & Josephson, 1972).

There seemingly is a sex and age differential that is associated with strengths and weaknesses among individuals. (Generally speaking, strength is correlated with an individual's ability to withstand illness, whereas weakness is correlated with an individual's heightened susceptibility.) For example, strength has been related to the male species. In the United States females are generally regarded as weaker than their male counterparts, and this sex weakness is generally perceived as women being more prone to illness primarily because of functional blood loss and anatomical differences. Certain age groups have also been related to individual strength and weakness. Infants and unborn fetuses are considered the weakest of all and are perceived to be at the mercy of the mother's behavior, including prenatal behavior. During pregnancy harmony and moderation are the key to a healthy baby; thus the pregnancy period carries the greatest taboos among most cultural groups. For example, some Mexican Americans, Amish, Hutterites, and both Whites and Blacks in the South subscribe to the doctrine of maternal moderation in pregnancy (Bauer, 1969). It is even believed that the mother's emotional state during pregnancy may affect the baby, particularly in the case of pity, fear, mockery, or hate. For example, some southern Black Americans believe that feelings of hate for a particular individual may cause the baby to resemble that person, or that a child could be subjected to seizures if the mother saw someone having a seizure and felt pity. Some Blacks, southern Whites, and Mexican Americans also believe that when a pregnant woman makes fun of someone with a physical affliction, the baby may be born with the same affliction, thus punishing the mother for lack of charity (Snow, 1981).

Since some cultural groups believe in a direct connection between the body and the forces of nature, it is important for the nurse to recognize the relevance of natural phenomena such as phases of the moon, positions of the planets, and seasons of the year. In the rural South there is a dependence on natural signs to regulate behavior. Some of these people rely on the *Farmer's Almanac* to guide such events as planting crops, setting hens' eggs, destroying weeds, weaning babies, and going fishing. The *Almanac* is consulted for many health needs, such as the best time to extract teeth or to have teeth filled (according to the *Almanac,* the best time to have teeth extracted is during the increase of the moon and the best time to have teeth filled is during the moon's decrease). The *Almanac* may also be used to pick the optimal time to have surgical procedures done. The nurse must keep in mind that the *Almanac* is not only used by rural Southern people; in Northern urban areas many Black pharmacists will give *Almanacs* as gifts to their customers for the New Year. Interestingly, the first *Almanac* is reported to have been written by a physician in 1897.

It is also important for the nurse to remember that many people from diverse cultural groups use the zodiacal signs to manipulate health regimens but do not mention this to health professionals for fear of being laughed at. Use of zodiacal signs illustrate how external forces are brought to bear on the individual; these signs are the basis for a lively practice of self-medication, dietary regulation, and behavior modifications. The nurse should keep in mind that some of these practices are harmful, some are neutral, and some are beneficial. For example, it would be extremely detrimental for a patient in need of a lifesaving surgical procedure to wait for a full moon to have the procedure done. It is important for the nurse to devise training programs that will teach patients to manipulate behaviors and interpret zodiacal signs in a way that will maintain health and prevent illness and disease.

In a study of the folk medicine system, it may become obvious that this system reflects a view of the world as a dangerous place, where the individual must be constantly on guard against nature, other individuals, and possible punishment from God. This world view teaches the individual that it is best to look out for oneself and that mistrust is wiser than trust.

The presence of an alternate medical (folk medicine) system that is different from, and at the same time possibly in direct conflict with, the Western medical system can serve to complicate matters. It not only becomes a matter of offering health care in the place of no health care, or offering superior health care in lieu of inferior health care, but the nurse must keep in mind that persons from diverse cultural backgrounds have deeply ingrained beliefs about how to attain and maintain health. These beliefs, which may be linked to the natural and supernatural worlds, may adversely affect the physician-patient and nurse-patient relationships and thus influence the individual's decision to follow or not follow prescribed treatment regimens. The nurse might correctly assume that when a low-income Black American, southern White, Puerto Rican, or Mexican American individual does arrive for professional health care, every home remedy known to the patient has already been tried. It is important for the nurse to ascertain what the patient has been doing to combat the illness. If the home remedy is harmless, it is best left in the treatment plan and the nurse's own suggestions added. However, harmful practices must be eliminated. One of the best ways for the nurse to eliminate harmful practices is to inquire whether or not the practice has worked. If the patient assumes that it has not worked, the nurse can simply suggest that something else be tried. If the patient perceives that a harmful practice is beneficial, then the nurse must provide education that will illuminate the dangers of this harmful practice.

Nurses have recently begun to explore the relationship of person and environment in nursing research. An exploratory study by Pyles (1989) related Etzioni's compliance theory to satisfaction by nursing employees in a school of nursing. Data from the study indicated that a normative power structure in the school and the resultant moral involvement profile in the faculty were compatible for an organization such as a university, which displays cultural goals. In a more clinical study Gould (1989) studied 112 elderly residents in three metropolitan nursing homes. The data suggested that life satisfaction is an indicator of well-being, which is useful as a measure of quality of care because of its linkage to health. The data additionally indicated that bonding develops between institutionalized elderly persons and their caregivers, which precludes the drive for self-determination. Thus the data provided an explanation of why lower-income elderly persons demonstated high levels of life satisfaction in spite of low levels of perceived influence over the institutional environment.

SUMMARY

Health may be viewed as a balance between the individual and the environment. Health practices and the actions individuals take when sick are affected by how the environment is viewed. Thus issues of environmental control are an important concern when the nurse interacts with the patient in a health care setting. To provide culturally appropriate care, the nurse should not only respect the individual's unique beliefs, but should also have an understanding of how these beliefs can be used to promote optimal health in the patient's environment.

CASE
STUDY

Martha Brown is a 27-year-old woman who lives in northern Kentucky in a small cabin in the hills. The cabin has no indoor plumbing, and she resides with her husband and six small children. The public health nurse makes a home visit after three of the children have been diagnosed by the school nurse as having lice. While the nurse is explaining the use of Rid (lice treatment) to the mother, she notes that Mrs. Brown has a persistent cough that she states she has had for 2 years. The nurse notes that the cough is productive, that Mrs. Brown looks emaciated, and that her color is extremely ashen. She tires easily. Although health insurance is a benefit of her husband's job in a nearby mine, Mrs. Brown's children were born at home and she has never had a complete physical. When asked why she has not gone to a nearby free health clinic, Mrs. Brown replies, "Sickness is God's will and he will cure me if he wants to. Anyway, my family comes first, and I don't have the time. Besides, doctors can't be trusted. My Aunt Jane went to one once, and she died the next week."

STUDY
QUESTIONS

1. Based on the fact that Mrs. Brown is Appalachian and taking into consideration the fact that every individual is unique, decide whether Mrs. Brown is more likely to be "being" oriented or "doing" oriented in regard to activity orientation.
2. Decide what the relational orientation is for Mrs. Brown based on her reply to the public health nurse about why she has not sought treatment.
3. Based on Mrs. Brown's reply to the public health nurse and on the fact that she is Appalachian, what people-to-nature orientation is she likely to have?
4. Decide, on the basis of Mrs. Brown's comment and the fact that she is Appalachian, what view of human nature she is likely to hold.
5. List at least three reasons why Mrs. Brown might be apprehensive about seeking medical help.

REFERENCES

Bauer, W.W. (1969). *Potions, remedies, and old wive's tales.* New York: Doubleday.

Bauwens, E., & Anderson, S. (1988). Social and cultural influences on health care. In M. Stanhope & J. Lancaster (Eds.), *Community health nursing: Process and practice for promoting health* (2nd ed., pp. 89-108). St. Louis: C.V. Mosby.

Brunswick, A.F., & Josephson, E. (1972, Oct.). Adolescent health in Harlem. *American Journal of Public Health, 72* (suppl.), 7-47.

Chrisman, N.J. (1977). The health seeking process. *Culture and Medicine in Psychiatry, 1,* 351-377.

Dunn, F.L. (1975). Transcultural Asian medicine and cosmopolitan medicine as adaptive systems. In E. Leslie (Ed.), *Asian medical systems: A comparative study* (p. 135). Berkeley: University of California Press.

Elling, R.H. (1977). *Socio-cultural influences on health care.* New York: Springer Publishing.

Fabrega, H. (1971). Medical anthropology. In B.J. Siegel (Ed.), *Biennial review of anthropology.* Stanford, Calif.: Stanford University Press.

Giuffra, M. (1987). Sociocultural issues. In J. Haber, P. Hoskins, A. Leach, & B. Sideleau (Eds.), *Comprehensive psychiatric nursing* (3rd ed.). New York: McGraw-Hill.

Gould, M. (1989, Nov. 14). *The relationship of perceived social-environmental factors and functional health status to life satisfaction in the elderly.* Paper presented at the Sigma Theta Tau international conference, Indianapolis.

Greene, L., & Johnston, F. (1980). *Social and biological predictors of nutritional status, growth, and development.* New York: Academic Press.

Haber, J., Hoskins, P., Leach, A., & Sideleau, B. (Eds.). (1987). *Comprehensive psychiatric nursing.* New York: McGraw-Hill.

Henderson, G., & Primeaux, M. (1981). *Transcultural health care.* Reading, Mass.: Addison-Wesley.

Kay, M. (1978). Clinical anthropology. In E.E. Bauwens (Ed.), *The anthropology of health* (pp. 3-11). St. Louis: C.V. Mosby.

Kleinman, A., Eisenberg, L., & Good, B. (1978). Culture, illness and care. *Annuals in Internal Medicine, 88,* 251-258.

Kluckhohn, K., & Strodtbeck, F. (1961). *Variations in value orientations.* New York: Row, Peterson.

Morganstern, J. (1966). *Rites of birth, marriage, death, and kindred occasions among the Semites.* Chicago: Quadrangle.

Morley, P., & Wallis, R. (1978). *Culture and curing.* London: Peter Owen.

Pillsbury, B. (1982). Doing the month: Confinement and convalescence of Chinese women after childbirth. In M. Kay (Ed.), *Anthropology of human birth.* Philadelphia: F.A. Davis.

Pyles, C. (1989, Nov. 13). *Power compatibility profile in a school of nursing.* Paper presented at the Sigma Theta Tau international conference, Indianapolis.

Rittenbaugh, C. (1978). Human foodways: A window on evolution. In E.E. Bauwens (Ed.), *The anthropology of health.* St. Louis: C.V. Mosby.

Rotter, J.B. (1966). Generalized expectancies for internal versus external control of reinforcement. *Psychological Monographs, 80*(1), 1-28.

Rotter, J.B. (1975). Some problems and misconceptions related to the construct of internal versus external control of reinforcement. *Journal of Consulting and Clinical Psychology, 43,* 56-67.

Snow, L.F. (1981). Folk medical beliefs and their implications for the care of patients: A review based on studies among Black Americans. In G. Henderson & M. Primeaux (Eds.), *Transcultural health care.* Reading, Mass.: Addison-Wesley.

Spector, R. (1989). Culture, ethnicity, and nursing. In P. Potter & A. Perry (Eds.), *Fundamentals of nursing: Concepts, process, and practice* (pp. 74-91). St.Louis: C.V. Mosby.

Weaver, T. (1970). Use of hypothetical situations in a study of Spanish-American illness referral systems. *Human Organisms, 29,* 141.

Williams, C., & Jelliffe, D. (1972). *Mother and child health: Delivering the services.* London: Oxford University Press.

....

CHAPTER 7

Biological Variations

BEHAVIORAL OBJECTIVES

After reading this chapter, the nurse will be able to:

1 Articulate biological differences among individuals in various racial groups.

2 Relate the importance of knowledge of biological differences that may exist among individuals in various racial groups to the provision of health care by the nurse.

3 Describe nursing implications that may arise when providing care for individuals in different cultural and racial groups.

4 Describe nutritional preferences and deficiencies that may exist among persons in different cultural groups.

5 Explain how psychological characteristics may vary from one culture to another.

6 Explain how susceptibility to disease may differ among individuals in different racial groups.

It is a well-known fact that people differ culturally. Cultural differences are evident in communication, spatial relationships and needs, social organizations (family, kinships, and tribes), time orientation, and ability or desire to control the environment. Less recognized and understood are the biological differences that exist among people in various racial groups. It is becoming more evident to nurses that a body of scientific knowledge does exist about biological cultural differences. References to and information about biocultural differences are mushrooming in the literature and have resulted in a field of study known as biocultural ecology (Bennett, Osborne, & Miller, 1975), which has as its major focus the study of human adaptation and homeostasis. The purpose of biocultural ecology is to transcend the fragmentation inherent in the separation of culture, human biology, and ecology/environment. Biocultural ecology studies diverse human populations by means of this three-way interaction system and focuses on specific, localized individuals and populations within a given environment. Data relative to all the variables significant to people within a racial group are essential for complete understanding of the people. Not only are no two persons alike, but no two cultural or racial groups are alike, and all phenomena relative to both individuals and cultural or racial groups must be understood.

While the significance of biocultural ecology concepts has existed in other disciplines, such as sociology and medical anthropology, the nursing literature has only recently documented the importance of this field for nurses. A focus on transcultural issues that began in the mid-1960s with the impetus of nurses such as Madeleine Leininger (1970) has helped nurses to develop cultural insights and a deeper appreciation for human life and values from a cultural perspective. However, in spite of the introduction of transcultural nursing concepts, to date, the nursing literature remains scanty on biological variations existing among people in various racial groups. The strongest argument for including concepts on biological variations in nursing education and subsequently nursing practice is that scientific facts about biological variations can aid the nurse in giving culturally appropriate health care. Nurses who care for people transculturally need to be cognizant of certain basic biological differences in order to give nonharmful and competent care.

The majority of nurses in the United States have been educated in a system of nursing practice based on biological baselines of the dominant White race. Because studies on biological baselines in growth and development, nutrition, and other biological phenomena have been conducted using White subjects, standardized norms available to the nurse do not recognize biological variations existing among different racial groups. That people in various racial groups differ tremendously is evidenced externally and is related to biogenetic variations that have occurred internally. Therefore values uniracially normed are inappropriate when applied across racial groups. In the United States, White-standardized values for factors related to growth and development, nutrition, and susceptibility to disease are often applied to Blacks, Orientals, and American Indians. Therefore significant deviations from the norm that may be labeled "nonnormal" might be more appropriately labeled "non-White" (Overfield, 1977). In fact, biological variations among racial groups are so diverse that multiple dimensions are encompassed.

DIMENSIONS OF BIOLOGICAL VARIATIONS

A direct relationship exists between race and body structure, skin color, other visible physical characteristics, enzymatic and genetic variations, electrocardiographic patterns, susceptibility to disease, nutritional preferences and deficiencies, and psychological characteristics. Differences among people in various racial groups in each of these areas are discussed in the following sections.

Body Structure

One category of difference between racial groups is body structure, which includes both body size and shape. Newborn body proportions differ among racial groups. Although research on this topic remains scanty, it has been postulated that newborn body proportions appear to be genetically programmed to conform to the pelvic shape of the mother (Overfield, 1977).

In regard to body structure and size, the face is perhaps one of the most fascinating areas of the body because it has many parts that combine to make the whole. The face tends to be the one prominent area that can visibly categorize people by race. For example, eyelids vary from racial group to racial group. In some racial groups the eyelids droop over the cartilage plate above the eye, and in other racial groups the eyelids do not droop. The epicanthic fold, another variation of the eyelids, is found predominantly in persons with Oriental characteristics but may be present in other racial groups.

Ears are another fascinating part of the face because they have a variety of shapes. Earlobes can be free and floppy, or attached close to the face as if the intent were to make sure the lobe stayed in place. Earlobes that are free and floppy are very handy for attaching earrings. When earlobes are attached, they are the least defined, and the wearing of objects such as earrings may be difficult.

Noses come in all sizes and shapes; however, nose size and shape correlate directly with one's racial ancestry. It has been postulated that small noses were an evolutionary result of living in cold climates, for example, the classic Oriental nose. On the other hand, noses with high bridges were a result of living in climates that were dry, for example, the classic Iranian and American Indian noses. People who lived in moist, hot climates developed broad, flat noses such as those found on Africans and American Blacks (Overfield, 1977).

Teeth offer another important variation in body size and shape. Tooth size, which is important because the teeth help shape the size of the lower face, varies among racial groups. For example, Australian aborigines have the largest teeth in the world, as well as four extra molars. Orientals and Black Americans have very large teeth, whereas White Americans have very small teeth. People with very large teeth tend to have their jaws projecting beyond the upper part of the face. This projection tends to be a normal variation and not an orthodontic problem. There is also a tendency among some racial groups for fewer numbers of teeth. For example, some racial groups do not have a third molar or maxillary lateral incisors. Peg teeth are sometimes a step in the evolutionary process that facilitates the presence or absence of a particular type of tooth (Overfield, 1977).

As teeth vary among racial groups, so do tongues. The most common variances are scrotal tongues, which occur in 5% of the population in some racial groups; geographic tongues, which occur in 3% of the population in some racial groups; and fissured tongues, which occur in 5% to 40% of the population in some racial groups (Witcop et al., 1963). The mandibular or palatine torus is also of concern to the nurse when inspecting the mouth. The torus is a bony protuberance, and the palatine torus occurs on the midline of the palate, whereas the mandibular torus occurs as a lump on the inner side of the mandible near the second molar. Tori are fairly common, with palatine tori occurring in up to 25% of the population in most racial groups studied. Mandibular tori occur in 7% of Whites, 2% of Blacks, and 40% of Orientals (Jarvis, 1972).

Another variation in body size and structure is attributable to muscle size and mass. In certain racial groups specific muscles are absent altogether. The peroneus tertius muscle, which is found in the foot, and the palmaris longus muscle, which is found in the wrist, are absent in individuals in some racial groups. However, muscle absence in general does not appear to be more prevalent in any particular racial group; nor does absence of a particular muscle correspond with absence of another muscle.

There have been numerous studies conducted regarding inheritability of stature (Overfield, 1985). In general, the conclusions are that people by virtue of race vary in height and that in the United States Black and White Americans are the tallest, American Indians are either similar in height or a few inches shorter than Mexican Americans, and Asian Americans are the shortest. Individuals of higher socioeconomic status in all ethnic groups are taller (Overfield, 1985).

In regard to physical growth and developmental rates, Blacks are generally advanced, whereas Orientals are generally retarded when these groups are compared with White norms.

Skin Color

When working with people from diverse cultural backgrounds, the nurse should have an understanding of how different races evolved in relation to the environment. Biological differences noted in skin color may be attributable to the biological adjustments a person's ancestors made in the environment in which they lived. For example, it has been scientifically postulated that the original skin color of humans on earth was Black (Overfield, 1977). Further postulations suggest that White skin was the result of mutation and environmental pressures exerted on persons living in cold, cloudy northern Europe. The mutation is thought to have occurred because light skin was better able to synthesize vitamin D, particularly on cloudy days. It is thought that Black skin became a neutral trait in climates where protection from the sun and heat of the tropics was not a factor (Overfield, 1977, 1985).

Skin color is probably the most significant biological variation in terms of nursing care. Nursing care delivery is based on accurate patient assessment, and the darker the patient's skin, the more difficult it becomes to assess changes in color. When caring for patients with highly pigmented skin, the nurse must first establish the baseline skin color, and daylight is the best light source for doing so. If possible, dark-skinned patients should always be given a bed by a window in order to provide access to sunlight. When daylight is not available to assess skin color, a lamp with at least a 60-watt bulb should be used.

To establish the baseline skin color, the nurse must observe those skin surfaces that have the least amount of pigmentation, which include the volar surfaces of the forearms, the palms of the hands, the soles of the feet, the abdomen, and the buttocks. When observing these areas, the nurse should look for an underlying red tone, which is typical of all skin, regardless of how dark its color. Absence of this red tone in a patient may be indicative of pallor. Additional areas that are important to assess in dark-skinned patients include the mouth, the conjunctiva, and the nail beds. Generally speaking, the darkness of the oral mucosa correlates with the patient's skin color. The darker the skin, the darker the mucosa; nevertheless, the mucosa is lighter than the skin.

The nurse must be aware that oral hyperpigmentation can occur on the tongue and the mucosa and is a condition that can alter the value of the oral mucosa as a site for observation. The occurrence of oral hyperpigmentation is directly related to the darkness of a person's skin. Oral hyperpigmentation appears in 50% to 90% of Blacks, as compared with 10% to 50% of Whites. Another important consideration for the nurse is the appearance of a hard palate, because it takes on a yellow discoloration, particularly in the presence of jaundice. The hard palate is frequently affected by hyperpigmentation in a manner similar to that of the oral mucosa and the tongue. The nurse should also assess the lips, because they may be helpful in assessing skin color changes (such as jaundice or cyanosis). It is important for the nurse to remember, however, that the lips of some Black people have a natural bluish hue (Rouch, 1977). Thus it is important for the nurse to have established the baseline color of the lips if they are to be of value in detecting cyanosis (Branch & Paxton, 1976).

It is also important for the nurse to establish the normal color of the conjunctiva when working with persons from transcultural populations. The conjunctiva will reflect the color changes of cyanosis or pallor and is a good site for observing petechiae. Another excellent source for determining the presence of jaundice is the sclera. The nurse should first establish a baseline color for the sclera, because the sclera of dark-skinned persons often has a yellow coloration due to subconjunctival fatty deposits. A common finding of persons with highly pigmented skin is the presence of melanin deposits or "freckles" on the sclera.

The final area of assessment should be the nail beds. The nail beds are useful when one is attempting to detect cyanosis or pallor. In dark-skinned persons it is difficult to assess the nail beds because they may be highly pigmented, thick, lined, or contain melanin deposits. Regardless of color, for baseline assessment, it is important for the nurse to note how quickly the color returns to the nail beds after pressure has been released from the free edge of the nail (Rouch, 1977). A slower return of color to the nail beds may be indicative of cyanosis or pallor. It is also difficult to detect rashes, inflammations, and ecchymosis in dark-skinned persons. It may be necessary to palpate rashes in dark-skinned persons, since rashes may not be readily visible to the eye. When palpating the skin for rashes, the nurse should note induration and warmth of the area.

Other Visible Physical Characteristics

In addition to looking for changes in pallor and cyanosis, it is important for the nurse to note other aberrations in the skin. For example, mongolian spots may be present on the skin of Black, Asian, Native American, or Mexican American newborns. Mongolian spots are bluish discolorations that vary tremendously in size and color and are often mistaken for bruises. Another aberration that is more common in Blacks than in other racial groups is keloids. These ropelike scars represent an exaggeration of the wound-healing process and may occur as a result of any type of trauma, such as surgical incisons, ear piercing, or insertion of an intravenous catheter.

Enzymatic and Genetic Variations

The basic genetic makeup of an individual is determined from the moment of conception. At the moment of conception, among other things, the upper limits of achievement are set; the "map," so to speak, is drawn. In other words, a person can be only what he or she is genetically determined to be. More specifically, growth and development cannot go beyond what the genes make possible. An individual will not grow 1 inch taller than genetic structure allows regardless of the amount of exercise or vitamins consumed. By the same token, an individual will be no more intelligent than genetic structure allows, despite the amount of tutoring or special schooling the individual receives (Burt, 1966; Lorton & Lorton, 1984).

In medical terms, a person's race represents his or her genetic makeup. Although race may be irrelevant in some situations, knowing the racial predisposition to a certain disease is often helpful in evaluating patients and diagnosing their illness, as well as in assessing risks (Divan, 1989). The genetic and enzymatic predisposition to certain diseases is discussed in this chapter under Susceptibility to Disease; lactose intolerance and G-6-PD deficiency are discussed under Nutritional Deficiencies.

The incidence of dizygote twinning is highest in Blacks, occurring in 4% of births. Dizygote twinning occurs in approximately 2% of births in Whites and in 0.5% of births in Asians (Bulmer, 1970).

Some research interpretations (Jensen, 1969, 1974, 1977) have indicated that the small but persistent differences between the average intelligence quotients (IQs) of Black children and those of White children reflect a genetic difference. Jensen (1969) claimed to have controlled for variables, including income and education. He reported that he found a difference in IQ, which he believed to be indicative of a genetic difference. Others have refuted Jensen's claim (Kamlin, 1974). In 1977 Jensen conducted a study of children between the ages of 5 and 16 in the rural South (Jensen, 1977), in which analysis of the data suggested that the IQs of Black children, but not those of White children, drop substantially as they grow older. Jensen believed that this contrast between Blacks and Whites possibly meant that the decrement in IQ was genetically determined. This has not been supported by research by others.

Drug Interactions and Metabolism

Reactions to drugs vary with race. There is some evidence suggesting that drugs are metabolized by different races in different ways and at different rates (Echizen, Horai, & Ishizaki, 1989). For example, Zhou et al. (1989) demonstrated that Chinese subjects are more sensitive to the cardiovascular effects of propranolol than are White subjects.

In the body there are three classes of reactions to foreign chemicals or drugs: hydrolysis, conjugation, and oxidation (Kalow, 1982). The following are examples of reactions to specific drugs.

Isoniazid is a drug commonly used to treat tuberculosis. There are two ways in which people will react to metabolize this drug: they will inactivate it either very slowly or very rapidly. Those persons who inactivate this drug very slowly are at risk for developing peripheral neuropathy during therapy (Vessell, 1972). Rapid inactivation of this drug occurs in 40% of Whites, 60% of Blacks, 60% to 90% of American Indians and Eskimos, and 85% to 90% of Orientals (Vessell, 1972). Pyridoxine is given with Isoniazid, and the doses are spaced at larger intervals for slower reaction during treatment for tuberculosis.

Primaquine is metabolized by oxidization and is used in the treatment of malaria. When this drug is given to individuals who lack the enzymes necessary for glucose metabolism of the red blood cells, hemolysis of the red blood cells occurs. Approximately 100 million people in the world are affected by this particular enzyme deficiency and thus are unable to ingest Primaquine. Approximately 35% of Black Americans have this particular enzyme deficiency.

Succinylcholine is a muscle relaxant used during surgery. It is inactivated by hydrolysis by the enzyme pseudocholinesterase. In most individuals it is rapidly inactivated, but some individuals have the atypical form of the enzyme and suffer prolonged muscle paralysis and an inability to breathe following administration of the drug. Black Americans, Orientals, and American Indians are at risk for having pseudocholinesterase deficiency. In Whites the risk is slightly higher than in these groups, and in some Jews and Alaskan Eskimos the risk is considerably greater; one out of 135 Alaskans is unable to metabolize the drug succinylcholine normally (Kalow, 1972; Vessell, 1972).

The rate of alcohol metabolism is another drug reaction that appears to have racial variance. Studies have indicated that American Indians and Orientals experience marked facial flushing and other vasomotor symptoms after ingesting alcohol as compared with their White and Black counterparts, who experience less severe reactions. There are two different enzymes involved in alcohol metabolism, both of which are variations of alcohol dehydrogenase (ADH): a high-activity type of ADH, which converts alcohol to acetaldehyde rapidly, and a low-activity variant, which converts it slowly (Kalow, 1972). The enzyme involved in metabolism of acetaldehyde to acetic acid also has several varieties, including acetaldehyde dehydrogenase one through four. Acetaldehyde dehydrogenase one (ALDH I) is considered normal; other types are considered deficient in their ability to metabolize acetaldehyde (Goedde, 1983).

Electrocardiographic Patterns

A common finding in Black Americans, particularly in Black men, is the occurrence of inverted T waves in the precordial leads of the electrocardiogram. This aberration is a normal variant in the Black population but would suggest a pathological condition if found in other racial groups, for example, Whites.

Susceptibility to Disease

Tuberculosis

Another category of differences between racial groups is susceptibility to disease. The increased or deceased incidence of a particular disease may be genetically determined. For example, some American Indians have a tuberculosis incidence that is 7 to 15 times that of non-Indians; Black Americans have a tuberculosis incidence three times higher than that of White Americans (Williams, 1975); and urban American Jews are the most resistant to tuberculosis (Overfield, 1977). The increased susceptibility of Blacks to tuberculosis may be a result of their tendency toward overgrowth of connective tissue components concerned with protection against infection, since tuberculosis is a granulomatous infection (Polednak, 1971).

Susceptibility to disease may also be environmental or a combination of both genetic and environmental factors. The evidence suggests that tuberculosis can occur in response to both socioenvironmental and psychological stress factors. In a classic study of patients in Seattle, Holmes et al. (1957) found that environmental factors appeared to be relevant in relation to the onset of tuberculosis. In the study, data in the life experiences of each patient were plotted for a 12-year period preceding hospitalization. Analysis of the data revealed that in the majority of patients there was a gradual increase in experiences that were perceived by the individual as significant and stressful. The combination of stressful life experiences and personal perception resulted in a psychological crisis situation that was evidenced in the 2-year period preceding hospitalization. Further analysis of the data done by Holmes et al. suggested that patients who are poorly equipped to deal with social relationships, especially when a lot of tension is present, may be at risk for tuberculosis.

Blood groups, RH factor, and disease

Blood groups also differentiate people in certain racial groups. A prevalence for type O blood has been found among American Indians, with some incidence of type A blood and virtually no incidence of type B blood. Almost equal incidences of types A, B, and O blood are found in Japanese and Chinese people, with the AB blood type found in only about 10% of the Japanese and Chinese population. American Blacks and Whites have been found to have equal incidences of A, B, and O blood types. The predominant blood types of American Blacks and Whites is A and O, with fewer incidences of AB and B types.

Statistically, persons with type O blood are at a greater risk for duodenal ulcers, whereas persons with type A blood are more likely to develop cancer of the stomach. In addition, there is some evidence that women with type O blood have a diminished chance of getting thromboembolitic disease, particularly when taking birth control pills, than women with other ABO blood types (Jick et al., 1969).

The negative RH factor in blood is most common in Whites, much rarer in other racial groups, and apparently absent in Eskimos (Lewis, 1942). Because there are at least 27 different antigens in the RH system, this system is complex and difficult to understand. Of clinical significance is the D antigen because it is more immunogenic than any other RH antigen and is usually the antigen involved in hemolytic disease of the newborn. When antigen D is present, the term *RH-positive* is used. Approximately 85% of persons in the world have RH-positive blood. The term *RH-negative* is used when antigen D is absent. Persons with the RH-negative factor who are exposed to RH-positive blood form RH antibodies. After continued exposure to RH-positive blood, the RH antibody will bind to corresponding antigens on the surface of red blood cells, which contain the RH antigen. Ordinarily RH antibodies do not fix complement. As a result, there is no immediate hemolysis, such as occurs with ABO incompatibility. Rather, RH-antigen red blood cells are broken down rapidly by macrophages in the spleen, resulting in a conversion of hemoglobin to bilirubin, which causes jaundice. Thus the multigravidus woman with the RH-negative factor who has an RH-positive mate will be more likely to produce babies who are susceptible to jaundice. This condition can be prevented if the woman is monitored appropriately during the course of the pregnancy and treatment initiated during fetal development.

Diabetes

Other conditions that appear to have biocultural or racial prevalence include diabetes mellitus, hypertension, sickle cell anemia, and systemic lupus erythematosus (SLE). Reportedly there is a high incidence of diabetes mellitus in certain American Indian tribes, including the Seminole, Pima, and Papago. However, diabetes is thought to be quite rare among Alaskan Eskimos (Westfall, 1971). Diabetes mellitus is a major health problem in America, with an incidence of over 6 million diagnosed cases. The incidence of diabetes mellitus is so widespread that it is postulated that for every person with diagnosed diabetes, there is another person who remains undiagnosed (Carter Center of Emory University, 1985). There are three types of diabetes: insulin-dependent diabetes mellitus (IDDM), non-insulin-dependent diabetes mellitus (NIDDM), and gestational diabetes mellitus (GDM). IDDM has a peak incidence between the ages of 10 and 14 years, apparently affects boys at a somewhat higher frequency than girls, has a higher incidence in Whites, and accounts for 10% to 20% of cases (Krolewski & Warram, 1985). NIDDM dramatically increases with age, has a higher frequency in women, has a higher incidence in non-White persons (particularly Hispanics and Native Americans), and accounts for 80% to 90% of cases (Carter Center of Emory University, 1985). GDM has been reported in 20% of all pregnant woman and increases with maternal age but is not affected by race or culture (Rifkin, 1984).

Hypertension

The incidence of hypertension has been reported to be significantly higher in American Blacks than in American Whites. The onset by age is earlier in American Blacks, and the hypertension is more severe and associated with a higher mortality among Black Americans. It has been postulated that 35% of American Blacks over age 40 are hypertensive (Tipton, 1974). In a study with a random sample of adults aged 18 to 79, 9% of non-Blacks and 22% of Blacks were found to be hypertensive according to standards set by the World Health Organization, wherein hypertension is indicated when a diastolic blood pressure of 95 mm Hg or greater is evidenced (Boyle, 1970). In another study done by the Chicago Health Association, the analysis of the data confirmed previous findings of a higher prevalence rate for hypertension among Black Americans in all age groups than for White Americans. Further analysis of the data suggested an equal prevalence of hypertension among both sexes in the Black race and an increased incidence with advancing age (Merck, Sharp, & Dohme, 1974). However, contrasting opinions suggest than hypertension occurs slightly more often in men than in women (Phipps, Long, & Woods, 1987).

A diagnosis of hypertension is confirmed when there is a consistent systolic blood pressure level above 140 torr and a consistent diastolic blood pressure level above 90 torr. Reportedly, as a result of this definition, hypertension is of concern for more than 60 million Americans. Many individuals who are hypertensive remain symptom free for a long time; thus researchers at the National Heart, Lung, and Blood Institute have estimated that more than 50% of persons with hypertension do not know that they are hypertensive. Hypertension continues to be the major cause of heart failure, kidney failure, aneurysm formation, and congestive heart failure. Primary hypertension is evidenced in 90% of reported cases, whereas only about 10% of reported cases are classified as secondary. The diagnosis for primary hypertension may be supported when the following risk factors are present:

1. Positive family history
2. Increased sensitivity to the renin-angiotension system
3. Obesity
4. Hypercholesteremia
5. Hyperglycemia

6. Smoking
7. Abnormal sodium and water retention

The diagnosis for secondary hypertension is made when the following causes are present (Phipps, Long, & Woods, 1987):

1. Coarctation of the aorta
2. Pheochromocytoma (a catecholamine-secreting tumor)
3. Cushing's disease
4. Chronic glomerulonephritis
5. Toxemia from pregnancy
6. Thyrotoxicosis
7. Effects of certain drugs such as contraceptives
8. Collagen disease

Primary hypertension affects more American Blacks than American Whites. Researchers at the National Health Examination Survey indicated that in the 24- to 34-year age-group, 3.6% of non-Black men and 12.5% of Black men have primary hypertension, as well as 2.3% of non-Black women and 8.6% of Black women. According to this study, these figures appear to rise steadily with age and at all age levels are conspicuously higher for Blacks. Thus the overall ratio of Blacks to non-Blacks for incidence of primary hypertension is estimated to be 2:1. In addition, primary hypertension is thought to be more severe for Blacks regardless of age level. The death rate for primary hypertension at all age levels up to 85 years of age is higher in Blacks than in non-Blacks. It was reported that men between the ages of 24 and 44 have a mortality as a result of primary hypertension of 14.8% for Blacks and 1% for non-Blacks. In this same age-group female mortality as a result of primary hypertension was reported to be 12.3% for Blacks and 0.8% for non-Blacks (Merck, Sharp, & Dohme, 1974). These data indicate that American Blacks succumb to primary hypertension almost 15 times more often than do non-Blacks. Furthermore, the death rate for hypertension is probably an underestimation. The nurse must be aware of significant risk factors for hypertension in order to assist in early detection and continued maintenance and treatment. Early detection and continued maintenance and treatment for hypertension can aid in reducing the mortality.

Sickle cell anemia

The most common genetic disorder in the United States is sickle cell anemia. Sickle cell anemia or the trait for sickle cell anemia occurs predominantly in the Black American population. It has been projected that 50,000 Black Americans have sickle cell anemia (Wyngaarden & Smith, 1985). Sickle cell anemia or the trait also occurs in people from Asia Minor, India, the Mediterranean, and the Caribbean area, although to a lesser extent than has been reported in American Blacks. Sickle cell is characterized by chronic hemolytic anemia and is a homozygous recessive disorder. In sickle cell anemia the basic disorder lies within the globin of the Hb, where a single amino acid (valine) is substituted for another (glutamic acid) in the sixth position of the beta chain. It is thought that this single amino acid substitution alters profoundly the properties of the Hb molecule; Hb S is formed instead of normal Hb A as a result of the intermolecular rearrangement. The normal oxygen-carrying capacity of the blood is found in Hb A. As a result of deoxygenation, however, there is a change in solubility of protein, which causes the Hb molecules to lump together, causing the cell membrane to contract, with the resultant sickle cell shape.

The affected cells have a shortened life span of 7 to 20 days, which is profoundly different from the life span of normal cells, which is 105 to 120 days. Hb SA is the heterozygous state and is often an asymptomatic condition referred to as sickle cell trait.

Sickle cell anemia is thought to have occurred for many years in Africa along the Nile river valley as an adaptive disease. In Africa this disorder was thought to produce resistance from malaria transmission by the *Anopheles* mosquito (Williams, 1975). In Africa sickle cell anemia or the trait affects approximately 10% of the Black population, and the death rate before the twenty-first year of life has been 100% in those affected with the disease. Before full recognition of the clinical significance of sickle cell anemia in America, the death rate was almost of the same magnitude as that in Africa. Today in America, as a result of improved and comprehensive care, as well as early recognition of the crisis of the disease, persons with sickle cell disease are found to live through their third and fourth decades of life.

A differential diagnosis for sickle cell anemia should be made for all Black persons who (1) have chronic anemia of undetermined origin, (2) demonstrate an increased susceptibility to infections, or (3) have unexplained attacks of joint, bone, or abdominal pain. Making the diagnosis of sickle cell anemia is done in the laboratory through a technique called hemoglobin electrophoresis. Hemoglobin electrophoresis provides a definitive diagnosis. In addition to hemoglobin electrophoresis, a complete history including a physical examination and laboratory data base should be done. The laboratory data base should include a complete blood cell count (CBC) with a differential and reticulocyte count, electrolytes, blood urea nitrogen (BUN), glucose, direct bilirubin, and a urinalysis (Satcher & Pope, 1974). In addition, radiographs of the chest, abdomen, and bones are indicated if there is evidence of pain or fever. However, a bone scan is preferable.

For persons with sickle cell anemia the indications for prompt admission to a hospital include (Leffall, 1974):

1. A vaso-occlusive pain crisis that does not respond to analgesics within 4 hours of administration
2. An aplastic crisis
3. Splenic sequestration, a life-threatening condition that requires immediate admission to the intensive care unit for continuous observation and therapy
4. A hyperhemolytic crisis, which can occur if the hemoglobin and hemotocrit levels continue to drop
5. Infections indicated by a temperature greater than 101° F or a white blood cell count greater than 15,000 (However, viral, ear, nose, and throat infections may not indicate admission for pediatric patients.)
6. Thromboembolic phenomena in the lungs, cerebrum, and long bones
7. Pregnancy, which indicates an increased risk

A common problem associated with sickle cell anemia is drug use and abuse. At the Martin Luther King, Jr., Hospital, a team of health professionals working through the National Sickle Cell Center were involved in the care of patients with sickle cell anemia. Their work revealed three kinds of problems (Satcher, et al., 1973):

1. Patients with sickle cell anemia were typically stereotyped as drug abusers by many health professionals.
2. The delay in seeking medical care during a sickle cell crisis was due to the patient's desire to tolerate pain and avoid drug dependence.
3. Drug abuse in patients with sickle cell anemia was found in those patients with severe and disabling conditions. These patients required drugs so frequently that they often became mentally and physically dependent.

It is important that the nurse be able to identify early signs of sickle cell crisis and teach the patient to recognize symptoms when they occur. The nurse should impress on the patient the significance of early recognition and treatment of crisis symptoms. Ongoing surveillance of signs and symptoms of sickle cell crisis can promote appropriate treatment and perhaps decrease early death.

Systemic lupus erythematosus

SLE is a chronic disease of unknown cause that affects organs and systems individually or in a variety of combinations. The disease affects women 8 to 10 times more often than it does men. The age distribution for the disease spans from 2 to 97 years of age. SLE was named after the classic butterfly rash. This rash is erosive in nature and thus "likened to the damage caused by a hungry wolf" (Rodnan & Schumacher, 1983). This disease was once thought to be relatively rare and always fatal. However, with the advent of better techniques for recognition, the disease has come to be thought of as fairly common, and its course can be controlled by corticosteroids. Even today, however, some patients do die as a result of lesions that affect major organs or as a result of secondary infections. Although the etiology for the disease is still unknown, three major causative factors are being investigated. One possibility for the causation of this disease is an aberration of the immune system, which causes immune complexes containing antibodies to be deposited in tissue. This deposit therefore causes tissue damage. The second possibility for the causation of this disease is the presence of a viral infection that is caused by or results from some immunological abnormality. The third possibility for the causation of this disease is that both of the above factors combine to produce the disease. In addition, some drugs are known to induce lupuslike syndromes. These drugs include procainamide (Pronestyl), isonicotinic acid hydrazide (INH, Isoniazid), and penicillin (Rodnan & Schumacher, 1983).

As previously indicated, SLE was thought to be a very rare disease. However, because of sophisticated detection procedures, researchers now postulate that this is not a rare disease—its incidence has been estimated to be 2.6 per 100,000 population. Although it is more frequent in Blacks than in non-Blacks, it is reported to be extremely rare among the Asian population.

The nurse who understands that signs and symptoms of arthritis may be indicative of SLE, especially when combined with weakness, fatigue, and weight loss, can assist in early detection. In addition, the nurse should look for symptoms of sensitivity to sunlight, including the development of a rash or symptoms of fever or arthritis as a result of exposure to sunlight. The butterfly lesions of SLE generally appear over the cheeks and bridge of the nose. These lesions are often bright red and may extend beyond the hairline, thus causing alopecia (loss of hair), particularly above the ears. Lesions may also be noted on the neck and may spread slowly to the mucous membranes and other tissues of the body. These lesions generally do not ulcerate; however, they do cause degeneration and atrophy of tissues. Other clinical findings may also be present, depending on the organs involved, and include glomerulonephritis, pleuritis, pericarditis, peritonitis, neuritis, and anemia. The most severe manifestations of SLE are renal and neurological in nature.

Laboratory tests used to diagnose SLE may need to be specific to the organs involved, for example, proteinuria, abnormal cerebrospinal fluid, or radiographic evidence of pleural reactions. Before the advent of the LE-cell preparation, or what is commonly referred to as the LE-cell test, the diagnosis was made by the presentation of the butterfly rash and systemic complications, and the prognosis for the patient was generally fatal. However, as a result of the LE-cell test and other sensitive tests, including the antinuclear antibody (ANA) or the antinuclear factor (ANF) test, patients with more varied symptomatology have been confirmed earlier. Thus through early detection appropriate treatment has been initiated. Patient teaching by the nurse should include instructions on the need for appropriate exercise, appropriate balance of rest and activity, and the necessity of avoiding direct exposure to sunlight. As indicated earlier, SLE is a disease with prevalence among some racial groups, and the nurse who recognizes the biocultural significance of the disease is more apt to give culturally appropriate nursing care.

AIDS

According to the Surgeon General's Report (1987), one fact that is emerging with clarity is the increasing incidence of acquired immunodeficiency syndrome (AIDS) among Blacks and Hispanics. In the United States 1 of every 8 Americans is Black, but among Americans with AIDS 1 of every 4 is Black. These numbers reflect the fact that 24% of the total cases reported thus far involve Black persons. In the United States 1 of every 12 Americans is Hispanic, but 1 of every 7 Americans with AIDS is Hispanic.

Nutritional Preferences and Deficiencies

Another category of differences among cultural groups is nutritional preferences and deficiencies.

Nutritional preferences

Nutritional preferences include habits and patterns. When it comes to food choices, people are creatures of habit (Zifferblatt, Wilbur, & Pinsky, 1980). The term *habit* connotes inflexibility, although people do change their habits for many reasons. The term *food patterns* is more descriptive of food choices. Many factors are associated with the formation of food patterns and preferences. Food patterns are developed during childhood as a result of family life-style and ethnic or cultural, social, religious, geographic, economic, and psychological components. All of these variables influence an individual's attitudes, feelings, and beliefs about certain foods. However, the paramount factors that seem to determine food choices are cultural and ethnic in nature. Adults in a particular culture set the tone for cultural food patterns, which establish the foundation for a child's life-long eating customs regarding the timing of meals, the number of meals per day, foods acceptable for specific meals, methods of preparation, dislikes and likes, and table manners. Children develop over time a sense of stability and security in regard to certain food patterns and attitudes about certain foods.

Schwerin, Stanton, and Smith (1982) indicated that distinct and discrete patterns of consuming foods in different combinations or forms exist, and that for the most part these patterns have remained consistent over the past decade. For example, many southern Americans would routinely choose grits as a food but would not routinely choose lentils. However, American diets are becoming more homogeneous because of many factors, including transportation, advertising, mobility, economic status, methods of production, and appreciation of other people's cultural heritage (Katz, Hediger, & Valleroy, 1974; Pangborn, 1975; Riggs, 1980; Saldana & Brown, 1984).

Some people, based on their culture, have not been traditionally known to make food choices solely on the basis of nutritional and health values of food. For example, one of the most nutritious vegetables, based on nutritional density, consumed in the United States is broccoli; however, broccoli ranks twenty-first among vegetables consumed. On the other hand, the tomato, which is the most commonly eaten vegetable in the United States, ranks sixteenth as a source of vitamins and minerals (Farb & Armelagos, 1980).

When people relocate, they carry established food habits to the new location, but these habits are retained only if the foods are available in the new location and are affordable. Foods in various cultures have different prestige or status. For example, beef and certain seafoods, such as lobster, are regarded as high-status foods among people in the United States. Hindus from India consider cows to be sacred and therefore do not eat beef. In seafaring countries seafoods have no status value, since they are common. Foods obtain their status rating from various factors, including religious beliefs, availability, cost, cultural values, traditions, and/or because a highly respected individual has endorsed it. Even today, in many cultures men and their opinions regarding food preferences are more highly regarded than women and their opinions. In fact, in certain cultures men are so highly regarded that they are served meals first, before women and children. As a result of this practice, women and children may receive insufficient quantities and less varieties of foods.

Food also has symbolic meaning, in some cultures, that has nothing to do with nutritious value. In these cultures eating becomes associated with sentiments and assumptions about oneself and the world (Chang, 1974; Farb & Armelagos, 1980). Food becomes symbolic to people not only because of religious connotations, but also because it can be used as a reward. For example, a mother who gives a child candy or ice cream as a reward for good behavior may be reinforcing that food as a good food. On the other hand, a mother who serves a particular food (for example, broccoli or cabbage) and says she is doing so because of bad behavior may be reinforcing that food as a bad food and/or punishment.

Food patterns and nutrition among Black Americans. Food patterns among Black Americans are not that significantly different from those of non-Blacks living in the same geographic area. However, distinct differences do exist for Black Americans living and raised in the North as compared with those living and raised in the South. Blacks, as a cultural group, are in the lower socioeconomic groups, which may precipitate nutritional problems. As a result of nutritional deficiencies Black Americans tend to have medical problems that are somewhat different from those of White Americans. As mentioned earlier, hypertension is a medical problem that is twice as great among Blacks as among Whites. Another medical problem, particularly in women, that has been linked to food patterns and selections is obesity. Soul foods, which are generally cooked for long periods of time and are well seasoned, may also contribute to many of the medical problems that Blacks encounter. Taking their roots from southern Blacks who saw their preparation as economical, soul foods include:

Name of food	Region	Type of food	Description
Poke salad	Southern U.S.	Wild greens	Prepared with spicy seasoning and fat-back
Collard greens	Southern U.S.	Garden raised	Prepared with spicy seasoning and fat-back
Fatback	Southern U.S.	Pork fat	Prepared from loin of pig
Chicken wings	Southern U.S.	Chicken	Prepared by frying with spicy seasoning
Chitterlings	Southern U.S.	Meat	Intestines of young pigs that are boiled or fried
Hog maws	Southern U.S.	Meat	Stomach of pig
Grits	Southern U.S.	Grain	Hulled and coarsely ground corn that is boiled and simmered
Hoppin' John	Southern U.S.	Combination	Black-eyed peas and rice
Dandelion greens	Southern U.S.	Wild greens	Prepared with spicy seasoning and fat-back
Ribs	Southern U.S.	Pork meat	Prepared with spicy seasoning and slow heat

A cultural pattern that has been established among Black pregnant women is the consumption of non-food items (pica), which supposedly originated because of nutritional needs. Another common practice among children under 3 years of age, pregnant women, and some men is the eating of earthy substances such as dirt or clay. This practice is known as geophagy and is practiced mainly in the lower socioeconomic groups. For many years in African society the biological need for calcium, iron, and other minerals, especially by pregnant and lactating women, was partially met by eating clays that were high in nutrients. An analysis of some clays has revealed significant amounts of calcium, magnesium, potassium, copper, zinc, and iron, which are the same substances that have been prescribed for pregnant and lactating women in modern societies (Farb & Armelagos, 1980). Africans who were brought to the United States as slaves continued to eat clay, which is still bought in some areas of the South and shipped to relatives in the North. However, geophagy leads to iron deficiency, mainly because clay inhibits the absorption of iron, potassium, and zinc (Halsted, 1968). It is believed that geophagy is both a cause and a consequence of anemia. In areas where clay is not readily available, laundry starch is sometimes substituted, although it can irritate the stomach and is almost completely lacking in valuable minerals.

There are many clinical implications for the nurse in meeting the nutritional needs of Black Americans, who normally have lower hemoglobin and hematocrit levels than non-Blacks (Dalman, Bar, & Allen, 1978; Garn, Ryan, & Abraham, 1980). Although these lower hemoglobin and hematocrit levels are thought to be partially caused by genetics, some studies suggest that nutritional factors may also be responsible (Jackson et al., 1983). Another clinical implication for the nurse who cares for Black Americans is that of lactose intolerance. Many Black Americans are lactose intolerant but can tolerate such milk products as buttermilk, yogurt, fermented cheese, and small quantities of milk. In addition certain nutrients known to be low in the

Black American diet include iron, calcium, and vitamin A. Another clinical implication for Black Americans is the high incidence of hypertension, which may necessitate a low-sodium diet. Since Black Americans habitually use large amounts of salt and other spicy seasonings, special attention needs to be given to the importance of seasoning foods to make them acceptable and at the same time limiting the use of salt.

Food patterns and nutrition among Puerto Ricans. Many Puerto Ricans, like persons from other Latin American cultures, subscribe to the theory of "hot" and "cold." The major differentiation for Puerto Ricans is that they classify diseases as hot and cold, and foods and medications as hot, cold, and cool. Both Indian and Spanish influences are reflected in Puerto Rican native dishes. Foods enjoyed by Puerto Ricans include:

Name of food	Type of food	Description
Acerola	Fruit	Barbados cherry
Arroz bianco	Grain	Enriched white rice
Bacalao	Meat	Salted codfish
San cocho	Combination	Soup prepared with meat and viandas
Safrito	Seasoning	Specially treated tomato sauce
Viandas	Vegetable	Starchy tropical vegetables that include plantains, green bananas, and sweet potatoes

The common fare of Puerto Ricans is rice cooked grainy and dried, and red or white beans stewed with bacon or olive oil, garlic, and onions. Another common fare is safrito, which is a tasty mixture of tomatoes, green peppers, sweet chili peppers, onions, garlic, oregano, and fresh coriander cooked together in lard or vegetable oil and used as a relish to season foods. Other foods eaten regularly in Puerto Rico include a variety of foods such as viandas (starchy vegetables, including plantains, sweet potatoes, and green bananas) and cassava, bread fruit, acerola, mango, avocado, corn, okra, chayotes, and tubers. The acerola, which is also called the West Indian or Barbados cherry, is the highest known source of vitamin C. The acerola contains 1000 mg of vitamin C per 100 g portion. Many of the food items that are common in the United States are very expensive because they have to be imported. Chicken, pork, and beef, which are normally fried, are usually limited in the diet because of their cost. Eggs are generally used as the main dish and may be served as omlettes. Milk is a very popular food item in Puerto Rico but is seldom drunk as a beverage. The intake of milk is thought to be low in native Puerto Rico because of its cost. A popular beverage is cafe con leche, which is a combination of coffee with 2 to 5 ounces of milk. This beverage constitutes the largest portion of milk that is consumed. For the most part, foods are cooked for very long periods of time, or they are fried. Lard and salt pork are commonly used to flavor many dishes. One food item that has an exaggerated reputation for being nutritious and is often given to children and lactating women is malt beer.

There are many clinical implications for the nurse in meeting the nutritional needs of Puerto Ricans whether native or American. Pregnant Puerto Rican women have a high incidence of megaloblastic anemia and therefore should be instructed to increase their intake of foods that are high in folic acid (Parker & Bowering, 1976). For the patient who needs to control carbohydrate intake, the nurse needs to instruct the patient about the necessity of counting viandas as bread exchanges. The nurse also needs to be aware that the diet of Puerto Ricans who have moved to mainland cities may lack variety because of the inability of some Puerto Ricans to afford the native island foods that they were accustomed to getting previously. Therefore the nurse and the patient should look for acceptable food items that are comparable in health value.

Food patterns and nutrition among Cubans. A major portion of the Cuban diet includes cut-up vegetables, stews, and casseroles that have been flavored with sage, parsley, bay leaves, thyme, cinnamon, curry powder, capers, onions, cloves, garlic, and saffron. An integral part of Cuban food preparation is saffron, which is so heavily used in the Cuban diet that some dishes are considered anemic looking and unpalatable unless they have a deep golden saffron hue. Chicken, fish, or meat soup is served at least once a day, before each major meal. Salad is also served every day, along with fried foods, especially fish, poultry, and eggs. Most Cuban people eat rice and beans of many different varieties. While fruits and vegetables are plentiful, most Cuban refugees state that fruits and vegetables are not consumed on a regular basis (Gorden, 1982). The typical breakfast of Cuban people consists of coffee and bread. Some Cuban adults drink a lot of strong coffee and rum. Foods enjoyed by Cubans include such food items as:

Name of food	Type of food	Description
Guava	Fruit	Small yellow or red sweet tropical fruit
Plantains	Fruit	Banana-like fruit that tastes like sweet potatoes and is boiled or fried

There are many clinical implications for the nurse in meeting the nutritional needs of Cuban people. The nurse needs to be aware that in most Cuban diets calcium intake is normally low; therefore the nurse should instruct the patient to incorporate some cheese and milk into the diet. In addition, the nurse should advise the patient to replace fried foods with other methods of food preparation, such as boiling or broiling. In addition, the patient should be advised that long cooking periods for some foods such as pork is beneficial.

Food patterns and nutrition among Native Americans. A problem for Native Americans living on reservations that is as prevalent today as it was in the past is food scarcity and a lack of food variety. For Native Americans fresh fruits, vegetables, and meats are very expensive, if these items are available at all. Traditional foods may vary among tribes; however, the basic Native American diet consists of corn, beans, and squash. A status food for most tribes is corn. Chili pepper is widely used among tribes because it adds spice to the diet and is considered to be a good source of vitamin C. On some reservations and particularly among some tribes, diets are considered to be very poor, supplying less than two thirds of the recommended daily allowances for one or more nutrients (Miller, 1981). The diets tend to be inadequate in calories, calcium, iron, iodine, riboflavin, and vitamins A and C (Owens et al., 1981).

Poor nutrition has been directly related to several leading causes of death among Native Americans, including heart disease and cirrhosis of the liver. Diabetes is three times more common among some Native American tribes (Miller, 1981). Native Americans have the highest reported prevalence of NIDDM (type II diabetes mellitus). In the Pima tribe hyperinsulinemia reflects a resistance to insulin action (Nagulesparan, Savage, & Knowler, 1982). Among some Native American tribes there is a prevalence for low hemoglobin values and mild thyroid deficiencies (Interdepartmental Commission on National Defense and Division of Indian Public Health [ICND & DIPH], 1964). Foods enjoyed by Native Americans include:

Name of food	Type of food	Description
Prickly pear	Fruit	Fruit of cactus

There are many clinical implications for the nurse in meeting the nutritional needs of Native American people. The nurse needs to recognize that the diets of most Native American tribes tend to be inadequate in protein, calcium, and vitamins C and A, which may be due to unavailability or economics. Another problem found among Native American tribes is the prevalence of lactose deficiency. The nurse should advise the patient to consume foods, other than milk, that are high in calcium and riboflavin.

Food patterns and nutrition among Japanese persons. Most Japanese dishes are ideally suited for American life because they are economical and nutritious. Japanese people take great pride in the visual effect of foods that they prepare. In the Japanese culture the arrangement of food, color contrasts, and even shape are considered to be as important as the cooking and seasoning of a particular food. In addition, the rules for picking up chopsticks, holding bowls and teacups, and eating soups are traditions that are well established and regularly observed. These traditional rules of etiquette are as important to the Japanese people as the preparation of the food.

Most of the foods are cooked on a hibachi (a small grill) by broiling, steaming, and stir frying. It is thought in the Japanese culture that stir frying preserves vitamins because the food is cooked only briefly. Meat, which is very expensive in Japan, is stretched with vegetables. Fish is used in some fascinating ways, such as being served raw. A common fare of the Japanese people is soybean products, which are considered to be an important source of protein, and tofu is used extensively. In the Japanese culture salads are rarely served with meals, and bread is often replaced by rice or noodles. The Japanese people have a tendency to use extraordinary flavors when cooking, such as wheat germ powder, which is called ajinomoto. Another important seasoning in Japanese cooking is soy sauce. The common beverages included in the Japanese diet among adults are unsweetened green tea (which is the national beverage), beer, and sake (rice wine). Milk is often included in the children's diet in the Japanese culture but is rarely used by adults. Foods enjoyed by the Japanese people include:

Name of food	Type of food	Description
Ajinomoto	Grain—wheat germ	Wheat germ
Sake	Beverage	Rice wine
Sashimi	Meat	Raw fish
Shoyu	Seasoning	Soy sauce
Tempura	Combination	Deep-fried seafoods and vegetables
Tofu	Vegetables	Soybean curds

There are many clinical implications for the nurse in meeting the nutritional needs of Japanese people. A common clinical problem found among the Japanese people is lactose intolerance. The nurse working with a Japanese patient should advise the patient to consume sources of calcium other than milk, such as tofu. The nurse should also advise the patient to use enriched rice and to avoid washing the grains before cooking to preserve the nutrient value. When working with a Japanese patient on a sodium-restricted diet, the nurse should teach the patient to measure the amount of soy sauce used and to avoid eating the many types of pickles that are ordinarily eaten. Another important clinical implication that the nurse should be cognizant of is the high incidence of stomach cancer among Japanese people, which has been associated with the high intake of raw fish among Japanese people (Qureshi, 1981). Raw fish is thought to carry the risk of infestation with fish tapeworms (Goldman, 1985) and has been associated with outbreaks of gastroenteritis (Morse, Guzewich, & Hanrahan, 1986).

Food patterns and nutrition among Koreans. Just as in other Oriental cultures, the main staple of the Korean diet is rice, which is mixed with other grains. The Korean people generally mix rice with barley, millet, and red beans because it is thought that a diet consisting of only white rice causes health problems. Most Korean people eat three meals daily, which are of equal proportions. Before cooking, foods are cut into small pieces to facilitate the use of chopsticks. Soups containing seaweed, meat, or fish are always served. One of the most popular condiments in Korea is ginseng; the Korean people believe that ginseng has roots resembling the human fetus, is a panacea for curing illnesses regardless of age or sex, and is an aphrodisiac.

Korea is a country that is surrounded on all three sides by water; thus fish products are plentiful and account for 85% of the nation's animal protein intake. Almost every conceivable kind of fish is served, whether raw, freshly steamed, or salted and dried. One of the most expensive food items in Korea is eggs, since they are scarce. The preferred meat of the Korean people is beef, which is prepared by marinating it with lots of sugar to provide a crispy coating. Kimchi involves one of the most nutritious preservative processes available in Korea and does not require refrigeration. Kimchi is prepared with chopped vegetables that are highly seasoned, salted, and fermented underground or in a special earthenware container. Kimchi can also be prepared from naturally grown vegetables such as cabbage, turnips, cucumbers, and other seasonable vegetables that are soaked in salt water overnight and seasoned the next day with garlic, scallions, ginger, and hot pepper. Kimchi is fermented without disturbance for at least 1 month and is best after 2 or 3 months.

Many vegetables are grown in Korea; thus Korean people serve both fresh vegetables and a lot of kimchi routinely. Vegetables are never overcooked and are seasoned with red and black pepper, garlic, sesame seed oil, and soy sauce. Since Korea is a country surrounded by water on three sides, seaweed is plentiful and is a food item that is highly prized for its nutritive value. In the Korean culture seaweed is a must for the expectant mother. A common fare in Korea is noodles made from rice flour. A Korean diet consists of many products made from soybeans, such as soy sauce, soybean paste, bean sprouts, bean curds, and soy milk. The dairy products of Korea include bean curd and soy milk. Because Korea is a densely populated country, there is no room for a dairy industry; thus milk is very expensive and scarce and is therefore served only to children. Because milk is so scarce, babies are often weaned from the breast as late as 2 years of age.

Fresh fruits are readily available in Korea and include apples, peaches, strawberries, pears, watermelons, blackberries, pomegranates, currants, and cherries. Fruit is generally served with each meal. Pastries such as cakes and pies are usually not served with meals; however, they can be found in many small specialty shops.

The national beverage of Korea is made from ginseng; Korea has never been a tea-drinking nation. Another beverage that usually accompanies a Korean meal is barley water, which is served cold in the summer and warm in the winter. Barley water is prepared with grains that stick to the pan after the rice for the meal has been removed. To this rice a cup or two of water is added, and the liquid is allowed to simmer slowly while the meal is being eaten; it is then served after the meal. Foods enjoyed by the Korean people include:

Name of food	Type of food	Description
Barley water	Beverage	Prepared from leftover rice grains
Ginseng	Condiment	Spice
Kimchi	Combination	Vegetables that are highly seasoned, salted, and fermented underground for 1 to 3 months

There are many clinical implications for the nurse in meeting the nutritional needs of Korean people. To date, the medicinal properties of ginseng have been poorly researched (Barna, 1985). However, it is thought that the long-term abuse of ginseng may be a contributing factor of hypertension. Other, less frequently seen adverse reactions from the long-term abuse of ginseng include nervousness, sleeplessness, skin eruptions, morning diarrhea, edema (Siegel, 1979), and irregularities in blood glucose levels ("Ginseng," 1980). The nurse who works with Korean American patients must keep in mind that in the United States rice is not commonly mixed with other grains, as is practiced in Korea. To increase the nutritive value of rice, the patient should use whole-grain or enriched rice.

Since Korean people are accustomed to the taste of seaweed, which is expensive, the nurse should encourage the patient to substitute seaweed with stronger-tasting greens such as turnip greens, kale, and mustard greens. Lactose intolerance is a common problem among adults in Korea. Thus the nurse should encourage the patient to substitute other dairy products for fresh milk, such as cottage cheese, yogurt, and aged cheese, as well as the nondairy product tofu. For a diabetic Korean patient, a sugar substitute may be dissolved in hot water and poured over meat that is broiled until the crispy texture has been achieved (Maras & Adolphi, 1985). While kimchi is a zesty accompaniment to plain, broiled foods, it is not readily available in the United States; therefore, a Mexican salsa may be used as a substitute (Maras & Adolphi, 1985).

Food patterns and nutrition among Middle Eastern people. The Middle East is composed of nine separate countries around the eastern Mediterranean sea: Greece, Turkey, Lebanon, Syria, Iraq, Iran, Israel, Jordan, and Egypt. These nine countries are bound together by foods and certain attitudes about foods. The common staple of the Middle Eastern people is lamb and goat. Because of the climate and the lack of suitable pasture land, beef is not favored in the Middle Eastern countries. In most Middle Eastern countries, dolma, a very popular meat dish, is often served. Dolma is made of ground meat mixed with rice, herbs, and spices and then wrapped in leaves or stuffed in vegetables. Since these nine countries are surrounded by the eastern Mediterranean seaboard, all varieties of saltwater and freshwater fish, shellfish, and roe are served. In some of the Mediterranean countries bound by religious tradition, some foods are restricted. For example, many Moslems avoid eating pork and wild birds; the main dish of the Moslem people is vegetables and legumes.

For most Middle Eastern people, bread is the staple of life; for every mouthful of food, most Middle Eastern people eat a mouthful of bread (Valassi, 1962). A meal without bread is unthinkable for most Middle Eastern people. Bread is generally homemade, fresh, and warm, and the more compact dark bread is preferred to refined white bread. Pilaf is a festive dish that is served in the entire Middle East. Other common fares of the Middle Eastern countries include beans and lentils, which rank directly behind bread and rice.

In the Middle East boiled beans are served cold with olive oil dressing and lemon juice. In addition, a variety of vegetables, both cooked and raw, are served. Seasonings commonly used by Middle Easterners in food preparation include onions, fresh tomato paste, olive oil, and parsley. There are more than 120 ways of preparing eggplant, which is a favorite of most Middle Easterners.

Baklava is one of the most popular and best-known sweets in the Middle East. However, sweets are generally served only on holidays or during social calls. Unlike Americans, Middle Easterners seldom serve sweets as desert. Instead, a bowl of fresh fruit consisting of cucumbers, guavas, mangoes, citrus fruits, dates, figs, pomegranates, or bananas is the usual desert. Cooking fats used in Middle Eastern cooking include olive and sesame oil, butter, and gee, which is a clarified butter made from goat's, sheep's, or camel's milk. Middle Easterners use animal fat to cook foods when the dish is to be eaten hot and oils when the dish is to be eaten cold. Meals are not considered tasteful and well prepared unless a large quantity of fat is used. The popular spices in the Middle East include mint, oregano, and cinnamon. The most popular herb is garlic. The exception to this is found in Iran, where garlic is considered vulgar. Olives in many shapes and colors are popular.

Milk is not commonly served to adults; however, it is given to children. Yogurt is considered to be a supreme health food that cures many ills, confers long life and good looks, prolongs youth, and fortifies the soul. Yogurt is served in many foods; for example, it is mixed with diced cucumbers and is used as a topping for rice, fried vegetables, and deserts. Thin yogurt that has been diluted with water is considered safer, less perishable, and more thirst quenching than milk. A specialty cheese served by Greek people is feta, a white cheese made from sheep's or goat's milk.

Wine is a forbidden drink in the Moslem faith. Other than Christians and Jews, many Near Easterners do not drink alcoholic beverages of any kind. Every meal is ended with coffee or tea; however, coffee takes precedence most of the time. The exception to this is found in Iran, where the favorite drink is tea served hot and sweet. Foods enjoyed by Middle Eastern people include:

Name of food	Culture	Type of food	Description
Baklava	Greek	Desert	Layered pastry made with honey
Bulgur	Middle Eastern	Grain	Granular wheat product with nutlike flavor
Dolmades	Greek	Combination	Grape leaves stuffed with beef
Feta	Greek	Dairy product	Soft, salty, white cheese made from sheep's or goat's milk
Kibbeh	Middle East	Meat	Fresh, raw lamb, ground and seasoned, similar to meat loaf
Moussaka	Greek	Combination	Meat and eggplant casserole
Phyllo	Greek	Grain	Paper-thin pastry for meat, vegetables, cheese and egg dishes, and pastries

There are many clinical implications for the nurse in working with people from the Middle East. Because fresh milk is not normally consumed by adults from most Middle Eastern countries, the protein and calcium content of the diet needs to be increased. The nurse should encourage the Middle Eastern patient to substitute fresh milk with yogurt, since it is a favorite of most Middle Eastern people. White cheese, cottage cheese, and aged sharp cheese can also be substituted for fresh milk. For the patient on a carbohydrate-restricted diet, the nurse must remember that since bread is high in carbohydrates, it should be restricted or eliminated from the diet. The elimination of bread from the diet of persons in cultures where bread is a main staple is difficult. However, the nurse must stress to the patient the importance of reducing carbohydrate intake. Since fat is used in large quantities to add taste to meals, the amount of fat in the diet could pose problems for patients on low-calorie, diabetic, or low-fat diets. For patients on sodium-restricted diets, feta cheese and olives should be eliminated from the diet.

Nutritional deficiencies

Racially related nutritional deficiencies include lactose intolerance and glucose-6-phosphate dehydrogenase (G-6-PD) deficiency. Lactose intolerance, or intolerance to milk, is a relatively common condition that is considered normal in many ethnic groups. It is found in over 66% of Mexican Americans and is very common in Black Americans, some American Indian tribes, Orientals, and Ashkenazic Jews (Bayless, 1975; Burns & Neubort, 1984; Kisch, 1953). In fact, it has been reported to be found in approximately 90% of adult Blacks, American Indians, and Orientals. While lactose intolerance is very common among these racial groups, it is reported to be much less common among Whites of northern European extraction, with only 5% to 15% of this population having the disorder. Yet the statistical significance reported among Whites of northern European extraction indicates that this condition is more than a rare phenomenon.

The cause of lactose intolerance is an insufficient amount of lactase, the enzyme responsible for converting the nonabsorbable milk sugar, lactose, into the absorbable sugars glucose and galactose. With lactase deficiency, any undigested lactose will remain in the small intestine, where, because of its osmotic capacity, it draws water. When the lactose reaches the colon, it begins to combine acetic acid and hydrogen gas, which results in the symptoms of lactose intolerance: cramping, flatulence, abdominal bloating, and diarrhea. These symptoms are dose related, meaning that they occur only if the person ingests more food containing lactose than the person's supply of available lactase can metabolize. Foods containing large amounts of lactose include milk, yogurt, and milk chocolate. Of these food items, nonfat dry milk contains the most lactose. Foods containing moderate amounts of lactose include cream, cottage cheese, and most cheeses. Even unlikely foods such as dried soup, cookies made from prepared mixes, cold cuts, and bread and butter contain small amounts of lactose ("When Patients," 1976).

The nurse must be cognizant of foods that can cause lactose intolerance symptoms, particularly when working with persons who are extremely lactose intolerant. For the majority of patients, treatment of this condition is usually a matter of restricting lactose-containing foods rather than eliminating them altogether. An adult who is advised to restrict milk and milk products but otherwise eat a well-balanced diet should not need any nutritional supplements. However, for pregnant or lactating women, nutritional supplements (for example, calcium tablets) may be necessary. Lactose intolerance does not generally develop until after childhood; children who are lactose deficient should be encouraged to eat aged cheeses, since the aging process changes lactase to lactic acid. In addition, some physicians may recommend a soy-bean-based milk substitute, as well as vitamins and calcium supplements. Even for the adult lactose-deficient patient, the astute nurse can suggest alternatives to milk products, such as cheese aged over 60 days. The nurse should be aware that telling the patient to drink milk may not necessarily be good advice for many adults in the world and should give special consideration to the pregnant or lactating woman in light of the fact that most racial groups with the exception of Whites cannot tolerate milk in adulthood (Bayless, 1975).

G-6-PD deficiency is another enzyme deficiency disorder that is more prevalent in certain racial or ethnic groups. While it is more prevalent in certain groups, these groups may have different forms of the deficiency. Williams (1975) reported that the type A variety, which moves rapidly on starch-gel electrophoresis, is found in 35% of American Blacks who have the deficiency. The slower-moving type B variety is found in 65% of Blacks who have the deficiency and in nearly all non-Blacks who have the deficiency. However, all forms affect males more than females because the genetic inheritance is carried on the X chromosome. The Canton/Chinese disorder of G-6-PD is another form that has been found among the Chinese population and the people of Southeast Asia. The incidence of the Canton-Chinese form ranges from 2% to 5% (Williams, 1975). Still another form of G-6-PD deficiency is the Mediterranean variety, which is the most clinically severe type. This form of G-6-PD deficiency affects up to 50% of male Greeks, Sardinians, and Sephardic Jews.

G-6-PD is an enzyme constituent of the red blood cells and is involved in the hexose monophosphate pathway, which accounts for 10% of glucose metabolism of the red blood cells. Under normal circumstances the proportion of glucose metabolized through this pathway may increase greatly if the cells are subjected to oxidants causing metabolic stress. The result is the formation of increased methemoglobin and degradation of hemoglobin. In addition, certain medications tend to overwhelm the protective mechanism, especially when older red blood cells are involved, because of a decline in G-6-PD activity with the aging of these cells. Red blood cells with a genetically determined deficiency of G-6-PD are unable to withstand lesser oxidative stresses, and, as a result, a hemolytic process ensues that precipitates a significant anemia. In the presence of certain conditions G-6-PD-deficient red blood cells hemolyze; thus hemoyltic anemia is the clinical manifestation of this disorder.

Conditions that precipitate hemolytic anemia in susceptible persons include the administration of certain drugs such as quinine, aspirin, phenacetin, chloramphenicol, probenecid, sulfonamides, and the thiazide diuretics. The presence of infection and the ingestion of fava beans (also called broad or horse beans) are also linked to the precipitous onset of hemolytic anemia. The fava bean is a dietary staple in some of the Mediterranean countries such as Greece and those of North Africa. Favism, a condition induced by ingesting the fava bean, is one of the most severe forms of G-6-PD hemolysis. G-6-PD deficiency has also been related to an adaptive process that has prevented malaria. The discerning nurse should assist the patient in identifying substances that are likely to precipitate hemolytic episodes. In addition, the patient should be taught to exercise caution to prevent serious infections from ensuing. G-6-PD deficiency is a condition that remains asymptomatic until an exposure occurs. The nurse must understand that hemolytic episodes are the result of culturally related nutritional habits, and geographic and environmental location.

Psychological Characteristics

Gaitz and Scott (1974) have indicated that although cultural factors may influence mental health scores in research studies, such scores are not indicative of whether one cultural group has more or fewer incidences of mental illness than another. There are many different definitions of mental health, one of which postulates that a person is mentally healthy when there is a balance in the person's internal life and adaptation to reality. Thus it can be determined that normal behavior is relative to a specific culture and that different psychological characteristics are promoted by each culture. Other variables that influence mental health include family relationships, child-rearing practices, language, attitudes toward illness, and social and economic status.

Some cultural groups have a low socioeconomic status, which consequently affects mental health. For example, some Mexican Americans have a low socioeconomic status in terms of substandard housing, education, physical health, political influence, communication, and social exclusion. The concept of social exclusion must be considered as a contributing factor in the failure of any particular cultural group to assimilate the culture of the wider society. Broad exposure to other life-styles, cultures, environments, and ideas facilitates an understanding and flexibility on the part of an individual when dealing with other people or when solving problems. Feelings of insecurity may also be related to cultural background. For example, psychological adjustment may be difficult for an American Indian who has lived on a reservation and goes to a college where there are few other Indians. The difficulty in adjustment may be attributable to the fact that this person has lived in an isolated environment in which there is a failure to become assimilated into the mainstream of society. Therefore it is important to take into consideration both ethnicity and economic factors when assessing mental health status.

There has been no consistent attack on problems of mental illness around the world. While no continent or island area has been immune from mental illness, the study of mental illness in relation to culture has been restricted and often localized. There may have been a hesitancy to study cultures and mental illness because of possible implications of racism (Griffith & Griffith, 1986). Some authorities cite that psychiatry has also not seriously discussed the possibility that racism may be a manifestation of an individual psychological disorder (Poussaint, 1975). In any case, research on mental illness on a broad world perspective has been seriously lacking.

While research, for the most part, is lacking, some interesting cultural data and implications are available in the studies that have been reported. Not only do mental illnesses seem to vary among cultures, but treatment does as well. In Japan psychiatric institutions are small, whereas in the United States they are large. Societies also have differing demands on individuals emerging from the treatment milieu. Not only do hospitals and treatment milieus differ around the world, but also the paths into illness show a different topography in each culture. Variations in class identity or in the pace of acculturation of class segments may produce differences in deviant types. Similarly, personalities seem to vary among persons from different geographic regions. There is some evidence that the cultural backgrounds and forms of illness vary apart from the question of how these illnesses are treated. For example, stresses placed on a traditional Chinese family are different from those placed on Hindus and Malays (Opler, 1959).

Lawson (1986) reported findings suggesting that racial and ethnic differences exist in the clinical presentations of psychiatric disorders. Significant racial differences have been noted among proposed biological markers for various psychiatric disorders, such as serum creatinine phosphokinase, platelet serotonin, and HLA-A2 determinations. Racial and ethnic differences in response to psychotropic medication, such as higher blood levels of the drugs found among Asians, affect dosage requirements and potential side effects. All of these developments underline the importance of considering ethnic and racial factors in caring for psychiatric patients.

In the United States the incidence of mental illness has been found to vary among certain racial groups. For example, posttraumatic stress disorder (PTSD) has been studied among Vietnam veterans. Because of racism in the military and racial and social upheaval in the United States during the Vietnam War years, as well as limited opportunities for Blacks in the postwar period, Black veterans of the Vietnam War often have harbored conflicting feelings about their wartime experiences. Black veterans have been found to suffer PTSD at a higher rate than White veterans. Diagnosis, as well as treatment, of PTSD among Blacks is complicated by a tendency to misdiagnose Black patients, by the varied manifestations of PTSD, by patients' frequent alcohol and drug abuse, and by medical, legal, personality, and vocational problems (Allen, 1986).

Also, in the United States there is evidence that schizophrenia has been consistently overdiagnosed and affective disorders underdiagnosed, particularly among Blacks and lower socioeconomic groups (Gurland, 1976; Taylor & Abrams, 1978; World Health Organization, 1976). General causes of such misdiagnoses include overreliance on the classic thought disorder symptoms pathognomonic of schizophrenia and, for affective disorders, lack of clearly defined boundaries between normal and abnormal mood, as well as failure to realize that patients with affective illness can manifest cognitive thought processes. In addition, according to Jones and Gray (1986), misdiagnoses among Blacks result from such factors as cultural differences in language and mannerisms, difficulties in relating between Black patients and White therapists and staff, and the myth that Blacks rarely suffer from affective disorders. The effects of cultural and racial differences on baseline behaviors and symptomatology have thus far received little consistent attention. Research is needed to investigate more closely how the general diagnostic problems in psychiatry affect certain racial groups. Research is also needed on how cultural and racial differences may affect diagnosis. Finally, baselines behaviors and symptomatology for racial groups need to be established.

Meinhardt and Vega (1987) have reported that most studies of utilization of mental health services by ethnic groups have used parity as a measure of whether members of ethnic groups are receiving a fair share of services. The level of services is assumed to be adequate if the percentage of ethnic group members in the treatment population is the same as the group's percentage in the general population. However, service planning based on achieving parity fails to consider that some groups may have higher levels of need than others. Equitable care between ethnic and racial groups based on need is another issue that mental health professionals are addressing (Lopez, 1981).

A better understanding of the differences among various cultures in the area of mental health and treatment for mental illness will enable culturally appropriate mental health care. Griffith and Griffith (1986) have pointed out that mental health professionals should give more consideration to the fact that cultural issues such as racism can cause psychological injury. It is evident from the increasing quantities of literature on culture and mental health that there is a growing awareness among health professionals that care for patients with mental problems must be culturally appropriate and that cultural factors do affect mental health. While rice and tea may not be the most potent tools of modern psychiatry, they may play an important role in making psychiatric care acceptable to the acutely disturbed Asian or Pacific American psychiatric patient (Lu, 1987). It is important for the nurse to study what is available about the population groups being served and to consider the important differences that may be required in the care provided. Not only must the nurse appreciate that caring for patients from different cultural groups may require different care methods, but the nurse must also assist other mental health workers in being sensitive to differing care needs.

CASE STUDY   Sarah Jennings is a 21-year-old Black, married woman and the mother of a 12-month-old daughter. Mrs. Jennings was diagnosed at age 11 as having sickle cell anemia. For the last 3 years, she has remained largely asymptomatic. She is admitted to the hospital in sickle cell crisis. Her admitting complaints include severe joint pains in both the upper and lower extremities, a temperature of 101.8° F, and shortness of breath. On physical examination, the nurse notes that Mrs. Jennings has coarse rales in the base of both lungs, and that her lips are cyanotic and dry. Her nail beds are also cyanotic, and when they are blanched, capillary refill is slow. Initial laboratory examination reveals a hemoglobin of 8 g/dl. During the nursing history taking, it is revealed that Mrs. Jennings has also had problems drinking milk and eating certain dairy products for most of her adult life.

STUDY QUESTIONS
1. List at least two contributing factors for Mrs. Jennings' sickle cell anemia that relate to biological variations by race and ethnic heritage.
2. List at least one other racial group with a predisposition for sickle cell crisis.
3. List the basic etiology of sickle cell anemia.
4. List at least two other conditions that Mrs. Jennings could be at risk for developing because of her race and ethnic heritage.
5. Describe at least two differences noted when assessing the skin color of dark-skinned individuals.

REFERENCES

Allen, I. (1986). Posttraumatic stress disorder among Black Vietnam veterans. *Hospital and Community Psychiatry, 37*(1), 55-60.

Barna, P. (1985). Food or drug? The case of ginseng. *Lancet, 2,* 548.

Bayless, T. (1975). Lactose and milk intolerance: Clinical implications. *New England Journal of Medicine, 292*(5), 1156-1159.

Bennett, K.A., Osborne, R.H., & Miller, R.J. (1975). *Biocultural ecology: Annual review of anthropology.* Palo Alto: Calif.: Annual Reviews.

Boyle, E. (1970). Biological patterns in hypertension by race, sex, body weight, and skin color. *JAMA, 213,* 1637-1643.

Branch, M., & Paxton, P. (1976). *Providing safe nursing care for ethnic people of color.* East Norwalk, Conn.: Appleton-Century-Crofts.

Bulmer, M. (1970). *The biology of twinning in man.* New York: Oxford University Press.

Burns, E., & Neubort, S. (1984). Sodium content of koshered meat (letter). *JAMA, 252*(21), 2960.

Burt, C.L. (1966). The genetic determination of difference in intelligence: A study of monozygote twins reared together and apart. *British Journal of Psychology 57,* 137-153.

Carter Center of Emory University. (1985). Closing the gap: The problem of diabetes mellitus in the United States. *Diabetes Care, 8,* 391-401.

Chang, B. (1974). Some dietary beliefs in Chinese folk culture. *Journal of the American Diet Association, 65*(4), 436.

Dalman, P.R., Bar, G.D., & Allen, C.M. (1978). Hemoglobin concentration in White, Black and Oriental children: Is there a need for separate criteria in screening for anemia? *American Journal of Clinical Nutrition, 31*(3), 377.

Divan, D. (1989). Letter to the editor. *The New England Journal of Medicine, 321*(4), 259.

Echizen, H., Horai, Y., & Ishizaki, T. (1989). Letter to the editor. *The New England Journal of Medicine, 321*(4), 258.

Farb, P., & Armelagos, G. (1980). *Consuming passions: The anthropology of eating.* Boston: Houghton Mifflin.

Gaitz, C., & Scott, J. (1974). Mental health of Mexican Americans: Do ethnic factors make a difference? *Geriatrics, 1*(11), 113-110.

Garn, S., Ryan, A.S., & Abraham, S. (1980). The Black-White difference in hemoglobin levels after age, sex, and income matching. *Ecology of Food Nutrition, 10*(2), 69.

Ginseng. (1980). *Medical Letter Drugs Therapy, 22*(17), 72.

Goedde, H. (1983). Population genetic studies on aldehyde dehydrogenase isoenzyme deficiency and alcohol sensitivity. *American Journal of Human Genetics, 35,* 769.

Goldman, D.R. (1985). Hold the sushi (letter). *JAMA, 253*(17), 2495.

Gorden, A.M. (1982). Nutritional status of Cuban refugees: A field study on the health and nutrition of refugees processed at Opa Locka, Florida. *American Journal of Clinical Nutrition, 35*(3), 582.

Griffith, E., & Griffith, E. (1986). Racism, psychological injury, and compensatory damages. *Hospital and Community Psychiatry, 37*(1), 71-75.

Gurland, B. (1976). Aims, organization, and initial studies of the cross-national project. *International Journal of Aging and Human Development, 7,* 283-293.

Halsted, J.A. (1968). Geophagia in man: Its nature and nutritional effects. *American Journal of Clinical Nutrition, 21*(12), 1384.

Holmes, T.H., et al. (1957). Psychosocial and psychophysiological studies of tuberculosis. *Psychosomatic Medicine, 19,* 134-143.

Interdepartmental Commission on National Defense and Division of Indian Public Health (ICND & DIPH). (1964). *Fort Belknap Indian Reservation: Nutrition survey.* Washington, D.C.: U.S. Public Health Service.

Jackson, R.T., Sauberlich, H.S., Skala, J.H., et al. (1983). Comparison of hemoglobin values in Black and White male U.S. military personnel. *Journal of Nutrition, 113*(1), 165.

Jarvis, A. (1972). Minor orofacial abnormalities in an Eskimo population. *Oral Surgery, 33,* 417-427.

Jensen, A.R. (1969). How much can we boast IQ and scholastic achievement? *Harvard Education Review, 29,* 1.

Jensen, A.R. (1974). Cumulative deficits: A testable hypothesis? *Developmental Psychology, 10,* 996.

Jensen, A.R. (1977). Cumulative deficit in IQ of Blacks in the rural South. *Developmental Psychology, 13,* 184.

Jick, H., et al. (1969). Venous thromboembolic disease and ABO blood type. *Lancet, 1,* 539-542.

Jones, B., & Gray, B. (1986). Problems in diagnosing schizophrenia and affective disorders among Blacks. *Hospital and Community Psychiatry, 37*(1), 61-65.

Kalow W. (1972). Pharmacogenetics of drugs used in anaesthesia. *Human Genetics, 60,* 415-427.

Kalow, W. (1982). The metabolism of xenobiotics in different populations. *Canadian Journal of Physiological Pharmacology, 60,* 1-19.

Kamlin, L.J. (1974). *The science and politics of IQ.* New York: John Wiley & Sons.

Katz, S.H., Hediger, M.L., & Valleroy, L.A. (1974). Traditional maize processing techniques in the New World. *Science, 184,* 765.

Kisch, B. (1953). Salt poor diet and Jewish dietary laws. *JAMA, 153*(16), 1472.

Krolewski, A., & Warram, G. (1985). Epidemiology of diabetes mellitus. In A. Marble et al. (Eds.), *Joslin's diabetes mellitus* (12th ed.). Philadelphia: Lea & Febiger.

Lawson, W. (1986). Racial and ethnic factors in psychiatric research. *Hospital and Community Psychiatry, 37*(1), 50-54.

Leffall, L.D. (1974). Cancer mortality among Blacks. *CA: A Cancer Journal for Clinicians, 24,* 42-46.

Leininger, M. (1970). *Nursing and anthropology: Two worlds to blend.* New York: John Wiley & Sons.

Lewis, J.H. (1942). *The biology of the Negro* (Chicago University Monographs in Medicine). Chicago: University of Chicago Press.

Lopez, S. (1981). Mexican Americans' usage of mental health facilities: Underutilization reconsidered. In A. Baron (Ed.), *Explorations in Chicano psychology.* New York: Praeger.

Lorton, J., & Lorton, E. (1984). Human development through the life span. Belmont, Calif.: Brooks/Cole.

Lu, F. (1987). Culturally relevant inpatient care for minority and ethnic patients. *Hospital and Community Psychiatry, 38*(11), 1126-1127.

Maras, M.L., & Adolphi, C.L. (1985). Ethnic tailoring improves dietary compliance. *Diabetes Education, 11*(4), 47.

Meinhardt, K., & Vega, W. (1987). A method of estimating underutilization of mental health services by ethnic groups. *Hospital and Community Psychiatry, 38*(11), 1186-1190.

Merck, Sharp, & Dohme. (1974). *Hypertension handbook for clinicians.* Westpoint, Pa.: Author.

Miller, M.B. (1981). Supplementing and adding variety to the diets of Indians on a reservation in Minnesota. *Journal of the American Dietetic Association, 78*(6), 626.

Morse, D.L., Guzewich, J.J., & Hanrahan, J.P. (1986). Widespread outbreaks of clam- and oyster-associated gastroenteritis. *New England Journal of Medicine, 314*(11), 678.

Nagulesparan, M., Savage, P.J., & Knowler, W.C. (1982). Increased in vivo insulin resistance in nondiabetic Pima Indians compared with Caucasians. *Diabetes, 31*(11), 952.

Opler, M. (Ed.). (1959). *Culture and health.* New York: Macmillan.

Overfield, T. (1977). Biological variations. *Nursing Clinics of North America, 12*(1), 19-27.

Overfield, T. (1985). *Biologic variations in health and illness: race, age and sex differences.* Reading, Mass.: Addison-Wesley.

Owens, G.M., Garry, P.J., Seymore, R.D., et al. (1981). Nutrition studies with White Mountain Apache pre-school children in 1976 and 1969. *American Journal of Clinical Nutrition, 34*(2), 266.

Pangborn, R.M. (1975). Cross-cultural aspects of flavor preferences. *Food Technology, 29*(6), 34.

Parker, S.L., & Bowering, J. (1976). Folacin in diets of Puerto Ricans and Black women in relation to food practices. *Journal of Nutrition Education, 8*(2), 73.

Phipps, W.J., Long, B.C., & Woods, N.F. (1987). *Medical surgical nursing: Concepts and clinical practice,* St. Louis: C.V Mosby.

Polednak, A. (1971). Connective tissue responses in Negroes in relation to disease. *American Journal of Physical Anthropology, 41,* 49-57.

Poussaint, A.F. (1975). Interracial relations. In A.M. Freedman, H.I. Kaplan, & B.J. Sandock (Eds.), *Comprehensive textbook of psychiatry* (2nd ed., Vol 2). Baltimore: Williams & Wilkins.

Qureshi, B.A. (1981). Nutrition and multi-ethnic groups. *Royal Social Health Journal, 101*(5), 187.

Rifkin, H. (Ed.). (1984). *The physician's guide to type II diabetes (NIDDN): Diagnosis and treatment.* New York: The American Diabetes Association.

Riggs, S. (1980). Tastes of America: Regionality. *Institutions, 87*(12), 76.

Rodnan, G., & Schumacher, H. (1983). *Primer on the rheumatic diseases* (8th ed.). Atlanta: Arthritis Foundation.

Rouch, L. (1977). Color changes in dark skin. *Nursing '77, 7*(1), 48-51.

Saldana, G., & Brown, H.E. (1984). Nutritional composition of corn and flour tortillas. *Journal of Food Science, 49*(4), 202.

Satcher, D., & Pope, L. (1974). *Emergency evaluation and management of persons with sickle cell disease.* Bethesda, Md.: National Institutes of Health.

Satcher, D., et al. (1973). *Sickle cell counseling: A committee's study and recommendations.* New York: National Foundation—March of Dimes.

Schwerin, H.S., Stanton, J.L., Smith, J.L., et al. (1982). Food, eating habits, and health: A further examination of the relationships between food eating patterns and nutritional health. *American Clinical Nutrition, 35*(Suppl. 5), 1319.

Siegel, R.K. (1979). Ginseng abuse syndrome: Problems with the panacea. *JAMA, 24*(15), 614.

Surgeon General. (1987, April). Speech to the media and the nation on AIDS.

Taylor, M.A., & Abrams, B. (1978). The prevalence of schizophrenia: A reassessment using modern diagnostic criteria. *American Journal of Psychiatry, 135,* 945-948.

Tipton, D. (1974, May). Physiological assessment of Black people. In *Care of Black patients* (X428.1). A group of papers presented at a conference on care of the Black patient, sponsored by Continuing Education in Nursing, University of California, San Francisco.

Valassi, K.V. (1962). Food habits of Greek Americans. *American Journal of Nursing, 11*(3), 240.

Vessell, E. (1972). Therapy-pharmacogenetics. *New England Journal of Medicine, 287*(18), 904-909.

Westfall, D. (1971, Nov.). Diabetes mellitus among the Florida Seminoles. *HSMHA Health Reports, 86,* 1037-1041.

When patients can't drink milk. (1976, Aug.). *Nursing Update,* pp. 10-12.

Williams, R.A. (Ed.). (1975). *Textbook of Black related disease.* New York: McGraw-Hill.

Witcop, E., et al. (1963). Oral and genetic studies of Chileans 1960: 1. Oral anomalies. *American Journal of Physical Anthropology, 21,* 15-24.

World Health Organization. (1976). *Schizophrenia: A multinational study.* Geneva: World Health Organization Press.

Wyngaarden, J.B., & Smith, L.H. (Eds.). (1985). *Cecil textbook of medicine.* Philadelphia: W.B. Saunders.

Zifferblatt, S.M., Wilbur, C.S., & Pinsky, J.L. (1980). Understanding food habits. *Journal of American Diet Association, 76*(1), 9.

Zhou, H.H., Koshakji, R.J.P., Silberstein, D.J., Wilkinson, G.R., & Wood, A.J.J. (1989). Racial differences in drug response: Altered sensitivity to and clearance of propranolol in men of Chinese descent as compared with American Whites. *New England Journal of Medicine, 320,* 565-570.

PART TWO

APPLICATION OF ASSESSMENT AND INTERVENTION TECHNIQUES TO SPECIFIC CULTURAL GROUPS

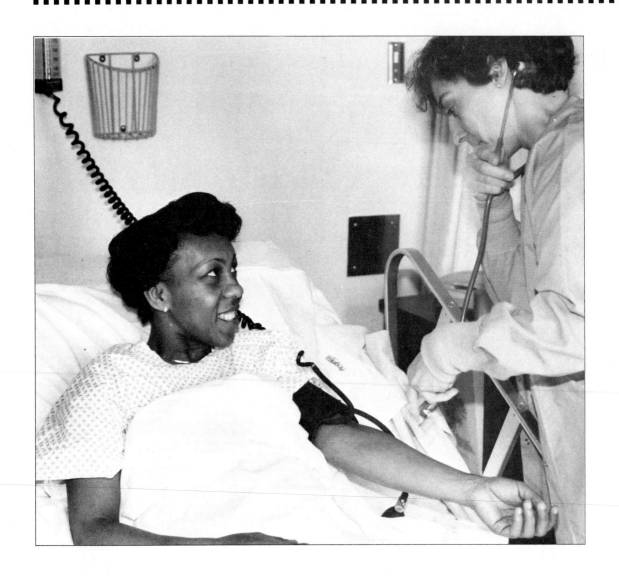

■ ■

CHAPTER 8

Black Americans

Brenda Cherry and Joyce Newman Giger

BEHAVIORAL OBJECTIVES

After reading this chapter, the nurse will be able to:

1 Identify ways in which the Black American culture influences Black individuals and health-seeking behaviors.

2 Recognize the need for an in-depth understanding of variables that are common within and across cultural groups in order to provide culturally appropriate nursing care when working with Black Americans.

3 Recognize physical and biological variances that exist within and across Black American groups in order to provide culturally appropriate nursing care.

4 Develop a sensitivity and an understanding for communication differences evidenced within and across Black American groups in order to avoid stereotyping and to provide culturally appropriate nursing care.

5 Develop a sensitivity and an understanding for psychological phenomena that influence the functioning of a Black American when providing nursing care.

In a time when people are seeking to become more culturally aware, it is important to note distinctions in terminology regarding cultural groups. This is certainly true of Black Americans. Some Black American individuals and groups are encouraging the use of the term *African Americans,* whereas others are encouraging the use of the term *Black Americans*. The term *African Americans* is used to refer to a cultural heritage that is a combination of both African and American. On the other hand, the term *Black Americans* is thought to place more focus on biological racial identity than on cultural heritage. For the purposes of this book, we have chosen the term *Black Americans* because it is commonly used in the literature.

OVERVIEW OF BLACK AMERICANS

According to the U.S. Census Bureau, there are approximately 26,488,218 Black Americans residing in the United States, who represent approximately 11.7% of the American population (*Statistical Abstracts,* 1988). During the seventeenth and eighteenth centuries Black Americans came to the United States under the system of slavery. Therefore Black Americans may be the only cultural and ethnic group who reside in the United States today who did not immigrate to this country voluntarily. (Although they did not come to this country voluntarily, indentured servants of majority age could elect to go to prison or indenture themselves for a period of 7 years to resolve their debt [Friedlander, 1966; Stanhope and Lancaster, 1988]. Unlike the descendants of indentured servants, Black Americans are the descendants of people who came to this country in bondage.) Even today, the cultural roots of Black Americans are entrenched in the Black American experience. According to Bloch (1983), it is the Black life experience that has established what has become known as the Black view of the external world. The Black life experience has shaped the internal attitudes and the belief systems of Black Americans, and it continues to influence interactions of Black Americans with persons from other cultural groups.

Some of the health problems noted particularly in Black Americans are thought to be the result of varying genetic pools and hereditary immunity. However, many of these problems have been found to be more closely associated with economic status than with race. Three intervening and reinforcing variables include poverty, discrimination, and social and psychological barriers. These three intervening and reinforcing variables are thought to be so profound in effect on Black Americans that they tend to keep these individuals from using the health care services that are available. These variables may also explain the fact that morbidity and mortality rates are higher among Black Americans. While underrepresented in the total population, Blacks remain overrepresented among the health statistics for life-threatening illness. The life expectancy for Blacks continues to lag behind that for Whites: the life expectancy for Blacks is 69.5 years as compared with 75.3 years for Whites (*Statistical Abstracts,* 1988). Black Americans also have a higher infant mortality rate (18.4 per 1000 live births in 1984) as compared with that of White Americans (9.4 per 1000 live births in 1984) (National Center for Health Statistics, 1985).

COMMUNICATION

Communication is the matrix for thought and relationship between all people regardless of cultural heritage (Murray, 1987). Verbal and nonverbal communication are learned in cultural settings. Difficulties arise if a person does not communicate in the way or manner prescribed by the culture because the individual cannot conform to social expectation. Communication, therefore, is basic to culturally appropriate nursing care.

Dialect

Dialect refers to the variations within a language. Black Americans speak English; however, there are widespread differences in the way English is spoken between Blacks and other ethnic and cultural groups. Different linguistic norms evolve among groups of people who are socially or geographically separated. Social stratification alters the nature and frequency of intracommunication between groups. When social separation, by factors such as ethnic origin or class, is responsible for the origin and perpetuation of a particular dialect, the dialect is referred to as a stratified dialect. When differences in dialect emerge as a result of geographic separation of people, the dialect is referred to as regional or geographic dialect.

Origins of Black dialect in the United States

Accurate and reliable data concerning the different dialects spoken by a vast majority of Black Americans is not available to the public or to educators (Turner, 1948). The study of pidgins and creole language has facilitated an intelligent study of Black English and the notable differences between Black English and Standard English (Hymes, 1970). Research into the languages of Brazilians of African descent, as well as Haitians, Jamaicans, and the present-day Black inhabitants off the seacoasts of South Carolina and Georgia, indicates a correlation of structural features of several of the languages spoken in parts of West Africa, as well as a similarity to the English spoken by Whites in the United States (Hymes, 1970).

The first Africans who were brought to the United States as slaves were systematically separated during transportation, and this separation continued on arrival. As a result, there was a combination of the various African languages with the languages of other cultural groups in the New World, such as the Dutch, the French, the English, etc. This combination of the different African languages with the other different languages fostered a need for a "common language" for all Blacks, which ultimately led to the restructuring of grammar of all language, including English. This process is referred to as pidginization and creolization. Pidgin English is not a language but a dialect.

Pidgin tends to be simple in grammar and limited in vocabulary. Typically in communities where pidgin is spoken, its use is limited to trade purposes, task-oriented activities, and communication between cultural or ethnic groups (Hymes, 1970). When pidgin dialect undergoes internal expansion and extension of use, the results are creolization. It is from the pidgin dialect that the Creole language was born. In the United States a number of Creole dialects developed and are still in existence today, particularly in the rural south in such places as New Orleans, Louisiana; Hattiesburg and Vicksburg, Mississippi; and Mobile, Alabama. Furthermore, the migration of Blacks from the South saw the development of pidginization and creolization in some northern cities such as New York, Chicago, and Detroit. Evidences of past migration and its effect on dialect and Black English remain obvious even today.

Language usage

The dialect that is spoken by many Blacks is sufficiently different from Standard English in pronunciation, grammar, and syntax so as to be classifed as "Black English." The use of Standard English versus Black English varies among Blacks and in some instances may be related to educational level and socioeconomic status, although this is not always the case. The use of Standard English by Black Americans is important in terms of social and economic mobility. However, the use of Black English has served as a unifying factor for Blacks in maintaining their cultural and ethnic identity. It is not uncommon for some Black Americans to speak Standard English when serving in a professional capacity or when socializing with Whites and then revert back to Black English when interacting in all-Black settings. Some Black Americans who have not mastered Standard English may feel insecure in certain situations where they are required and expected to use Standard English, and when confronted with such situations, they may become very quiet, with the result that they may be labeled hostile or submissive.

Pronunciation of Black English

There is a tendency for users of Black dialect to pronounce certain syllables and/or consonants somewhat differently. For example, *th*, as in *the, these,* or *them,* may be pronounced as *d*, as in "de," "des," and "dem" (Dillard, 1972; Wolfram & Clark, 1971). In Black English there is also a tendency to drop the final *r* or *g* from words; thus *father* or *mother* becomes "fatha" or "motha." The words *laughing, talking,* and *going* are pronounced "laughin," "talkin," and "goin" without the *g*. Speakers of Black English may also place more emphasis on one syllable as opposed to another; for example, *brother* may be pronounced "bro-tha." In addition, the final *th* of words is pronounced as *f* in Black English; thus *bath, birth, mouth,* and *with* are pronounced "baf," "birf," "mouf," and "wif."

Copula deletion of the verb *to be* is a common omission in some environments; for example, the speaker of Black English might say, "He walking" or "She at work" in contrast to the Standard English, "He is walking" or "She is at work." Black English speakers may also use the unconjugated form of the verb *to be* where Standard English speakers would use the conjugated form. An example of this would be, "He be working" in contrast to the Standard English, "He is working."

In Standard English every verb is in sequence and must be marked as either present or past tense. However, in Black English only past-tense verbs need to be marked. For example, in Black English the *s* marking the present tense may be omitted; thus "He go" or "She love." Attempts to correct this can result in phrases such as "I goes" and "We loves."

Speakers of Black English may also omit the possessive suffix. For example, in Black English one might say, "Richard dog bit me" or "Mary dress," in contrast to the Standard English, "Richard's dog bit me" or "Mary's dress" (Dillard, 1972).

Speakers of Black English also have some words that are classified as slang. These words are different from slang words used in other dialects and may or may not convey the same meaning. For instance, Blacks may use the word *chilly* or *chillin* to infer sophistication, whereas a White individual may use the word *cool* or *groovy* to convey the same meaning. Some Blacks may use the verb *to fix* to denote planned actions, for example, "I'm fixin to go home," whereas the user of Standard English would say, "I am getting ready to go home."

The speech of some Black Americans is very colorful and dynamic. For these persons, communication also involves body movement (kinesis). Some Blacks tend to use a wide range of body movement, such as facial gestures, hand and arm movements, expressive stances, handshakes, and hand signals, along with verbal interaction. This repertoire of body movements can also be seen in sports and in dance, which is the highest communicative form of body language.

Some Black Americans will use sounds that are not words to add expression to their conversation or to music, such as *oo-wee* or *uh huh,* which have analogies in some of the Gullah languages from West Africa but not in English (Jones, 1968a).

The term *signifying* describes an approach wherein one attempts to chide or correct someone indirectly. For example, one might correct someone who is not dressed properly by saying, "You sure are dressed up today."

A large majority of Black Americans use Black English in a systematic way that can be predictably understood by others; thus Black English cannot, nor should not, be regarded as substandard or ungrammatical. It is estimated that approximately 80% of Black Americans use Black English at least some of the time (Dillard, 1972).

Implications for Nursing Care

The nurse must develop a sensitivity to communication variances as a prerequisite for accurate nursing assessment and intervention in multicultural situations. In all nursing environments the potential for misunderstanding the patient is accentuated when the nurse and the patient are from different ethnic groups. Perhaps the most significant and obvious barrier occurs when two persons speak different languages. However, the nurse must be cognizant of the fact that barriers to communication exist even when individuals speak the same language. The nurse may have difficulty explaining things to a patient in simple, jargon-free language in order to facilitate the patient's understanding. The nurse must develop a familiarity with the language of the patient, since this is the best way to gain insight into the culture. Every language and dialect is special and has a unique way of looking at the world and at experiences (Kluckhohn, 1972). Every language also has a whole set of unconscious assumptions about the world and life. According to Kluckhohn (1972), people see and hear what the grammatical system of their language makes them sensitive to perceive.

The nurse who works with Black American patients may find that although the language is the same, the perception of what message is being sent and received by the nurse and the patient may be different. Therefore it is of the highest priority for the nurse who is working with Black Americans, particularly those who speak Black English, to understand as much of the context of the dialect as possible.

The nurse must bear in mind that Black English cannot be viewed as an unacceptable form of English. Thus it is important for the nurse to avoid labeling and stereotyping the patient. The nurse should avoid chiding and correcting the speech of Black Americans, since this behavior can result in the patient's becoming quiet, passive, and, in some cases, aggressive or hostile. On the other hand, while the nurse should attempt to use words common to the patient's vocabulary, mimicking the patient's language can be interpreted as dehumanizing. For example, if a nurse were to say "dem" for *them,* or "dese" for *these,* the patient may perceive this as ridicule.

When working with persons who speak Black English, the nurse must keep in mind that the patient may use slang to convey certain messages. However, slang terms often have different meanings between individuals and especially between cultural groups. For example, a Black patient's response to questioning about a diagnostic test, "It was a real bad experience," may actually mean that it was a unique and yet positive experience. The nurse working with this patient will need to clarify the exact meaning of the word *bad.* In Black English the word *bad* is often used for the exact opposite, in other words, *good.* In another example, a Black patient who states that the medication has been taken "behind the meal" may mean the medication has been been taken after eating. A nurse may interpret *behind* to mean *before* rather than *after,* since the dictionary definition states that *behind* means "still to come." The nurse must be cautious about interpreting particular words each time a Black individual uses certain terminology.

It is essential that the nurse identify and clarify what is happening psychologically and physiologically to the Black patient. When possible, the nurse should substitute words commonly understood by the Black patient for more sophisticated medical terms. When this is done, the nurse will find that the Black patient is more receptive to instructions and more cooperative. Stokes (1977) offers a list of terms commonly used by nurses and equivalent words used by some Blacks:

Conditions (medical/Black English)	Functions (medical/Black English)
Diabetes/sugar	Constipation/locked bowels
Pain/miseries	Diarrhea/running off, grip
Syphilis/bad blood, pox	Menstruation/red flag, the curse
Amemia/low blood, tired blood	Urinate, urine/pass water, tinkle, peepee
Vomiting/throw up	

The nurse must remember that some Black Americans place a great deal of importance on nonverbal elements of communication and that the verbal pattern of some Black patients may differ significantly from that of a non-Black nurse. It is also important for the nurse to remember that the words used by some Black patients may be the same as those used by the nurse but have different, idiosyncratic meanings. When working with Black patients, the nurse must also remember that eye contact, nodding, and smiling are not necessarily essential or direct correlates that the Black patient is paying attention (Sue, 1981).

SPACE

According to Hall (1966), the degree to which people are sensorially involved with each other, along with how they use time, determines not only at what point they feel crowded or have a perception that their personal space is collapsing inwardly, but the methods for alleviating crowding as well. For example, Puerto Ricans and Black Americans are reported to have a much higher involvement ratio than other cultural groups such as German Americans or Scandinavian Americans. It is believed that highly involved people, such as Black Americans, require a higher density than less involved people. However, highly involved people may at the same time require more protection or screening from outsiders than do people with a lower level of involvement.

To understand the variable of space, it is essential to understand time and the way it is handled, because the variable of time influences the structuring of space. According to Hall (1966), there are two contrasting ways in which people handle time, monochronic and polychronic and each affects the way in which an individual perceives space. People with low involvement are generally monochronic, because such individuals tend to compartmentalize time; for example, they may schedule one thing at a time and tend to become disoriented if they have to deal with too many things at once. On the other hand, polychronic individuals tend to keep several operations going at once, almost like jugglers, and these individuals tend to be very involved with each other.

Implications for Nursing Care

The nurse who works with Latin Americans, Africans, Black Americans, or Indonesians may feel somewhat uncomfortable because these cultures generally dictate a much closer personal space when personal and social spaces are involved (Sue, 1981). Since some Black Americans are perceived as polychronic individuals, it is important for the nurse to remember that polychronic individuals tend to collect activities.

When polychronic individuals interact with monochronic individuals, some difficulties may be experienced because of the different ways in which these individuals relate to space and to each other. An example of a difficulty encountered between monochronic and polychronic individuals is when monochronic individuals become upset or angry because of the constant interruptions of polychronic individuals.

Some monochronic individuals believe that there must be order to get things done. On the other hand, polychronic individuals, such as some Black Americans, do not believe that order is necessary to get things done. The nurse who works with Black Americans must keep in mind that to reduce polychronic effects, it is necessary to reduce multiple activity involvements on the part of the patient. The nurse can accomplish this by separating activities with as much screening and scrutiny as necessary (Hall, 1966). One goal of nursing intervention should be to help the patient structure activities in a ranked order that will produce maximal benefits for the patient.

SOCIAL ORGANIZATION

Social organization refers to how a cultural group organizes itself around particular units (such as family, racial or ethnic group, and community or social groups). Most Black Americans have been socialized in predominantly Black environments. Historically, because of legalized segregation, Black Americans were separated or isolated from the mainstream of society. Consequently, Black Americans are the only cultural group in the United States that has not been assimilated into the mainstream society. Even today, Black Americans maintain separate and in most cases unequal life-styles as compared with other Americans. Evidence of the failure to assimilate on the part of Black Americans is seen in the existence of predominantly Black neighborhoods, churches, colleges and universities, and public elementary and high schools.

Historical Review of Slavery and Discrimination

Patterns of discrimination have existed in the United States since the inception of slavery. With the inception of slavery came the foundations of attitudes and beliefs that were and continue to be the pillars that support the institution of racism. Racism, discriminatory practices, and segregation combined have produced insularity or separatist feelings and attitudes on the part of some Black Americans. As a result, Black Americans are often accused of having more separate and more insular patterns of communication, which have restricted some Black Americans from participating in the wider White society. Thus some Black Americans prefer to maintain themselves within their own group. Accordingly, this insularity has promoted the retention of culturally seeded beliefs that differ from the beliefs held by the dominant culture. Leininger (1978) noted that every cultural group has unique beliefs that influence their attitudes regarding health. These beliefs tend to determine the type of behavior and health care practices that a particular cultural group views as appropriate or inappropriate. In other words, the attitudes and beliefs regarding health and illness vary in the United States between Blacks and Whites and even among Black Americans themselves.

Attitudes, beliefs, values, and morals are the basic structural units of any culture. Culture is an outward manifestation of a way of life; it is dynamic and fluid, and ever evolving. The family is the basic social unit of most cultures and is the means by which culture is passed down from one generation to the next. The inception of slavery in the United States precipitated the beginning of the destruction of the transplanted African culture. In Africa Black Africans had been accustomed to a strictly regulated family life with rigidly enforced moral codes. The family unit was closely knit, well organized, connected with kin and community, and highly functional for the economic, social, psychological, and spiritual well-being of the people (Jones, 1968b). The family was the center of African civilization.

The destruction of the African family began with the capture of slaves for transplantation to the New World, which began in 1619. As slaves were captured, the young, healthy, men, women, and children were forcibly removed from their families and tribes. This separation continued as these slaves journeyed to the New World because they were placed on ships without regard for family unity, tribe, or kinship. On the arrival of the slaves in the United States, this systematic separation of individuals from families continued.

The cruelest form of emasculation of the Black Africans, now Americans, was the breeding of slaves for sale. Infants and children were taken from their mothers and sold as chattel. Marriage between slaves was not legally sanctioned and was generally left to the discretion of the owners. Some slave owners assigned mates when slaves reached breeding age. Others would not permit their slaves to marry a slave from another plantation. Most slave owners sold husbands, wives, and children without consideration for family ties. The children that were produced of the slave union belonged to the slave owner, not to the parents. The Black American family in the United States during slavery lacked autonomy because the family members were someone else's property. The parents was unable to provide security or protection for their children. Husbands were unable to protect their wives. In a documentary of the lives of 75 Black women, Angelou (1989) describes the heartbreaking tenderness of Black women and the majestic strength they had to survive the subjugation and horror of the slavery experience.

Changing Roles of the Black American Family

Under the system of slavery in the United States, the role of the Black man as husband and father was obliterated. The Black man was not the head of the household, nor was he the provider or the protector of his family. Instead, he was someone else's property. Under the system of slavery, the Black man remained powerless to defend his wife and children from harm, particularly when they were beaten or sexually assaulted by the White overseer or owner, or by any White person. The Black male slave was often referred to as "boy" until he reached a certain age, at which point he became "uncle." The only crucial function for the Black man within the Black family was siring children.

In the United States under the system of slavery, the Black woman became the dominant force in the family. She was forced to work side-by-side with her male counterpart during the day and additionally had the responsibility of caring for family members at night. The Black woman was forced to bear children for sale and to care for other children, including those of the slave owner. Some Black women during slavery were also forced to satisfy the sexual desires of any White man, and any children born out of this union were also considered slaves. If the Black woman had a husband, he was merely her sexual companion and was referred to as her "boy" by the slave owner and by White society in general. The inception of slavery, the division of the African family and subsequently the African American family, and the subordinate role of the Black man all played a significant part in the establishment of the female-dominated household that exists even today in the United States.

Even after slavery was abolished in the United States, the destructive forces against the Black family persisted. Today, the residual effects of slavery are still evident in some parts of the country. After slavery was abolished and during the emancipation period and the years that followed, the Black American man was either denied jobs or given tasks that were demeaning and dehumanizing. From the time of the abolition of slavery until the mid-1960s, Black Americans in some parts of the country were attacked, lynched, and murdered. Sexual attacks on Black American women also continued. Such actions further served to drive some Black American men away from their families. Thus there was further weakening of the family and subsequently of the Black male role (Bullough & Bullough, 1982). In spite of the discriminatory practices and the continued hostile attacks against Blacks, some Black American families nevertheless were able to establish themselves. As these Black families were able to develop a secure economic status, they began to establish schools, churches, and other social organizations.

Characteristics of the Black American Family

In the United States there are basically two types of family structures: the male-headed (patriarchal) family structure and the female-headed (matriarchal) family structure. According to the U.S. Department of Commerce, Bureau of the Census (1982), 47.1% of Black families in the United States are female headed, and according to Covell and Turnbull (1982), as many as 59% of Black families are female headed. In contrast, 13.9% of White families and 23% of Hispanic families are female headed. The fact that approximately half of the Black families in the United States are female headed is due in part to factors related to and carried over from slavery. For example, the Black family has not been able to overcome deficits related to education and income. According to the U.S. Department of Commerce, Bureau of the Census (1982), the average income for Black men as compared with men in other cultural groups with similar skills and educational levels is significantly lower. Black men with 9 to 11 years of education earned $15,000 a year in 1980, as compared with their White counterparts, who earned approximately $18,200. The salary of a Black man with a 4-year college degree was comparable to the salary of a White man with only 9 to 11 years of education ($18,200). Even the number of Blacks (female or male) obtaining a high school education or a college degree is significantly lower than that of their White counterparts. For example, in a recent analysis the high school dropout rates for Black Americans was 18%, as compared with 12% for Whites and 3% for Asians; the number of Blacks (female or male) who attended college was 27.7%, as compared with 31.8% for Whites (*Statistical Abstracts,* 1988).

Implications for Nursing Care

Even today, the Black family is often oriented around women; in other words, it is matrifocal. This has implications for the nurse because within the Black family structure the wife and/or mother is often charged with the responsibility for protecting the health of the family members. The Black woman is expected to assist each family member in maintaining good health and in determining treatment if a family member is ill. This has both positive and negative effects, since Black patients often enter the health care delivery system at the advice of the matriarch of the family. The nurse must recognize the importance of the Black woman in disseminating information and in assisting the patient in making decisions. While the Black family may be matrifocal, it is nevertheless essential to include the Black man in the decision-making process.

Some Black families are composed of large networks and tend to be very supportive during times of crisis and illness. Large-network groups can have both positive and negative effects on wellness, illness, and recovery behaviors. In a study done by Jackson, Neighbors, and Gurin (1986), it was found that network size was positively related to distress: the more informal helpers there were, the higher the distress score on the instrument used in the survey. One conclusion of the study is that network size is not a good measure of perceived social support. According to the study, the more serious the problem, the more people within the network are consulted for help, but the more people consulted does not necessarily reduce the severity of the problem; rather, an individual with an acute illness may spend so much time seeking assistance within the network that necessary and timely treatment is delayed. The nurse should include all the members of the network in the planning and implementation of health care. This is essential, because some members of the network may provide advice or care that could be detrimental to the patient. For example, a Black patient who is admitted with an electrolyte imbalance and is brought laxatives from home by a relative may have additional electrolyte problems when the laxatives are taken without consulting members of the health care team. In this case the nurse must emphasize the importance of the nurse's role in providing health care. Once the family develops a feeling of trust, the nurse is more likely to be consulted should perceived health needs arise; for example, the patient needs a laxative.

TIME

Time is a concept that is universal and continuous. All emotional and perceptual experiences are interrelated with the concept of time. The perception of time is individual and is determined by cultural experiences (Hall, 1976). In the United States, time has become the most important organizing principle of the dominant culture (Hall, 1976). The majority of individuals of the dominant culture are time conscious and very future oriented; they make it a common practice to "plan ahead" and "save for a rainy day." Time has become very important and comparable to money in the American society. Doing things efficiently and faster has become the American way.

It is impossible to characterize Black Americans and their perceptions of time as one way or the other, since Black Americans, just as individuals from other cultural groups, vary according to social and cultural factors. Some Black Americans who have become assimilated into the dominant culture are very time conscious and take pride in punctuality. These individuals are likely to be future oriented and believe that saving and planning are important. They are likely to be well educated and to hold professional positions, although this is not always the case, since some Blacks who are not well educated and do not hold professional jobs still value time and have hopes for the future (they are likely to encourage their children to seek higher education and to save for the future) (Poussaint & Atkinson, 1970).

On the other hand, some Black Americans react to the present situation and are not future oriented; it is their belief that planning for the future is hopeless because of their previous experiences and encounters with racism and discrimination. They believe that their future will be the same as their present and their past (Poussaint & Atkinson, 1970). These individuals are likely to be jobless or have low-paying jobs. Educational levels may vary from junior high school to college degrees among persons who share this belief. Such individuals are unlikely to value time; thus they do not value the concept of punctuality and may not keep appointments or may arrive much later than the scheduled time. It is the belief of some Black Americans that time is flexible and that events will begin when they arrive. This belief has been translated down through the years to imply an acceptable lateness among some Black Americans of 30 minutes to an hour. This perception of time can be traced back to West Africa, where the concept of time was elastic and encompassed events that had already taken place, as well as those that would occur immediately (Mbiti, 1970).

Finally, some Black Americans have a future-oriented concept of time because of their strong religious beliefs. These individuals may be from all socioeconomic and educational levels. It is their belief that life on earth, with all of its pain and suffering, is bearable because there will be happiness and lack of pain after death. Black Americans who hold this belief plan their funerals and even purchase their grave plots long before their deaths (Smith, 1976).

Implications for Nursing Care

Since some Black Americans perceive time as flexible and elastic, it is essential for the nurse to include the patient and family in the planning and implementation of nursing care. When planning nursing care with the patient and family, the nurse should emphasize events that have flexibility where time is concerned, such as morning care and bathing. On the other hand, the nurse must also emphasize events that have no flexibility where time is concerned and where delay in doing something, such as taking time-released medications or medications for certain conditions, would have serious implications for the patient's well-being. For example, a patient with high blood pressure must be made to understand that the medication must be taken as and when prescribed, not when and as desired. A medication missed today cannot be made up by taking double the amount tomorrow. As another example, an insulin-dependent diabetic patient cannot delay the time periods between meals.

Some Black Americans are perceived as individuals with present time orientations. Such persons may have a more flexible adherence to schedules and may believe that immediate concerns are more relevant than future concerns. Because appointment schedules may lack meaning, the nurse must emphasize the importance of adhering to the appointment schedule. If the nurse knows a particular patient has a pattern of arriving late, the nurse may advise the patient to arrive for scheduled appointments at least half an hour early. For the nurse who works with patients who are focused on the present, it is essential to avoid crisis-oriented rather than preventive nursing (Sue, 1981).

ENVIRONMENTAL CONTROL
Health Care Beliefs

In the United States the system of health care beliefs and practices are extremely complex and diverse among cultural groups. Variations in health care beliefs and practices cross ethnic and social boundaries. These variations are evidenced even within families. Culture influences individual expectations and perceptions regarding health, illness, disease, and symptoms related to disease. Accordingly, culture, cultural beliefs, and cultural values influence how one copes when confronted with illness, disease, or stress (Anderson & Bauwens, 1981).

In the United States a distinction between illness and disease has been made by anthropologists and sociologists (Staples, 1976). *Illness* has been defined as an individual's perception of being sick, which is not necessarily related to the biomedical definition of *disease*. *Disease* has been defined as a condition that deviates from the norm. Thus illness may exist in the absence of disease and vice versa (Staples, 1976). Norms used to determine a disease condition, using Western standards, have for the most part been taken from studies conducted on White subjects. Thus when these norms are applied to other cultural groups, such as Black Americans, the norm values may be meaningless and lead to erroneous conclusions. For example, to receive a 2 for color on the Apgar scoring system for newborns, the infant most be completely pink. Another example of a Western norm expectation is that an inverted T wave may be an ominous, pathological finding. However, in the case of Black Americans such a finding should be the expectation, rather than being perceived as ominous and pathological. Also, growth as related to body size and physique is often normed by White Western standards. Thus Black Americans, who mature at an earlier age and typically have larger physiques than those of their White counterparts, may be perceived as being either overweight or oversized when White Western norms are applied.

Health care beliefs and the Black family

Blacks in the United States are a highly heterogeneous group; thus it is impossible to make a collective statement about their health care beliefs and practices. Many health care beliefs that are exhibited by Blacks in the United States are derived from their African ancestry (Smith, 1976). For example, in West Africa, where a vast majority of Black Americans originated, man was perceived as a monistic being, that is, a being from which the body and soul could not be separated (Smith, 1976). Man was also perceived as a holistic individual with many complex dimensions. Religion was interwoven into health care beliefs and practices. (West Africans continue even today to believe that illness is a natural occurrence resulting from disharmony and conflict in some area of the individual's life.) Since life was centered around the entire family, illness was perceived as a collective event and subsequently a disruption of the entire family system. The traditional West African healers always involved the individual's entire family in the healing process, even when the disorder was thought to be somatic in origin. Thus the traditional West African healer based treatment on the premise of wholeness, the necessity for reincorporation of the patient into the family system, and involvement of the entire family system in the care and treatment of the individual (Smith, 1976).

Perception of illness

In the United States some Blacks perceive illness as a natural occurrence resulting from disharmony and conflict in some aspect of an individual's life. This belief is a cultural value that has been passed down through the generations to American Blacks as a result of West African influences and tends to involve three general areas: (1) environmental hazards, (2) divine punishment, and (3) impaired social relationships (Snow, 1977). An example of an environmental hazard would be injuries due to being struck by lightening or being bitten by a snake. Divine punishment would include illnesses or diseases that the individual would attribute to sin. Impaired social relationships may be caused by such factors as a spouse leaving or parents disowning a child (Snow, 1977).

Another belief held by some Black Americans is that everything has an opposite. For every birth, there must be a death; for every marriage, there must be a divorce; for every occurrence of illness, someone must be cured (Snow, 1978). Some Black Americans may not be able to distinguish between physical and mental illness and spiritual problems, and as a result may present themselves for treatment with a variety or combination of somatic, psychological, and spiritual complaints (Smith, 1976). For example, a patient may present real symptoms of an ulcer but may relate the symptoms to past sins or grief over a financial loss. The patient desires assistance not only for the somatic disorder, but also for the psychological and spiritual complaints.

Blacks who share mainstream attitudes about pain may respond to pain stoically out of a desire to be a perfect patient. This means that they tend not to "bother" the nurse by calling for attention or for pain medication. For such patients the nurse must make it clear that the patient has a right to relief from pain. On the other hand, some Black patients exhibit a different form of stoicism. Hard experience has convinced them that trouble and pain are God's will. In this case the nurse needs to help the patient understand that pain retards healing and is medically undesirable (LoBiondo-Wood, Zimmerman, & Gaston-Johansson, 1989).

Folk Medicine

Folk medicine is germane to many cultural and ethnic groups. Individuals from all aspects of society may use folk medicine either alone or in conjunction with a scientifically based medical system. The importance of folk medicine and the level of practice vary among the different ethnic and cultural groups, depending on education and socioeconomic status (Bullough & Bullough, 1982). In contrast to the scientifically based health care system in the United States, folk medicine is characterized by a belief in supernatural forces. From this perspective health and illness are characterized as natural and unnatural.

According to Snow (1983), it matters whether a Black American comes from a rural background when it is necessary to select health care providers. Some Black Americans who were reared in the rural South may have grown up being treated by folk practitioners and may not have encountered a physician until they reached adulthood. Therefore these people are more likely to turn to a neighborhood folk practitioner when they become ill. According to White (1977), folk medicine is still used within the Black community because of humiliation encountered in the mainstream health care system, lack of money, and lack of trust in health care workers. Today, some Black Americans go to physicians in order to get prescribed medications, not because they feel the physician is superior in knowledge or training (Murray, 1987).

Witchcraft, voodoo, and magic are an integral aspect of folk medicine (McKenzie & Chrisman, 1977). Natural events are those that are in harmony with nature and provide individuals who believe in and practice folk medicine with a certain degree of predictability in the events of daily living. Unnatural events, on the other hand, represent disharmony with nature, so that the events of day-to-day living cannot be predicted (Snow, 1983). Another aspect of the folk medicine system is a belief in opposing forces, or the belief that everything has a opposite, as discussed under Perception of Illness (for every birth, there must be a death, etc.). Also incorporated into the system of folk medicine is the belief that health is a gift from God, whereas illness is a punishment from God or a retribution for sin and evil (Snow, 1983). This concept is evidenced by the belief held by some Black Americans that if a child is born with a physical handicap, it is a punishment from God for the past wrongdoings of the parents. In this way, sins of the father and mother are passed on for retribution by the children (Snow, 1983). Such beliefs are not limited to Black Americans but are also found among other cultural groups in the United States; for example, some Mexican Americans believe that illness is a punishment for some sin or misdeed (Snow, 1983).

Practice of Black folk medicine

There are still some Black Americans in the rural South and in the urban northern ghettos who practice folk medicine based on spirituality, including witchcraft, voodoo, and magic (McKenzie & Chrisman, 1977). Some of these individuals may also use the orthodox medical system. Historically, such cities as New Orleans and Baton Rouge, Louisiana, were very much voodoo oriented, and such beliefs were held not only by Blacks, but by members of other cultural groups as well. Even today, the Black folk medicine system is practiced by the high-ranking voodoo queen in some Louisiana cities. The Louisiana Voodoo Society is a carryover from a combination of Haitian and French cultural influences (Mitchel, 1978). Voodoo and witchcraft are not restricted to Louisiana, but are also practiced in such places as the Georgia sea islands, which are just off the the coast of Savannah. Interestingly enough, some of the inhabitants of the Georgia sea islands remain pure-blooded descendants of West African ancestry. Even today, some inhabitants of the Georgia sea islands have refused to intermarry with members of other cultural groups, thus maintaining the tradition of "pure-blooded" lineage (Wolfram & Clark, 1971). Pure-blooded descendants of West Africans are also found off the coast of South Carolina. Some of these people speak Gullah (an admixture of various African languages) and tend to isolate themselves when possible from the mainstream of society (Wolfram & Clark, 1971).

Black folk medicine system defined

In the system of Black folk medicine, illness is perceived as a natural or unnatural occurrence. A natural illness may occur because of an exposure to the elements of nature without protection (such as a cold, the flu, or pneumonia). Natural illnesses occur when dangerous elements in the environment enter the body through impurities in food, water, and air. However, the words *natural* and *unnatural* are connoted to mean more or less than the dictionary definitions of these words. For example, cancer, which is linked to such environmental hazards as smog, cigarette smoke, toxic waste, and other chemical irritants would be considered a natural illness in a professional medical system. However, those persons who share beliefs in Black folk medicine might view cancer as an unnatural illness, perceiving it as a punishment from God or a spell cast by an evil person doing the work of the devil (Snow, 1974). Persons who share beliefs in the Black folk medicine system may not readily acknowledge the fact that cancer, for example, may be caused by environmental factors such as cigarette smoking; thus they may continue smoking even after being diagnosed.

As indicated above, unnatural illnesses are perceived as either a punishment from God or the work of the devil. This is in contrast to the dictionary definition of illness as an unhealthy condition of the body or mind (*Webster's*, 1984).

Types of folk practitioners

Jordan (1975) identified distinct types of folk practitioners. The first type is the "old lady" or the "granny," who acts as a local consultant. This individual is knowledgeable about many different home remedies made from certain spices, herbs, and roots that can be used to treat common illnesses. Another duty of this individual is to give advice and make appropriate referrals to another type of practitioner when an illness or a particular medical condition extends beyond her practice (Jordan, 1975). The second type of practitioner is the "spiritualist," the most prevalent and diverse type of folk practitioner. This individual attempts to combine rituals, spiritual beliefs, and herbal medicines to effect a cure for certain illnesses and/or ailments. The third type of practitioner is the voodoo priest or priestess. In some West Indies islands, the voodoo person can be a man, whereas in some rural southern areas of the United States, the voodoo person must be a woman and may inherit this title only by birthright and a perceived special gift (Snow, 1974).

In contrast to the type of voodoo priest or priestess found in some West Indies islands and in some rural or urban southern U.S. areas is the type of voodoo priest or priestess found in some larger urban areas such as Chicago; Queens or Jamaica, New York; or Los Angeles. In these cities the voodoo folk practitioner may be either male or female, does not have to inherit the right to practice by virtue of bloodline, and does not have to possess significantly powerful gifts (Snow, 1974). Historically, the voodoo priestess found in cities such as New Orleans must possess certain physical characteristics; that is, she must be Black, and, more specifically, she must be of mixed ancestry, either an octoroon (a person of one-eighth Black ancestry) or a quadroon (a person of one-fourth Black ancestry) if her powers are to be superior (Snow, 1974).

Even today, some southern and northern Blacks still turn to one of these three types of practitioners when seeking medical advice. Educational level or socioeconomic status does not appear to alter or affect how some Black Americans perceive folk practitioners. Similar views are shared by some members of other cultural groups. In the summer of 1988, newspaper articles throughout the United States carried the story that the first lady of the United States refused to make any moves or to allow her husband, the president of one of the most powerful countries in the world, to make decisions unless an astrologist was consulted.

Witchcraft: an alternative form of folk medicine

The practice of witchcraft is quite widespread and is not limited to the parameters of the United States. Various degrees of witchcraft are practiced in countries throughout the world. In addition, the practice of witchcraft is not limited to any one particular cultural group. Persons who believe in witchcraft believe that it can be used not only to cure illness or disease, but also to cause illness or disease. For example, strokes, dementia, and some gastrointestinal disorders may be perceived by some persons who believe in witchcraft to be the direct result and/or influence of witchcraft (Henderson & Primeaux, 1981).

The practice of witchcraft is based on the belief that there are some individuals who possess the ability to mobilize the forces of good and evil. These abilities are based on the principles of sympathetic magic, which underlie many of the beliefs of folk medicine practice. The basic premise of sympathetic magic is that everything in the universe is connected. There is a direct connection between the body and the forces of nature. Interpretation and direction of events are accomplished by understanding these connections. Sympathetic magic is categorized into contagious and imitative magic. The basic premise of contagious magic is the perception that physically connected objects can never be separated; therefore any actions against the parts constitute an action against the whole (Henderson & Primeaux, 1981). Individuals who practice witchcraft may use a piece of clothing or nail clippings from someone to cast an "evil" spell or to protect the individual. The basic premise of imitative magic is that like follows like, or that one will imitate what one desires to achieve. For example, a knife placed under the bed will cut pain; an evil charm put on when the moon is waxing will increase the moon.

A recurring theme in the practice of witchcraft is that of animals being in the body. Lizards, toads, snakes, and spiders are thought to be the most common types of intruders. These animals are dead and pulverized and are generally thought to enter the body via food or drink. It is not uncommon for persons who believe in witchcraft to refuse to eat or drink food prepared by someone they believe may have put a hex on them. Individuals who believe that such a spell has been cast on them may present themselves at health care facilities with symptoms described as "reptiles crawling over the body or snakes wiggling in their stomach." Some of these individuals may also share the belief that the physician is powerless to help them once they have been "hexed" (Jordan, 1979).

Perceptions concerning folk medicine and other alternative medical solutions

The prevalence of the belief in and the use of folk medicine remedies and other alternative forms of health care is not fully understood (Jacques, 1976). It is impossible to generalize or postulate how widespread the use of folk medicine remedies is among Black Americans. However, evidence does exist that some Black Americans throughout the entire country do believe in and practice folk medicine, as well as other alternative forms of health care such as witchcraft, voodoo, and spiritualism (Snow, 1983). There is also evidence to support the notion that different levels of folk medicine are practiced (Jacques, 1976). The boundaries of folk healers for some Black Americans may also vary. For example, "the granny type of folk healer" may only possess the skills and knowledge to cure simple illnesses or aliments. In contrast, a "witch doctor" is thought to possess supernatural powers that allow the "casting out of such things as animal demons" (Jordan, 1979). In addition, Black folk medicine practitioners may have titles different from those of folk practitioners found in other cultural groups in the United States, such as " conjure doctor," "underworld man," "father divine," "the root doctor," and the " root worker" (Jacques, 1976).

Origins of Black folk medicine

Black folk medicine practices in the United States can be traced back to regions of West Africa (Smith, 1976). There are also influences on Black folk medicine that originated in other countries such as Haiti, Jamaica, and Trinadad (Smith, 1976). Because of slavery, there was a blending of various African tribes, particularly in slave states and/or cities such as New Orleans, Louisiana, and Savannah, Georgia, with other cultural groups such as the French, the Creoles, and the Indians. Various folk medicine practices found among some Black Americans in the North, as well as the South, have been handed down from generation to generation. Even today, the consistent use of some form of Black folk medicine continues, indicating that these practices have withstood the test of time and are presumed to be valid, although no empirical data exist that would indicate the validity and/or reliability of such practices.

Rationale for the use of Black folk medicine

Some Black Americans choose to use folk medicine because of tradition, whereas others have made this choice based on previous discriminatory practices and unfair treatments that existed throughout some regions of the United States in years past. In this regard, the delivery of health care services were not exempt from "Jim Crow" laws, which were legally sanctioned until the mid-1960s throughout the South. However, the northern regions of the United States also were not exempt from such discriminatory practices in regard to health care. This is evident in the passage of the Hill-Burden Act in 1946, which was not abolished until 1966 with the passage of the Federal Medicare Act (Bullough & Bullough, 1982).

The Hill-Burden act, also known as the Hospital Construct Survey Act, provided federal grants for the construction of hospitals, private and public, that admittedly did not service Blacks. Under this law, hospitals, whether public or private, were allowed to discriminately service populations based on race. In addition, these same hospitals were allowed to continue these discriminatory practices in regard to hiring and staffing patterns. From such practices were born the all-Black hospitals, which were found not only in the South but in the North as well. Inclusions and exclusions for purposes of rendering health care services to those persons in need were left to the proprietors of the hospital. Thus patterns of admission and service to Black Americans varied throughout the country without regard to regional locale. In some northern and western states admission to and service by some hospitals remained theoretically open to all races on equal terms, whereas in other states the courts upheld the rights of hospital proprietors to segregate as they saw fit.

This discriminatory practice was dramatically emphasized by the deaths of two famous Black Americans: Bessie Smith, in 1937, and Charles Drew, in 1950. Bessie Smith was a legendary "blues" singer who was critically injured in an automobile accident while traveling from Jackson, Mississippi, to Memphis, Tennessee. White attendants at the scene of the accident surmised correctly that Smith had a severed right arm and therefore needed immediate medical attention. The attendants took Smith to a hospital designated as "all white," and the administrators at the hospital refused to treat her despite the severity of her injuries. The ambulance attendants were forced to take Smith to Memphis, were she could be treated. On arrival, Smith was in profound shock, having lost a great quantity of blood. It has been said that despite Bessie Smith's obvious fame and the great admiration shown her by millions of fans, both Black and White, the fact that she was Black ultimately caused her death (Albertson, 1982).

Charles Drew, a surgeon, discovered blood plasma and developed the procedure for blood plasma transfusion. Even today, people throughout the world, regardless of race, benefit from his discovery. However, despite his profoundly important contribution to the medical field, the discovery of blood plasma was of no benefit to Drew when he, like Smith, was involved in an automobile accident and similarly was refused treatment in an "all white" hospital. Although Drew was responsible for the technique of blood plasma transfusion, it was not used to save his life because he was taken to a hospital that legally had the right to refuse him treatment.

Black folk medicine therefore took roots not only as an offshoot of African cultural heritage, but as a necessity when Black Americans could not gain access to the traditional health care delivery system. Furthermore, some Black Americans turned to Black folk medicine because they either could not afford the cost of medical assistance or were tired of the insensitive treatment by caregivers in the health care delivery system (Bullough & Bullough, 1972). Today Black Americans have access to the health care delivery system through legal channels. Some Black Americans still refuse to use the system, however, citing reasons such as past experiences, the escalating cost of health care, and the sometimes insensitive treatment on the part of non-Black caregivers in regard to the physiological and psychosocial differences evidenced among Blacks.

Some Black Americans have a strong religious orientation, and most Black Americans belong to the Protestant faith. Although folk medicine and folk practices are widely documented in the literature as being common practices for the treatment of illnesses among Black Americans, the most common and frequently cited method of treating illness remains prayer (Spector, 1979). According to Snow (1977), many of her informants found it impossible to separate religious beliefs from medical ones.

Implications for Nursing Care

Cultural health practices are often considered efficacious, neutral, or dysfunctional (Pillsbury, 1982). Practices that are considered efficacious are recognized by Western medicine as beneficial to health, regardless of whether they are different from scientific practice. Practices that are regarded as beneficial by the nurse should be actively encouraged. The nurse should keep in mind that a treatment plan that is congruent with the patient's own beliefs has a better chance of being successful. For example, some Black Americans believe that certain herbs and spices are essential in the treatment of certain disequilibriums in the body. In this case herbal tea could be used in place of water and might be just as beneficial for the treatment of specific conditions such as dehydration. Neutral practices (such as putting a knife under the bed to cut pain) are considered to be of no significance one way or the other to the health of an individual. Dysfunctional health practices are viewed as harmful from a health point of view. For example, it is considered a dysfunctional health practice in Western medicine to use sugar and over-refined flour excessively. Dysfunctional health practices found among some Black Americans include such practices as using boiled goat's milk and cabbage juice for stomach infection.

Since some Black Americans tend to equate good health with luck or success, an illness may be viewed as undesirable and equated with bad luck, poverty, domestic turmoil, or even unemployment. As indicated previously, illnesses may be classified as natural or unnatural. Natural illnesses occur because a person is affected by natural forces without adequate protection. The nurse may be able to help the patient more readily understand how these natural illnesses, such as colds and flu, can be avoided. Unnatural illnesses, which are thought to be the direct result of evil influences, are much more difficult for the nurse to combat. If the nurse has a patient who believes that unnatural illness has resulted from witchcraft or voodoo or is a punishment from God, it may be very difficult to convince the patient that a treatment can be implemented that will minimize or eliminate the problem. For example, a patient may view breast cancer as a punishment from God. In this instance the patient should be encouraged to seek medical treatment because unnecessary delay can have serious consequences. While the nurse may not subscribe to cultural healing beliefs, it is essential that the nurse recognize their existence and their importance for some Black American patients. It is also important for the nurse to remember that effective nursing care cannot be implemented until the nurse acknowledges certain cultural health beliefs that have an impact on the patient's behavior and recovery.

Among some Black Americans it is believed that the maintenance of health is strongly associated with the ability to read the signs of nature. Subsumed in this belief is the idea that natural phenomena such as the phases of the moon, the seasons of the year, and planetary positions all either singly or in combination affect the human body and human physiological functioning. Some Black Americans believe that the best days to wean babies, for example, or to have dental or surgical procedures done, can be found in the *Farmer's Almanac* (Snow, 1974). To the nurse such beliefs may seem peculiar; however, the nurse must acknowledge the existence of such beliefs before culturally appropriate nursing care can be given. The nurse must also recognize that while some of these beliefs may be helpful, others may be neutral, and still others may be extremely dangerous for the patient. The nurse must be able to sort beliefs into these three categories and be able to assist the patient in recognizing beliefs that may be dangerous.

Some Black Americans believe that cultural healing remedies help a person psychologically in dealing with discomfort. However, when these things fail, they believe a physician should be consulted. These same Black Americans may also believe that the nurse should recognize these cultural beliefs and use remedies based on these beliefs that prove to be helpful to the patient (Bloch, 1976a). When a Black patient does arrive for professional health care, the nurse might assume that the patient has tried all the cultural healing remedies known. While doing the initial assessment, the nurse needs to find out what the patient has been using at home to minimize illness symptoms. This initial assessment will assist the nurse in determining whether these home remedies will interact or interfere with orthodox medical approaches. If the patient has been using harmless home remedies, they may be kept for use in the patient's treatment. Other harmless remedies might be added to the patient care plan at the patient's suggestion (Bloch, 1976a).

Religion for some Black Americans has functioned primarily as an escape mechanism from the harsh realities of life. The Black church functions to promote self-esteem among its membership. The Black church also acts as a curator for maintaining the culture of many Black Americans. Therefore the nurse cannot overlook the importance of the Black minister and the Black church in the recovery of the patient. If there is no Black minister within the hospital facility, the nurse should feel free to contact the patient's own minister. It is essential for the nurse to remember that the Black minister can essentially bridge the gap between the Black patient and other health care workers because the Black minister understands the rituals, folk ways, and mores of Black Americans (Smith, 1976).

BIOLOGICAL VARIATIONS

Until recently, the education of health care practitioners was based on the biopsychosocial characteristics of the dominant White culture. The lack of an in-depth understanding of biological and cultural differences resulted in less than optimum health care for persons who were not members of the dominant culture. When providing care to Black patients, the nurse must realize that racial differences involve more than skin color and hair texture. Black people have distinctive genotypes and phenotypes that characterize them as a racial group and as different from other racial groups. Moreover, the nurse must understand that Blacks also have ethnic and cultural differences that distinguish them from other ethnic and cultural groups.

Birth Weight

The mean birth weights of Black and White infants in the United States differ, with Black infants weighing approximately 240 g less than White infants. When controls for income level, maternal age, smoking, and marital status are made, Black infants still weigh less. At birth, Black infants are 2 cm shorter and 0.7 cm smaller in circumference than White infants (Pratt, Jones, & Seigal, 1977). It is clear that prematurity, which is defined as a birth weight under 2500 g, is twice as common for Blacks as for Whites (Morton, 1977), and it has been suggested that the definition for prematurity be lowered from 2500 to 2200 g for Blacks (Morton, 1977). The length of the gestational period for Blacks tends to be 9 days shorter than that for Whites, and a slowing down of gestational growth occurs in Black infants after 35 weeks. Before 35 weeks of gestation, Black infants are usually larger than White infants (Pratt, Jones, & Seigal, 1977). The reasons for these differences in birth weights remain vague.

Growth and Development

There is a tendency for Black children to mature faster than White children. Today Black children are more mature at birth in both the musculoskeletal and the neurological systems (Falkner & Tanner, 1978). Neurologically Black children tend to be more advanced until about the age of 2 or 3 years, and in the musculoskeletal system they tend to be more advanced until puberty (Roche, Roberts, & Hamell, 1978). The differences in skeletal maturity are attributed to genetic and environmental factors.

Body size, height, weight, bone length, and body structure of Blacks and Whites have been extensively studied in the United States. Studies done by Abraham, Clifford, and Najjar (1976) revealed that the average height and weight of Black and White men aged 18 to 74 are approximately the same; White men tend to be 0.5 cm taller than Black men. The average height for Black and White women is the same; however, Black women are consistently heavier than White women at every age, and between the ages of 35 and 64 they are typically an average of 20 pounds heavier than their White counterparts

Body Proportion

The body proportions of Blacks differ from those of Whites, Orientals, and American Indians. There are definitive differences in bone length that are obvious on study. Blacks have shorter trunks than Whites and tend to have longer legs than Whites, Orientals, and American Indians. Black men tend to have wider shoulders and narrower hips than Orientals, who tend to have narrow shoulders and wide hips. The long bones of Blacks are significantly longer and narrower than those of Whites (Farrally & Moore, 1976). The bones of Blacks are also denser. Black men have the densest bones, followed by Black women, White men, and finally, White women, who have the least bone density of the two races. The greater bone density explains why osteoporosis is rare in Blacks and why White women have a greater incidence of osteoporosis. Bone curvature also varies among the different races. The femurs of American Blacks are markedly straight as compared with those of American Indians, whose femurs are anterially convex, and those of Whites, who have intermediate curvature. This characteristic appears to be genetically determined, but weight also seems to be a factor, since obese Blacks and Whites tend to demonstrate more curvature than other individuals (Gilbert, 1977).

Body Fat

The amount and distribution of body fat is another area where there are marked differences by virtue of race and ethnic group. The racial differences are mostly related to socioeconomic status. Persons from the lower socioeconomic class tend to have more body fat than those from the middle class, and persons from the middle class tend to have more body fat than those from the upper class. There is some evidence suggesting that fat distribution varies according to race. Black people tend to have smaller skin fold thickness in their arms than Whites, but the distribution of fat on the trunk is similar for both Whites and Blacks (Bagan, Robson, & Soderstrom, 1971). Whites have a larger chest volume than Blacks; hence they have greater vital capacity and forced expiratory volume (Oscherwitz, 1972). Blacks, on the other hand, have a larger chest volume than American Indians and Orientals and thus greater vital capacity and forced expiratory volume than members of these racial groups (Oscherwitz, 1972).

Skin Color

Skin color, or pigmentation, is the most distinguishing physical difference among the various races and is determined by melanin. All people have some melanin, but some racial groups have more melanin than others. The greater the amount of melanin that an individual has, the darker the skin pigmentation will be. The skin color of persons who are classified as Blacks may range from "white" to very dark brown or perhaps even black. Melanin provides protection from the effects of the sun; thus Blacks and other dark-skinned individuals have a lower incidence of skin cancer. Blacks do get sunburned, but not as easily as Whites (Overfield, 1985).

The skin coloring should be uniform, but areas that are not exposed to the sun may be lighter, such as the buttocks, abdomen, and thorax. The exceptions to this rule for Black people are the skin folds in the groin, the genitalia, and the nipples, which tend to be darker than the rest of the body. (An old wives' tale suggests that to determine the true color of a newborn infant, one should look at the ears, which tend to be darker at birth than the rest of the body.) With the exception of the areas just mentioned, hypopigmentation and hyperpigmentation (unless it is a birthmark) are abnormal (Bloch, 1983). Pigmentation of the lips, nail beds, palmar surfaces, creases of the hands, and plantar surfaces and creases of the feet may vary, as does skin coloring. The range of coloring for the lips of Black Americans may vary from pink to plum colored. The palmar and plantar surfaces may range from light pink to dark pink to a brownish color, and the creases may range from dark pink to dark brown, depending on the amount of pigmentation (Bloch, 1976b). The gums may have areas of hyperpigmentation, and the sclera may have scattered areas of brown pigmentation that appear to be freckles.

Mongolian spots are a common variance found in Black infants. They are migratory leftovers of melanocytes that have lingered in the lumbosacral region at a greater than normal depth, which accounts for their dark blue-green appearance. Mongolian spots occur in 90% of Blacks, 80% of Orientals and American Indians, and only 9% of Whites (Jacob & Walton, 1976). Normally found on the buttocks, thighs, ankles, and arms, mongolian spots usually disappear in the first year of life and should not be mistaken for a bruise.

Birthmarks appear to be most common in Black individuals, occurring in 20% of Blacks as compared with 2% to 3% of Whites, Mexicans, and American Indians. These pigmented marks appear as sharply demarcated macules that vary from light tan to dark brown, depending on the skin color. They may be present anywhere on the body (Overfield, 1985).

Black skin is also more susceptible to an overgrowth of connective tissue in response to injury, or keloid formation. Keloids are raised areas of scar tissue that can result from minor injuries such as skin tears or punctures, from more major injuries such as burn injuries or traumatic lacerations, or from surgical incisions (Rook, 1970).

Normal, healthy skin should be warm, dry, and elastic. There should be a red glow present in Black skin. Color changes associated with abnormal conditions are rashes, which may be difficult or impossible to detect in the individual who is darkly pigmented. Darkly pigmented lips and nail beds with melanin deposits make nursing assessment even more difficult. When possible, the nurse should become familiar with the patient's normal coloring in order to establish a baseline. The skin assessment should be done in a well-lighted room. Sunlight is the best lighting, and if artificial lighting is used, it should be nonglaring (Bloch & Hunter, 1981). When assessing the darkly pigmented individual for specific color changes such as pallor, jaundice, or cyanosis, the nurse should inspect the conjunctiva and oral membranes of the buccal mucosa. Jaundice also appears as a yellowish discoloration of the sclera if it is not pigmented. The mucous membranes of the buccal mucosa, and the palmar and plantar surfaces may also be inspected for yellow discoloration.

The nurse may also rely on palpitations and the patient's history to detect the presence of bruises in the darkly pigmented patient. The nurse should use the dorsal surface of the hand to assess for areas of increased warmth, as well as tenderness. Questioning should include a history of recent trauma. The petechiae cannot be readily visualized on the dark-skinned individual. The nurse should inspect the sclera for dark blue spots. The patient history should include questioning about symptoms of conditions in which petechiae would be present. Palpitation and the patient history may also be used to detect the presence of a macular rash on the patient who is dark skinned (Bloch, 1983).

Enzymatic Variations

Biochemical variations and their effects on health vary according to race. As with other racial variations, biochemical variations are attributed to genetic factors and environmental influences. Lactose intolerance is a well-known condition that is correlated with race: 90% of African Blacks and 75% of American Blacks are affected with lactose intolerance (McCrackin, 1971). Individuals with lactose intolerance lack the enzyme to convert lactose to glucose and galactose, and as a result, gastrointestinal symptoms of bloating, cramping, and diarrhea occur. The condition is genetically transmitted, although the specific gene has not been identified (Johnson, Cole, & Abner, 1981). There appears to be two periods in life during which symptoms occur: during infancy shortly after weaning and during the teen years or early 20s. The condition is diagnosed on the basis of signs or symptoms that occur after the ingestion of milk or other products containing lactose, and treatment consists of having the individual avoid these products, with appropriate substitution of other products. The nursing implications for nurses caring for Black patients include (1) knowledge of the condition and its prevalence among Blacks and (2) education of patients with the condition to avoid products containing lactose. The education of these patients should include encouraging them to read labels and make appropriate food substitutions (Bloch, 1974).

AIDS (HIV) Risk

A recent study reported in *Scope*, a publication of the Institute of Black Chemical Abuse (1989), involving 633 heterosexual intravenous drug abusers in San Franciso revealed the rapid spread of human immunodeficiency virus (HIV) infection in the Black community. Twelve percent of the entire sample was found to be seropositive. However, 26% of the Black subjects tested seropositive, as compared with 10% of the Hispanics and 6% of the Whites studied. The entire sample group studied was 59% male; 41% female; 52% White; 29% Black, and 20% Hispanic and "other" racial groups. The study found a strong correlation between intravenous cocaine use and a sharply increased risk for HIV infection. Daily intravenous cocaine users, 35% of whom were HIV antibody positive, were nearly six and a half times more likely to be infected than drug users who did not inject cocaine. Some of the reasons suggested for this greater frequency were the greater frequency with which users inject the drug, the "shooting gallery" setting in which injection typically takes place (which encourages the sharing of needles), and the method most commonly used, which involves the drawing of a greater quantity of blood into the needle on average than is normally done with other intravenous drugs. The percentage of Black intravenous cocaine abusers who reported sharing their "works" with other Black users was found to be substantially higher than the percentage of White users who reported sharing needles with other Whites. This study also verified other research findings that high-risk behaviors tend to cluster together and that behavioral factors, rather than biological variables, account for the racial differences in HIV infection rates (Institute of Black Chemical Abuse, 1989).

Psychological Characteristics

Some studies depict the pattern of interaction in the Black family as being pathological and unstable. Findings from one study suggest that if there is stability in the Black family, it is due to the presence of a controlling, domineering mother. The pathological family interaction that occurs in some Black American families is said to affect the male son so profoundly that in later life he is unable to adjust to the role of husband and father. Consequently, in unstable Black families the Black male is unable to form mature, lasting relationships with others *(Culture of Poverty Revisited)*. In studies done on Black male alcoholics it was found that these individuals have the lowest scores on tests of personality integration, with a more passive and compliant coping style than any other ethnic group of male alcoholics (Carroll, Klein, & Santo, 1978). It is thought that this passive and compliant coping style was rooted in the slavery era. During slavery, Black mothers were forced to teach their male children to be passive if they were to survive the authority of the slave master, because to be "uppity" meant possible physical punishment or even death. Today, it would seem essential that the Black male display the same survival skills because the authority figure still remains (police, educators, employers, etc.).

In a study done on Black boys from father-absent homes, it was found that dependency and a passive coping style were evident among these boys (Barclay & Cusumano, 1967). Other studies suggest that boys from father-absent homes tend to be more dependent on their peer groups, display fewer aggressive behaviors, have lower self-esteem, and are more likely to display overt masculine behavior. In some studies looking at psychological issues of father-absent homes, social class appeared to be an intervening variable. A more deleterious effect on sex role orientation was found in boys who lived in father-absent homes before the age of 5 (Covell & Turnbull, 1982). Because there is a probability of a Black child being reared in a female-headed household, it has become necessary for Black mothers to encourage masculine traits in their sons. In an earlier study it was found that mothers who encouraged masculine traits in their sons had more of an impact in father-absent homes than in father-present homes (Biller, 1969).

Some social scientists and health care providers contend that Black Americans are at risk for the development of mental health problems. Corrective steps have been taken to alleviate the development of mental health problems; however, the mental health system continues to struggle to meet the emotional needs of Black Americans (Snowden, 1982; Snowden & Todman, 1982). Bullough and Bullough (1982) reported that admission rates to mental health hospitals are higher and the hospital stay is longer for Black Americans than for any other ethnic group in America. However, it was found that when socioeconomic status was carefully controlled, psychosis rates among Whites and Blacks appeared similar.

Chemical abuse

Alcoholism is one of the number one health problems in the Black community, contributing to reduced longevity. There are high incidences of acute and chronic alcohol-related diseases among Blacks, such as alcoholic fatty liver; hepatitis; cirrhosis of the liver; heart disease; cancers of the mouth, larynx, tongue, esophagus, and lung; and unintentional injuries and homicide (Ronan, 1987).

Harper and Dawkins (1976) reported that of 16,000 articles on alcohol abuse published from 1944 to 1974, only 77 included references to Blacks and only 11 were specifically about Blacks. King (1982) reported that most studies between 1977 and 1980 reported only on patterns of alcohol use. Only one study (Stalls, 1978) explored racial differences in patterns of alcohol metabolism. Stalls (1978) found an increasing incidence of alcohol abuse among Black youth and women, with serious implications for fetal alcohol syndrome. Drinking appeared to peak in the 16- to 23-year-old range, and, among women, drinking was highest for divorced women under the age of 45. Brisbane (1987) noted that women who drank were typically under the age of 45, employed, and considered themselves middle class. Williams (1986) noted a contradiction in the high incidence of alcohol-related diseases and drinking patterns reported in Blacks; when age and socioeconomic levels were controlled, Blacks actually abstained more, drank less frequently, and consumed less alcohol than their White counterparts. Black women were the exception, with 11% of Black women drinking heavily as compared with 4% of White women.

Several causes of alcohol abuse and misuse in Black America have been identified in the literature. A primary factor is economics. Many Black men drink as a result of unemployment, which leads to depression and frustration because of the inability to meet financial commitments. Williams (1986) concluded that unemployment is correlated with a high risk for alcohol problems among Blacks. Availability is also a factor (Parker & Harman, 1978). Brown and Tooley (1989) have reported that in Los Angeles there are approximately three liquor stores per city block. Black peer pressure is also reported as a contributing factor; peers expect heavy drinking, and brand names and quantity are often status identifiers. Finally, heavy alcohol use may be related to a desire to escape unpleasant feelings. Sterne and Pittman (1972) have also pointed out themes that seem to be present in Black American alcohol use. They linked being paid on the weekend to Saturday relaxation and thus drinking. A second theme is the prevalence of taverns in the Black community that serve as social centers. Finally, alcohol appears to be used as an escape from personal problems.

Black Americans are less likely to seek treatment for problem drinking than any other ethnic group in America (Lawson & Lawson, 1989). Research suggests that several areas must be addressed to increase the likelihood of successful treatment outcomes. The first step is to get the Black alcoholic into a treatment program. Programs that are located within the community and that are accessible to public transportation are more likely to be used, except by the upwardly mobile Black American, who is more likely to seek private services outside the community. The Black church can, and in some instances does, serve a dual role in this first step because it can provide a facility and at the same time act as a referral source. Most Black churches are centrally located within the Black community, and even as members relocate, they tend to maintain their roots in the Black church. Also, prayer has been associated with the treatment modality and overall success rate for the recovering alcoholic. The church continues to be the mainstay of the Black family, and, rather than seeking outside help for alcoholism, the family often attempts to resolve problems by going to the minister. Some Blacks have reported that they stopped drinking before seeking professional help because of their spirituality, which assisted with the transition (Brisbane, 1987; Hudson, 1986; Knox, 1986; Westermeyer, 1984).

When treating the recovering alcoholic, the nurse must remember that the family can often provide assistance in the form of shelter, food, money, or clothing. The extended family may also take on counseling roles that close relatives find too painful (Brisbane & Womble, 1986).

The nurse must also have an awareness of the socioeconomic context and its impact on intrapsychic processes. The elimination of stereotypical bias by both the nurse and the patient and the inclusion of social values and traditions are necessary to maximize intervention, give culturally appropriate nursing care, and affect recovery rates (Institute of Black Chemical Abuse, 1988).

Posttraumatic stress disorder

A number of studies have been conducted that suggest that minority Vietnam veterans have experienced a greater degree of maladjustment following the Vietnam War than their White counterparts (Allen, 1986; Laufer, Gallops, & Frey-Wouters, 1984). Some of these studies have given a variety of reasons for this, including the fact that minorities felt more conflict about participating in war because they had less to gain than persons in the dominant culture, such as Whites. Another reason postulated by the researchers was the fact that minorities were more likely to be identified with the enemy, who was also different in skin color from White Americans. Perhaps the most significant reason for posttraumatic stress disorder (PSTD) among minority Vietnam veterans was that fact that the status of minorities declined in the United States during the turbulence of the 1960s at the same time that Blacks were fighting for America in Vietnam (Allen, 1986; Laufer et al., 1981).

A more recent study by Penk et al. (1989) has also found that among Vietnam combat veterans, Black Americans appeared to be more maladjusted than their White counterparts. One conclusion of this study is that ethnicity emerges as a significant parameter in studies of PSTD, but the exact contributions of ethnicity have not been explained fully by current findings on the subject. Many researchers have postulated that significant increases noted in PSTDs seen in Black Vietnam veterans may be due in part to the fact that during the Vietnam War years (1964 to 1975) Blacks suffered the major loss of a leader (through the assassination of Martin

Luther King, Jr., in 1968) and experienced the racial conflicts evidenced by rioting in Washington, D.C., Watts, and other cities throughout the country (Karnow, 1983).

Other psychological characteristics

The psychiatric literature on psychological characteristics of Blacks and treatment of Blacks by mental health professionals is colorful and controversial. The psychiatric literature has reported increased psychopathological disorders among Blacks (Pasamanick, 1964). Anatomical, neurological, and endocrinological differences have been cited as signs of Black inferiority (Thomas & Sillen, 1972; Tobias, 1970). Research has been done on Blacks that would not have been considered for other ethnic groups; for example, in the well-publicized Tuskegee project, Black men with syphilis were intentionally denied treatment without being informed of their disease (Cave, 1975; Jones, 1982). Research on intelligence quotients (IQs) has been used to support statements of genetic inferiority and justify social policies such as selective immigration laws and school segregation (Hirsch, 1981). Such psychological research has added to racial stereotyping and bias among some mental health professionals.

According to Meyers and Weissman (1980-1981), some differences in phobias have been found between Blacks and Whites. Robins et al. (1981) noted that the lifetime prevalence rate of acrophobia was significantly higher for Blacks than for Whites. Vernon and Roberts (1982) found that Blacks, as compared with Whites, had a significantly lower lifetime rate of both major and minor depression but had a rate of bipolar depression that was twice that of Whites. A possible explanation for the discrepancy in findings is the lack of national data on racial differences in diagnostic analogs. It is now widely accepted that on the MMPI (Minnesota Multiphase Personality Inventory) Blacks tend to score higher on the paranoia and schizophrenia scales than Whites because the instrument was not standardized on a Black population (Bell & Mehta, 1981; Gynther, 1981; Jones, Gray, & Parson, 1981). When standardized diagnostic systems are used today, Blacks do not differ from Whites in the prevalence of most psychiatric disorders. Robins et al. (1981) and Meyers and Weissman (1980-1981) have reported finding no significant race differences for schizophrenia or affective disorders (Adebimpe, 1981; Lawson & Lawson, 1989; Mukherjee, Shukla, & Woodle, 1983; Spurlock, 1985).

Snow (1978) found that a belief in witchcraft was shared by a third of the Black patients who were treated at a southern psychiatric center. Blacks who believe they have a folk illness may use the services of a root worker, reader, spiritualist, or voodoo priest. It is important for the nurse to know that the patient may have used the services of a folk practitioner before or in conjunction with scientific mental health therapy. Wintrob (1973) has promoted the idea that individuals with a belief in folk remedies such as root work or obeah may regard scientific treatment only as palliative, because curing the total condition requires neutralization by a specially skilled folk healer. Wintrob (1973), Kreisman (1975), Weclew (1975), and Sandoval (1977) have suggested that mental health professionals should attempt to complement use of scientific medicine with folk practices for patients who believe mental disorders are attributed to folk causes.

Implications for Nursing Care

The best reason for including the concept of biological variations in nursing practice is that knowledge of scientific facts aids the nurse in giving culturally appropriate care. It is also essential for the nurse who cares for people from other cultures to know certain biological concepts, not only in order to give culturally appropriate nursing care, but also to give nonharmful nursing care.

Important biological variations that the nurse should be aware of are related to body size, birth weight, and body proportion. It is important for the nurse who works with Black children to remember that Black children at birth tend to weigh less and be shorter than their White counterparts, and that these variations may be due in part to socioeconomic status. Therefore the nurse, whether in a hospital or a clinic setting, must carefully evaluate growth status in terms of height and weight for Black children. Although some nurses think that since growth charts are White normed, the charts lack implications for Black children, serious deviations can have implications for intervention for nutritional deficiencies. These variations between Black and White children may continue as the child grows. For example, Black preschoolers are neurologically more advanced than their White counterparts. In addition, Black children tend to have less subcutaneous fat than White children but are taller and heavier by the age of 2 (Owen & Lubin, 1973). The fact that Black preschoolers are taller and heavier may indicate a need for appropriate patient teaching about nutritional needs of the growing child.

Since the average weight for a Black woman is consistently higher than for her White counterpart at every age, it is important for the nurse to teach Black patients the value of serving nutritiously sound meals. In addition, the nurse must emphasize the importance of exercise, not only to maintain ideal weight, but also for cardiovascular purposes.

It is essential that the nurse develop a sensitivity for and familiarity with physical features that are common to Blacks, as well as Black-related illnesses and diseases. If the nurse is unable to develop a familiarity with physical features common to Blacks and to Black illnesses or diseases, the nurse cannot possibly hope to recognize or diagnose conditions that may cause disequilibrium in the body. In addition, the nurse must be prepared to deal promptly, efficiently, and appropriately with clinical variables that are common to all Black patients and yet have significant variability in some Black patients, such as hypertension or sickle cell anemia.

There is no clear correlation between hypertension and obesity in Blacks, as there is with other ethnic groups such as Whites. On the other hand, there appears to be a direct correlation between the amount of skin pigmentation and the frequency of hypertension. Therefore, since it has been suggested that there is a direct relationship between skin pigmentation and hypertension, the nurse should emphasize the need for the Black patient to undergo hypertension screening (Boyle, 1970).

Since glucose-6-phosphate dehydrogenase (G-6-PD) deficiency, a hematological problem present in 35% of Black Americans, is a prevailing problem among Black Americans today, it is essential that the nurse stress the importance of the fluorescent spot test as a screening tool to diagnose this deficiency. The nurse can serve as a patient advocate and insist or mandate that this test be a routine part of laboratory testing for all Black patients. Also, precautions should be taken to eliminate the transfusion of G-6-PD–deficient blood, particularly in transfusions for infants (Beutler, 1972). In addition, the nurse should exercise precaution when planning diets for Black patients, particularly Black infants, since they may be lactose intolerant. In the case of lactose intolerance the nurse should plan diets that take into account the substitution of milk and milk products by more compatible products with the same nutritional value (Bloch, 1981).

SUMMARY

It is important for the nurse to remember that if help is requested in regard to a Black patient, it generally will come from within the family system, and that it is important to include the family system when planning and implementing nursing care. Failure to include the family in the planning and implementation of nursing care may result in failed interventions. The nurse who is attempting to help the patient problem solve also needs to remember that problem solving tends to be action oriented; the Black patient may become impatient if it appears that nothing is actually happening to alleviate the present problem (Bloch, 1983).

In caring for the Black patient, the nurse must recognize and acknowledge the patient's racial, cultural, and ethnic background, since it is in these areas that the patient's experiences take place. Not only is it important for the nurse to consider necessary adjustments in patient care when the patient is from a different racial origin, but it is also important that the racial origin of the nurse be considered. In a classic and innovative study by Remington and DaCosta (1989), the effects of ethnocultural differences between supervisor and caregiver are dramatically illustrated. The nurse who denies or does not believe race is not a factor denies a significant part of the patient's being.

*CASE STUDY**   William Boyd is a usually energetic 15-year-old boy who lives with his mother and father and six brothers and sisters in southern Georgia. Today William has come to the local health care clinic with his mother, complaining of severe abdominal and joint pains. William tells the clinic nurse that the pain started this afternoon while playing ball with his friends. The nurse observes that William appears scared and is "doubled over" with pain, crying out, "Momma, my belly is killin' me." William's mother tells the nurse that William has "tired blood," which the nurse interprets to be sickle cell disease. William's mother states that William's recent health has been good except for a "chest cold a couple days ago."

On examination, the nurse notes that William is a poorly developed 15-year-old with a somewhat short trunk and long extremities. The nurse also notes that William has a peculiar "cone" shape to his head. William's skin is hot and dry, with an oral temperature of 100.6° F and dry mucous membranes. The abdomen is firm and very tender, especially in both upper quadrants. William complains of pain in his upper and lower extremities, as well as in his back and chest.

A blood smear is used to confirm William's sickle cell disease, and the diagnosis of sickle cell crisis is made by the clinic physician. William is admitted to the hospital with orders for intravenous fluids for hydration and narcotic analgesics for pain. William's mother makes arrangements to sleep in his hospital room at night.

William is discharged 4 days after admission.

*Case study by Dale Moore, B.S.N., R.N.

CARE
PLAN

Nursing Diagnosis   Pain related to sickle cell crisis due to thrombotic episode.

Patient Outcome

Patient will convey relief of pain with alleviating measures.

Nursing Interventions

1   Evaluate pain level and treat with analgesics as ordered.
2   Teach patient reason for pain and explain plan of care to reduce pain.
3   Assess patient's fear and assist patient
with reducing fear.
4   Encourage patient to ask for pain medication as needed.
5   Encourage proper hydration to promote
circulation.

Nursing Diagnosis   Infection, potential for, related to sickle cell anemia.

Patient Outcome

Patient will understand risk factors associated with the potential for infection and
will incorporate measures to reduce the
potential for infection.

Nursing Interventions

1   Provide patient with a nutritionally balanced diet.
2   Assess past history of infections, especially respiratory tract infections.
3   Instruct and encourage proper personal
hygiene.
4   Stress importance of adequate rest and
sleep.
5   Teach importance of avoiding persons
with respiratory tract infections.

Nursing Diagnosis   Anxiety related to acute sickle cell crisis.

Patient Outcome

Patient's anxiety will be reduced with effective teaching, pain control, and reassurance.

Nursing Interventions

1   Allow for one family member to remain
in room with patient as desired.
2   Provide patient with frequent reassurance and comfort measures.
3   Provide patient with a calm and quiet
environment.
4   Help patient realize a sense of security.
5   Involve patient's family in his care.

Nursing Diagnosis   Tissue perfusion, altered, related to sickle cell crisis.

Patient Outcome

Patient will recognize factors/situations that
impair tissue perfusion and adjust life-
style to promote increased tissue perfusion.

Nursing Interventions

1   Maintain proper hydration.
2   Avoid environmental situations conducive to dehydration.
3   Reduce possible trauma-causing situations.

4   Instruct patient to wear warm clothing in cool environments.
5   Construct an exercise program specific to patient's needs.
6   Discourage prolonged periods of immobilization.

Nursing Diagnosis   Growth and development, altered (potential for), secondary to sickle cell disease.

Patient Outcome

Patient will exhibit an understanding of and participate in activities that promote normal growth and development.

Nursing Invertentions

1   Assess patient's understanding of importance of proper rest and nutrition.
2   Assist patient in developing an exercise program compatible with sickle cell disease.
3   Explore patient's feelings about himself.
4   Provide patient with an opportunity to explore hobbies and activities to help personal growth and development.
5   Allow patient the opportunity to show personal independence by involving him in care decisions.

Nursing Diagnosis   Communication, impaired verbal, related to cultural differences in dialect, resulting in possible misinterpretation of terms on the part of health care providers.

Patient Outcome

Effective communication between patient, patient's family, and health care providers will be established.

Nursing Interventions

1   Establish rapport with patient and family members.
2   Make use of culturally appropriate dialect while reinforcing appropriate terms.
3   Determine meaning of the dialect used (e.g., "tired blood" for anemia).
4   Avoid criticizing dialect used by patient and his family.
5   Spend appropriate amount of time with patient and his family to ensure that the proper meaning of unfamiliar words and terms is understood.
6   Communicate in an unhurried, relaxed manner.
7   Show respect when talking to family members by using "Mr.," "Mrs.," "Ms.," along with the last name.

Nursing Diagnosis Coping, ineffective family: compromised, related to stress resulting from hospitalization of a family member.

Patient Outcome	*Nursing Interventions*
Family will more effectively deal with stress after conversing with health care workers about expected outcome of patient's acute illness and planned treatment.	1 Assess family's understanding of patient's hospitalization. 2 Determine family's usual source of strength. 3 Assess family's spiritual and/or religious background and its importance. 4 Spend time with family members, listening to their concerns. 5 Ensure family members that they will be kept abreast of any changes in patient's condition. 6 Involve family members in patient's care as appropriate. 7 Make arrangements for one family member to spend the night in patient's room.

STUDY QUESTIONS

1. List the cause for the intense pain associated with sickle cell crisis.
2. Why is it important for the nurse to get a detailed health history for other members of William's family?
3. What measures might the nurse undertake to help William maintain his self-concept?
4. What are the dangers associated with sickle cell crisis?
5. List several strategies that may help health care providers communicate better with Blacks.
6. Describe ways in which health care providers may show sensitivity and acceptance of Black folk health care practices.
7. Compare and contrast the social organization of Blacks, especially in the South, from the 1940s to the present.
8. List several practices from ancient African ancestry that are part of modern nursing philosophy.
9. Describe the importance of folk medicine practices and folk healers to Black Americans in the rural setting.

REFERENCES

Abraham, S.J., Clifford, L., & Najjar, M.F. (1976, Nov.). Height and weight of adults 18-74 years of age in the United States. *Advancedata, 3,* 1-18.

Adebimpe, V. (1981). Overview: White norms and psychiatric diagnosis of Black patients. *American Journal of Psychiatry, 138,* 279-285.

Albertson, C. (1972). *A night in the life of Bessie Smith.* New York: Steine & Day.

Allen, I.M. (1986). Post-traumatic stress disorder among Black Vietnam veterans. *Hospital and Community Psychiatry, 37,* 55-61.

Anderson, S.V., & Bauwens, E.E. (1981). *Chronic health problems: Concepts and application.* St. Louis: C.V. Mosby.

Angelou, M. (1989). Maya Angelou (personal interview and portrait). In B. Lanker (Ed.), *I dream a world: Portraits of Black women who changed America.* New York: Stewart, Tabori, & Chang.

Bagan, M., Robson, J., & Soderstrom, R. (1971). Ethnic differences in skin fold thickness. *American Journal of Clinical Nutrition, 24,* 864-868.

Barclay, A., & Cusumano, D.R. (1967). Father absence, cross sex identity, and field-dependent behavior of male adolescents. *Child Development, 38,* 343-350.

Bell, C., & Mehta, H. (1981). The misdiagnosis of Black patients with manic depressive illness: Second in a series. *Journal of the National Medical Association, 73,* 101-107.

Beutler, E.H. (1972). Glucose-6-phosphate dehydrogenase deficiency In W.J. Williams (Ed.), *Hematology* (pp. 291-308). New York: McGraw-Hill.

Biller, H.B. (1969). Father absence, maternal encouragement, and sex role development in kindergarten boys. *Child Development, 40,* 539-546.

Bloch, B. (1974, May 3-4). A look at nursing intervention and Black patient care. In B. Bloch (Coordinator), *Care of the Black patient on the job: An on the job look at health care needs of the Black patient.* Conference presented by Continuing Education in Nursing, University of California, San Francisco, School of Nursing, San Francisco.

Bloch, B. (1976a). *Health care from a minority viewpoint.* Upublished study. University of California, San Francisco, School of Nursing, San Francisco.

Bloch, B. (1976b). Nursing intervention in Black patient care. In D. Luckraft (Ed.), *Black awareness: Implications for Black patient care* (pp. 27-35). New York: American Journal of Nursing Company.

Bloch, B. (1981). Black Americans and cross-cultural counseling experiences. In A.J. Marsella & P.B. Pedersen (Eds.), *Cross cultural counseling and psychotherapy.* New York: Pergamon Press.

Bloch, B. (1983). Bloch's assessment guide for ethnic/cultural variations. In M.S. Orque, B. Bloch, & L.S.A. Monrroy, (Eds.), *Ethnic nursing care: A multicultural approach* (pp. 49-75). St. Louis: C.V. Mosby.

Bloch, B., & Hunter, M. (1981). Teaching physiological assessment of Black persons. *Nurse Educator, 6,* 24-27.

Boyle, E., Jr. (1970). Biological pattern in hypertension by race, sex, body weight, and skin color. *JAMA, 213,* 1637-1643.

Brisbane, F.L. (1987). Divided feeling of Black alcoholic daughters. *Alcohol Health and Research World, 12,* pp. 48-50.

Brisbane, F.L., & Womble, M. (1986). Afterthoughts and recommendations. *Alcoholism Treatment Quarterly, 2*(3-4), 249-270.

Brown, F., & Tooley, J. (1989). Alcoholism in the Black community. In G. Lawson & A. Lawson (Eds.), *Alcohol and substance abuse in special populations.* Rockville, Md.: Aspen.

Bullough, V.L., & Bullough, B. (1982). *Health care for the other Americans.* East Norwalk, Conn.: Appleton-Century-Crofts.

Carroll, J.F., Klein, M.I., & Santo, Y. (1978). Comparison of the similarities and differences in the self-concepts of male alcoholics and addicts. *Journal of Consulting Clinical Psychology, 46,* 575-576.

Cave, V. (1975). Proper uses and abuses of the health care delivery system for minorities with special reference to the Tuskegee syphilis study. *Journal of the National Medical Association, 67,* 82-84.

Covell, K., & Turnbull, W. (1982). The long term effects of father absence in childhood on male university students' sex-role identity and personal adjustment. *Journal of Genetic Psychology, 141,* 271-276.

Culture of poverty revisited. (no date). New York: Mental Health Committee against Racism.

Dillard, J.L. (1972). *Who speaks Black English: Its history and usage in the United States.* New York: Random House.

Falkner, F., & Tanner, J. (1978). *Human growth I: Principles and prenatal growth.* New York: Plenum Press.

Farrally, M., & Moore, W. (1976, July). Anatomical differences in the femur and tibia between Negroids and Caucasians. *American Journal of Physiology and Anthropology, 43*(1), 63-69.

Friedlander, W. (1966). *Introduction to social welfare* (2nd ed.). Englewood Cliffs, N.J.: Prentice Hall.

Gilbert, B.M. (1977). Anterior femoral curvature: Its probable basis and utility as a criterion for racial assessment. *American Journal of Physical Anthropology, 45*(3), 601-604.

Gynther, M. (1981). Is the MMPI an appropriate assessment device for Blacks? *Journal of Black Psychology, 7,* 67-75.

Hall, E.T. (1966). *The hidden dimension.* New York: Doubleday.

Hall, E.T. (1976). *Beyond culture.* New York: Anchor Books.

Harper, F., & Dawkins, M. (1976). Alcohol and Blacks: Survey of periodical literature. *British Journal of Addiction, 71,* 327-334.

Henderson, G., & Primeaux, M. (1981). *Transcultural health care.* Reading, Mass.: Addison-Wesley.

Hirsch, J. (1981). To "unfrock the charlatans." *Sage Race Relations Abstracts, 6,* 1-65.

Hudson, H.L. (1986). How and why Alcoholics Anonymous works for Blacks. *Alcoholism Treatment Quarterly, 2*(314), 11-29.

Hymes, D. (Ed.). (1970). *Pidginization and creolization of languages.* London: Cambridge University Press.

Institute of Black Chemical Abuse. (1988). *Annual report.* Minneapolis: Author.

Institute of Black Chemical Abuse. (1989, spring). *Scope.* Quarterly publication of the Institute of Black Chemical Abuse, Minneapolis.

Jackson, J., Neighbors, H., & Gurin, G. (1986). Findings from a national survey on Black mental health: Implications for practice and training. In National Institute of Mental Health: *Mental health research and practice in minority communities.* Rockville, Md.: U.S. Department of Health and Human Services.

Jacob, A.H., & Walton, R.G. (1976). Incidence of birthmarks in the neonate. *Pediatrics, 58,* 218-222.

Jacques, G. (1976). Cultural health traditions: A Black perspective. In M.F. Branch & P.P. Paxton (Eds.), *Providing safe nursing care for ethnic people of color.* East Norwalk, Conn.: Appleton-Century-Crofts.

Johnson, R., Cole R., & Abner F. (1981). Genetic interpretation of social/ethnic differences in lactose absorption and tolerance. *Human Biology, 53*(1), 1-3.

Jones, B., Gray, B., & Parson, E. (1981). Manic-depressive illness among poor urban Blacks. *American Journal of the National Medical Association, 72,* 141-145.

Jones, L. (1968a). *Black music.* New York: William Morrow.

Jones, L. (1968b). The myth of a Negro literature. *Home: Social Essays.* London.

Jones, L. (1982). *Bad blood: The Tuskegee syphilis experiment.* New York: Free Press.

Jordan, W.C. (1975). Voodoo medicine. In R.A. Williams (Ed.), *Textbook of Black related diseases* (pp. 115-138). New York: McGraw-Hill.

Jordan, W.C. (1979). The roots and practice of voodoo medicine in America. *Urban Health 8,* 38-48.

Kamin, L.J. (1974). *The science and politics of IQ.* Hillsdale, N.J.: Lawrence Erlbaum.

Karnow, S. (1983). *Vietnam: A history.* New York: Viking Press.

King, L.M. (1982). Alcoholism—Studies regarding Black Americans: 1979-1980. *Alcohol and Health Monograph 4: Special Population Issues,* pp. 385-407.

Kluckhohn, C. (1972). The gifts of tongues. In L.A. Samover & R.D. Porter (Eds.), *Intercultural communication: A reader.* Belmont, Calif.: Wadsworth.

Knox, D.H. (1986). Spirituality: A tool in the assessment and treatment of Black alcoholics and their families. *Alcoholism Treatment Quarterly, 2*(3-4), 313-343.

Kreisman, J. (1975). The curandero's apprentice: A therapeutic integration of folk and medical healing. *American Journal of Psychiatry, 132,* 81.

Laufer, R.S., Gallops, M.S., & Frey-Wouters, E. (1984). War stress and trauma: The Vietnam veterans experience. *Journal of Health and Social Behavior, 18,* 236-244.

Laufer, R.S., Yager, T., Frey-Wouters, E., Donnellan, J., Gallops, M., & Stenbeck, K. (1981). *Legacies of Vietnam.* Washington, D.C.: U.S. Government Printing Office.

Lawson, G., & Lawson, A. (1989). *Alcoholism and substance abuse in special populations.* Rockville, Md.: Aspen.

Leininger, M. (1978). *Transcultural nursing.* New York: John Wiley & Sons.

LoBiodo-Wood, G., Zimmerman, L.M., & Gaston-Johansson, F.J. (1989, April 2). *Pain descriptors selected by different ethnic groups.* Paper presented at the 13th Annual Midwest Nursing Research Society Conference, Cincinnati.

Mbiti, J. (1970). *African religions and philosophies.* New York: Anchor Books.

McCrackin, R. (1971). Lactose deficiency: An example of dietary evaluation. *Current Anthropology, 12*(4-5), 479-517.

McKenzie, J., & Chrisman, N. (1977). Healing herbs, gods, and magic. *Nursing Outlook, 25*(5), 325-327.

Meyers, J., & Weissman, M. (1980-1981). *The prevalence of psychiatric disorders (DSM-III) in the community: 1980-1981.* Unpublished manuscript.

Mitchel, F. (1978). *Voodoo medicine: Sea islands herbal remedies.* Berkley, Calif.: Reed, Cannon, & Johnson.

Morton, N.E. (1977). Genetic aspects of prematurity. In D.M. Reed & F.J. Stanley (Eds.), *Epidemiology of prematurity.* Baltimore: Urban & Schwarzenberg.

Mukherjee, S., Shukla, S., & Woodle, J. (1983). Misdiagnosis of schizophrenia in bipolar patients: A multiethnic comparison. *American Journal of Psychiatry, 140,* 1571-1574.

Murray, R. (1987). *Psychiatric/mental health nursing.* East Norwalk, Conn.: Appleton & Lange.

National Center for Health Statistics (1985, Sept.). *Monthly Vital Statistics, 34*(Suppl. 2).

Oscherwitz, M. (1972). Differences in pulmonary function in various racial groups. *American Journal of Epidemiology, 96*(5), 319-327.

Overfield, T. (1985). *Biologic variations in health and illness: race, age and sex differences*. Reading, Mass.: Addison-Wesley.

Owen, G.M., & Lubin, A. (1973). Anthropometric differences between Black and White preschool children. *American Journal of Diseases in Children, 126,* 168.

Parker, D., & Harman, M. (1978). The distribution of consumption model of prevention of alcoholic problems: A critical assessment. *Journal of the Study of Alcohol, 39,* 377-399.

Pasamanick, B. (1964). Myths regarding prevalence of mental disease in the Negro. *Journal of the National Medical Association, 58,* 6-17.

Penk, W., Robinowitz, R., Black, J., Dolan, M., Bell, W., Dorsett, D., Ames, M., & Noriega, L. (1989). Ethnicity: Post-traumatic stress disorder (PTSD) differences among Black, White, and Hispanic veterans who differ in degrees of exposure to combat in Vietnam. *Journal of Clinical Psychology, 45*(5), 729-735.

Pillsbury, B. (1982). Doing the month: Confinement and convalescence of Chinese women after childbirth. In M. Kay (Ed.), *Anthropology of human birth*. Philadelphia: F.A. Davis.

Poussaint, A., & Atkinson, C. (1970). Black youth and motivation. *Black Scholar, 1,* 43-51.

Pratt, M.W., Jones, Z.L., & Seigal, N.L. (1977). National variations in prematurity (1973-1974). In D.M. Reed & F.J. Stanley (Eds.), *The epidemiology of prematurity* (pp. 53-74). Baltimore: Urban & Schwarzenberg.

Remington, G., & DaCosta, G. (1989). Ethnocultural factors in resident supervison: Black and White supervisors. *American Journal of Psychotherapy, 43*(3), 343-355.

Robins, L., Helzer, J., Crougham, J., & Ratcliff, K. (1981). National Institutes of Mental Health diagnostic interview schedule: Its history, characteristics and validity. *Archives of General Psychiatry, 38,* 381-389.

Roche, A.F., Roberts, J., & Hamell, P.V. (1978). Skeletal maturity of youths 12-17 years of age: Racial, geographic and socioeconomic disproportions. *National Health, 11*(167), 1-98.

Ronan, L. (1987). Alcohol-related health risks among Black Americans. *Alcohol Health and Research World, 12,* 36-39.

Rook, A. (1970). *Racial and other genetic factors in dermatology*. Philadelphia: F.A. Davis.

Sandoval, M. (1977). Santeria: Afro-Cuban concepts of disease and its treatment in Miami. *Journal of Operational Psychiatry, 8*(52).

Smith, J.A. (1976). The role of the Black clergy as allied health care professionals in working with Black patients. In D. Luckraft (Ed.), *Black awareness: Implications for Black care* (pp. 12-15). New York: The American Journal of Nursing Company.

Snow, L.E. (1974). Folk medical beliefs and their implications for care of patients: A review based on studies among Black Americans. *Annuals of Internal Medicine, 81,* 82-96.

Snow, L.E. (1977). Popular medicine in a Black neighborhood. In E.H. Spicer (Ed.), *Ethnic medicine in the Southwest*. Tucson: University of Arizona Press.

Snow, L.E. (1978). Sorcerers, saints, and charlatans: Black folk healers in urban America. *Culture, Medicine, and Psychiatry, 2,* 69.

Snow, L.E. (1983). Traditional health beliefs and practice among lower class Black Americans. *Western Journal of Medicine, 139*(6), 820-828.

Snowden, L. (1982). *Reaching the underserved: Mental health needs of neglected populations*. Newbury Park, Calif.: Sage Publications.

Snowden, L., & Todman, P.A. (1982). The psychological assessment of Blacks: New and needed developments. In E.E. Johns & S.J. Korchin (Eds.), *Minority mental health* (pp. 193-226). New York: Praeger.

Spector, R.E. (1979). *Cultural diversity in health and illness*. East Norwalk, Conn.: Appleton-Century-Crofts.

Spurlock, J. (1985). Psychiatric states. In R.A. Williams (Ed.), *Textbook of Black-related diseases*. New York: McGraw-Hill.

Stanhope, M., & Lancaster, J. (1988). *Community health nursing*. St. Louis: C.V. Mosby.

Stalls, F.A. (1978). Racial differences in alcohol metabolism. *Alcohol Clinical and Experimental Research, 2*(1), 10.

Staples, R. (1976). *Introduction to Black sociology*. New York: McGraw-Hill.

Statistical abstracts of the United States. (1988). Washington, D.C.: U.S. Department of Commerce, Bureau of the Census.

Sterne, M., & Pittman, D.J. (1972). *Drinking practices in the ghetto.* St. Louis: Washington University Social Science Institute.

Stokes, L.G. (1977). Delivering health services in a Black community. In A.M. Reinhardt & M.B. Quinn (Eds), *Current practice in family-centered community nursing* (Vol. 1; pp. 51-65). St. Louis: C.V. Mosby.

Sue, D. (1981). *Counseling the culturally different: Theory and practice.* New York: John Wiley & Sons.

Thomas, A., & Sillen. (1972). *Racism and psychiatry.* New York: Brunner/Mazel.

Tobias, P. (1970). Brain-size, grey matter, and race: Fact or fiction. *American Journal of Physical Anthropology, 32,* 3-26.

Turner, L. (1948, April). Problems confronting the investigation of Gullah. *American Dialect Society Publications, 9,* 78-84.

U.S. Department of Commerce, Bureau of the Census. (1982, May). *Current population reports, divisions and states: 1980.* 1980 Census of Population, Doc. No. P.C. 80-51-1. Superintendant of Documents. Washington, D.C., U.S. Government Printing Office.

Vernon, S., & Roberts, R. (1982). Use of the SADS-RDC in a triethnic community survey. *Archives of General Psychiatry, 39,* 47-52.

Webster's ninth new collegiate dictionary. (1984). Springfield Mass.: Merriam-Webster.

Weclew, R. (1975). The nature, prevalence, and level of awareness of "curanderismo" and some of its implications for community health. *Community Mental Health Journal, 11,* 145.

Westermeyer, J. (1984). The role of ethnicity in substance abuse. In B. Stimmel (Ed.), *Cultural and sociological aspects of alcoholism and substance abuse* (pp. 9-18). New York: Haworth Press.

White, E.H. (1977). Giving health care to minority patients. *Nursing Clinics in North America, 12,* 27-40.

Williams, M. (1986). Alcohol and ethnic minorities: Native Americans—An update. *Alcohol Health and Research Works, 11*(2), 5-6.

Wintrob, R. (1973). The influences of others: Witchcraft and rootwork as explanations of behavior disturbances. *Journal of Nervous and Mental Disorders, 156,* 318.

Wolfram, W.A., & Clark, H. (Eds.). (1971). *Black-White speech relationships.* Washington, D.C.: Center for Applied Linguistics.

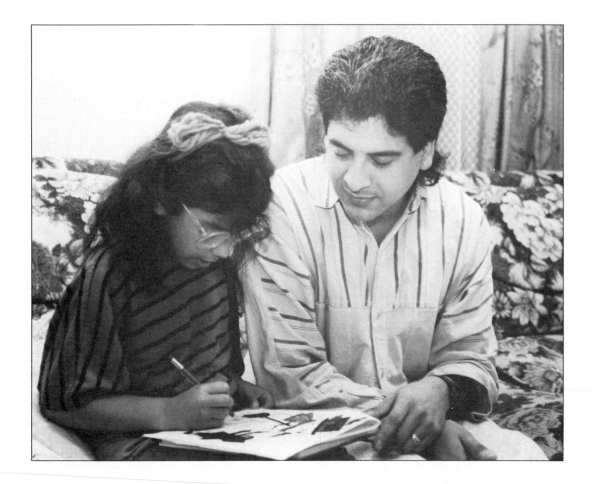

■ ■

CHAPTER 9

Mexican Americans

Joan Kuipers

BEHAVIORAL OBJECTIVES

After reading this chapter, the nurse will be able to:

1 Discuss the impact of Spanish language usage by Mexican Americans in adapting to the mainstream U.S. culture.

2 Explain the distance and intimacy behaviors of Mexican Americans.

3 Describe the organization of the Mexican American family unit.

4 Explain the Mexican American orientation to time.

5 Identify Mexican American beliefs regarding the ability to control the environment.

6 Describe how the "hot-cold" beliefs of Mexican Americans influence their health and illness beliefs.

7 Explain the health care beliefs, diseases, and practices within the *curanderismo* folklore system.

8 Identify the biological variations of Mexican Americans.

9 Identify implications or precautions for providing effective nursing care to Mexican Americans.

OVERVIEW OF MEXICO AND MEXICAN AMERICANS

Mexico, or what is commonly referred to as the United Mexican States, is a country in the southern part of North America. Mexico consists of 31 states and a federal district. The boundaries of Mexico extend southward from the United States to Guatemala and Belize in Central America. The western coast of Mexico borders on the Pacific Ocean, which includes the Gulf of California and the Gulf of Tehuantepec. The eastern coast of Mexico fronts on the Caribbean Sea and the Gulf of Mexico, which includes the Bay of Campeche. Mexico, which includes several outlying islands, has a total area of 761,604 square miles and is the third largest Latin American nation after Brazil and Argentina. Mexico is about a fifth the size of the United States.

Geographically there is a similarity between the southwestern United States and northern Mexico. Today, because of the geographic closeness, some Mexican Americans move back and forth between Mexico and the United States. This allows them to remain in contact with their families and native customs. Mexican Americans moved northward from Mexico into the southwestern section of the United States, where the majority still reside in Texas and California. Most Mexican Americans have rural agricultural backgrounds (U.S. Department of Commerce, Bureau of the Census, 1979). However, it is difficult to generalize about geographic location and the occupational background of people in this ethnic group. The diversity in Mexican Americans ranges from rural villagers in New Mexico and Colorado (Saunders, 1954; Weaver 1970), to agricultural laborers in Texas (Rubel, 1966), to low-income residents in Arizona, to urban lower-class individuals in California (Clark, 1970). Just as the people are diverse, so are the many studies that represent different populations of Mexicans and offer differing definitions of Mexican Americans. Therefore any discussion of Mexican Americans is further complicated by the problem of precisely defining this population. In the early years of the United States, Mexican Americans helped establish many southwestern cities and taught the settlers skills in mining, farming, and ranching. Thus unlike many other immigrants, most Mexican Americans have remained close to their homeland.

Mexican Americans are the second largest minority in the United States, with approximately 10,500,000 persons (Garcia, 1988). Persons in this ethnic group most commonly refer to themselves as Mexican American or Chicano. Many Mexican Americans can trace their ancestry back to early Indian groups that developed great Mexican civilizations before the arrival of the Spanish explorers. Mexican Americans are a blend of both Indian and European cultures. When the Spaniards came to Mexico in 1519, they found Indians who were skilled in writing, mathematics, astronomy, painting, sculpture, and architecture. Indian pottery, metalwork, and textiles were very highly developed for the time period. The Spaniards attempted to convert the Indians to Christianity and in so doing destroyed the native culture, which was soon replaced by Spanish customs and culture.

Some Mexican Americans have come across the border into the United States seeking higher wages and better working conditions. Many, however, have experienced dehumanizing discrimination in education, jobs, and housing. Skin color, language differences, and Spanish surnames have all contributed to discrimination. For Mexican Americans, feelings of isolation, persecution, and discrimination have in some instances resulted in acute paranoid reactions and posttraumatic stress disorders (PTSDs) (Cervantes, Snyder, & Padilla, 1989; Rivera, 1978).

"Cultural uniqueness" is not academic nomenclature for Mexican Americans. The phrase is used to describe physical, emotional, and behavioral distinctions unique to many Mexican Americans (Chavez, 1986). Unlike European immigrants who often hasten to absorb the culture found in the United States, many Mexican Americans have not. Mexican Americans to this day try to retain a cultural identity within the dominant population (Chavez, 1986). In *Megatrends,* John Naisbitt (1982) states that "none of the new groups individually can begin to match the numbers and the potential influence of Spanish-speaking Americans." Concepts such as *machismo* (manliness), *confianza* (confidence), *respeto* (respect), *verguenze* (shame), and *orgullo* (pride) predominate in the culture, and traditional gender and family roles continue to be part of the heritage that separates Mexican Americans from other cultural groups.

While some Mexican Americans are well educated (Favazza, 1983), according to Bonilla (1973), the educational achievement of most Mexican Americans is extremely low. For example, in the early 1970s the average Mexican American child completed only a seventh grade education; only 27% of Mexican Americans completed high school; and only 2.5% of Mexican American men and 1% of Mexican American women graduated from college (*Statistical Abstracts,* 1988). In 1986 Mexican Americans who had less than 5 years of schooling encompassed a total population of 15.5%: in the 25- to 34-year-old age-group, approximately 6% had less than 5 years of schooling; in the 35- to 44-year-old age-group, 10.2% had less than 5 years of schooling; in the 45- to 64-year-old age-group, 17.5% had less than 5 years of schooling; and in the 65-year-old or older age-group, 33.1% had less than 5 years of schooling. In contrast, in 1986 Mexican Americans who had completed 4 years of high school or higher education encompassed a total population of 37.6%: in the 25- to 34-year-old age-group, 54.7% had completed high school or more; in the 35- to 44-year-old age-group, 47% had completed high school or more; in the 45- to 64-year-old age-group 33.5% had completed high school or more; and in the 65-year-old or older age-group, approximately 9.8% had completed high school or more (*Statistical Abstracts,* 1988). Gradually Mexican Americans have learned the English language, and as they have begun to speak English more fluently, the level of education has increased. Consequently, problems of some Mexican Americans are dissipating as they become more active in seeking solutions to poor housing, jobs, and discrimination.

A major issue for some Mexican Americans is lack of citizenship. Lack of citizenship is a barrier to gaining education, skills, stable jobs, decent living conditions, and government benefits. For Mexican Americans who are illegal aliens, there frequently is tension regarding discovery and deportation back to Mexico. Preoccupation with possible discovery and deportation for illegal aliens serves to further augment the symptoms of PTSD (Cervantes, Synder & Padilla, 1989).

The plight of the illegal alien has been expanded since enactment of the Immigration and Reform and Control Act of 1986 (Gelfand & Bialik-Gilad, 1989). In an attempt to control illegal immigration into the United States, employers are now required to verify citizenship status within 24 hours after hiring an employee. Sanctions are being placed against employers who fail to meet this requirement or who hire illegal aliens knowingly. Noncitizens who apply for public assistance funds must verify that they are not undocumented aliens. It is now very difficult for these people to obtain health care except from church-related agencies. Because of diagnostic related group requirements, hospitals are not as willing to treat uninsured, indigent people. Also, undocumented aliens do not qualify for Medicare or Medicaid funds. It is feared that as this group ages without adequate health care, chronic and costly medical conditions will develop. Because of employer sanctions, aliens are being forced into lower-paying jobs, which limit even more their ability to support the costs of their own health care needs or those of their aged relatives. The illegal alien is subject to isolation and abuse. The immigration officers have more power than previously to go after the aliens, so that much energy is involved in evading detection (West & Moore, 1989).

Most Mexican Americans who live in large cities cannot afford good housing because they lack work skills and therefore have low-paying jobs. They often live in crowded, substandard housing with limited access to quality health care facilities and city services (Garcia, 1988). Other Mexican Americans are migrant farm workers who move around the country seeking work when crops are to be harvested. They often encounter unsanitary living conditions and poor wages.

Mexicans are noted for their celebration of holidays. Many Mexican Americans have continued to celebrate Mexican holidays in addition to the holidays celebrated by other Americans. During the celebration of the Mexican Christmas called *Las Posadas,* the children are fond of breaking a pinata, a papier-mache container filled with candy and gifts. Other important holidays are *Cinco do Mayo* (May 5) and Guadalupe Day (December 12), which is Mexico's most important religious holiday. Affluent Mexican Americans often spend significant amounts of money on special food and drink, decorations, and fireworks for a holiday festival. Holidays provide an opportunity for Mexican Americans to share with others.

COMMUNICATION

Spanish, the primary language for many Mexican Americans, is the third most commonly used language in the world and one of the six languages used by the United Nations (Monrroy, 1983).

Dialect or Pattern

The Spanish language is spoken in many dialects; Mexican Americans who have an Indian heritage may speak 1 of more than 50 dialects. Fortunately, however, most of the words spoken have the same meaning (Monrroy, 1983). Differences in dialect may be found in certain communities. Dialects may also be identified by their proximity to the Mexican border.

Touch

Adult Mexican Americans can be characterized as tactile in their relationships. Although female Mexican Americans may initiate more tactile behavior in communicating, there is a contradiction where modesty is concerned. There is a strong social value that women do not expose their bodies to men or even other women. During a pelvic examination a Mexican American female patient may express "feeling hot" because of the embarrassment from the examination (Brownlee, 1978). Some Mexican Americans will even avoid touching their own genitalia (Clark, 1970). While religious beliefs may explain lack of birth control, extreme discomfort with certain areas of the body may also explain why some Mexican American women avoid the use of a diaphragm. Men also have strong feelings about modesty and may feel threatened if expected to have a complete physical examination (Murillo, 1978). This modesty may explain the reluctance to use condoms on the part of some Mexican American men (Monrroy, 1983).

Context

When being interviewed, Mexican Americans may engage in "small talk" before approaching the business of the interview. It is important for the nurse to remember that small talk will often facilitate accomplishing nursing objectives for the interview and is therefore not a "waste of time."

Murillo (1978) has noted that in communicating with others, the Mexican American uses diplomacy and tactfulness; there is also pride in verbal expression, which is likely to be elaborate and indirect. Direct confrontation and arguments are thought to be rude and disrespectful. Self-disclosure is reserved for those whom the individual knows well. The Mexican American may appear agreeable on the surface regarding an issue because of the value of courtesy. However, later the nurse may be surprised and disappointed because agreements are not being carried out. Kidding is seen as rude, depreciating, and offensive and is likely to generate a negative response (Monrroy, 1983). In communicating, all the physiological senses are used, such as smelling, tasting, touching, feeling, and hearing. Intensified use of the senses in communication has been related to the Mexican American's love of sounds, bright colors, action, and even spicy food (Murillo, 1978).

Kinesics

Eye behavior is important to Mexican Americans, especially when children are involved. *Mal ojo* ("evil eye") is a folk illness described as a condition that affects infants and children (Dorsey & Jackson, 1976) and occurs because an individual who is thought to possess a special power voluntarily or involuntarily injures a child by looking at and admiring but not touching the child (Foster, 1978). With this condition the child cries, develops a fever, vomits, and loses appetite. This disorder may be prevented by touching or patting a child when admiring the child. The way the spell is broken is for the individual who has given the "evil eye" to touch the child. Therefore it is important for the nurse to touch the child when giving care, since in the minds of Mexican Americans this action can both prevent and treat the illness.

English as a Second Language

Most Mexican Americans can also speak some English. However, the inability to speak English fluently has led to a high failure rate for school-age Mexican Americans. Lack of language fluency has also limited the ability to improve job status and in turn the quality of life. Laosa (1975) reported that the longer Mexican immigrants stay in the United States, the less likely they are to retain the mother language. This probably is most directly attributable to the fact that English is the language used in schools and at work. Increasing attention is being given to the need for bilingual education for Mexican American students, and, as a result, more Mexican Americans are becoming bilingual.

Communication by Mexican Americans is also complicated by the phenomenon that many Mexican Americans go on to develop a language that blends English and Spanish. Mexican American adults use this blended form of language more often than children do. Consequently, a nurse who may know both English and Spanish may still have difficulty understanding this blended language.

Some Mexican Americans still use English selectively. In an extensive study on language loyalty among various ethnic groups residing in the United States, it was found that Spanish remains the most persistent of all foreign languages. Thus because of its persistent use, Spanish seemingly has the greatest prospects of survival (Fishman, 1967). While other ethnic groups have become disillusioned with the use of their mother tongue, Mexican Americans have been more likely to retain their mother language in succeeding generations in the United States. Even today, some fluency in Spanish characterizes most Mexican Americans at all income levels. Another reason for the persistence of Spanish among Mexican Americans is that in the United States the mass media for information and entertainment is permeated with Spanish. Today Spanish accounts for approximately 66% of the total foreign language broadcasting in the United States.

It is not uncommon for people who speak different languages to use each language in different contexts or for different purposes. Perhaps the most frequent situation is that of Mexican Americans who use English in their work and Spanish at home or with their friends (Marcos, 1988). There are several rather isolated villages in northern New Mexico where the only English spoken is for official occasions such as conferring with a government agency. Because of the remoteness of these communities, these Mexican Americans may retain the use of Spanish as their principal language.

Implications for Nursing Care

Because some Mexican Americans rely on Spanish to communicate with other people, it is very frightening for them to participate in the American health care system, and it is frustrating for the nurses giving them care. More student nurses need to be recruited from this ethnic group, especially in the cities of the South and West. Nursing programs would be enhanced if students were required to take courses in foreign languages, since patients could be encouraged to communicate in the language most comfortable to them.

It is important for the nurse to remember that language is a cultural factor that influences health care practices. The nurse who works with bilingual Mexican Americans must remember that often under stress these persons may revert to their first language, Spanish. The nurse should avoid scolding the patient who communicates in Spanish. Rather, the nurse should emphasize that the nurse can be more helpful if the patient communicates in the language that both the nurse and the patient understand. When this is not possible because of high levels of stress on the part of the patient, the nurse should look to translators who may be available within the agency or in the community at large. Family members may provide invaluable assistance both in reducing stress and in translating the patient's needs. Using family members could also promote the building of trust in the nurse in order to facilitate compliance on the part of the patient.

Understanding the impact of bilingualism on the patient also requires appreciation of the dimension of language independence—the capacity to acquire, maintain, and use two separate language codes, each with its own lexical, syntactic, phonetic, semantic, and ideational components. Many Mexican Americans who are proficient in both Spanish and English operate parallel language codes, each with its own associations between message words and events in their ideational system (Marcos & Alpert, 1976). A good example of language compartmentalization can be found in the saying of Emperor Charles V: "To God I speak in Spanish, to women in Italian, to men in French, and to my horse in German" (*Oxford Dictionary,* 1980). In certain situations a patient may speak to his or her family in Spanish, to the nurse in English, and, when extremely stressed, to both family and nurse in a combination of both English and Spanish. This tendency for bilingualism can become extremely alarming for the patient, as well as for health care providers.

It is also important for the nurse to keep in mind that Mexican Americans tend to describe emotional problems by using dramatic body language. In addition, research has shown that when Mexican Americans are interviewed in English, or across their language barrier, they are usually judged by experienced clinicians as showing a more severe degree of symptomatology than when they are interviewed in their mother tongue (Favazza, 1983; Marcos et al., 1973).

The nurse must guard against the use of idioms and abstractions when dealing with patients who do not completely understand the language. It is also important to avoid responding to the patient in a joking manner. For example, a nursing assistant working with a Mexican patient who needed a bath jokingly used the phrase "dirty Mexican." The patient reported this to the nursing supervisor, stating that this was a racial comment and therefore fell under the state statutes against patient abuse. The nursing assistant countered that the phrase was used in a nonharmful manner to conjole the patient into taking a bath, since he was dirty. When working with a Mexican American patient who lacks understanding of the language, statements using slang or colloquialisms should be avoided, since they may be interpreted literally.

SPACE

Kluckhohn (1976) categorized people and the modalities of relationships as individualistic, collateral, or lineal. Some Mexican Americans are categorized as both collateral and lineal, implying that there may be a patron-peon system such as a boss-worker relationship or a family-versus-individual relationship.

Mexican Americans value physical presence, including the presence of family members. It is important for Mexican Americans to see relatives face-to-face, to embrace, touch, and just be with each other (Keefe, 1984). Mexican Americans as a group demonstrate a great need for group togetherness. Ford and Graves (1977) found that when Mexican American second graders related to others, there was closer interpersonal distance and more touching among girls. Touching was of longer duration when spatial parameters were closer. Boys tended to be less tactile when relating to others. It is believed that this pattern of socialization begins with the parent-child relationship and continues into adulthood. During the early years the parents are permissive, warm, and caring with all their children. However, in later years, the girls remain much closer to home and are protected and guarded in their contacts. In contrast, the boys are allowed to be with other boys in informal social groups where they develop their machismo (Murillo, 1978).

Implications for Nursing Care

Despite the fact that Mexican Americans like consistent, close relationships and physical touching, female nurses should always assist a male physician in examining a female patient and guard against exposing body parts other than those that are the focus of the examination (Murillo-Rohde, 1977). Male patients may refuse to allow a complete examination because of their modesty.

The nurse who plans care delivery for Mexican American patients must keep in mind that Mexican Americans may resist care provided by those perceived as being different or from a different ethnic background (Monrroy, 1983). Some Mexican Americans may also have cultural biases that prohibit care being administered by persons of the opposite sex. For example, a male student nurse was assigned to a Mexican American patient in labor. This assignment precipitated problems because the patient, husband, and family were all very uncomfortable, since "only her husband should see her like that." It was necessary to change the assignment in order to provide care.

SOCIAL ORGANIZATION

The foundation of the Mexican community is the nuclear family (parents and children). It is generally believed that Mexican Americans are familistic. For some Mexican Americans familism has been perceived as curtailing mobility by sustaining emotional attachment to people, places, and things. In the Mexican American culture, familism has been identified as the prime cause not only of low mobility, but also of resistance to changes of all kinds. For Mexican Americans, familism, along with a special assigned male role, is a source of collective pride. Nevertheless, Mexican Americans are believed to be deterred from collective and individual progress because of familism.

For Mexican Americans extended family relationships have special significance, and the family is perhaps the most significant social organization (Murillo, 1978). The major dominating theme of the traditional Mexican American family is the need for collective achievement of the family as a group. Thus the need for family collectivity and other family needs supersede the needs of individual members. Also, any dishonor or shame that may occur for an individual member is considered a reflection on the entire family. The Mexican American family takes pride in family endeavors and generally does not seek help from outsiders to solve problems or meet needs. Mexican American families place a great deal of value on having many relatives live nearby. The local extended family is tightly integrated, has frequent face-to-face encounters, and provides one another with mutual aid (Keefe, 1984). Lantican and Corona (1989) have reported that Mexican Americans have a mean network size of 5.78, which may include in-laws, grandparents, and a substantial number of relatives. Some 69% of the Mexican Americans studied reported that most of their support was provided by immediate family members. One interesting aspect of this study revealed that for the Mexican American primigravidas studied, pregnancy was most likely to be discussed with the husband first. There are frequent expressions of affection, trust, and respect among kin. Members of extended families are concerned about how their behaviors and actions will affect (either positively or negatively) their families. The Mexican American patient who is hospitalized often desires the presence of the family. Families, as well, come to the hospital expecting to be there and to be part of the decision-making process.

Although most Mexican Americans have nuclear families that live separately, it is not uncommon for the extended family or other relatives to live in the same household (Miller, 1986). According to Chavez (1986), new immigrants (especially those who are undocumented) tend to live in a multiple family arrangement, which offers the advantages of social and economic support. As the length of residency increases and the family becomes more financially independent, the nuclear family tends to find a singular arrangement for its household.

Within the family the father has the dominant role, assuming responsibility for being head of the house and the decision maker (Monrroy, 1983). For the male family member, there is a strong sense of machismo that is not compatible with the loss of self-esteem or authority. The wife/mother of the family has a primary role of keeping the family cohesive. Although the mother may influence family decisions, she does not have a dominant role in the family. Increasing numbers of Mexican American women are finding work outside the home. Women who live in a rural setting often help with the family farming activities. Divorce is uncommon, but stable out-of-wedlock relationships are not unusual in the lower socioeconomic levels.

The entire family may contribute to the financial welfare of the family. Parental control in Mexican American families is strong. Older children contribute by caring for younger family members or animals, or by helping with the production of food or other family enterprises. Children in migrant families often earn money by working along with other family members. The elderly are respected and live with married children if they are not self-sufficient. The elderly also pass down cultural and folk medicine beliefs.

An important institution in the Mexican heritage is the Catholic practice of *compadrazgo,* or coparenthood (godparenthood), which was introduced to Mexico by the Spaniards. Godparents accept coresponsibilities for a child along with the parents. This kinship begins with the baptism of the child and continues throughout the life cycle; it is used for religious purposes and also becomes an important resource for coping with life stressors (Kemper, 1982). Frequently, a godparent is chosen from a higher socioeconomic level, which enables the child to have social resources that are more extensive than what the family could provide.

Valdez (1980) found that Mexican American families of a lower socioeconomic class tended to show more ethnic identification than those of a higher socioeconomic class. This phenomenon served to provide support for Mexican Americans of lower socioeconomic classes and a more positive adaptation to the mainstream U.S. culture.

Implications for Nursing Care

Of primary importance for the nurse caring for Mexican American patients is the concept that family values and roles are paramount to the patient's treatment and recovery. The nurse should remember that the male head of the family should be consulted in health care decision making for other family members. It is also important that the nurse include the entire family, both immediate and extended members, in the assessment, planning, and implementation of nursing care if treatment is to be effective (Hough, 1985). Rather than viewing a large family who wishes to be with the patient as an annoyance and frustration to staff, the nurse should discuss with the family how visits can be planned in such a way that care can still be delivered and the patient can obtain needed rest. Murillo-Rohde (1977) has suggested that nurses use the family to help with the patient's care. She says the family could feed, bathe, or walk the patient, thus decreasing the anxiety and guilt of the family and the patient.

In addition, the nurse could be relieved of some of the work load. Allowing the family to participate in the patient's care builds trust and respect and encourages compliance and support for discharge planning and teaching.

When the nurse is experiencing difficulty in getting a patient to follow a particular medical regimen, the nurse may suggest that the patient solicit the opinions of other family members regarding proposed actions. Suggesting family consultation will demonstrate that the nurse understands the importance of the family in regard to health matters. Furthermore, the nurse's actions should help to build a relationship of trust between the nurse and the patient.

When caring for a younger patient, the nurse may encounter the *compadrazgo,* or godparent, who provides important support to the child and family. The godparent may want to assume some of the care of the patient because of a sense of divine responsibility for the child's welfare. Allowing this to take place can serve to reduce fear and anxiety and enhance adjustment to the health care facility.

TIME

Mexican Americans are usually characterized as having a present orientation of time and being unable or reluctant to incorporate the future into their plans. An example of this orientation is that some Mexican Americans may spend several years' savings on an important religious festival. Also, the Mexican custom of the siesta in some ways represents the belief that rest (or the present) has a priority over continued work that could produce monies to safeguard the future. Individuals with this present orientation of time may appear to lack practical concern about the future or the need for deferring gratification to a future time. Many investigators believe that this orientation restrains Mexican Americans from upward social mobility. In addition, some regard the present orientation of time as a barrier to assimilation and integration into the mainstream of American culture.

Khoury and Thurmond (1978) found few differences in the time perceptions of Mexican American and Anglo-American college students, despite the fact that the Mexican American students in the study were still maintaining cultural ties with the Mexican American culture. However, these findings cannot be generalized to Mexican Americans who are more immeshed in their culture and less educated.

Implications for Nursing Care

It is important for the nurse to remember that personal ethnocentric attitudes toward time may negatively affect the planning of care for patients with a different time orientation. Since Mexican Americans have been characterized as being present time oriented, these patients may not share the nurse's attitude concerning matters related to time, particularly if the nurse is from a future-oriented cultural group. It is also important to remember that a Mexican American patient may be late for an appointment not because of reluctance or lack of respect, but because the patient may be more concerned with a current activity than he or she is with planning ahead to be on time. This concept, known as elasticity, implies that future-oriented activities can be recovered but present-oriented activities cannot.

Since Mexican Americans are likely to be present time oriented, the nurse may experience difficulties in planning and implementing health care measures such as long-term planning. In addition, the nurse may experience difficulties in explaining why and when medications should be taken. When working with a patient who has a condition such as hypertension, it is important for the nurse to emphasize the effects of this condition, as well as short-term problems that can occur if the medication is not taken on time. Emphasis on short-term problems is more likely to be beneficial, since it is more likely to get results.

Since Mexican Americans are present time oriented, their perceptions and understanding of acute and chronic illness may be affected. Mexican Americans may first seek out the most accessible and affordable care, which may be folk healing with a folk practictioner.

ENVIRONMENTAL CONTROL
Locus of Control

Mexican Americans are more likely to believe in an external locus of control than are persons in the dominant culture. This belief that the outcome of circumstances is controlled by external forces is conveyed socially. Some Mexican Americans perceive life as being under the constant influence of the divine will. There is also a fatalistic belief that one is at the mercy of the environment and has little control over what happens. Associated with this view is the belief that personal efforts are unlikely to influence the outcome of a situation; thus some Mexican Americans do not believe that they are personally responsible for present or future successes or failures. This belief may precipitate feelings of hopelessness regarding future and positive change.

Impact on personal control

Transcultural studies have found that people with a belief in external control can be expected to have more distress as a outcome of this view (Hough, 1985). On the other hand, Mirowsky and Ross (1984) noted that distress was not observed in the Mexican culture as an outcome of a belief in an external locus of control. Mirowsky and Ross suggested that although distress can result from strong family ties, it is offset by the family's strong support and responsibility to the individual. A consequence of strong family ties is that the individual may have a greater feeling of personal control, which in turn deters anxiety.

Health Care Beliefs

The cultural belief in external locus of control influences the manner in which some Mexican Americans view health. Some Mexican Americans believe that health may be the result of good luck or a reward from God for good behavior. For some Mexican Americans health represents a state of equilibrium in the universe wherein the forces of "hot," "cold," " wet," and "dry" must be balanced. (This concept is thought to have originated with the early Hippocratic theory of health and the four humors. According to the Hippocratic theory, the body humors—blood, phlegm, black bile, and yellow bile—vary in both temperature and moisture (Harwood, 1971), and persons who subscribe to this theory believe that health exists only when these four humors are in balance. Thus health can be maintained by diet and other practices that keep the four humors in balance.) Illness, on the other hand, is believed to be misfortune or bad luck, a punishment from God for evil thoughts or actions, or a result of the imbalance of hot and cold or wet and dry.

Theory of Hot and Cold and Perception of Illness

One category of disease is hot and cold imbalance, wherein illness is thought to be caused by prolonged exposure to hot or cold; to cure the illness, the opposite quality of the causative agent is applied to assimilate the hot or cold. Included in this category are illnesses that, rather than being caused by temperature itself, are associated with hot or cold aspects of substances found in medicines, elements, air, food, and bodily organs (Richardson, 1982). Treatment is focused on such things as suggestions, practical advice, prayers, or indigenous herbs, with the goal of reestablishing balance (Ruiz, 1985).

Headaches may have a causative agent that is thought to have a hot or cold quality. If the causative agent for a headache is thought to have a hot quality, then cold herbs may be placed on the temples to absorb the heat; if the causative agent is thought to have a cold quality, then hot herbs are applied (Ingham, 1970). As another example of hot and cold imbalance, a person who has eaten unripened fruit may complain that "the cold of the fruit has gotten me in the stomach" (Currier, 1966).

Other illnesses such as paralysis, rheumatism, and earaches are thought to be caused when cold *aires* enter the body. These illnesses are principally disabling in nature and are painful (Currier, 1966). People are thought to be more susceptible to cold *aires* when going from a warm place to a cold place, or when they have just eaten, because eating is thought to cause a warm state. When people with these illnesses have a high fever, a hot poultice is administered to the legs to draw the fever out of the head to the cool legs. The origin of these cold *aires* is thought to be in dark places such as river bottoms, ant hills, and caves, particularly those dark places "where the devil lives." The cure for *los aires* is for the individual to be cleansed with hot herbs and eggs and then covered with cigarette smoke (Ingham, 1970). Cleansing may also be done with black and red clay whistle dolls and combined with an offering of hot black chicken, unsalted mole, tamales, alcohol, and cigarettes that is made to an ant hole. These practices are also described as witchcraft.

While cold is thought to harm the body from without, excesses of heat developed from within the body itself and extending outward are believed to be related to such diseases as cancer, rheumatism, tuberculosis, and paralysis (Wilson & Kneisl, 1988; see box on p. 197). The focus of heat in the body is the stomach, whereas the head, arms, and legs are thought to be cool. Hot illnesses such as skin ailments and fever may be visible to the outside world.

Many of the disorders due to hot and cold imbalances are digestive in nature. This is related to the fact that an imbalance of hot and cold foods is thought to be damaging and suggests that to ensure good health, both hot and cold foods must be taken into the body (Currier, 1966). The quality of the food eaten determines whether diarrhea is a hot or cold condition. If the stool is green or yellow, the diarrhea is hot and the remedy is cold tea, whereas if the stool is white, the diarrhea is cold and the remedy is hot tea.

Hot and cold are also associated with other aspects of life. Symbolically, cold is

HOT-COLD CONDITIONS AND THEIR CORRESPONDING TREATMENT

Hot conditions

Fever
Infections
Diarrhea
Kidney problems
Rashes
Skin ailments
Sore throat
Liver problems
Ulcers
Constipation

Cold conditions

Cancer
Pneumonia
Malaria
Joint pain
Menstrual period
Teething
Earache
Rheumatism
Tuberculosis
Colds
Headache
Paralysis
Stomach cramps

Hot foods

Chocolate
Cheese
Temperate-zone fruits
Eggs
Peas
Onions
Aromatic beverages
Hard liquor
Oils
Meats such as beef, waterfowl, mutton
Goat's milk
Cereal grains
Chilipeppers

Cold foods

Fresh vegetables
Tropical fruits
Daily products
Meats such as goat, fish, chicken
Honey
Cod
Raisins
Bottled milk
Barley water

Hot medicines and herbs

Penicillin
Tobacco
Ginger root
Garlic
Cinnamon
Anise
Vitamins
Iron preparations
Cod-liver oil
Caster oil
Aspirin

Cold medicines and herbs

Orange flower water
Linden
Sage
Milk of magnesia
Bicarbonate of soda

Adapted from Wilson, H., and Kneisl, C. (1988). *Psychiatric Nursing*. Reading Mass.: Addison-Wesley.

related to things that menace the individual, whereas hot is related to warmth and reassurance. In addition to air, water is seen as a source for cold. If an individual has participated in an activity that is considered hot, this person will not go near water, because of its association with death (at death, blood is believed to be turned into water). The effort to balance hot and cold forces in the Mexican American belief system reflects the relationship between the individual and the environment. It is an symbolic attempt to attain a social order that is equitable (Ingham, 1970).

Theory of Hot and Cold and Effects on Growth and Development

Hot and cold have symbolic significance for the nature and process of reproduction. During pregnancy a woman may be advised not to consume hot foods. On the other hand, during menstruation or after childbirth a woman might be told to avoid cold foods or taking a bath. Infertility is associated with a "cold" womb, lack of intimacy, and rejection. A pregnant woman is thought to have an especially warm body, and to dissipate the warmth, she should bathe often and take short walks (Currier, 1966). The idea that warmth relates to intimacy follows in the relationship of mother and child. If a pregnant mother rejects her child, she is subject to an emotionally based disease called *bilis,* which can cause the infant to have chronic headaches and permanent injury. This suggests that the child may display chronic malnutrition, which Currier (1966) relates to a lack of affection and support. Nursing of the child is also related to hot and cold characteristics. A diminished milk flow is thought to result from coldness, whereas warmth is thought to increase the flow. An excess of warmth causes the child to become ill, because the milk curdles and becomes indigestible.

During the first year of life, a child is kept physically close to the mother either by being wrapped in her shawl or by sleeping in a bed next to her. When the child is weaned and starts walking, the mother deprives the child of this physical contact; and when the child experiences the cold floors and lack of physical attachment, he or she may experience rage and depression. This condition is related to a lack of support and physical warmth (Currier, 1966).

Folk Medicine

The belief that health is a matter of chance and controlled by forces in nature is the basis of folk medicine. Folk medicine as practiced by Mexican Americans combines elements of the European Roman Catholic view and that of the original Indians of Mexico. These beliefs have led to unique ways of accounting for physical and mental illnesses, their consequences, and unique methods of dealing with illnesses. This belief and practice system regarding health care is indigenous to the Mexican American community and is known as *curanderismo* (Rivera & Wanderer, 1986). Within this folk medicine system, the *curandero* is the folk healer. The *curandero* views illness from a religious and social context, rather than the medical-scientific perspective of the dominant Western society.

The concept of balance dominates much of the Mexican American world view regarding the cause and treatment of illness. Good health infers that one is in proper balance with God, as well as the family, fellow men, and the church (Weclew, 1975). Illness is often believed to be a result of an imbalance in the social or spiritual aspects of life.

Types of folk practitioners

Operating within the *curanderismo* folklore system of beliefs and practices are several levels of healers. The first healer sought out is a member of the family; if the case is or becomes more complicated, healers within the community are sought out. Several levels of folk healers are described here, beginning with the lowest level, the family healer.

Family folk healer. The first person to be consulted at the time of illness is a key family member who is respected for her knowledge of folk medicine. This individual may be a wife/mother, grandmother, or revered elderly relative. The healing practices are passed down in the family from mother to daughter. If the patient does not improve, there is usually an intermediary person who directs the patient to the *curandero*.

Jerbero. The *jerbero* is a folk healer who specializes in using herbs and spices for preventive and curative purposes. This person grows and distributes herbs and spices, and explains how to use them effectively (Richardson, 1982).

Curandero/curandera. The more serious physical and mental/emotional illnesses are brought to the *curandero* (folk healer). If the practitioner is a woman, she is referred to as a *curandera*. The *curandero* perceives life as being under the consistent influence of the divine will. People are thought to be born as sinners, with death being the result of their sins. The central focus of these healers' treatment is relieving patients of their sins. Suffering is seen as a component of illness, and death is seen as failure to be cured of sin (Ruiz, 1985). The *curandero* believes that water, food, and air are important to the maintenance of health. Imbalance of these elements, imbalance between God and man, and imbalance between hot and cold are thought to contribute to illness.

Weclew (1975) and Ness and Wintrob (1981) have reported that *curanderos* see patients with a wide range of both physical and psychological symptoms, such as gastrointestinal distress, back pain, headache, fever, depression, anxiety, irritability, fatigue, hostility, shame, guilt, sexual problems, alcoholism, and the common folk diseases. The diagnosis is made after a thorough assessment of all aspects of the patient's life, including the family and even the supernatural. The treatment is provided in a room in the *curandero's* home that is decorated with much religious paraphernalia. Treatments used include massage, diet, rest, suggestions, practical advice, indigenous herbs, prayers, magic, and supernatural rituals. Although *curanderos* use white magic, there are times when, because the cure is difficult, they resort to black magic.

The *curandero,* who is believed to have the "God given" gift of healing and is a full-time specialist, is often consulted before medical contact is made or may be consulted concomitantly with a medical contact. The effectiveness of *curanderos* seems to be in their ability to use their personality and healing regalia to encourage hope and trust on the part of the patient. The beliefs and practices of this healer are supported by the family and the community, which tends to strengthen the patient's sense of control over the situation. *Curanderos* are often preferred over the medical community because they are personal, less dehumanizing, know the family, and are an integral part of the whole Mexican American community. *Curanderos* in most cases have power over witches because they are believed to heal through the power of God.

Brujos/brujas (witches). This level of healers may not be sought out until other forms of healing have been tried. The practitioners of witchcraft utilize several kinds of magic. Black magic is practiced by both male witches *(brujos)* and female witches *(brujas),* and red magic and green magic are thought to empower a witch to solve love problems by assuming an animal form. As mentioned previously, white magic is practiced by a *curandero,* is considered good magic, and is used in folk healing (Wanderer & Rivera, 1986).

A motive for witchcraft may be hatred, jealousy, or envy. To cure, witches may use food or drink, imitative magic (such as dolls), evil air, or animal metamorphosis to bewitch (Wanderer & Rivera, 1986). There are many superstitions adhered to in this healing mode; for example, the keeping of black animals protects against witchcraft.

Health and folk beliefs specific to children

In addition to the childhood illnesses thought to be caused by *aires,* several other folk-defined childhood illnesses are well known in the literature on *curanderismos* (Rivera & Wanderer, 1986).

Caida de la mollera.   *Caida de la mollera* refers to a fallen fontanel in infants caused by a fall, by bouncing the child roughly, or by removing the nipple from the baby's mouth with too much force. This is viewed as an imbalance between the fontanel and the palate that blocks the passage of foods and liquids. Associated with *caida de la mollera* are the symptoms of inability to suck or grasp the nipple, vomiting, diarrhea, fever, restlessness, and crying spells.

Before seeking out a physician, mothers often seek out older women in the community who seem to know how to treat this problem. The following remedies have been noted by Ruiz (1985): pressing against the palate from inside the mouth, praying, applying eggs to the head and then pulling hairs, and holding the child with the head down. Reinert (1986) has noted that this condition is usually caused by severe dehydration, and correct medical treatment with intravenous fluids is essential.

Mal ojo ("evil eye").   As mentioned earlier, *mal ojo* occurs when an individual who is thought to possess a special power admires or covets the child of another and looks at but does not touch the child. *Mal ojo* at times is associated with witchcraft and black magic. This condition causes the symptoms of headaches, high fever, crying, diarrhea, restlessness, irritability, loss of weight and sleep, and sunken eyes (Rivera & Wanderer, 1986; Ruiz, 1985). The cure for the problem is to mix a hen's egg with water and place this under the head of the child's bed. This supposedly drives the bad influence out of the child's body. Another remedy is to have the person thought to be the source of the "evil eye" touch the afflicted individual. It is thought that the child will deteriorate, with severe coughing and vomiting, and possibly die if not treated. Families are known not to bring children with this problem to physicians because they fear the physician will misdiagnose the child and the child's condition will worsen.

Folk-related diseases of both children and adults

Susto (magical fright).   *Susto* is caused by a frightening experience or event and leads to the temporary loss of one's spirit from the body. This condition may even affect an unborn child if the mother is frightened. *Susto* is associated with childhood epilepsy, is seen more often in females, and if left untreated is believed to develop into tuberculosis or even be fatal. Symptoms of *susto* include crying, insomnia, anorexia, restlessness, nightmares, stomachache, diarrhea, high fever, and being afraid of just about anything.

Susto is treated by getting the patient on the floor, outstretching the hands, and then having a healer sweep the patient with indigenous herbs while praying. This treatment attempts to get the individual's spirit back into the body (Rivera & Wanderer, 1986; Ruiz, 1985).

Empacho. Patients suffering from *empacho* are believed to have a chunk of food that they are unable to pass, causing a lot of abdominal pain. They are taken to an older woman who possesses the knowledge to treat this problem. To diagnose the illness, the patient is held face down by the skin of the back. During this procedure, if a crack is heard, the diagnosis is *empacho* and the following treatment is instituted: body massages around the back and waist are given to restore the body's balance of hot and cold, which in turn, allows the food chunk to pass through the intestine (Ruiz, 1985).

Religious Views

Roman Catholicism is the prominent religion practiced by Mexican Americans. Common religious practices are baptism, confirmation, communion, weddings, and funerals. During times of crisis, Mexican Americans may rely on the priest and family for prayers. When a family member is ill, rituals that are practiced include promise making, offering candles, visiting shrines, and offering prayers (Logan & Semmes, 1986). The religious views are heavily influenced by the folk beliefs.

The Mexican American who is Roman Catholic may have beliefs that are influenced by ancient Indian practices of witchcraft and voodoo. As a result, the Mexican American may believe in demons. Incorporated in this system is a belief in witchcraft practices to manipulate evil forces (Wanderer & Rivera, 1986). Wanderer and Rivera (1986) have noted that in the Mexican American community witchcraft is called *brujeria* and is seen as a magical or supernatural illness and occasionally as an emotional illness. *Brujeria* has no scientific basis and is thought to be precipitated by opponents using the evil forces of hexes and spells. Symptoms of *brujeria* include paranoia, delusions, hallucinations, a feeling of being controlled by another person, mania, perverted and fitful behavior, depression, suspicion, and anxiety. Motives for witchcraft include envy, vengeance, hatred, and jealousy. (Kiev, 1968; Madsen & Madsen, 1969).

Implications for Nursing Care

The belief that the outcome of circumstances is controlled by external forces can influence compliance with health care. This belief may influence Mexican Americans to be less compliant in regard to nursing care because they believe that they do not have much control over their lives. This perspective may impact negatively on the acceptance of wellness programs in the U.S. health care system, such as smoking cessation, addiction programs, prenatal care, and chronic disease treatment. Because the Mexican American healing system of *curanderismos* incorporates religious beliefs, some Mexican Americans may also feel they are more in touch with the divine will, and therefore the origin and healing of illness, when they enter the health care system. The nurse should understand that Mexican Americans will have more respect for the caregiver who accepts the spiritual and folk basis of their health beliefs.

The healers in the folk medicine system are people with whom the Mexican Americans have established relationships and with whom they can easily communicate. These healers know and can treat the folk illnesses that the uninitiated health care worker may not recognize. It is helpful for the nurse to understand the respect this culture has for the *curandero,* who is often consulted simultaneously with the physician or nurse. The long-term goal of a nurse working within a Mexican American community should be to understand the folk medicine beliefs and to try to establish a relationship with the *curandero* in hopes of influencing acceptance and understanding of the rationale for modern health care practices, and thereby gaining the community's confidence.

The nurse should recognize that the *curandero* is involved in relieving people of their sins in order to experience healing, and that a spiritual perspective is usually an integral part of the U.S. health care system. One might compare the healer's influence in this ethnic group to that of the clergy in the dominant U.S. society wherein mutual cooperation is focused on meeting patients' spiritual and physical needs. Mexican American patients also need to be encouraged to practice their Roman Catholic religious beliefs and to receive supportive visits from the clergy. Acknowledging the patient's reliance on the folk health care system, as well as on their religious beliefs and medical assistance, will promote a more holistic focus for nursing care.

It is important to recognize the strong influence of hot and cold imbalance in folk beliefs. Some of these healing beliefs and practices are practical, such as massage, prayer, listening, or the application of cold for a fever. However, some practices can lead to missed clues for serious conditions that will not respond to these remedies, such as serious diarrhea, vomiting, dehydration, parasites, or malnutrition in children. For example, the nurse should suspect that malnutrition in a 1-year-old child may be due to the practice of disengaging the child from the mother at the time of weaning. Teaching the mother about the child's physical and emotional needs may improve the malnutrition. When dealing with children, Leininger (1978) warns the nurse to touch the children so that if the parents fear the "evil eye," the cultural remedy of touch will cure the condition.

Beliefs regarding hot and cold characteristics will impact on how the patient accepts some of the treatment plan. The nurse should note how the patient is accepting treatment, and if there is noncompliance, the nurse should talk with the patient and family to determine if the basis for noncompliance is folk beliefs. For example, the nurse might inquire if the condition is considered a hot or cold disease. The patient may have some definite beliefs about this and about whether the medical treatment can restore the hot-cold balance within the body. If the treatment is in contradiction to folk beliefs, the nurse should use solid scientific evidence to support the importance of the treatment. One can expect the older patient or first-generation immigrant to be more attached to these beliefs; therefore focusing health teaching on younger family members may be more useful in establishing compliance.

In dealing with folk-related diseases, the nurse needs to understand perceived causes for these conditions, for example, environmental influences, such as *caida de la mollera* or *empacho,* or evil influences, such as *mal ojo* or *susto.* Since these diseases are considered indigenous to the culture, they are usually seen and treated first by the *curandero.* Patients coming to the nurse's attention with these conditions probably have had these symptoms for a while and have already been treated unsuccessfully by the *curandero*. The nurse's physical assessment needs to be thorough. Rather than showing disrespect for the folk healer, the nurse should develop the relationship with the patient in such a way as to maintain the support of the folk healer.

BIOLOGICAL VARIATIONS
Skin Color

The skin color of Mexican Americans can vary from a natural tan to dark brown. Persons with lighter color have more Spanish ancestry, whereas darker-skinned persons have more Indian ancestry. It is more difficult to recognize vasodilation or vasoconstriction in the darker-skinned patient, in whom vasoconstriction and anemia are manifested as an ashen color rather than a bluish coloration. The mongolian spots (areas of darker skin found on the sacral area) found on infants usually disappear by age 4. The hair of Mexican Americans is usually dark and may be curly and woolly, straight, or wavy (Monrroy, 1983).

Susceptibility to Disease

There are several categories of diseases with high incidence in Mexican Americans. Reinert (1986) has cited a report from the state of Texas, Special Committee on Diabetes Service, saying that in Mexican Americans not only is the incidence of diabetes five times the national average, but complications are frequent. In a study using census figures from 1969 to 1971 and 1979 to 1981, Stern et al. (1987) reported less decline in the death rates of Mexican American men from total ischemic heart disease and myocardial infarction than in the death rates of other men. Hypertension is also found with increased prevalence among Mexican Americans (Ailinger, 1982). Pernicious anemia, most often seen in the elderly, has been shown to occur in those of Latin American origin at a younger age than in White patients (Carmel, Johnson, & Weiner, 1987). There is evidence that socioeconomic status has a strong effect on hemoglobin and hematocrit levels and that the poor have lower hemoglobin and hematocrit levels than do middle- and upper-class individuals. There is also some evidence that given similar socioeconomic conditions, Mexican Americans tend to have higher hemoglobin and hematocrit levels than do their White counterparts (Overfield, 1985). Hispanic patients in the Southwest were found to have a poorer prognosis with melanomas because they arose from the palms, sublingual regions, mucous membranes, and soles; were more advanced in stage; occurred in older people; and metastasized. (Black, Goldhahn, & Wiggins, 1987).

It is essential for the nurse working with Mexican Americans to realize that approximately 85% of the health problems common to Mexican Americans involve communicable diseases (Anthony-Tkach, 1981), including respiratory tract infections, diarrhea, skin disorders, nutritional problems (particularly during the first year of life), macroscopic parasitosis, and amebiasis. One of the most severe medical problems facing nations throughout the world is tuberculosis, which is thought to occur in areas where there are crowded living conditions, low income, substandard housing, and inadequate health care. As an infectious disease, tuberculosis is common throughout the world, since a vast majority of the people live in poverty. In the United States the population that is most at risk for the incidence and transmittal of tuberculosis includes newly arrived immigrants, such as Asians, Mexicans, and Puerto Ricans; refugees; migrant workers; and homeless or street people (Brunner & Suddarth, 1988; Hood & Jackson, 1989). Because of the high prevalence of tuberculosis in Mexico, it is thought that Mexican Americans may have a predisposition to a higher prevalence of tuberculosis than other Americans (Anthony-Tkach, 1981).

In Mexico the life expectancy at birth has increased from 35 to 62 years over the last four decades. For every child between the ages of 1 and 4 who dies in the United States, approximately 23 die in Mexico (U.S. Department of Commerce, Bureau of the Census, 1987). One of the leading causes of death among children is malnutrition. Approximately 50% to 75% of the Mexican population suffer from malnutrition. While the problem of malnutrition in Mexico is thought to be primarily economic, it may also have an educational component. The nurse needs to make an assessment of the potential need for nutritional education among Mexican American patients.

The two leading causes of death in Mexico are pneumonia and gastrointestinal diseases that are related to bacteria and parasites. Accidents and violence are thought to be the third leading cause of death among Mexicans, and cardiovascular disease is thought to be the fourth leading cause of death (Anthony-Tkach, 1981).

In a recent study of 19 low-income Mexican American women diagnosed as having non-insulin-dependent diabetes mellitus, Luyas (1989) found that the patients or their informants explained diabetes onset in terms of economic and family problems, whereas health providers explained diabetes onset mainly in biological terms. This study illustrates the importance of knowing the patient's perspective on a medical diagnosis in order to provide culturally appropriate and sensitive nursing care.

Psychological Characteristics

According to Reinert (1986), Mexican Americans often encounter serious health problems resulting from the stress of coping with poverty. These problems include being overweight and an increased risk for suicide. Because of their belief that alcohol consumption is a way of celebrating life, alcohol is consumed in all aspects of life and contributes to the increased incidence of accidents and violence. Arrendondo et al. (1987), in reviewing the literature, found that for Mexican Americans, alcoholism is possibly the most crucial health problem. Research on substance abuse among Hispanics indicates that alcohol is the most frequently abused intoxicant. Edmondson (1975) has suggested that Mexican American adult men have an alcoholism rate that is significantly higher than the national norm for other American men. Other researchers have also reported high levels of alcoholism within the American Hispanic community (Garcia, 1976; Ruiz, Vasquez, & Vasquez, 1973.) Men are most often affected, because the male role may be correlated with being able to ingest large amounts of alcohol. The family pride protects this behavior as long as the man provides for the family. Some research has been reported that indicates that children who have alcoholic parents or grandparents are at higher risk for alcoholism because of their physiological relationship (Lawson, Ellis, & Rivers, 1984). Arrendondo et al. (1987) noted that Mexican Americans have a higher death rate from illnesses related to chronic alcohol consumption, such as cirrhosis of the liver.

In a study on the prevalence of psychiatric disorders, Karno et al. (1987) reported that Mexican Americans had fewer drug abuse problems than non-Hispanics. Other research has found, however, that when rates of substance abuse are considered among Mexican Americans, marijuana is the second most abused drug, with heroin and cocaine being the third most abused drugs (Eden & Aguilar, 1989). Inhalants are also frequently abused among young Hispanics (Eden & Aguilar, 1989).

Some studies have indicated that there is less incidence of mental illness among Spanish-speaking people. This is thought to be because there are fewer role conflicts in Mexican American families, since the rules of behavior of the culture are clearly defined (Murillo, 1978). In Mexican American families, the family may also serve as a buffering mechanism that encourages individual members to share and thereby reduces anxiety and stressful situations. The Mexican American's view of the world also enables some Mexican Americans to blame external forces for failures, thereby reducing guilt. Mexican Americans are also unlikely to seek treatment in hospitals and other clinical facilities for mental illnesses. Mexican American women have been found to have slightly more dysthymic disorders, panic disorders, and phobias than other women (Murillo, 1978). Social and cultural differences between the Mexican American and the dominant American society appear to be a recurring theme among Mexican American patients with symptoms of psychological disorders. Feelings of social isolation may serve to increase personal feelings of isolation. It is important for the nurse to be aware of self-image problems that are socially created and those that are more personal in nature. Knowledge of these factors will assist the nurse in making the diagnosis and planning nursing care that will help lower the patient's psychological risk.

Implications for Nursing Care

Nurses must be aware that cultural differences are important to patient care and therefore must be considered when providing care. A health intervention that opposes a particular cultural practice may not be successful even if it is considered a good health measure. For nursing care to be effective, the nursing and health measures implemented must be considered culturally relevant. This same awareness must be developed by the nurse in regard to biological variations. A nurse who lacks understanding of biological variations may actually contribute to the promotion of ill health.

It is important for the nurse to recognize that the informal health care system in Mexico is generally composed of several elements, one of which is self-medication. In the early 1980s in Mexico, just as in the United States, prescriptions were required for all medications such as antibiotics and steroids. However, during this time the sale of drugs in Mexico was uncontrolled with the exception of narcotics, barbiturates, and other addictive drugs. The pharmacist was, in effect, the chief physician's surrogate, and many Mexican American immigrants have been accustomed to receiving medication from a pharmacist without a prescription. In addition, some Mexican Americans consider medication to be always necessary and may not believe their illness is being treated unless a particular medication is ordered.

The massive scale to which self-medication is practiced in Mexico is potentially dangerous (Anthony-Tkach, 1981). To illustrate this point, in 1974 an outbreak of typhoid fever that was thought to be the worst incidence in the century occurred in and around the area surrounding Mexico City. The causative agent was identified as chloramphenicol-resistant *Salmonella typhi*. Health officials in Mexico City believed that the indiscriminate use of antibiotics may have caused the organism to become resistant to the effects of chloramphenicol. It is important for the nurse to assess whether a Mexican American patient with a communicable disease is practicing self-medication for treatment. The assessment of the potential for self-medication, as well as close follow-up, may be beneficial in reducing the drug-resistant causative organisms that can ensue from self-medication. The nurse who works with Mexican American patients with communicable diseases needs to emphasize that communicable diseases are preventable and that prompt care is essential to reducing exposure to, as well as morbidity and mortality from, communicable diseases.

When working with the Mexican American patient, the nurse should be knowledgeable about the effects of the bacillus Calmette-Guérin (BCG) as opposed to the purified protein derivative (PPD) skin test for tuberculosis. BCG is a strain of *Mycobacterium bovis* that is widely used in countries with a high incidence of tuberculosis, such as Mexico. When an individual is inoculated with BCG and then later given a PPD skin test, there generally is an intense reaction to the combination of the BCG and the PPD, resulting in possible skin necrosis and subsequent scarring of the infected area (Anthony-Tkach, 1981). Therefore the nurse who works with Mexican American patients must ascertain whether the patient has had a tuberculosis skin test and, if so, whether the test was the BCG. If the nurse is in doubt as to whether or not the tuberculosis skin test was the BCG, the nurse should recommend that the patient have a chest radiograph instead of the skin test.

Treatment of chemical dependency among Mexican Americans is a major challenge because of three central factors that inhibit treatment: integration of alcohol consumption within the Hispanic culture, the psychology of the Spanish culture, and the family dynamics of the traditional Hispanic. Drinking behavior is so ingrained in the Mexican culture that social functions ranging from baptisms to funerals generally include the serving of alcoholic beverages (Arrendondo et al., 1987). Drinking occurs among Mexican Americans when the individual is coping with negative feelings, as well as when the individual is experiencing positive feelings. The nurse must remember that the fatalistic element of Hispanic psychology helps to incorporate and at the same time augment drinking problems among Mexican Americans. When a drinking problem is described by a Mexican American in an intake interview, it may be followed by the patient saying, "That's life" or "This is our cross to bear." For the most part, this external locus of control serves to block the identified alcoholic, and the family as well, from assuming a more active role in the recovery process.

Rather than seeking outside professional help for the treatment of alcohol abuse, Mexican Americans may collaborate with the *curandero* in treating the alcoholism or may try self-medication. The nurse needs to assess whether the patient who is a substance abuser is using a *curandero* or is self-medicating with other drugs, because the use of a *curandero* or self-medication may further intensify the problem. The nurse also needs to assess carefully whether a patient with a drug abuse problem would be best suited for individual, group, or family therapy. This determination can only be made after a thorough intake interview. Because the Mexican American family is built on a system of family orientation, it is thought that perhaps the best mode of treatment for Mexican Americans is family therapy. The initial purpose of family therapy for Mexican American substance abusers should be to evaluate the family's influence on the patient's chemical dependency problems. The nurse should incorporate both the nuclear and the extended family in the evaluation.

To plan safe and effective, individualized nursing care for members of the Mexican American community that is appropriate and congruent with their life-styles and cultural beliefs, nurses must know and understand the cultural patterns and belief systems of this ethnic group (Murillo-Rohde, 1977).

It is important for the nurse to remember that Mexican Americans differ from other cultural groups in their expression of symptoms and in how the ill person is perceived and treated by others. For example, in the Mexican American culture, epilepsy carries a far lesser social stigma than in other ethnic and cultural groups. Mexican Americans incorporate Hippocratic explanations when describing this particular disease and believe it is caused by a physical imbalance; thus treatment is reported to be medicinal and herbal in nature (Kiev, 1972).

SUMMARY

One of the most important roles of the nurse in caring for the Mexican American patient is that of teacher. Teaching should begin with an assessment of the patient's ability to communicate and understand. This will guide the nurse in deciding what other family members need to be included in the teaching process. The home situation needs to be carefully evaluated to adapt care to the reality of the living situation. Instruction should include all aspects of the patient's condition and treatment. It should be communicated in simple, concrete terms with ample opportunity to raise questions and validate understanding. There should be continuous evaluation of learning by questioning and return demonstrations, and problem solving should be encouraged. Throughout this process the nurse continues to build a trusting relationship with the patient so that follow-up care will be maintained. This helps ensure that the patient will seek out medical care before future situations get out of control.

The Mexican American community in the United States is rich in cultural beliefs and values. This group has adhered to these beliefs and values more than other minority groups. Because this group is growing rapidly in size and now is gradually moving to areas of the country other than the Southwest, more nurses will be coming into contact with Mexican Americans through community and health care systems. Mexican Americans present many opportunities and challenges to the health care system and to nursing in particular. By understanding the cultural diversity unique to Mexican Americans and accepting their beliefs, especially those relating to health care, the nurse can plan effective, individualized care.

---

*CASE STUDY** George Garcia, a 23-year-old migrant farm worker, and his wife, Anita, age 20, bring their 4-month-old daughter to the emergency room of a small community hospital. They speak only broken English. They have another small child with them, as well as two older women. They are very worried about the infant, who they say has been unable to retain feedings of diluted cow's milk. Now, because of poor sucking and increased sleeping, the infant has not had anything by mouth for the past 24 hours. When asked, the parents indicate that the infant has had only three wet diapers since yesterday. The nurse notices that the infant's eyes are sunken, she is listless, and the fontanels are depressed. When asked, the parents say the infant has been sick for 3 or 4 days. One of the older women makes a pushing up motion with her hand as she points to the infant's mouth. Further assessment reveals a rectal temperature of 103° F. The family has not taken the temperature at all in the past 3 to 4 days. Skin turgor is good; mucous membranes are tacky. There has been no diarrhea. The infant's heart rate is 120 and regular, but thready. Respirations are 12 per minute at rest. The infant does not cry during rectal temperature taking or when touched with a cold stethoscope.

---

*I wish to acknowledge Stacie Hitt, R.N., M.S.N., for assistance in developing the case study and care plan.

CARE
PLAN

Nursing Diagnosis   Fluid volume deficit related to diarrhea.

Patient Outcome	*Nursing Interventions*
Infant will exhibit signs of adequate hydration.	1 Offer appropriate fluids as tolerated. 2 Maintain accurate record of intake. 3 Weigh daily. 4 Assess all parameters (e.g., vital signs, skin character). 5 Apply urine collection device if indicated. 6 Measure urine volume and specific gravity.

Nursing Diagnosis   Nutrition, altered: less than body requirements.

Patient Outcome	*Nursing Interventions*
Infant will consume and retain appropriate number of calories per weight per day.	1 Gradually reintroduce foods as indicated. 2 Observe infant's response to feedings. 3 Describe feeding behavior.

Nursing Diagnosis   Diarrhea resulting in alteration in bowel elimination as evidenced by hypoactive bowel sounds.

Patient Outcome	*Nursing Interventions*
Infant will resume normal peristaltic and elimination patterns.	1 Record fecal output: number, volume, characteristics. 2 Observe and record presence of associated signs: tenesmus, cramping, vomiting.

Nursing Diagnosis   Body temperature, altered.

Patient Outcome	*Nursing Interventions*
Infant will regain and maintain a body temperature within normal limits.	1 Reduce environmental temperature. 2 Place infant in lightweight clothing and bed linen. 3 Encourage cool liquids. 4 Take rectal temperature every 4 hours.

Nursing Diagnosis   Sensory alteration as evidenced by listlessness.

Patient Outcome	*Nursing Interventions*
Infant will respond to a full range of stimuli.	1 Record intervals of sleep and wakefulness; observe infant's level of activity when awake. 2 Assess ease of arousal. 3 Encourage family to participate in holding/caring/talking with patient.

Nursing Diagnosis   Communication, impaired verbal, related to foreign language barriers.

Patient Outcome	*Nursing Interventions*
Family will be able to communicate basic needs and understanding of infant's condition and care.	1 Assess language spoken best by family. 2 Assess family's ability to comprehend English. 3 Talk slower than normal to family. 4 Use gestures or drawings for clarity. 5 Be careful to touch children after looking directly at them. 6 Make a conscious effort to address father when explaining care. 7 Show respect to older women. 8 Obtain a fluent, consistent translator.

Nursing Diagnosis   Health maintenance, altered, related to lack of health information.

Patient Outcome	*Nursing Interventions*
Family will demonstrate understanding and ability to perform skills necessary for care of infant at home.	1 Determine information family needs. 2 Determine folklore beliefs related to health care. 3 Initiate the teaching. 4 Determine influence older women have on family's health care beliefs. 5 Determine equipment needed for home care. 6 Seek social service referral. 7 Seek assistance from agencies.

STUDY QUESTIONS

1. Which family member is likely to make the decision about whether to allow the infant to be hospitalized?
2. What might the nurse do to encourage the best communication with this family?
3. What kinds of data should be obtained in the history?
4. What folk disease does the family likely believe the infant has?
5. How should the nurse explain to the family why the infant needs to be hospitalized?
6. Why would it be advantageous for the nurse to touch both the infant and the other child while relating to them?
7. How could the nurse show acceptance of the folk remedies that may have already been tried with the infant?
8. The infant is admitted to the hospital. What could be expected in terms of family visitation?
9. What teaching goals should the nurse have for this family?

REFERENCES

Ailinger, R. (1982). Hypertension knowledge in a Hispanic community. *Nursing Research, 31*(4), 207-210.

Anthony-Tkach, C. (1981). Care of the Mexican-American patient. *Nursing and Health Care, 2,* 424-427.

Arrendondo, R., Weddige, R., Justice, C., & Fitz, J. (1987). Alcoholism in Mexican-Americans: Intervention and treatment. *Hospital and Community Psychiatry, 38*(2), 180-183.

Black, W., Goldhahn, R., & Wiggins, C. (1987). Melanoma within a southwestern Hispanic population. *Archives of Internal Medicine, 123*(10), 1331-1334.

Bonilla, E.S. (1973). Ethnic and bilingual education for cultural pluralism. In M.D. Stent, W.R. Hazard, & H.H. Rivlin (Eds.), *Cultural pluralism in education: A mandate for change* (pp. 115-122). East Norwalk, Conn.: Appleton-Century-Crofts.

Brownlee, A.T. (1978). *Community, culture, and care*. St. Louis: C.V. Mosby.

Brunner, L., & Suddarth, D. (1988). *Textbook of medical-surgical nursing*. Philadelphia: J.B. Lippincott.

Carmel, R., Johnson, C., & Weiner, J. (1987). Pernicious anemia in Latin Americans is not a disease of the elderly. *Ethnology, 147*(11), 1995-1996.

Cervantes, R., Snyder, S., & Padilla, A. (1989). Posttraumatic stress in immigrants from Central America and Mexico. *Hospital and Community Psychiatry, 40*(6), 615-619.

Chavez, N. (1986). Mental health services delivery to minority populations: Hispanics—a perspective. In M. Miranda & H. Kitano (Eds.), *Mental health research and practice in minority communities*. Rockville, Md.: National Institute of Mental Health.

Clark, M. (1970). *Health in the Mexican American culture*. Berkley: University of California Press.

Currier, R. (1966). The hot-cold syndrome and symbolic medicine. *Ethnology, 5*(3), 251-263.

Dorsey, P., & Jackson, H. (1976). Cultural health traditions: The Latino-Chino perspective. In M.F. Branch & P.P. Paxton (Eds.), *Providing safe nursing care for ethnic people of color* (pp. 41-80). Norwalk, Conn.: Appleton-Century-Crofts.

Eden, S., & Aguilar, R. (1989). The Hispanic chemically dependent client: Considerations for diagnosis and treatment. In G. Lawson & A. Lawson (Eds.), *Alcoholism and substance abuse in special populations*. Rockville, Md.: Aspen.

Edmondson, H.A. (1975, Feb. 7). *Mexican American alcoholism and deaths at L.A.C. and U.S. Medical Center*. Testimony before the Subcommittee on Alcoholism to the California State Health and Welfare Committee.

Favazza, A. (1983). Cultural factors in diagnosis and treatment. In *ACP psychiatric update*. New York: Medical Information Systems.

Fishman, J. (1967, April). Bilingualism with and without diglossia: Diglossia with and without bilingualism. *Journal of Social Issues, 23*, 29-38.

Ford, J., & Graves, J. (1977). Differences between Mexican-American and White children in interpersonal distance and social touching. *Perceptual and Motor Skills, 45*(3, Pt. 1), 779-785.

Foster, G. (1978). Relationship between Spanish and Spanish American folk medicine. In R.A. Martinez (Ed.), *Hispanic culture and health care: Fact, fiction, folklore* (pp. 183-202). St. Louis: C.V. Mosby.

Garcia, D. (1988). Mexican Americans. In W. Nault (Ed.), *World Book Encyclopedia* (pp. 446-449). Chicago: World Book.

Garcia, L. (1976, Feb. 4). *Spanish speaking alcoholism problems and needs*. Testimony before the Subcommittee on Alcoholism and Narcotics to the U.S. Senate, Washington, D.C.

Gelfand, D., & Bialik-Gilad, R. (1989). Immigration reform and social work. *Social Work, 34*(1), 23-27.

Harwood, A. (1971). The hot-cold theory of disease. *JAMA 216*(7), 1153-1158.

Hood, L., & Jackson, N. (1989). Caring for the patient with TB. *Advancing Clinical Care, 4*(4), 14-18.

Hough, R. (1985). Life events and stress in Mexican-American culture. In *Stress and Hispanic mental health: Relating research to service delivery* (pp. 110-146). Rockville, Md.: U.S. Government Printing Office.

Ingham, J. (1970). On Mexican folk medicine. *American Anthropologist, 72*(1), 76-87.

Karno, M., Hough, R., Burnam, M., Javier, R., Escobar, J., Timbers, D., & Boyd, A. (1987). Psychiatric disorders among Mexican Americans and non-Hispanic Whites in Los Angeles. *Archives of General Psychiatry, 44*(8), 695-700.

Keefe, S. (1984). Real and ideal extended familism among Mexican Americans and Anglo Americans: On the meaning of "close" family ties. *Human Organization, 43*(1), 65-70.

Kemper, R. (1982). The compadrazgo in urban Mexico. *Anthropological Quarterly, 55*(1), 17-30.

Khoury, R., & Thurmond, G. (1978). Ethnic differences in time perception: A comparison of Anglo and Mexican Americans. *Perceptual and Motor Skills, 47*(3, pt. 2), 1183-1188.

Kiev, A. (1968). *Curanderismo: Mexican American folk psychiatry*. New York: Free Press.

Kiev, A. (1972). *Transcultural psychiatry*. New York: Free Press.

Kluckhohn, F. (1976). Dominant and variant value orientations. In P.J. Brink (Ed.), *Transcultural nursing: A book of readings* (pp. 63-81). Englewood Cliffs, N.J.: Prentice Hall.

Lantican, L., & Corona, D. (1989, Nov. 14). *A comparison of the social support networks of Filipino and Mexican-American primigravidas.* Paper presented at the Sigma Theta Tau International Conference, Indianapolis.

Laosa, L. (1975). Bilingualism in three United States Hispanic groups: Contextual use of language by children and adults and their families. *Journal of Educational Psychology, 67*(5), 617-627.

Lawson, G., Ellis, D.C., & Rivers, P.C. (1984). *Essentials of chemical dependency counseling.* Rockville, Md.: Aspen.

Leininger, M. (1978). *Transcultural nursing: Concept, theory, and practice.* New York: John Wiley & Sons.

Logan, B., & Semmes, C. (1986). Culture and ethnicity. In B. Logan & C. Dawkins (Eds.), *Family centered nursing in the community* (pp. 112-113). Reading, Mass.: Addison Wesley.

Luyas, G. (1989, Nov. 14). *An explanatory model of diabetes by Mexican American woman.* Paper presented at the Sigma Theta Tau International Conference, Indianapolis.

Madsen, W., & Madsen, C. (1969). *A guide to Mexican witchcraft.* Mexico: D.F. Minutiae.

Marcos, L.R. (1988). Understanding ethnicity in psychotherapy with Hispanic patients. *American Journal of Psychoanalysis, 48*(1), 35-42.

Marcos, L.R., & Alpert, M. (1976). Strategies and risks in psychotherapy with bilingual patients: The phenomenon of language independence. *American Journal of Psychiatry, 133,* 1275-1278.

Marcos, L.R., Alpert, M., Urcuyo, L., & Kesselman, M. (1973). The effect of interview language on the evaluation of psychopathology in Spanish-American schizophrenic patients. *American Journal of Psychiatry, 130,* 549-553.

Miller, F. (1986). The people. In B. Cayne, & B. Holland, (Eds.), *Encyclopedia Americana* (pp. 819-830). Danbury, Conn.: Grolier.

Mirowsky, J., & Ross, C. (1984). Mexican culture and its emotional contradictions. *Journal of Health and Social Behavior, 25*(1), 2-13.

Monrroy, L.S.A. (1983). Nursing care of Raza/Latina patients. In M.S. Orque, B. Bloch, & L.S.A. Monrroy (Eds.), *Ethnic nursing care: A multicultural approach* (pp. 115-148). St. Louis: C.V. Mosby.

Murillo, N. (1978). The Mexican American family. In C.A. Hernandez, M.J. Haug, & N.N. Wagner (Eds.), *Chicanos: Social and psychological perspectives* (pp. 15-25). St. Louis: C.V. Mosby.

Murillo-Rohde, I. (1977). Care for all colors. *Imprint, 24*(4), 29-32, 50.

Naisbitt, J. (1982). *Megatrends.* New York: Warner Books.

Ness, R., & Wintrob, R. (1981). Folk healing: A description and synthesis. *American Journal of Psychiatry, 138*(11), 1477-1481.

Overfield, T. (1985). *Biological variations in health and illness.* Reading, Mass.: Addison-Wesley.

Oxford dictionary of quotations (p. 140). (1980). New York: Oxford University Press.

Reinert, B. (1986). The healthcare beliefs and values of Mexican-Americans. *Home Healthcare Nurse, 4*(5), 23-27, 29-31.

Richardson, L. (1982). Caring through understanding: Part 2. Folk medicine in the Hispanic population. *Imprint, 29*(2), 21, 72-77.

Rivera, G., & Wanderer, J. (1986). Curanderismo and childhood illnesses. *The Social Science Journal, 23*(3), 361-372.

Rivera, J. (1978). *The new faces of racism: The Chicano case.* Report to the Association for Huanist Sociology.

Rubel, A. (1966). *Across the tracks: Mexican Americans in a Texas city.* Austin: University of Texas Press.

Ruiz, P. (1985). Cultural barriers to effective medical care among Hispanic-American patients. *Annual Review of Medicine, 36,* 63-71.

Ruiz, P., Vasquez, W., & Vasquez, K. (1973). The mobile unit: A new approach in mental health. *Community Mental Health Journal, 9,* 18-24.

Saunders, L. (1954). *Cultural difference and medical care.* New York: Russell Sage Foundation.

Statistical abstracts of the United States. (1988). Washington, D.C.: U.S. Department of Commerce, Bureau of the Census.

Stern, M., Bradshaw, B., Eifler, C., Fong, D., Hazuda, H., & Rosenthal, M. (1987). Secular decline in death rates due to ischemic heart disease in Mexican Americans and non-Hispanic Whites in Texas, 1970-1980. *Circulation, 76*(6), 1245-1250.

U.S. Department of Commerce, Bureau of the Census. (1979). Population characteristics: Persons of Spanish origin in the United States. *Current Population Reports,* Series P-20, 339, Washington, D.C.: Author.

Valdez, A. (1980). *Ethnic maintenance among Mexicans and Puerto Ricans*. Report to Southwestern Sociological Association.

Wanderer, J., & Rivera, G. (1986). Black magic beliefs and white magic practice: The common structures of intimacy, tradition and power. *The Social Science Journal, 23*(4), 419-430.

Weaver, T. (1970). Use of hypothetical situations in a study of Spanish-American illness referral systems. *Human Organisms, 29,* 140.

Weclew, R. (1975). The nature, prevalence, and level of awareness of "curanderismo" and some of its implications for community mental health. *Community Mental Health Journal* 11(2), 145-154.

West, M., & Moore, E. (1989). Undocumented workers in the United States and South Africa: A comparative study of changing control. *Human Organization, 48*(1), 1-9.

Wilson, H., & Kneisl, C. (1988). *Psychiatric nursing*. Reading, Mass.: Addison-Wesley Publishing Co.

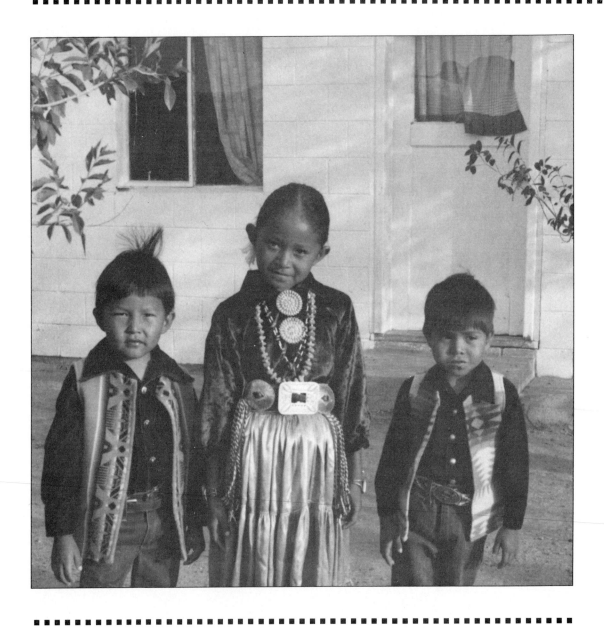

■■■

CHAPTER 10

Navajo Indians

Catherine E. Hanley

BEHAVIORAL OBJECTIVES
After reading this chapter, the nurse will be able to:

1 Identify ways in which the Navajo culture influences Navajo individuals and health-seeking behaviors.

2 Recognize physical and biological variances that exist in and across Navajo groups in order to provide culturally appropriate care.

3 Develop a sensitivity and understanding for communication differences as evidenced within and across Navajo groups in order to avoid stereotyping and to provide culturally appropriate nursing care.

4 Develop a sensitivity and understanding for psychological phenomena that influence the functioning of a Navajo person when nursing care is being provided.

5 Describe the impact of traditional Navajo folk medicine and the relationship to health-seeking behaviors.

OVERVIEW OF THE NAVAJO INDIANS

Archeological evidence places Navajos in the Gobernador Canyon area of northwestern New Mexico by the late 1400s or early 1500s. By the early 1600s some Navajos had migrated as far as the Black Mesa country of northern Arizona (Iverson, 1981). The first written historical observations of the Navajo have been attributed to Arate Salmeron (1626) and Father Benavides (1630).

According to Iverson (1981), the various Pueblo peoples exerted a tremendous influence on the evolution of the Navajo culture in the new region. There is historical evidence suggesting that the Navajos and Pueblos were at times foes. However, Brugge (1968) suggested a number of instances wherein Navajo and Pueblo villages allied themselves against the Spanish and other outside groups, and Young (1961) also concluded that the Navajos and the Pueblos existed together in a more peaceful rather than hostile relationship. Regardless of whether the Pueblos and the Navajos lived peacefully or not, the Pueblos probably did influence change in the Navajo lifestyle in some critical ways. For example, the Navajos have a matrilineal clan system that exists even today and dictates that a Navajo Indian inherits the clan and thus the lineage from the mother (Iverson, 1981). The implication is that people from the same clan are considered relatives with varying responsibilities to one another.

For the Western Pueblos the clan traditions were strong, and it is probable that they influenced the Navajos in the direction of clan formation (Iverson, 1981). In addition, the Pueblo people were very sedentary and had agricultural ways that undoubtedly also had some effect on the Navajos. As a consequence of these influences, the Navajos gradually adopted a way of life that was significantly less nomadic, with less emphasis on hunting, than that of other Apachean groups. Seemingly, the Navajos learned trades such as weaving, pottery making, silversmithing, and the art of agriculture from the Pueblo people in route to the Southwest (according to Iverson [1981], the Navajos credit "Spiderwoman" with their instruction in weaving). Differences existed in that Pueblo men traditionally were weavers, whereas Navajo men very rarely became weavers.

During the sixteenth, seventeenth, and eighteenth centuries, the Navajo people underwent tremendous expansion, cultural acquisition, and social change. According to Young (1961), the Navajos have always had a great capacity to absorb and elaborate on cultural traits adopted from other people. For example, the Pueblo weaving tradition is responsible for producing the Navajo blanket, which is unmistakenly the product of the *Diné* (the Navajo word for "chosen people"). The language, although distinctively Navajo, was learned by other Indians; however, few Navajos attempted to master a foreign tongue (Young, 1961). The Navajo people lived freely within the beautiful lands of their forefathers, located between the Four Sacred Mountains: Blanca Peak to the east, Mount Taylor to the south, San Francisco Peak to the west, and Hesperus Peak to the north. Four directional colors were associated with the Four Sacred Mountains: white with Blanca Peak, blue with Mount Taylor, yellow with San Francisco Peak, and black with Hesperus Peak. To understand the history of the Navajo people, it is important to understand the significance of the Four Sacred Mountains, which historically were considered the cardinal boundary peaks surrounding the Navajo country. Even today, Navajo people believe that the Four Sacred Mountains were gifts from the "Holy People"; therefore traditions, prayers, songs, and sacred trust are embodied in these mountains (Navajo Health Systems Agency, 1985).

Perhaps one of the most significant periods of Navajo history occurred during 1864, when over 9000 Navajo persons were captured in what is now known as Arizona and were forced to journey to Fort Sumner on the Bosque Rodondo Reservation in the then territory of New Mexico. During this long journey (known in Navajo history as the "long walk") and internment at Fort Sumner, over 2000 Navajo men, women, and children died of respiratory tract diseases, gastrointestinal disorders, and exhaustion.

It was during May 1868, the fourth year of their forced internment, that the Navajos' elected leader, Chief Barboncito, said to a Washington delegation appointed by President Andrew Johnson, "I hope to God you will not ask me to go to any other country except my own." In speaking these words, Chief Barboncito expressed the feelings, beliefs, traditions, and desires of the Navajo people. On May 28, 1868, the United States of America and the Navajo tribe entered into a treaty that was ratified on August 12, 1868, by President Andrew Johnson (*Treaty,* 1973).

After the signing of the 1868 treaty, the Navajos moved progressively in the direction of the Four Sacred Mountains. Gradual as it might have seemed, the call from the Four Sacred Mountains for the return to Navajo ways reflected the futuristic response of self-determination, self-governance, and self-actualization (Hanley, 1987). Although the treaty signed at Fort Sumner was not the first treaty but the eighth treaty made between the Navajo people and the United States in 22 years, it was historically significant because it led to their release from Fort Sumner and to the establishment of their first reservation at Fort Defiance, Arizona. (At that time Arizona was a separate territory; it became the forty-eighth state in 1912.) After the Navajo people were released from their internment at Fort Sumner, they began to develop a diversified economy. For the Navajo, stock raising was an important element of the economy, but not the only element. From early and later historical accounts, it appears that the Navajos have always been perceived as great farmers. A re-emerging question about the Navajo people concerns why the Navajos traditionally needed such a diverse economy; another reemerging question concerns why livestock took on a more essential role within the Navajo economy. The answers to these questions seemingly overlap and are mutually reinforcing: for the Navajo people a diversified economy made more thorough and efficient use of the different opportunities provided by various soils, altitudes, and vegetations.

Today, there are three different climatic zones for the Navajo people. The humid, or mountain, zones account for roughly 8% of the total Navajo area; the mesas and high plains, with their intermediate steppe climate, account for roughly 37% of the Navajo area; and the comparatively warm desert regions account for roughly 55% of the Navajo area. For the Navajo people winter temperatures in these regions range from an average minimum of 4° to 15° F in the humid zone, to 10° to 25° F in the steppe zone, to 11° to 30° F in the desert zone. Summer temperatures in these regions have an average maximum temperature ranging from 70° to 80° F in the humid zone, to 80° to 88° F in the steppe zone, to 100° F or higher in the desert. The average rainfall in all three areas is concentrated in the late summer period, which extends from July to September, with great variation in amount within each zone. The desert and humid zones each receive an additional 41% of precipitation in the form of winter snow. The soils in the Navajo region may be classified as excellent, good, or fair in terms of runoff, grass-producing ability, and erosion. Only about a third of the area is considered excellent or good in terms of soil productivity, and about 15% of the soil is unproductive, with little vegetative cover. The vegetation includes grassland, meadows, sagebrush, browse (shrub), and woodland (which is inaccessible and barren in some places); in the Navajo region the diversity is striking. More Navajo land is covered with coniferous timber than with sagebrush (Young, 1961).

It is thought that the conflicts between the Navajos and their neighbors were contributing factors to their economic diversification. For example, historical accounts suggest that as raiding by and against the Navajo people grew in intensity, it consequently complicated agricultural pursuits and led to an increased need for mobility. In addition, the steady growth of the Navajo population figured greatly into the economic diversification: as the Navajo tribe grew in number, so did the quantity of livestock. There were two principal periods of growth in regard to the Navajo tribe. The first period of growth came in the last years of the eighteenth century and in the early years of the nineteenth century prior to the Anglo-American campaign against the Navajos. The second principal period of growth followed the Navajo return from Bosque Redondo. It was during the first area of expansion that livestock was established as an economically important commodity (Brugge, 1964).

The spectacular growth of the Navajo population began during the post–Fort Sumner era. In 1870 the Navajo population numbered 15,000 (Boyce, 1942). By 1900 the Navajo population had grown to 21,000, and by 1935 the population had grown to 35,500 persons. The population has grown steadily ever since. In 1981 there were approximately 151,000 Navajo Indians, who resided primarily in basically rural areas on or near the 27,000-square-mile reservation that is located in the states of Arizona, New Mexico, Colorado, and Utah (U.S. Department of Commerce, Bureau of the Census, 1988), and by 1986 the Navajo population had grown to 171,097, making the Navajo tribe the largest Indian tribe in the continental United States.

Today in the United States, there are approximately 300 Indian tribes residing in 26 states, with most Native Americans residing in the western part of the United States as a consequence of the forced western migration of the tribes. Today, while many Native Americans remain on reservations and in rural areas, an equal number also reside in cities, especially in states such as Oklahoma, California, New Mexico, and Alaska (Henderson & Primeaux, 1981).

The Navajo tribe derives revenue from oil, coal, and uranium, and from federal grants and contracts. Nevertheless high unemployment rates continue to be a major problem among the Navajo people (Heraldson, 1988).

COMMUNICATION
Dialect and Style

The Navajo language is classified as "Athapaskan" because historically it is thought to have been derived from the languages used by the people of Lake Athapaskan in Northwest Canada. The Navajo language is also similar to the languages spoken by some people living in Alaska, some people on the northern coast of the Pacific ocean, and the people of the Apache tribe. These separate groups speaking a language similiar to the Navajo language are referred to as Athapaskans.

The language of the Navajo people involves a tonal speech in which inflections are of great importance. Every vowel and consonant are fully sounded regardless of how many times they are doubled or tripled in the same word. Vowels are often interchanged, creating several variations and meanings of the same word.

The Navajo language is thought to reflect the concept of the universe, which is constantly in motion. Within the Navajo language, position is defined as a withdrawal from motion. For example, a person speaking English says "on," whereas a Navajo person says something directly opposite in meaning for the word *on;* the Navajo speaker says, "at rest." Whereas an English speaker says, "I dressed" or "One dresses," the Navajo speaker says, "I moved into my clothes" or "One moves into clothes." The language directly parallels mythological thought in that not only is the language in motion, but so are cultural and spiritual heroes (Sobralske, 1985).

When Navajo people speak, most of the sentences contain the word *good*. For some Navajo people the word *good* may be defined as a favorable or desirable quality that promotes prosperity and happiness. Therefore the word *good* is synonymous with other words such as *agreeable, attractive,* or *beautiful (nizhonié)*. The concept of goodness is directly related to the ideology of health and is even found in the Blessingway healing ceremony. The Blessingway healing ceremony is viewed by the Navajos as a "good" event because the ceremony promotes everlasting harmony or perfection.

Even today, the majority of the Navajo people still speak the native language. Although many Navajo Indians are fluent in both the Navajo language and the English language, there are also many who do not speak English and therefore require the assistance of a Navajo interpreter when seeking or receiving health care. The Navajo language does not always have an equivalent single word for an English word; instead the language makes use of a description of all occurrences impacting on what is being said.

Until recently the Navajo language was unwritten. In World War II a special branch of the U.S. Marine Corps was developed for Navajos who served as Navajo code talkers. It has been estimated that this highly esteemed group saved millions of lives, since the enemy was unable to understand the Navajo language or infiltrate its code.

Touch

Instead of using the handshake practiced in the dominant culture, on meeting another person, Navajos extend their hand and lightly touch the hand of the person they are greeting. Other examples of the use of touch in the Navajo culture include the tradition of massaging a newborn baby as a bonding experience between mother and baby, and the tradition of giving a small gift and preparing a small feast for the family when the baby laughs for the first time because this token of esteem touches the heart of all of the people around the baby. Another example is the taboo against touching a dead person or animal killed by lightning, which is extended to touching articles associated with the deceased individual or animal involved. This traditional taboo is not extended to animals whose death resulted from natural causes.

Use of Silence and the Importance of Names

On initially meeting strangers, Navajo people may appear silent and reserved. Once the Navajo individual becomes familiar with the other person, warm behavior is usually demonstrated. In addition, when introducing themselves by name, Navajo people give honor to ancestors by stating the clan and the location of the home.

Kinesics

Kinesics practiced within the Navajo culture include the avoidance of eye contact. In dominant cultures found within the United States, eye contact is considered important and if not present may cause suspicion. However, the opposite is true in the Navajo culture, where eye contact is considered a sign of disrespect.

In earlier days the Navajo people frowned on pointing anything at another person; if pointing occurred, it was considered insulting. Some Navajos believed that an object being passed to another person should be held upright so that an end would not point at the other person.

Language Lateralization

In a study of language lateralization in Navajo reservation children, one group of Navajo children were tested by a researcher who spoke only Navajo (McKeever et al., 1989). Another group of Navajo as well as Anglo children were tested by a researcher who spoke only English. Findings from the study suggest that there appeared to be a strong right ear advantage for the Anglo group tested by the English-speaking researcher. A similar right ear advantage was found in the Navajo children when they were tested by the Navajo-speaking researcher, whereas the Navajo children tested by the English-speaking researcher revealed minimal, nonsignificant right ear advantage. Most of the research prior to this point has suggested that Navajos and other Native Americans have an absence of right ear advantage. The results of this study were found to be inconsistent with the view that Navajos and other Native Americans are right hemisphere dominant and thus have a left ear advantage as a function of the appositional mode of language and thought (McKeever et al., 1989).

Implications for Nursing Care

Because the Navajo language does not always have one single word that is similar to an English word, to do a nursing assessment and develop a nursing diagnosis, goals, and interventions, the nurse must remember that what is being said must be interpreted. Since some Navajo people do not speak English, it may be necessary to provide a person who is fluent in the Navajo language. When a Navajo interpreter is utilized, this person must be knowledgeable about medical terminology, as well as the cultural aspects of the Navajo life-style.

It is also important to note that the first encounter is not always made to deal with official matters; rather, it is meant to provide an opportunity for the nurse to become acquainted with the family and vice versa. Future rapport with the family is based on this consideration.

Navajo individuals who enter the profession of nursing may experience a cultural shock when care must be provided for a dying patient because of the taboo against touching a dead or dying person and items associated with death. Because of the taboos associated with death, some Navajo nurses may have a healing ceremony performed after contact with a dead person.

SPACE

Both time and space are bound one to another; therefore it must be remembered that the elimination of time alters spatial concepts (Hall, 1966). For some Navajo people there is no such thing as imaginary space. Space is so real a concept that it may not be located in any dimension other than real space. For example, space may not be located in the realm of thought; there is no abstract space. For the Navajo Indian a space such as that found in a room or a house is the same as a small universe (Hall, 1966).

For the Navajo people personal living space, or that of the traditional Navajo dwelling (hogan), is surrounded with many traditions and superstitions or taboos. The hogan is an open room with distinct functional areas. Many Navajo persons believe that shared space provides a spiritual security and a sense of trust. Sheepskins, with the head facing the fire, are used for sleeping. A wood-burning stove, situated center front with the vent pipe extending through the ceiling, provides a means of cooking food. Taboos associated with death in a hogan include the need to seal the entry, warning other Navajos to stay away, and frequently the need to abandon or burn the hogan when a death has occurred. Another event that renders a hogan unusable is lightning striking in close proximity to it; even wood from such a hogan is never used for any purpose by a Navajo, with the exception of a Navajo medicine man in relation to ceremonies. Before a new hogan is occupied, it is usually blessed by a hired Navajo medicine man, either by strewing pollen along the cardinal points or by having a formal ceremony performed. The hogan is so important to the Navajo culture that all Navajo ceremonies are performed within it. While the hogan is often crowded with members of both nuclear and extended families, the Navajo need for extension of space is demonstrated by the fact that miles often separate one hogan from another or one camp from another.

Implications for Nursing Care

Since personal space is so important and has no imaginary boundaries, it is important to remember that some Navajo patients may have difficulty adapting to situations that place them in spaces that are not familiar. It is important for the nurse to familiarize the patient with the space provided during hospitalization and when personal space is limited during health care administration. The nurse should be sensitive to the fact that a hospital might be totally strange or unfamiliar to some Navajo people, with new things and experiences such as different types of food, different buildings and equipment, different varieties of uniforms, different types of health professionals and support staff, and different types of communication. This is particularly true when Navajo patients are hospitalized off the reservation where Navajo interpreters are not available or when great distances from their home prevent visitation from their extended family.

The nurse may encounter other health concerns and problems related to life in the cramped environment of a hogan, for example, infectious diseases from the lack of indoor plumbing and water supply, and burns related to the indoor stoves. Lack of food and food storage may contribute to nutritional deficiencies. In addition, the distance that the nurse encounters between hogans has a public health implication, since isolation from the mainstream creates barriers in the delivery of health care. One main barrier is the lack of public transportation. Non-Navajo-speaking public health nurses cope with this barrier through the assistance of Navajo interpreters traveling as a team in a four-wheel-drive pickup truck over treacherous terrain and unpaved roads.

SOCIAL ORGANIZATION
Family

The Navajo culture is extremely family oriented, but the term *family* has a much broader meaning than just referring to the nuclear family of father, mother, and children. The biological family is the center of social organization and includes all members of the extended family. The Navajo people are traditionally a matriarchal society, which means that when a couple marry, the husband makes his home with his wife's relatives, and his family becomes one of several units that live in a group of adjacent hogans or other-type dwellings.

There is no set number or type of relatives limiting the extended family, and their focus is to help one another grow, to collaborate on resources that will provide an adequate livelihood, and to participate in daily life occurrences. Assistance with ceremonies, particularly those associated with birth, death, marriage, and/or sickness, is shared and has great importance. Usually a male family member looked on as having the greatest amount of prestige will rise as leader for the extended family and provide necessary direction. However, in settling issues, all sides are listened to, and the entire group determines the outcome.

The family is considered so important in the Navajo culture that to be without relatives is to be really poor; children learn from infancy that the family and the tribe are of paramount importance. With the Navajo people, being there for a family member is extremely important, and it is not unusual for many members of the extended family to come to the hospital and stay with the patient or in close proximity to the patient until the time of discharge. This is particularly true of mothers who have a child on the pediatric unit. All efforts should be made to provide overnight accommodations for the mother in the same room with her child if this not medically contraindicated.

Family roles and structure

Within the traditional nuclear family the mother is responsible for the domestic duties associated with the home. The father, on the other hand, is responsible for any outside work necessary to maintain the family and the home. Children are responsible for assisting both parents (Roessel, 1981). Within Navajo families children are viewed as assets, not liabilities. Navajo Indian children are rarely told they cannot do something, but are frequently told of the consequences of doing a particular thing (Primeaux, 1977). Children are encouraged by their parents and members of the extended family to live and learn by their decisions. Since the Navajo traditions are passed down by the elderly, Navajo children are taught to respect tradition and to honor wisdom (Primeaux, 1977).

Marriage

Even today, some Navajo marriages are still arranged. In any case, marriage and the family are considered the foundation of Navajo life. In Navajo society, women are expected not to excel or achieve more success than their husbands (Roessel, 1981). This is even the case among some Navajo nurses who may be cautious about excelling in the profession at the risk of their marriage. In earlier times divorce among traditional Navajos occurred when the wife placed her husband's belongings outside the hogan (Roessel,1981).

Traditional Navajo Dress

The dress of traditional Navajo women has been adapted from the dress of the Spaniards encountered during the internment of the Navajo people at Fort Sumner. The dress usually consists of long gathered calico skirts and brightly colored velveteen blouses. Because of the harsh terrain and large amount of walking done by Navajo women to get from one place to the other, sneakers and socks are the primary type of footwear.

Traditional Navajo men have adapted the western type of garb, which includes jeans, cotton western shirts, boots, and wide-brimmed hats. Both men and women commonly carry woolen blankets and wear large amounts of turquoise, coral, and silver jewelry, as well as ornate buttons and belts. Also, both men and women traditionally wear their long hair tied in a knot behind their head; the knot is covered with rows of white woolen yarn.

Religion

Historically, the Navajo people have been guided by sacred myths and legends that describe the tribe's evolution from inception to the present time. Supernatural beings portrayed in these stories symbolize the Navajo culture, in which religion and healing practices are blended with each other. Values and beliefs intrinsic to their culture and religion form the Navajo day-to-day living experiences.

Implications for Nursing Care

It is important for the nurse to remember that both the nuclear and the extended family are of paramount importance to the Navajo patient. Because the Navajo people view the family members as being responsible for each other, it is not uncommon for many relatives to come to the hospital to care for and about the Navajo patient. Restrictive hospital rules that allow only two visitors at a time or only immediate relatives have no meaning for some Navajo people. The nurse and other members of the health care team should be sensitive to the reality that hogans and camps are at times located a great distance from one another and that therefore visiting a sick relative in the hospital may necessitate travel for many miles, with other family sacrifices needed to obtain funding for this journey. Referral to appropriate available resources will have a positive impact on family-centered care. The presence of family members also provides an ideal opportunity for their inclusion in discharge-planning sessions. Flexibility in scheduling follow-up clinic appointments should also be considered.

Since the Indian kinship or clan system is unfamiliar to most nurses in the United States, it is important for the nurse to develop a sensitivity to and an understanding of the significance of Indian clanships. For example, not only does one inherit lineage from one's mother, but also it is not uncommon for a Navajo child to have several sets of grandparents, uncles, cousins, brothers, and sisters. Among the Navajo people first cousins may be treated as brothers and sisters, and great aunts and uncles as grandparents. The whole system of clanship may prove to be thoroughly confusing to the nurse, since several sets of grandparents, brothers, sisters, uncles, and aunts may show up at the hospital, all claiming close relationship to the patient.

TIME

The cultural interpretation of time has a temporal focus that views human life as existing in a three-point range that includes past, present, and future (Kluckhohn & Strodtbeck, 1961). Navajo Indians are viewed as being primarily present time oriented. However, it should be noted that some Navajo Indians are perceived as being both past- and present time oriented. The common orientation held in regard to the man-nature theme is a mixed perception that espouses that man is subjugated to nature and at the same time suggests that man should learn to live in harmony with nature. In a classic study done by Kluckhohn and Strodtbeck (1961), it was noted that the present time orientation was the preferred mode of time orientation for the population of Rimrock Navajos sampled. The findings of the study also suggested that past time orientation was somewhat more preferable than future time orientation but that the difference in preference was not statistically significant. In the study it was also noted that while some of the respondents preferred to be perceived as being subjugated to nature, the one significant preference was a perception of being in harmony with nature.

Implications for Nursing Care

Most people in the dominant culture in the United States are regulated by clocks and are therefore very time conscious. Future-oriented individuals may have a great deal of difficulty with some Navajo people because of their present time orientation. It is important for the nurse to remember that since Navajo Indians are perceived as being present oriented, time is viewed as being on a continuum with no beginning and no end (Primeaux, 1977). In some Indian homes there are no clocks, since Indian time is casual, present oriented, and relative to present needs that need to be accomplished in a present time frame. Since certain tasks are associated with present needs, it may be difficult for the nurse to counsel and advise a Navajo patient about crucial future events such as taking medications. The present time orientation of a Navajo patient may cause this person to eat two meals today, four meals tomorrow, no meals the next day, and three meals the day after. This becomes an important nursing implication if a patient is told to take the medicine with meals, particularly if the medication is to be taken three times a day. Another indication of the Navajo present time orientation is related to the failure to keep clinical appointments.

ENVIRONMENTAL CONTROL

Some Navajo Indians are perceived as having an external locus of control; while they believe that man is not subjugated to the effects of nature, they also believe that it is essential for man to live in harmony with nature and its elements. As mentioned earlier, in the classic study done by Kluckhohn and Strodtbeck (1961) it was noted that the Rimrock Navajos sampled preferred the orientation theme of "man in harmony with nature." One conclusion from the study was that some Navajo Indians had a mixed locus of control that was suggestive of both a "being"- and a "doing"-oriented culture.

In the past, self-esteem and a health-oriented locus of control have been postulated as predictors of attitudes and behaviors directly related to children's health. Lamarine (1987) conducted a study to measure the relationship between self-esteem, a health-oriented locus of control, and health attitudes of Navajo children in the fourth, fifth, and sixth grades. The analysis of the data suggests that there is a statistically significant relationship between self-esteem and positive attitudes toward health. In addition, the study found that self-esteem was a modest predictor of health attitudes and health behavior intentions among Navajo and Pueblo children.

A craniofacial team at the University of New Mexico Medical Center at Albuquerque, New Mexico, has been successful in the treatment of a large population of Navajos because of team awareness of the Navajo concept of health (Smoot et al., 1988). This understanding of the Navajo concept of health wherein man is viewed as being in balance with his environment (and therefore an understanding of the Navajo people's concerns with ghosts, "skinwalkers," and rules for orderly living) allowed team members to integrate the family, as well as the Navajo medicine man, into the care and treatment of children with craniofacial diseases. In addition, to provide culturally appropriate care, it was essential that the craniofacial team develop an understanding of traditional Navajo healing ceremonies and the need for special handling of disposed body parts during surgery.

Illness/Wellness Behaviors

Traditional Navajo concepts espouse the need for the Navajo people to be in harmony with the surrounding environment and with the family. Some Navajo Indians have a perception of health that is not limited to the physical body but encompasses congruency with the family, the environment, livestock, supernatural forces, and the community. To maintain spiritual health, some Navajo people believe it is essential to be in harmony with supernatural forces. Iverson (1981) concluded that health and religion cannot be separated within the Navajo world; rather, the linkage between traditional religion and healing ceremonies found among Navajo Indians is obvious.

Traditional Navajo concepts of health and disease have a fundamental place in the Navajo concept of man and his place in the universe. Native healing ceremonies encompass traditional Navajo medicine and general native healing practices, and form the foundation of Navajo culture. They are central to the attitudes, beliefs, values, and perceptions of the Navajo people.

Blessingway is the main philosophy from which over 35 major and minor ceremonial variations are derived. This Navajo practice attempts to remove ill health by means of stories, songs, rituals, prayers, symbols, and sand paintings (Sobralske, 1985). In the Blessingway ceremony the importance of family and clan members is emphasized in the healing process. The mother is considered particularly important because she can relate prenatal incidents of ill nature that affect health.

Native Healers

Navajo medicine men and medicine women spend many years learning their skills and serving as apprentices. There are several types of medicine men and women:

1. Diagnosticians, or those who diagnose illness or the cause of disharmony. Their title may be "crystal gazer" or "hand trembler," depending on the method used in diagnosing the patient.
2. Singers (*he'tah'li*), or those who perform and direct the elaborate and complex healing ceremonies.
3. Herbalists, or those specialized practitioners who use herbs to treat patients and who may also diagnose illness and causes of ailments.

Medicine men and medicine women have *jists,* or medicine bundles, containing symbolic and sacred items, including corn pollen, feathers, stones, arrowheads, and other instruments used for healing and blessing. Many of these sacred objects and plants are found on the sacred mountains that border the Navajo reservation and are gathered by medicine people only (Navajo Health Systems Agency, 1985).

There is great effort on the part of the Indian Health Service and the traditional

Navajo healers to work together in a collaborative and cooperative way. It is not uncommon to observe a medicine man or medicine woman in the hospital speaking with a physician regarding the care of a patient. When medically indicated, patients may also receive hospital passes to participate in a healing ceremony held outside the hospital. There has been a continued and sustained mutual respect on the part of these two groups for the expertise of the other (Navajo Health Systems Agency, 1985).

In 1984 the Navajo Health Systems Agency conducted a research study to investigate the types of traditional healing services being provided and the types of cultural orientation to traditional healing practices being provided for newly hired Indian Health Service care providers. The conclusions of the survey reiterated the need for continued and improved collaboration and cooperation between traditional medicine people and Western physicians. For example, serious cases of injury and illness are often referred to the hospital by medicine people, and physicians are known to send patients to medicine people when deemed appropriate, particularly in cases of psychological or behavioral disorders (Navajo Health Systems Agency, 1985).

Implications for Nursing Care

To a Navajo Indian the concept of *being* is a fundamental concept; as mentioned earlier, Navajos are considered more "being" oriented than achievement oriented. Individuals are perceived as being more important than possessions, wealth, or other material things. If something is perceived as good, it is only as good as its value to other people. It is important, therefore, for the nurse to remember that some Navajo Indians believe that goodness is found only when one is in complete harmony with the surrounding environment. The nurse should also keep in mind that if a Navajo person is to have the perception of being in harmony with the environment, the environment must be structured in such a way that harmony is promoted. If a nurse were to deny or not allow the patient the opportunity to achieve harmony with other people, animals, plants, nature, weather, and supernatural forces, the patient would not be able to obtain a sense of assuredness in relation to physical, social, psychological, and spiritual health.

It is important for the nurse to determine which cultural health practices are beneficial, neutral, or harmful to the patient in order to provide culturally appropriate care. If a cultural practice is considered either beneficial or neutral, the practice should be incorporated into the plan of care. However, if a cultural practice is considered harmful, the nurse should devise a teaching strategy that will assist the patient in developing an understanding of the implications of the practice on continued health maintenance. For example, after delivery the umbilical cord is taken from the newborn, dried, and buried near an object or place that symbolizes what the parents want for the child's future. Burial close to the home of the infant signifies the continued tie or relationship with the child's home and Mother Earth. Since this neutral practice does not negatively affect health care, it should be acknowledged, accepted, and incorporated into the plan of care. Also, to provide culturally appropriate nursing care, it is essential that the nurse respect the need for Navajo people to maintain traditional rituals even when hospitalized. For example, it would not be uncommon for a Navajo individual to sprinkle certain foods such as corn and cornmeal around the bedside during a curative ritualistic ceremony. The nurse who comes in the room and finds cornmeal around the bedside may initially be disturbed and insist that the family member remove it. However, the nurse should keep in mind that this cornmeal (as well as other rituals) is extremely important and that, since it does not have any negative health-related implications, it should be left at the bedside until the patient and the family desire its removal (Primeaux, 1977).

The U.S. government has passed a number of acts and implemented a number of programs specifically to address health-related issues among the Navajo people and their involvement in the determination of their health care. The 1975 Indian Self-Determination Act provides that any federal program serving the health needs of the Navajo people may be either self-determined or contracted for by the Navajo Tribe or its designee. Services contracted for must be comparable to or exceed existing services under the direction of federally operated programs such as the Indian Health Service. Through collaborative efforts the commitment to improve the health status of the Navajo population and to increase tribal involvement in health care management has been enhanced, reconfirmed, and extended to other components of health care (Hanley, 1987).

The basic authority for health care for American Indians and Alaskans is provided by the Snyder Act of 1921. The Bureau of Indian Affairs assumed responsibility as a federal branch for providing health care services for the Navajo people until 1954. In 1954 this responsibility was transferred to the Indian Health Service as a result of the U.S. Transfer Act of 1954. In 1967 the Navajo area of the Indian Health Service was established to address the health care needs of the Navajo people. Today, the Navajo area is 1 of 12 areas within the Indian Health Service and has its administrative location in Window Rock, Arizona.

BIOLOGICAL VARIATIONS

Many Native Americans continue to be faced with a number of health-related problems. Some of the contributing factors include the fact that many of the old ways of diagnosing and treating illness have not survived the migration and changing ways of most Native Americans. It has been estimated that at least a third of all Native Americans live in a state of absolute poverty. As a direct result of poverty and the compounded problems of lost skills and economic endeavors, as well as the increased complexity of disease entities, many Native Americans are in a health-related crisis. In addition, as a result of poverty, many illnesses and diseases are related to such factors as poor living conditions and malnutrition. Native Americans are thought to be at risk for tuberculosis, maternal and infant deaths, diabetes, and malnutrition.

In the past, Native Americans continuously had the highest infant mortality rate in the United States; however, the infant mortality rate for Indians in 1984 to 1986 (9.7 deaths per 1000 live births) was below the national level of 10.4 deaths per 1000 live births for all persons in the United States in 1985 (Indian Health Service, 1985). (The birth rate for Native Americans is almost double that of the general U.S. population.) While the neonatal death rate for Native Americans has been reduced, the postneonatal death rate is 2.3 times that for infants from the general U.S. population, including all other ethnic groups (Spector, 1985). The high postneonatal death rate is thought to be attributable to the marked incidence of diarrhea among young babies and to the harsh environment.

In 1986 the ratio of the age-adjusted death rate for the Indian population to that of the general U.S. population was 1.0. This figure includes all races and may indicate that American Indians are no longer dying at a faster rate than the U.S. population in general. American Indians still have higher rates of death from specific causes; for example, death rates from accidents and diabetes are more than twice those of the general population, and death rates from tuberculosis and liver diseases are more than three times as great as those of the general U.S. population (*Indian Health Service Chart Book Series,* 1988; Rhodes, 1989). The life expectancy at birth for most Native Americans is 71.1 years, which is an increase of at least 6 years from the expectancy figure for 1969 to 1971. However, while Native Americans have had an increase in life expectancy, their life expectancy still lags behind that for all other races in the United States (National Indian Health Board, 1984).

During the 3-year period from 1984 to 1986, the leading causes of death in the Native American population included (1) heart disease, (2) accidents, (3) malignant neoplasms, (4) cerebrovascular disease, (5) chronic liver disease, (6) diabetes, (7) pneumonia and influenza, (8) homicide, (9) suicide, and (10) chronic obstructive pulmonary disease (*Indian Health Service Chart Book Series,* 1988). In 1986 the leading causes of death among the Navajo population included (1) all accidents, including motor vehicle accidents; (2) heart disease; (3) malignant neoplasms; (4) pneumonia and influenza; (5) homicide; (6) chronic liver disease, including cirrhosis, and cerebrovascular disease; (7) suicide, congenital anomalies, and diabetes; (8) chronic obstructive pulmonary disease; (9) nephritis; and (10) septicemia (*Indian Health Service Chart Book Series,* 1988). The leading causes of hospitalization for Navajo patients during 1988 included (1) obstetrical deliveries; (2) all accidents, including motor vehicle accidents; (3) upper respiratory tract infections; (4) diseases of the genitourinary system; (5) ill-defined conditions; (6) mental disorders; (7) supplementary conditions; (8) disease of the circulatory system; (9) skin diseases; and (10) diseases of the endocrine system (*Indian Health Service Chart Book Series,* 1988).

Body Size and Structure

Navajo Indian children tend to have low length-for-age and high weight-for-length measures. These reference indicators are suggestive of the fact that among Navajo Indians there is a suboptimal nutritional status. There is a tendency for Navajo children with birth weights of less than 2500 g to be shorter, lighter, and thinner than children with birth weights of over 2500 g. In a study done by Peck et al. (1988), the analysis of the data suggests that much of the nutritional risk, as indicated by growth abnormality among Navajo infants, is most directly attributable to the persistent effects of intrauterine growth retardation and low birth weights.

Skin Color

Skin color is perhaps the most recognizable way in which people are categorized. While other surface characteristics subtly add to this categorization, skin color is perhaps one of the most obvious ways in which people vary across ethnic and cultural barriers. Skin color variability is caused by a pigment that is produced by the melanocytes located in the epidermal layer of the skin.

According to Wasserman (1974), the melanocytes have an origin in the neural crest, which is near the embryonic central nervous system and seemingly migrates into the fetal epidermis. It is this origin that explains the significance of pigmentation. Mongolian spots are therefore leftovers that somehow linger in the lumbar sacral region at a somewhat greater than ordinary depth, which causes the bluish effect seen on the skin surface. Mongolian spots are obvious in 90% of Blacks, 80% of Orientals and Native Americans, and 9% of Whites (Jacobs & Walton, 1976). Mongolian spots are commonly found on the buttocks and back, and occasionally on the abdomen, thighs, and arms. Mongolian spots appear so ominous on inspection that a nurse who is unfamiliar with this type of discoloration may easily mistake them for child abuse. It is the neural origin of melanocytes that explains the shape. Mongolian spots resemble neurons with dendritic appendages that insert themselves well up into the epidermal cells. These appendages inject melanosome granules containing melanin pigments into the epidermal cells (Szabo, 1975).

Dark-skinned individuals are seemingly protected from the effects of sunlight to a greater degree than are light-skinned individuals. One reason for this may be the dispersal of the melanosomes from the basal cells directly to the stratum granulosum. Therefore when inspecting the skin of Whites, Orientals, and American Indians, the nurse will find that malanosomes are incorporated singly (Szabo et al, 1969).

Other Visible Physical Characteristics

One visible physical difference that appears to be a startling finding for the nurse is the cleft uvula, wherein the uvula may be separated at the tip, thereby giving it a fishtail appearance. While this is the most common variation, the separation can also occur as a complete separation into two uvulas (Meskin, Gorlin, & Isaacson, 1964). While this condition is rare in Blacks and Whites, it reaches a frequency of about 10% in Orientals, and in some American Indian groups the frequency of a cleft uvula may be as high as 18% (Schaumann, Peagler, & Gorlin, 1970).

Another visible physical difference is related to age-related increases in earlobe creasing. A recent study of Eskimos, Navajos, and Whites done by Overfield and Call (1983) found no differences between the groups in the frequency of age-related earlobe creasing. However, findings from the study did suggest a difference in relation to age and onset of earlobe creasing across ethnic and cultural barriers. Whites were found to have earlobe creases at least a decade earlier than were Navajo Indians.

Enzymatic Variations

It has been suggested that lactose intolerance occurs among the majority of the populations of the world, affecting 94% of Orientals, 90% of African Blacks, 79% of American Indians, 75% of American Blacks, 50% of Mexican Americans, and 17% of American Whites (Bose & Welsh, 1973; Leichter & Lee, 1971; McCracken, 1971; Sowers & Winterfeldt, 1975).

Susceptibility to Disease

Tuberculosis

The role of socioeconomic factors in the incidence of tuberculosis, which include conditions such as overcrowding and poor nutrition, cannot be disregarded. However, ethnicity also appears to be an important factor in the incidence of tuberculosis. There have been numerous studies suggesting a high incidence of tuberculosis among Native Americans (Delien, 1951; Heath, 1980). The incidence of tuberculosis varies among tribes from a low of 2% for Apaches to 4.6% for Navajos (Reifel, 1949). In the 1980s the previously high incidence of tuberculosis among Native Americans was greatly decreased, but the incidence is still considered high compared with the general population.

Diabetes

Non-insulin-dependent, or type 2, diabetes mellitus is a major health problem for American Indians, occurring as early as the teens or early 20s. The earlier onset has led to an earlier onset of complications, as well as excessive mortality in the early and midadult years. Age-specific death rates for diabetes appear to be 3 to 4 times higher for American Indians between the ages of 25 and 54 as compared with the rest of the general U.S. population (U.S. Department of Health and Human Services, 1982). In addition, the complications from diabetes among American Indians are appearing with distressing frequency. The National Diabetes Advisory Board noted in May 1982 that complications such as amputations have a rate of occurrence 2 to 3 times that of the general U.S. population and a renal failure rate 20 times that of the general U.S. population. In a recent study of the Ute Indians, it was noted that the prevalence of diabetes among this tribe is 4 times the statewide rate and that the rate of diabetic neuropathy is at least 43 times that for the diabetic population in the general Utah population.

According to the U.S. Department of Health and Human Services (1982), 33% of outpatient visits in some facilities for Indian health services are for diabetes-related problems. In addition, in some Indian tribes the rate of newly diagnosed diabetes is as high as 25%. (It is interesting to note, however, that before the 1940s the incidence of diabetes among Indians was rare [Tom-Orme, 1984]). The highest prevalence rates of diabetes among Native Americans are found among the Pima Indians of Arizona, the Seneca Indians of Oklahoma, and the Cherokee Indians of North Carolina; the lowest rates are found in the Navajo, Hopi, and Apache Tribes (Tom-Orme, 1984).

It is uncertain as to why diabetes mellitus is so prevalent among American Indians. One hypothesis suggests that some Americans have a genetic predisposition for diabetes that is seemingly triggered by changes in dietary practices and increasing obesity (Neel, 1962). Another hypothesis, entitled the "thrifty gene" hypothesis, suggests that during the centuries when American Indians lived a migratory life, which was marked by periods of feast and famine, a "thrifty gene" developed as a result of natural selection. It has been proposed that this gene might have possibly affected carbohydrate metabolism and storage so that during times when food was readily available, carbohydrates could be more readily stored in the body to be used during periods of scarcity. This theory proposes that, even today, some American Indians continue to store carbohydrates in excess, but since periods of food scarcities or famine no longer occur in the propensity that they once did, American Indians tend to become obese, which ultimately leads to the development of diabetes (Boyle & Andrews, 1989).

Numerous studies have been done that support the ideology of American Indians having a predisposition for diabetes mellitus. In a study done by Sugarman (1989), 177 cases of gestational diabetes and 13 cases of preexisting diabetes were identified in a retrospective analysis of 4094 deliveries among Navajo Indian women. The findings of the study therefore suggest a prevalence of 4.6% for maternal diabetes in pregnancy. The study also noted that when women with preexisting diabetes or who had had documented gestational diabetes during a previous pregnancy were excluded, the prevalence of gestational diabetes was 3.4%. While each data source independently failed to identify 20% to 40% of diabetic pregnancies, more than 97% of cases were identified when the data sources were used collectively (Sugarman, 1989).

In a similar study, 181 pregnant Navajo women were screened for gestational diabetes (Massion et al., 1987). The findings of this study indicated that the 50 g oral glucose screening test was greater than 7.2 mmol/L or 130 mg/dl in 44 of the 181 subjects, or approximately 24.3% of the subjects tested. In addition, it was greater than 8.3 mmol/L or 150 mg/dl in 23 of the 181 subjects, or approximately 12.7%. Using standard oral glucose tolerance testing, the incidence of gestational diabetes in the study population was found to be 6.1% for all pregnancies. Therefore the study concluded that universal screening of gestational diabetes is recommended among Navajo Indian women because they are perceived as a high-risk population (Massion et al., 1987.

Sugarman and Percy (1989) noted an age- and sex-adjusted prevalence of non-insulin-dependent diabetes mellitus of 10.2% among approximately 76% of Navajo adults living on reservations. This figure was approximately 60% greater than the estimated prevalence of 6.4% for the general U.S. population. In addition, findings from the study suggest than Navajo people are overweight as compared with the general U.S. population (Sugarman & Percy, 1989).

O'Connor et al. (1987) conducted a cross-sectional study to assess the association of various demographics and medical care variables with metabolic outcomes in non-insulin-dependent diabetic Navajo subjects. In the study, the dependent variable was identified as metabolic control and was measured as the mean of all random plasma glucose values obtained at scheduled clinic visits for diabetes over a 2-year period. Using multivariant analysis, the researchers noted that better metabolic control was most strongly associated with compliance with appointments. In addition, the study noted an association between the mode of treatment and metabolic control.

Shigella

The resistance to trimethoprim-sulfamethoxazole (TMP-SMX) emerged among *Shigella* isolates from the Navajo reservation in the southwestern United States in 1985 and consequently was of paramount importance to health care workers (Griffin et al., 1989). In 1983 TMP-SMX resistance was noted at a rate of 3%; however, by 1985 this rate had increased significantly to 21%. The findings of the study indicated that all of the respondents who were studied and examined were resistant to ampicillin and streptomycin and had minimal inhibitory concentrations resistant to sulfamethoxazole. The findings also indicated that polyclonal highly TMP-SMX–resistant *Shigella* emerged through transfer of trimethoprim-resistant genes from aerobic bowel flora to endemic *Shigella* strains. Therefore the findings suggested that the use of antimicrobials can lead to symptomatic shigellosis.

Myocardial infarction

Klain et al. (1988) noted that the myocardial infarction attack rate for Navajo men had more than doubled in comparison with an earlier study the researchers had conducted. In addition, they noted that there was a gradual increase in myocardial infarctions among Navajo women. The study concluded that the majority of the Navajos who sustained acute myocardial infarctions were hypertensive (51%), diabetic (50%), or both (31%). However, it was noted that very few of the respondents in the study admitted that they smoked cigarettes.

Arthritis

There appears to be a high prevalence of arthritis, including rheumatoid arthritis, among selected American Indian tribes as compared with non-Indian populations (Hill & Robinson, 1969; Rosenberg et al., 1982). Rheumatoid arthritis was found at a rate of 6.8% in Chippewa Indians, and Wilkins et al. (1973) noted in a study done on Yakima Indians in Washington state that Chippewa women had an arthritis incidence of 3.4%. While it has been suggested that Navajo Indians have a unique form of arthritis, the findings of one study suggest that Navajos have the same type of arthritis as the rest of the population (Rate et al., 1980). Nurses should also be aware that there have been notable findings of arthritis in the presence of negative blood studies in the Navajo population. While it has been suggested that geographic location is one major contributing factor to the problem of arthritis, tribes that reside in one location and then move to another do not exhibit any changes in prevalence rates (Overfield, 1985).

Nutritional Preferences

Since there are more than 300 different American Indian tribes, American Indian dietary practices vary widely. However, it should be noted that contemporary American Indian diets combine foods indigenous to the areas with modern processed foods. Food practices are also influenced by tribal beliefs and practices, geographic area, and local availability of selected foods. In certain tribal areas where game and fish are plentiful, these foods are important food sources within the diet. While fruits, berries, roots, and wild greens are perceived to have important nutritional value, they are scarce in many federally defined Indian geographic regions. They are also scarce in large urban centers such as large cities except as they are found in season in supermarkets (Boyle & Andrews, 1989; U.S. Department of Agriculture, Food and Nutrition Service, 1984).

Foods preferred by many Navajos include meat and blue cornmeal. Milk, on the other hand, is usually not listed by Navajos as a preferred food, and this lack of preference for milk has contributed to protein malnutrition among Navajos. One study reporting protein malnutrition among elderly Navajo patients indicates that protein malnutrition is present and is more common in males, inpatients, and the aged elderly (Williams & Boyce, 1989). The importance of cultural dietary preferences among Navajos in relation to patient teaching has been identified by Koehler, Harris, and Davis (1989). According to these researchers, dietitians and nutritionists should be aware of the rich ethnic diversity that exists among Native Americans and use this knowledge accordingly in nutritional counseling.

After 6 months of ethnographic research, Wolfe and Sanjur (1988) conducted a study on 107 Navajo women who for the most part were in the food assistance program. With its primary purpose being to describe and evaluate the contemporary Navajo diet, the study was done on the basis of a 1-day dietary recall. Using data from this 1-day dietary recall, mean nutrient intakes were found to be below the recommended daily allowances for calcium, phosphorus, iron, and vitamin A. Analysis of the data also suggested that 63% of the women in the sample were overweight or obese. Although overall percentages of energy from fat, carbohydrates, and protein were closer to those recommended in the dietary allowances than were the percentages found in the general U.S. population, the fat intake appeared to be primarily saturated, and fiber intake was lower than the average for the rest of the general U.S. population. In addition, it was noted that among the Navajo women sampled in the study, traditional foods were infrequently consumed. Another significant finding suggested that women with higher incomes tended to have better diets. The study also noted that commodity foods supplied by the U.S. Department of Agriculture's food distribution program provided approximately 43% of caloric intake and 37% to 57% of the intake of all nutrients with the exception of fat and vitamin C for 72% of the population sampled. Thus a significant finding of the study was the important contribution that the food distribution program makes to the contemporary Navajo diet.

Alcohol Metabolism

For many years behavioral scientists have been searching for the biological reason why certain racial or ethnic groups such as Orientals and American Indians react differently to alcohol than do other racial or ethnic groups, and it has been noted that alcohol metabolism varies by virtue of ethnic heritage. For example, some Orientals and American Indians have reported physical symptoms such as profound facial flushing and other vasomotor symptoms after drinking alcohol. Wolff (1973) noted that most Whites do not experience similar symptoms. It has also been suggested that a high incidence of alcoholism is found in some ethnic groups such as American Indians, Blacks, and Whites (Klatsky et al., 1977). The conclusion of researchers studying differences in alcohol metabolism is that alcohol is first oxidized to acetaldehyde by the alcohol dehydrogenase (ADH) enzyme. At this point acetaldehyde is oxidized to acetic acid by acetaldehyde dehydrogenase (ALDH) (Stamatoyannopoulos, Chen, & Fukui, 1975). Two variants in the ADH enzyme have been noted: a high-activity variant that converts alcohol to acetaldehyde very quickly and a low-activity variant that converts alcohol to acetaldehyde slowly (Kalow, 1982). In addition, the ALDH enzyme is known to have a range of variability from ALDH1 through ALDH4. Normal variability is set at ALDH1, and deficiencies are noted in all the other types (Goedde et al., 1983). Approximately 85% to 90% of American Indians and Orientals have been found to have the high-activity variant of ALDH, which means that the alcohol they consume is rapidly converted to acetaldehyde. However, the next step, conversion of acetaldehyde to acetic acid, is delayed in 35% to 70% of American Indians and Orientals. It is because of these enzyme differences that a majority of American Indians and Orientals experience a rapid onset initially and thereafter a slow decrease in blood acetaldehyde levels (Goedde et al., 1983).

While attempts have been made to explain biological variations of metabolic absorption of alcohol in different racial or ethnic groups, it is not meant in this context to explain the causes of alcoholism. Alcoholism exists among Native Americans in very high percentages.

Psychological Characteristics

There appears to be one interesting racial difference in brain development in regard to cerebral speech lateralization differences noted among Orientals, American Indians, and other races. It has been suggested that Hopi, Navajo, and Japanese individuals either process linguistic information in both hemispheres or have right hemisphere dominance (Overfield, 1985; Scott, 1979). Among Navajo Indians this finding is very demonstrable, particularly when one is given a dichotic listening task. Navajo Indians appear to have a left ear advantage, which is suggestive of right cerebral hemisphere dominance, as opposed to their White counterparts, who have the usual right ear advantage suggestive of left cerebral hemisphere dominance. For the nurse who is working with an aphasic patient, possible racial differences in cerebral dominance cannot be overlooked (Overfield, 1985).

Implications for Nursing Care

It is important for the nurse to remember that while many researchers have implicated socioeconomic factors as a causative agent in tuberculosis, other researchers have related ethnicity to the high incidence of tuberculosis. Regardless of the etiological causation, nurses need to assist Navajo people in learning about the significance of tuberculosis. Teaching should be clear and should attempt to clarify any misunderstandings about tuberculosis. The nurse should use straightforward and easy-to-understand language. For example, the nurse might teach the patient and family how tuberculosis is spread and demonstrate how the organism can actually be seen through a microscope. The nurse should also make every effort to explain the symptoms of tuberculosis in simple terms so that the patient and family develop an understanding of the condition. For example, the nurse might begin by telling the patient and family that the symptoms begin with the patient beginning to lose weight, then developing a cough, and then finally starting to spit up blood. In addition, the nurse might lessen the anxiety created by the need for radiographs by saying that the taking of radiographs is just like the taking of photographs (Wauneka, 1962).

Harris et al. (1988) designed and tested a cardiovascular health education curriculum utilizing 215 fifth grade students from rural New Mexico, including Navajo, Pueblo, and Hispanic children. The teaching effort of the program was augmented by materials, examples, and exercises relevant to these particular cultures. The findings of the study suggested a significant increase in knowledge among these students about the cardiovascular system, obesity, tobacco use, and the necessity for exercise, nutrition, and habit change. The study concluded that a culturally oriented program can be valuable in promoting a healthy life-style in minority group children such as Navajo Indians.

SUMMARY

Today, the Navajo nation is a culture in transition. As changes occur in educational levels, employment, and environment, the Navajo people find themselves assimilating more with the dominant culture found in the United States. The need to be able to blend the traditional Navajo culture with the dominant culture found in the United States is creating conflict for some Navajo people. When providing health care to Navajo patients, nurses are being challenged to seek ways to bridge the gap between traditional cultural practices and Western medical practices in order to provide culturally appropriate nursing care.

*CASE
STUDY*   Mary Littlejohn, a 20-year-old Navajo Indian, is admitted to the hospital for a high-risk preg-nancy related to gestational diabetes. This is Mrs. Littlejohn's second pregnancy. She is mar-ried and has a 2-year-old daughter at home. She lives in a hogan with her daughter, husband, mother, father, and two aunts. There is no running water, electricity, or plumbing in the home. When Mrs. Littlejohn arrives at the hospital for admission, 12 of her family members are with her. Once she has been admitted to her room and is in bed, her grandmother sprin-kles cornmeal around her bed. When the nurse takes the patient's history, Mrs. Littlejohn re-lates that she had the same problem last time she was pregnant. Mrs. Littlejohn also relates to the nurse that she has felt tired and very weak, has had some spots before her eyes, and has had headaches. In addition, she has had to urinate very frequently at night and does not appear to be able to get enough water or food. The nurse notes on examination that the patient's blood pressure is 140/88, her temperature is 99.8° F, her pulse is 102, and her tongue appears coated. The laboratory test done at Mrs. Littlejohn's last clinic visit a week ago revealed that her serum glucose level was 160 mg/dl.

*CARE
PLAN*   ***Nursing Diagnosis***   Health maintenance, altered, related to high-risk pregnancy.

Patient Outcomes	***Nursing Interventions***
1 Patient and family will verbalize a desire to learn more about high-risk pregnan-cies, diabetes, gestational diabetes, and appropriate techniques to reduce symp-tomatology.	1 Identify with patient and family socio-cultural factors that influence health-seeking behaviors.
2 Patient and family will verbalize a will-ingness to comply with medical thera-peutic regimen to control gestational diabetes.	2 Determine patient's and family's knowl-edge level about diabetes, gestational diabetes, and implications for high-risk pregnancies.
3 Patient and family will verbalize an un-derstanding of the need to comply with routine, scheduled follow-up care to pre-vent an at-risk delivery.	

Nursing Diagnosis   Communication, impaired, related to sociocultural variables.

Patient Outcomes	***Nursing Interventions***
1 Family will be able to communicate per-sonal and family-related needs to health care personnel.	1 Assist family in developing adequate communication techniques to communi-cate feelings and anxieties to one another and to health care personnel.
2 Family will be able to communicate feel-ings about diabetes, gestational diabetes, and treatment regimen.	2 Assist family in developing the ability to determine discrepancies in communi-cated verbal and nonverbal behavior.
3 Each family member will be able to send precise, understandable messages to one another through appropriate verbal and nonverbal communication.	3 Assist family in developing appropriate language skills and nonverbal perception to decrease the possibility of faulty per-ception.

Nursing Diagnosis   Family processes, altered, related to gestational diabetes and high-risk pregnancy.

Patient Outcomes	*Nursing Interventions*
1 Family will participate in care and maintenance of patient.	1 Determine family's understanding of patient's condition.
2 Family will assist nurse in helping patient return to a high level of wellness.	2 Determine support systems available to family from external resources.
3 Family will verbalize difficulties encountered in seeking appropriate external resources.	3 Determine with family supportive networks of friends and extended family members.
	4 Involve family in care and management of patient.
	5 Encourage family to verbalize fears and anxieties.

STUDY QUESTIONS

1. List several factors that may contribute to diabetes among Navajo Indians.
2. Identify at least one reason why Mrs. Littlejohn's grandmother sprinkled cornmeal around her bed.
3. Describe at least two communication barriers encountered by nurses in the dominant society when providing care to some Navajo Indian patients.
4. Describe at least one health practice that Mrs. Littlejohn may adhere to that may be perceived as a negative health practice.
5. Describe the structure of the traditional Navajo family and the relationship to health-seeking behaviors.
6. Identify the possible negative effects of the environment and spatial relationships in a hogan on health and health-seeking behaviors.

REFERENCES

Bose, D.P., & Welsh, J.D. (1973). Lactose malabsorption in Oklahoma Indians. *American Journal of Clinical Nutrition, 26,* 1320-1322.

Boyce, G. (1942). *A primer of Navajo economic problems.* Mimeographed material. Window Rock, Ariz.: Navajo Service, Bureau of Indian Affairs.

Boyle, J., & Andrews, M. (1989). *Transcultural concepts in nursing care.* Glenview, Ill.: Scott, Foresman/ Little, Brown College Division.

Brugge, D. (1964). Navajo land usage: A study in progressive diversification. In C.S. Knowlton (Ed.), *Indian and Spanish adjustments to arid and semiarid environments.* Lubbock: Texas Technological College Committee on Desert and Arid Zone Research, Contribution No. 7.

Brugge, D. (1968, spring). Pueblo factionalism and external relations. *Ethnohistory,* pp. 191-200.

Delien, H. (1951). Continuity of program—A necessity of tuberculosis control among American Indians. *Lancet, 71*(4), 136-137.

Goedde, H., et al. (1983). Population genetic studies on aldehyde dehydrogenase isozyme deficiency and alcohol sensitivity. *American Journal of Human Genetics, 35,* 769-772.

Griffin, P.M., Tauxe, R.V., Redd, S.C., Puhr, N.D., Hargrett-Bean, N., & Blake, P.A. (1989). Emergence of highly trimethoprim-sulfamethoxazole-resistant *Shigella* in a Native American population: An epidemiologic study. *American Journal of Epidemiology, 129*(5), 1042-1051.

Hall, E. (1966). *The hidden dimension.* New York: Doubleday.

Hanley, C.E. (1983, Dec.). *Establishing a nursing network: A support system for nurses and nursing practices— Creative approaches to a quality nursing environment.* Paper presented at a symposium of the Arizona Hospital Association, Mesa, Ariz.

Hanley, C.E. (1987, April). *Changing patterns of health care on the Western Navajo reservation.* Unpublished thesis, American College of Healthcare, Chicago.

Harris, M.B., Davis, S.M., Ford, V.L., & Tso, H. (1988). The checkerboard cardiovascular curriculum: A culturally oriented program. *Journal of School Health, 58*(3), 104-107.

Heath, C. (1980). *A descriptive and evaluative study of the tuberculosis occurring in American Indians residing in Shannon and Washabaugh Counties, South Dakota, 1970 through 1978.* Thesis, University of Texas, Houston.

Henderson, G., & Primeaux, M. (1981). *Transcultural health care.* Reading, Mass.: Addison-Wesley.

Heraldson, S.S. (1988). Health and health services among the Navajo Indians. *Journal of Community Health, 13*(3), 129-142.

Hill, R.H., & Robinson, H.S. (1969). Rheumatoid arthritis and ankylosing spondylitis in British Columbia Indians. *Canadian Medical Association Journal, 100,* 509-511.

Indian Health Service. (1989). *The IHS Primary Care provider, 14*(10), 113-124.

Indian Health Service Chart Book Series. (1988). U.S. Department of Health and Human Services, Public Health Service, Indian Health Service.

Iverson, P. (1981). *The Navajo nation.* Westport, Conn.: Greenwood Press.

Jacobs, A.H., & Walton, R.G. (1976). Incidence of birthmarks in the neonate. *Pediatrics, 58,* 218-222.

Kalow, W. (1972). The metabolism of xenobiotics in different populations. *Physiology and Pharmacology, 60,* 1-9.

Klain, M., Coulehan, J.L., Arena, V.C., & Janett, R. (1988). More frequent diagnosis of acute myocardial infarction among Navajo Indians. *American Journal of Public Health, 78*(10), 1351-1352.

Klatsky, A., et al. (1977). Alcohol consumption among White, Black, or Oriental men and women: O'Kaisen-Permanente multiphasic health examination data. *American Journal of Epidemiology, 105*(4), 311-322.

Kluckhohn, F., & Strodtbeck, F. (1961). *Variations in value orientations.* Elmsford, N.Y.: Row, Peterson.

Koehler, K.M., Harris, M.B., & Davis, S.M. (1989). Core, secondary, and peripheral foods in the diets of Hispanic, Navajo, and Jemez Indian children. *Journal of American Dietary Association, 89*(4), 638-640.

Lamarine, R.J. (1987). Self-esteem, health locus of control, and health attitudes among Native American children. *Journal of School Nursing, 57*(9), 371-374.

Leichter, J., & Lee, M. (1971). Lactose intolerance in Canadian West Coast Indians. *Journal of Digestive Diseases, 16*(9), 809-813.

Littlehawk, J. (1979). Interview by Rachel Spector at Boston State College, Boston.

Massion, C., O'Connor, P., Gorab, R., Crabtree, B.F., Nakamura, R.M., & Coulehan, J.L. (1987). Screening for gestational diabetes in a high-risk population. *Journal of Family Practice, 25*(6), 569-575.

McCracken, R. (1971). Lactase deficiency: An example of dietary evolution. *Curriculum Anthropology, 12*(4-5), 479-517.

McKeever, W.F., Hunt, L.J., Wells, S., & Yazzie, C. (1989). Language laterality in Navajo reservation children: Dichotic test results depend on the language context of the testing. *Brain Language, 36*(1), 148-158.

Meskin, L.H., Gorlin, R.J., & Isaacson, R.J. (1964). Abnormal morphology of the soft palate: The prevalence of cleft uvula. *Cleft Palate Journal, 1,* 342-346.

National Indian Health Board. (1984). A research agenda for Indian health. *NIHB Reporter 3*(12), 4.

Navajo Health Systems Agency. (1985). *Report on traditional medicine survey.* Window Rock, Ariz.: Author.

Neel, J.V. (1962). Diabetes mellitus: A "thrifty" genotype rendered detrimental by progress. *American Journal of Human Genetics, 14,* 353-362.

O'Connor, P.J., Fragneto, R., Coulehan, J., & Crabtree, B.F. (1987). Metabolic control in non-insulin-dependent diabetes mellitus: Factors associated with patient outcomes. *Diabetes Care, 10*(6), 697-701.

Overfield, T. (1985). *Biologic variation in health and illness.* Reading, Mass.: Addison-Wesley.

Overfield, T., & Call, E.B. (1983). Earlobe type, race, and age: Effects on earlobe creasing. *Journal of American Geriatric Society, 31*(8), 479-481.

Peck, R., Marks, J., Kibley, M., Lee, S., & Trowbridge, F. (1988). Birth weight and subsequent growth among navajo children. *Public Health Reports, 33,* 88.

Primeaux, M. (1977). Caring for the American Indian patient. *American Journal of Nursing, 77*(1), 91-94.

Rate, R., et al. (1980). Navajo arthritis reconsidered. *Arthritis Rheumatism, 23*(11), 1299-1302.

Reifel, A. (1949). Tuberculosis among Indians of the United States. *Diseases of the Chest, 16,* 234-249.

Rhoades, E. (1989, Feb.). FY 1990 budget presentation to the Subcommittee of the Department of the Interior and Related Agencies, U.S. House of Representatives.

Roessel, R. (1981). *Women in Navajo society*. Rough Rock, Navaho Nation, Ariz.; Navajo Resources Center.

Rosenberg, A., et al. (1982). Rheumatic diseases in western Canadian Indian children. *Journal of Rheumatology, 9*(4), 589-592.

Schaumann, B.F., Peagler, F.D, & Gorlin, R.J. (1970). Minor orofacial anomalies among a Negro population. *Oral Surgery, 29*(4), 566-575.

Scott, S. (1979). Cerebral speech lateralization in the Native American Navajo. *Neuropsychologia, 17*(1), 89-92.

Smoot, E.C., Kucan, J.O., Cope, J.S., & Asse, J.M. (1988). The craniofacial team and the Navajo patient. *Cleft Palate Journal, 25*(4), 395-402.

Sobralske, M. (1985). Perceptions of health: Navajo Indians. *Topics in Clinical Nursing, 7*(3), 32-39.

Sowers, M., & Winterfeldt, E. (1975). Lactose intolerance among Mexican Americans. *American Journal of Clinical Nutrition, 28*, 704-705.

Spector, R. (1985). *Cultural diversity in health and illness*. East Norwalk, Conn.: Appleton-Century-Crofts.

Stamatoyannopoulos, G., Chen., S., & Fukui, M. (1975). Liver alcohol dehydrogenase in Japanese: High population frequency of atypical form and its possible role in alcohol sensitivity. *American Journal of Human Genetics, 27*, 789-796.

Sugarman, J.R. (1989). Incidence of gestational diabetes in a Navajo Indian community. *Western Journal of Medicine, 150*(5), 648-651.

Sugarman, J.R., & Percy, C. (1989). Prevalence of diabetes in a Navajo Indian community. *American Journal of Public Health, 79*(4), 511-513.

Szabo, G. (1975). The human skin as an adaptive organ. In A. Damon (Ed.), *Physiological anthropology*. New York: Oxford University Press.

Szabo, G., et al. (1969). Racial differences in the fate of melanosomes in human epidermis. *Nature, 222*, 1081-1082.

Tom-Orme, L. (1984). Diabetes intervention on the Uintah-Ouray reservation. In M. Carter (Ed.), *Proceedings of the Ninth Annual Transcultural Nursing Conference*. Salt Lake City: Transcultural Nursing Society.

Treaty between the United States of America and the Navaho tribe of Indians (1973). Las Vegas: KC Publications.

U.S. Department of Agriculture, Food, and Nutrition Service. (1984). *Native Americans: A guide for nutrition educators*. Washington, D.C.: U.S. Government Printing Office.

U.S. Department of Commerce, Bureau of the Census. (1988). *Census of population*. Washington D.C.: U.S. Government Printing Office.

U.S. Department of Health and Human Services, Public Health Service, National Institutes of Health. (1982). *Diabetes in the 80's*. Report of the National Diabetes Advisory Board. Washington, D.C.: U.S. Government Printing Office.

Wasserman, H.P. (1974). *Ethnic pigmentation: Historical, physiological and chemical aspects*. New York: Elsevier.

Wauneka, A. (1962). Helping a people to understand. *American Journal of Nursing, 62*(2), 88-96.

Wilkins, R., et al. (1973). HLA antigens in Yakima Indians with rheumatoid arthritis. *Arthritis Rheumatism, 25*(12), 1435-1439.

Williams, R., & Boyce, W.T. (1989). Protein malnutrition in elderly Navajo patients. *Journal of American Geriatrics and Sociology, 37*(5), 397-406.

Wolfe, W.S., & Sanjur, D. (1988). Contemporary diet and body weight of Navajo women receiving food assistance: An ethnographic and nutritional investigation. *Journal of American Dietary Association, 88*(7), 822-827.

Wolff, P. (1973). Dietary habits and cancer epidemiology. *Cancer, 43*, 1955-1961.

Young, R. (1961). The origin and development of Navajo tribal government. In R.W. Young (Ed.), *The Navajo yearbook* (Vol. 8, pp. 371-411). Window Rock, Ariz.: Bureau of Indian Affairs.

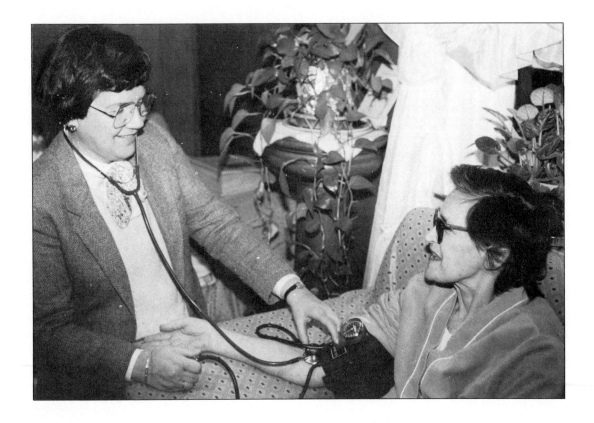

CHAPTER 11

Appalachians

Cynthia C. Small

BEHAVIORAL OBJECTIVES

After reading this chapter, the nurse will be able to:

1 Describe the communication style used by Appalachians..

2 Explain the Appalachian orientation to both time and space.

3 Explain the health care beliefs, values, behaviors, and medical and folk practices of persons from the Appalachian culture.

4 Describe how the attitude of Appalachians affects the use of conventional medical health care services.

5 Identify how beliefs of persons from Appalachia affect feelings of environmental control.

6 Develop a culturally sensitive care plan for persons from Appalachia or with an Appalachian background.

OVERVIEW OF APPALACHIA

Approximately 24 million people live in federally defined Appalachian regions spanning 1000 miles across 397 counties in 13 states, including Virginia, West Virginia, Kentucky, Georgia, Alabama, Tennessee, Maryland, New York, Mississippi, North Carolina, South Carolina, Ohio, and Pennsylvania (Durrance & Shamblin, 1976; Lewis, Messner, & McDowell, 1985; Tripp-Reimer & Friedl, 1977). It is hard to make numerical statements about Appalachia, since most statistical facts are tabulated on a statewide rather than a regional basis. However, it is possible to make some generalizations about the Appalachian region based on pooled data. For example, the population within the federally defined region is largely White, primarily of Scottish-Irish or British descent, and predominantly fundamental Protestant. For the most part, the Appalachian region is classified as a rural, nonfarming area. In Appalachian areas such as West Virginia, less than 10% of the population are in settlements of more than 2500 persons.

Predominant occupations found in many of the Appalachian regions include mining, timber, and textile industries. Steinman (1970) noted that the Appalachian population, rather than being characterized by a single condition, is noteworthy for geographic and sociocultural isolation. While people who are considered Appalachians generally reside in the Appalachian region, some Appalachians have migrated to various parts of the United States. Conversely, some mainstream Americans have also migrated to the Appalachian regions to work primarily in service-oriented professions; however, migration to the region does not in itself result in classification as an Appalachian.

Because of the isolation, lack of definitive physical characteristics, and low visibility of the people, the Appalachian subculture has been relatively overlooked as an American ethnic minority. This is in contrast to most minority groups, which have received a great deal of attention and tend to be outwardly distinguishable from the mainstream or majority of Americans. While Appalachians have been referred to as "mountaineers" or "hillbillies," they infrequently identify themselves by such classifications and have not tended to identify themselves as belonging to an ethnic or minority group. The largest operating unit of social organization among Appalachians tends to be the family; therefore the people tend to maintain a family group identity and loyalty as opposed to an Appalachian group identity.

The forefathers of many Appalachian persons came from such countries as England, Wales, Scotland, Germany, and France to seek religious freedom (Tripp-Reimer, 1982). Historically, this quest for freedom from oppression was made evident by the particular pattern in which the Appalachian people settled and by their use of space to distance themselves from outsiders. Although many of these individuals, who later would be termed Appalachians, were literate on arrival in America, formal education was stopped when the isolation from the mainstream of society began (Jones, 1983). It appeared that these Europeans who fled to the United States in search of religious freedom and solitude chose to reject the accouterments of civilization. Today, life in the wilderness and the continuing isolation of Appalachians, particularly southern mountaineers, has distinguished Appalachians from the mainstream of American society. For many Appalachians, continued isolation has led to a disparity not only in formal education, but in health status as well.

Because of their continued isolation, Appalachians have continued to be the brunt of discriminatory jokes, cartoon strips, and television programming depicting them as shiftless, lazy, irresponsible, toothless, and preoccupied with making "moonshine" and fighting to protect their family from intruders. As with much labeling of minority groups, this stereotyping has emphasized negative behaviors and perpetuates the continued isolation. However, the nurse must keep in mind that identification of Appalachians as a subcultural group, without the negative stereotyping, is essential, because a large majority of Appalachians do share similar values, beliefs, behaviors, and health care needs. It is also essential to identify Appalachians as a subcultural group because of the approximately 3.5 million Appalachian people who have migrated to major urban areas of the north central United States since 1950. People who have migrated from the Appalachian regions for the most part have remained at the poverty level and often tend to congregate with other persons from Appalachia, thus further perpetuating the Appalachian subculture in many areas (Tripp-Reimer, 1982).

Many Appalachian persons live in and around the Rocky Mountain terrain, and the roads to their homes are long, rough, steep, narrow, and often impossible to navigate. In addition, many of the homes are small and overcrowded, with inadequate plumbing and sewage systems, which promotes the spread of disease (Schwartz, 1973). Other contributing factors that augment poor health status among Appalachians include low-paying jobs, lack of employment, low educational attainment levels, and increased poverty levels. It is thought that the employment of Appalachians in coal mines and textile factories further increases the risk of respiratory disorders and other medical problems among these people.

COMMUNICATION

Appalachians are English-speaking people; however, the meaning of words used by Appalachians may differ from their meaning when used by individuals in the mainstream of American society. Also, in various Appalachian regions people use different dialects, some of which are quite dissimilar to Standard English both in vocabulary and pronunciation. A distinguishing feature of these various dialects is that they contain numerous items of Scottish or Elizabethan English heritage. Some of these distinctions are only minor variations in pronunciation and are rapidly learned, such as "deef" for *deaf,* "welks" for *welts,* "whar" for *where,* "hit" for *it,* "your'n" for *your,* and "heerd" for *heard.* In some Appalachian regions different dialects used by the people are similar to those of the cultural heritage. Other distinctions involve phrases that convey different meanings from the same phrases as they are used in Standard English (Dial, 1974). Thus phrases used by some Appalachians may be interpreted entirely differently by non-Appalachians. For example, an Appalachian person may say "running off," which may be interpreted by a non-Appalachian as "leaving home," "going on tour," or "running away," but for an Appalachian person this term implies diarrhea. While these examples of basic difficulties in communicating with Appalachian people are not indicative of a health threat, it is important for the nurse to remember that among Appalachians some folk beliefs are expressed in distinct idioms, which therefore have highly significant clinical application.

Snow (1976) concluded that one of the major concerns of southern folk medicine is the state of the blood. The characteristics or ranges of the blood for some Appalachians include thick to thin, good or bad, and high or low. Among Appalachians the characteristic of high or low is a measure of blood volume, and it is believed that the variations of high or low blood can be regulated through diet. If symptoms of high blood occur, such as headaches, vision problems, palpitations, and dizziness, certain foods and drinks are omitted and others are consumed. Significant clinical problems might arise if an Appalachian were told that there was a problem with "high blood pressure." The patient more than likely would interpret high blood pressure as "high blood," which would be harmful, because the Appalachian folk remedy for "high blood" is drinking brine from pickles or olives. The assumption behind drinking brine is that the excess blood volume will be drawn from the cells.

Appalachians are people oriented and are very accepting of other Appalachian persons who have health-related problems. This people-oriented value can be seen in the way in which individuals from the Appalachia communicate in regard to health problems. For example, it is unacceptable among Appalachians to use the term "crazy" in reference to an individual with a mental health deviation. However, it is acceptable to say that such an individual has "bad nerves" or is "quite turned." It is important for the nurse to be aware of differing language meanings when interacting with Appalachian persons in order to communicate effectively.

Some individuals from Appalachia tend to be nonverbal, using and relying on nonverbal communication techniques. Nonverbal communication techniques employed by some Appalachians include the avoidance of eye contact with the nurse or any other outside person to communicate needs (Finney, 1969). While avoidance of eye contact in other regions of the United States may be regarded as shyness, depression, or untruthfulness, to the Appalachian person, maintaining eye contact (or "staring") is perceived as being impolite or lacking good manners (Hicks, 1969). In addition, direct eye contact is viewed by some Appalachians as aggressive or hostile behavior (Murray & Huelskoetter, 1987). It is only when an Appalachian person becomes angry or upset that direct eye contact is observed in a relationship.

Many Appalachian persons tend to use a verbal pattern that is much more concrete than the patterns displayed by middle-class Americans, who tend to be more abstract. In other words, Appalachians tend to use fewer adverbs and adjectives, and less precise descriptions of emotions or discrete body sensations. For example, it would be quite difficult for the nurse to elicit from an Appalachian patient specific information on the type of pain experienced, that is, dull or sharp.

Appalachians are a private people who do not generally interfere in other people's business, because they do not want to offend anyone. Also, some Appalachians may tell others what they want to hear rather than what they should hear. Their intent is not to distort the truth but to avoid hurting another person's feelings.

Implications for Nursing Care

As the textile, mining, and lumber industries began to grow in the Appalachian regions, many Appalachian persons were stripped of their land and other natural resources. Therefore it became difficult for them to trust outsiders. Before positive interactions can occur between an Appalachian individual and an outsider, it is essential that a trusting relationship be established. One of the best ways to gain the confidence of an Appalachian individual is to use tact and to take the time to listen and talk about matters that relate to the individual and the family. It is also important that the nurse use the approach of dropping hints as opposed to giving orders. Another useful technique is to solicit the opinion and advice of the Appalachian person before taking any action. This technique is useful because it may increase the self-worth and self-esteem of the Appalachian person and because it promotes the feeling that the nurse considers the individual and his or her beliefs important.

Hicks (1969) reported that Appalachians demonstrate what is termed an "ethic of neutrality," which is evidenced in four behavioral imperatives: (1) avoiding aggression or assertiveness, (2) not interfering in another person's business unless requested to do so, (3) avoiding domination over other people, and, above all, (4) avoiding arguments but instead seeking agreement.

Again, the nurse should be aware that some Appalachians may tell nurses what they want to hear, rather than what they need to hear, thus augmenting the difficulties encountered when the nurse attempts to develop a culturally appropriate nursing care plan. Perhaps one reason for this is that most health care professionals in the Appalachian regions are more than likely to be cultural outsiders and may be viewed as being unfamiliar with the needs of the Appalachian people. Foreign-born nurses and physicians have an even greater difficulty establishing rapport with Appalachians because of language, skin color, and cultural differences. Regardless of the cultural heritage that a nurse may bring to the health care arena, it is essential that the nurse allow ample opportunity for establishing rapport and developing a working relationship with the patient. It is possible to do this by taking time to listen and to converse with the patient and family, using language that is understandable to them and at the same time soliciting, when possible, their advice (Lewis, Messner, & McDowell, 1985).

SPACE

Personal space is a very important concept to Appalachian individuals. For the most part, Appalachians have preferred to live apart from the rest of society in social and physical isolation. While this separation originally developed out of a desire to escape religious persecution, the desire for isolation persisted after migration to the United States, with Appalachian families living on small farms or homes some distance from their neighbors or "up the holler." Thus family relationships are often the only social contact.

Implications for Nursing Care

In contrast to the typical behavioral characteristic of Appalachians, which is to be family oriented and concerned with the well-being of others, when an Appalachian individual is ill, personal space collapses inwardly (Simpkins, 1974), meaning that the Appalachian person expects to be waited on and cared for by others. Thus the focus of both the individual and the members of the family is on the ill person. In a hospital setting this may create obstacles to planning and executing nursing care, since it is not unusual for a large number of family members to arrive with the patient and to expect to maintain close proximity with the patient throughout the duration of the hospitalization. This desire for close proximity is also evidenced when a patient is scheduled for a clinic appointment, even if the condition is perceived by the health care professionals as minor.

SOCIAL ORGANIZATION
Family

Appalachians are extremely family-oriented people (Jones, 1983). The nuclear and extended family are both very important to the Appalachian person. Relatives may even help an individual determine which job to take and which church to attend. Some Appalachians are so intensely loyal that they feel a personal responsibility for in-laws, nieces, and nephews, as well as other distant family members. Appalachians tend to place a greater importance on the extended family than do most middle-class Americans; the extended family is considered important regardless of the economic level of the individual. Thus relatives are sought for advice, validation, and support on all matters, particularly those pertaining to health and illness (*Culture of Poverty Revisited,* no date; Lafargue, 1980). For the Appalachian person, the consideration of the extended family is important because kinship groups are the major social-organizing force in the region. Therefore it is difficult to organize an entire community because some Appalachians do not consider the community a working level of social organization. Rather, these people perceive the most inclusive working level of social organization to be the extended family (Tripp-Reimer & Friedl, 1977).

The extensive ties to the nuclear and extended family are evident when a family member or relative becomes ill or dies in that members of the entire family may be absent from their jobs to be with the ill or dying relative during the duration of the crisis. This tendency to miss work because a family member is ill has a negative impact for some Appalachians at the work place. If a family member is chronically ill or if many members are ill, continued employment may be sacrificed for the "good" of the family (Jones, 1983). This intense loyalty for family members remains long after an Appalachian person has migrated from the region, and many supervisors in northern industries become frustrated with Appalachian employees when they are absent from their jobs because of the funeral of a cousin or other distant relative or because the employee needed to "take his wife to the doctor." This loyalty is also carried over into housing in northern areas; a landlord may find a property deserted with all personal belongings intact because the tenant had an urgent need to return to the Appalachian region to be with a sick relative.

Appalachian families are closely knit. It is not unusual for the family to take in relatives for long periods of time, thus creating or increasing the problem of overcrowding. This tendency to take in family members for an extended period of time is even seen in northern areas. In fact, one of the foremost problems found among Appalachians in northern cities is overcrowding because the Appalachian migrants take in relatives until they get a job or a place of their own. Appalachians are so fiercely loyal to their family that although the members of the immediate family may not approve of the taking in of additional relatives, it is difficult for them to ask the relative to leave. James Stills (1978) gives an excellent example of this type of familism in *A River of Earth:*

A father may bring in a relative regardless of whether or not there is food, and the mother may become so disgusted that she burns down the house and moves the family into a tiny smoke house in order to get rid of the relatives whom her husband could not ask to leave.

According to Stills, among Appalachians blood is very thick.

The Appalachian family is basically patriarchal (Murdock, 1971; Tripp-Reimer, 1982). The father is generally responsible for determining whether a family member should see a doctor. However, "grandmas" have a lot of clout in health care matters, especially if there is a concern about which home remedy is best to use for a particular illness. In the case of pregnancy, the family tends to become more cohesive and provide love and security to the expectant mother. Children are very important to the Appalachian family, and a great deal of importance is placed on having children. Having children implies that a man is "really a man" and that a woman is "fulfilled." Appalachians begin having children at an earlier age and tend to have very large families. Children are often cared for by the grandparents, particularly if both parents work. The children appear to have a sense of who they are and a greater sense of belonging.

Appalachian children are accepted regardless of what they do. For the most part, Appalachians do not wish to have their lives or the lives of their children influenced by mainstream America (Murray & Huelskoetter, 1987).

Elderly family members are respected and either live with their children or at a nearby location. The attitude among Appalachians toward the elderly is one of honor because the culture is transmitted through teachings passed down through the generations. Rowles (1983) found that spatial separation of the elderly from children when the children relocated generated critical dilemmas for the current generation of Appalachian elderly persons, who had difficulty reconciling fear of leaving the familiar environment (with its physical, social, and emotional support) with their desire to be close to the family. The study was based on a 4-year observation of elderly persons in a rural northern Appalachian community and was done primarily to explore the tensions between factors that reinforced inertia and factors that encouraged relocating to the homes of children residing outside the Appalachian region.

The Appalachian family prefers to be independent. At a time when most people hire others to fix their cars or build their homes, Appalachians take pride in doing things for themselves. This may explain the difficulty encountered by many Appalachian persons when it is necessary to ask for financial help or welfare. However, there are conflicting opinions on this issues. While some Appalachian professionals report that Appalachian people would rather work than accept welfare, some non-Appalachian professionals contend that Appalachian people do not like to work, are benefit oriented, and are basically unmotivated (Tripp-Reimer, 1982).

Religion

Appalachians tend to be very religious, not in the sense that they go to church regularly, but in the sense of value. Initially on arrival in the United States, many Appalachian persons were Presbyterians or Episcopalians, or belonged to some other formally organized denomination. However, these churches required educated clergy and a centralized organization, both of which proved to be impractical in the wilderness. As a result, locally autonomous sects sprang up and began to grow in the Appalachian regions. For the most part, these individualistic churches stressed the fundamentals of the faith and depended largely on local resources and leadership. Many social reformers have viewed the local sect churches found in the Appalachian regions as a hindrance to social progress. However, it has been said by some Appalachians that what these social reformers have failed to see is that the church has helped the Appalachian people and made life worth living in grim situations (Jones, 1983).

For the most part, religion has shaped the lives of the Appalachian people; at the same time, however, the Appalachian people have shaped their religion. Culture and religion are intertwined among Appalachians. Religion has became fatalistic for these people and for the most part stresses rewards in another life. There are few Appalachian atheists, because the harshness of the terrain seems to demand a spiritual belief in a life in the hereafter. The findings of a study on the effects of religious variables (Schiller & Levin, 1988) suggest that while it is difficult to isolate any consistent trends in regard to religious variables, low-ordered analysis would tend to suggest that because of their religious values, Jews are higher utilizers of health care than non-Jews. On the other hand, the findings of the study in regard to religion and health care utilization among Appalachians were inconclusive.

Implications for Nursing Care

It is important for the nurse to remember that since Appalachians tend to be family oriented, it is essential to solicit family opinions and attitudes in regard to health care. If the family's ideas and opinions are not incorporated into the plan of care, it is likely that the patient may not accept or value the health care services provided. The nurse must also keep in mind that regardless of the acuity level of the patient, it is possible that the entire family may congregate at one time to be with the patient to lend support. Rather than becoming frustrated by this situation, the nurse should utilize family members to improve patient teaching techniques. For example, if an Appalachian patient is admitted to the hospital for diabetes, not only should the patient be given instructions on diabetic care, but the family members should also be given the same level of instruction, since they can shape or alter the patient's perception of illness and Western medical treatment.

The nurse must also remember that since religion and culture are intertwined in most cases, it is important that an assessment of the patient's religious beliefs be done on admission to the health care system. Since some Appalachians tend to be very fundamental and fatalistic in their religious beliefs, it is essential that the nurse consider that this belief is an influencing variable that may determine whether or not a patient will elect to seek conventional medical advice.

TIME

Appalachians are considered present oriented. They believe that because tomorrow is not promised, they must live for today. Their life-style is laid-back and unhurried, and this is reflected in the inability of some Appalachians to adhere to a set schedule or time. For example, it is not uncommon for a patient to arrive 2 days early or 2 days late for a health clinic appointment. However, if the patient cannot be seen that day, he or she may never return.

In a comparison of time perceptions of Appalachians and time perceptions of non-Appalachian health care professionals, Tripp-Reimer (1982) found a marked difference in interpretations of time perceptions. The analysis of the data suggests that non-Appalachian professionals view present time orientation as a negative value. These professionals concluded that Appalachians have no concept of time, and that they lack the concepts and skills needed for both long- and short-term planning and frequently do not keep appointments. According to these professionals, present time orientation is so interwoven with the day-to-day routine of Appalachians that it is a wonder these people are able to get through a day. On the other hand, the Appalachian professionals concluded that Appalachians tend to live for today because they cannot be sure of what tomorrow will bring.

Another finding of the study was that Appalachians often miss appointments during the day because they are afraid of being fired if they take off from work. While these findings may not be representative of all people with present time orientation, they do illustrate the need for the nurse to be culturally sensitive when working with persons with present time orientation (Tripp-Reimer, 1982).

Implications for Nursing Care

Since some Appalachians have a present-oriented outlook, they tend to live at a more easygoing pace that facilitates an awareness of body rhythms as opposed to time schedules and clocks. Since Appalachians are present time oriented, it is best and often necessary for the nurse to spend a few minutes visiting "a spell" with the patient before an examination or treatment is to be done. While the nurse may be concerned about the time constraints and may not wish to engage in a time-consuming activity such as small talk, it is best to remember that present-oriented people, such as Appalachians, value such activities. Another consideration for the nurse is that it is quite common for some Appalachian patients to arrive for an appointment when the patient feels ready as opposed to when the appointment is scheduled. If a doctor or nurse refuses to see a patient because he or she is late, the patient and the patient's family may not utilize the services again. One way to facilitate the patient arriving at an appointment on time is to make the necessary transportation arrangements.

ENVIRONMENTAL CONTROL
Locus of Control

Appalachians tend to have an external locus of control. The dominant value orientation employed by Appalachians is a deviation from those value orientations held by many middle-class Americans, who have been classified as "doing" or achievement oriented. Appalachians, on the other hand, tend to be "being" oriented, which means that they tend to be oriented toward spontaneous activity and have a more relaxed pace of life. Simpkins (1974) concluded that the "being" orientation held by some Appalachians forms a "toot" work pattern; that is, they may work for a time and then engage in other activities to reestablish equilibrium. It is this "being" orientation, when coupled with the present time orientation, that tends to block a preventive orientation toward health care while promoting and enhancing a crisis orientation. Therefore it is very likely that the nurse's initial encounter with an Appalachian person may be an emergency situation, such as the delivery of an infant.

The external locus of control demonstrated by some Appalachians is viewed as one of fatalism and is thought to have a strong link to religion. Appalachians believe that God has control over their lives and that however things turn out, it is the "Lord's will." Also, they tend to see their rewards in the life to come. This orientation as developed by Kluckhohn and Strodtbeck (1961) is termed "man-to-nature." Some middle-class Americans believe that man has control over nature, whereas some Appalachians do not believe that they have control over their future. It is this fatalistic belief that results in the failure of some Appalachians to seek preventive medical advice. However, not all Appalachians respond to their fatalism in this manner. In a study by Ford (1967), the data suggest that although 70% of the Appalachians surveyed believed that the time of death is predetermined, more than 80% would seek medical care in the case of a dire illness.

The lineal-collateral relational orientation for some Appalachians possibly serves as the basis for some of the most dramatic deterrents to the use of health care services (see Chapter 6 on Environmental Control). The lineal-collateral orientation suggests that an individual's most significant relationships are with family-related groups, kinship groups, or close neighbors. Many middle-class Americans tend to seek self-actualization through their jobs and other personal involvements, whereas the Appalachian person tends to seek fulfillment through kinship and neighborhood interactions. Fatalism or fatalistic attitudes may cause individuals to become complacent with their condition or health problem and not attempt to improve their life or seek health care.

On the other hand, fatalistic attitudes may help the Appalachian person survive disappointments in life. Associated with this outlook of fatalism is the belief that an individual lives under certain rules and regulations in life; therefore the total belief system could be classified as fundamental and fatalistic.

Illness/Wellness Behaviors

The way in which the Appalachian person views health is influenced by beliefs in an external locus of control. The belief that life is controlled by nature is a major factor in the practice of folk medicine for some Appalachians and has led to some unusual ways of coping with illness. The Appalachian folk medicine system has folk healers commonly referred to as "granny women" or "herb doctors." These folk healers are used because they are familiar with the culture, because they are mountain people themselves, because they have a similar religious background, and, finally, because they are trusted. They use herbs such as ginseng, foxglove, and yellow root, which have all been shown to have some medicinal value. However, the strength of the drugs that are used in home remedies may be considerably weaker than the drugs used in pharmaceutical preparations (Lewis, Messner, & McDowell, 1985). Nevertheless, there is a tendency on the part of some Appalachians to utilize folk practitioners over physicians. In such cases an individual may actually stop taking medication prescribed by a physician and begin taking herbal medication.

The Appalachian view of illness differs from the traditional mainstream American view of illness. According to the Appalachian view, sickness is the will of God. Also, in the Appalachian view there is a very clear distinction between the role of the well (that is, as a self-sufficient mountaineer) and the role of the ill. The nurse should keep in mind that during illness personal space for some Appalachians has a tendency to collapse inwardly, resulting in a reversal of the role that is typically considered normal for the Appalachian individual (Simpkins, 1974).

The Appalachian region, even today, has a deficiency in health care resources and practitioners. However, even if resources were available, it is unlikely that some Appalachians would use them, since some Appalachians maintain a general distrust of health care organizations and professionals. A number of other reasons for lack of use of available services have been cited, including a general dislike of impersonal, formal relationships and a fear of being "cut on" or "going under the knife." Thus some Appalachians tend to seek conventional medical health care only when extreme situations arise.

Some Appalachians, like some other individuals in the mainstream of American society, will try home remedies when they first become ill. However, for some Appalachians this first stage of illness behavior is likely to last longer and consist of a wider range of therapeutic treatments such as herbal teas, poultices, and tonics. This can have serious untoward effects, since some Appalachian patients will wait a prolonged amount of time before seeking even a lay practitioner such as a "granny woman" or an "herb doctor" (Lewis, Messmer, & McDowell, 1985; Messmer, Lewis, & Webb, 1984). The lay practitioner will be consulted during the second stage of illness, and it is this delay in seeking conventional Western medical treatment that augments even the most minor physical ailments.

Horton (1984) found that the incidence of headaches in Appalachian women and backaches in Appalachian men is not within the normal patterns of medical statistics.

The findings of Horton's study further suggest that the Appalachian perception of disability is in marked contrast with that of the predominant society. It is a common belief among some Appalachians that disability is inevitable and accompanies age. Some Appalachians view all incapacity as disabling but believe that to be a "deserving" disabled person, one must be moral and physically active. The study also found that it is a common belief among Appalachians that good Christian members of the community are called as servants to minister to the disabled and their families. Therefore medical rehabilitation is not viewed as a viable option.

Nations, Camino, and Walker (1985) conducted a study to determine whether ethnomedical beliefs and practices play an important role in primary care. In their study, 33 of 73 patients from a rural Appalachian area who presented themselves to a university primary care internal medicine program had 54 ethnomedical complaints. Of the ethnomedical complaints presented, 24.1% were of high blood pressure, 22.2% were of feeling weak and dizzy, 16.7% were of "nerves," 5.6% were of "sugar," and 3.7% were of "falling out." These 33 patients had biomedical complaints as well, and the remaining 40 patients had biomedical complaints without evidence of ethnomedical complaints. No patients presented ethnomedical complaints alone. In the study, approximately two thirds of the patients consulted nonmedical personnel, including family members and friends, for their complaints, and at least 70% engaged in self-treatment prior to any clinical consultation. Those patients who presented ethnomedical complaints along with biomedical complaints sought advice from nonphysicians significantly more often than those patients who presented biomedical complaints only (with an alpha set of 0.02). However, no statistical differences were found in the self-treatment practices among the groups. Approximately 130 biomedical complaints were presented and recorded by the patient's physician; however, none of the 54 ethnomedical complaints was formally recorded. The high incidence of ethnomedical complaints among Appalachians and the failure of physicians to recognize these complaints mandate that health care providers be taught improved history-taking skills and the essentials of ethnomedical illnesses if culturally sensitive patient care is to be provided.

Health Care Beliefs, Diseases, and Practices within the Folklore System

Appalachians greatly depend on other family members to the point where it is difficult to consider hospitalization. Furthermore, Appalachians generally dislike hospitals, since it is their belief that one enters a hospital to die.

Appalachians have a tendency to be noncompliant in following medical regimens and treatment but expect to be helped directly when seeking episodic treatment in the medical system because of illness. For example, if the physician applies some ointment to a sore, the patient will generally be confident that help has been given. However, if the physician gives the ointment to the patient with instructions for use, along with a treatment plan, this may be viewed by the patient as a refusal to provide care.

Implications for Nursing Care

Since some Appalachians tend to have an external locus of control, which may foster a fatalistic attitude, it is essential that the nurse be willing to recognize that some less-than-conventional medical treatment can have beneficial effects. Those folk beliefs and practices that have neutral or beneficial effects should be incorporated into the plan of care. In the case where folk medicine beliefs and practices are not only inconsistent but may prove to be harmful, it is essential that the nurse provide health information that is congruent with the patient's frame of reference. The relevance of providing health information to Appalachians is evidenced in the findings of a study done by Chovan and Chovan (1985) to determine the ways in which men and woman cope with stressful situations. It was found that when coping responses were characterized in four modes—intrapsychic, inaction, direct action, and information seeking— Appalachian individuals used the information-seeking mode.

BIOLOGICAL VARIATIONS

Unsanitary conditions that were prevalent in the 1970s continue today in many Appalachian regions. Schwartz reported in 1973 that 60% of the houses in Appalachia had inadequate plumbing, only 1 out of 4 communities had a water system, and only 1 out of 8 communities had a sewage system. In 1985 Lewis, Messner, and McDowell (1985) reported living conditions for some elderly Appalachians that remained below standard by middle-class values, lacking running water, electricity, and indoor plumbing. Many Appalachian persons suffer from parasitic diseases that are more than likely related to the unsanitary conditions.

These conditions augment the water and air pollution that is further enhanced by the mining and textile industries. In addition, the crowding of large families and the intense poverty all serve to augment the prevalence of disease.

Susceptibility to Disease

Respiratory tract diseases

Mortality from tuberculosis is 50% higher than the national average among Appalachians (Ford, 1967). In addition, the incidence of other respiratory tract diseases such as pneumonia, influenza, and black lung disease is far greater than the national average. High-risk occupations such as mining, lumbering, and textile work all serve to increase the number of respiratory and other disabling physical health problems. Steinman (1970) reported an increased prevalence of early childhood diseases in a screening program in a rural area of Kentucky. For example, 30% of the children surveyed had upper respiratory tract diseases, 24% had hypochromic anemia, and 34% had ear ailments such as otitis media.

Coronary artery/coronary heart disease

The incidence of coronary artery/coronary heart disease among Appalachians has also been reported to exceed the national average (Ford, 1967). Leaverton, Feinleib, and Thom (1984) noted that among White men and women the recent decline in mortality from coronary disease has not been uniform by state; rather, some clustering in regard to coronary disease has emerged. When the data regarding certain Appalachian states were reviewed, there were similarities that tended to indicate a slower decline and thus a worsening of mortality from coronary heart disease.

Diabetes

Leichter et al. (1982) studied the social and economic impact of diabetes mellitus and its complications on the commonwealth of Kentucky and found that diabetes is a more serious public health problem than previously thought. According to the study, diabetes afflicts 4.4% of the population in Kentucky; borderline forms of diabetes affect an additional 2.4% of the population in Kentucky and appears to be especially prevalent in the Appalachian regions and in rural western Kentucky. In general, an average of 5.23% of all hospitalizations in Kentucky occur because the patient has diabetes.

Infant Mortality

Spurlock, Moser, and Flynn (1989) conducted a study to analyze differences in postnatal mortality rates between the southeastern Appalachian region of Kentucky and the remainder of the state. The primary purpose of the study was to identify factors related to increased infant mortality in the Appalachian region. The findings of the study suggest that the relative risk of postnatal death in the Appalachian regions studied as compared with the remainder of Kentucky was 1.38 (95% confidence = 1.15 to 1.65). Even when adjustments for birth weight, maternal age, and marital status of the parents were made, no appreciable effects on the risk ratio were evidenced. It was interesting to note, however, that adjustments for maternal education negated the increased risk of postnatal deaths among the Appalachian region births. When causes of postnatal deaths were examined, three specific disease groupings were found that were disproportionately represented among Appalachian region infants: sudden infant death syndrome, congenital malformations, and infections.

Nutritional Deficiencies

Ezell, Skinner, and Penfield (1985) studied the snacking patterns of adolescents selected from four metropolitian and three rural schools in eastern Tennessee. According to the study, 89% of the respondents surveyed ate at least one snack on the day of the survey, and boys and girls were similar in their snacking habits and patterns. Morning snacks, which more than likely were purchased from the school store or the school vending machine, included such items as candy and salty foods; afternoon and evening snacks included such items as bread and cereals; and carbonated beverages and deserts were popular during all time periods. The nutrients that were present in the lowest amounts in these snacks included iron, calcium, and vitamin A.

Skinner et al. (1985) also studied the snacking patterns of male and female adolescents in a southern Appalachian state. They noted that breakfast was skipped by 34% of the respondents and that 27% either skipped lunch or ate a snack-type lunch. The evening meal was eaten by 94% of the boys and 89% of the girls, and snacks accounted for about one third of the daily caloric intake. The mean intake of nutrients for girls indicated a deficiency in vitamin A, calcium, and iron at all of the meals throughout the day. The mean intake of nutrients, particularly iron, for boys was low at breakfast, lunch, and snacks.

Blondell (1988) studied urban rural factors associated with cancer mortality in Kentucky in order to develop a hypothesis on cancer prevention. The data from Blondell's study suggest that subsistence farming, where most of the farm produce is kept for home use rather than marketed, was the single best indicator of low overall cancer rates for males and females in rural and Appalachian Kentucky. The study also noted that the subsistence farming diet was based largely on milk and whole grains, which are reported to be rich in anticarcinogens, including selenium, magnesium, calcium, protease inhibitors, fiber, phenols, and allelopaths.

Psychological Characteristics

It is important for the nurse to be aware that people in Appalachia tend to define illness as a state requiring the presence of subjective symptoms. What is defined by others as mental illness may be referred to as a "case of nerves" (Tripp-Reimer & Friedl, 1977) or a person "getting old" or being "odd-turned" (Lewis, Messner, & McDowell, 1985). In other words, an elderly Appalachian seen as functioning quite normally in the hills by neighbors may be diagnosed as severely depressed if taken to a psychiatric clinic outside of Appalachia. Behaviors often associated with mental illness may be referred to by the Appalachian as laziness, immorality, or being "psychic" or criminal. Rather than psychiatric treatment or in fact any sort of medical treatment, Appalachians view the appropriate response for these problems as either toleration by the family or punishment by the legal system (Flaskerud, 1980).

Banziger and Foos (1983) conducted a study to determine the association between income factors such as welfare and unemployment and utilization of community mental health centers in rural Appalachia. A multiple regression analysis indicated that compared with other independent variables such as life satisfaction, demographics, and other personal and social factors, users of mental health care services were more likely to be recipients of food stamps. This relationship was noted to be considerably stronger when the more rural areas were separated out for analysis. Some relationship between employment and the need to use mental health services was also found. In a similar study done by Banziger, Smith, and Foos (1982), the relative predictive strengths of selected economic factors such as welfare, banking activity, and unemployment were reviewed for utilization of mental health services. A regression analysis indicated that economic factors did account for considerable variations in mental health factors. The findings also suggest that welfare is a primary factor and an excellent predictor of utilization of mental health services.

Critchley and Cantor (1984) did a study to question the authenticity of Charcot's original description of hysteria, which has come to be questioned in the popular media. The findings of this study suggest that it is possible to encounter florid forms of hysteria in culturally deprived communities such as those in Appalachian regions.

Implications for Nursing Care

Most of the health problems found in the Appalachian regions are partially the result of factors found in the environment, including occupational hazards specific to the region. Because of the remoteness of some of the areas, lack of available health care services, and poor sanitary conditions, some health problems that have been alleviated in the more progressive parts of the United States, such as tuberculosis, remain prevalent among the population in the Appalachian regions. Another factor that contributes to health-related problems in the Appalachian regions is that there are 34%

fewer physicians and 20% fewer dentists practicing in these areas than in other parts of the United States (Tripp-Reimer & Friedl, 1977). The limited number of licensed physicians and dentists has resulted in a major portion of primary health care being delivered by nurses. Nurses in Appalachian areas provide comprehensive family-oriented care, whether as nurse-midwives, school or community health nurse practitioners, or staff nurses in outreach clinics.

A recurrent theme among Appalachians is the lack of available health information and the desire for more health information on the part of the people. It is essential that the nurse devise health teaching plans and strategies for implementation that will reach across the Appalachian regions regardless of remoteness.

SUMMARY

The Appalachian people have a rich heritage that can offer the nurse and other health care providers insight into the cultural beliefs. For generations these cultural beliefs and values have been passed down and have persevered. In recent years, some Appalachians have moved to urban areas, and nurses and health care providers are now more likely to come in contact with Appalachian people through the conventional medical system. When working with persons from the Appalachian region, the nurse can employ some of the positive aspects inherent to the people, such as strength, independence, sensitivity, and faith, all of which will facilitate a therapeutic nurse-patient relationship. In addition, knowledge of the culture and acceptance of health care beliefs can both serve to assist the nurse in giving culturally sensitive, individualized nursing care.

CASE STUDY   Sarah James, an 89-year-old widow who lives alone next door to her son in Sweetwater, Tennessee, is seen at the clinic by the family clinical nurse specialist because she "feels bad." She arrives at the clinic with her three sons and their families, who are concerned because Sarah has been "running off" several times a day and will not eat. The clinical nurse specialist visits "for a spell" and then begins to take a health history. When the clinical nurse specialist asks what has brought Mrs. James to the clinic, the eldest son reveals that Sarah has "run off" six or seven times since yesterday and cannot drink her tea. Also, according to the eldest son, Mrs. James has not recently traveled out of Sweetwater, does not have proper refrigeration, and has recently eaten some "tater" salad that had set out all day in the hot weather. It is determined that the diarrhea is watery, brown, and nonodorous. Mrs. James has also had dry heaves but has not vomited and does not verbalize symptoms of pain.

Further assessment by the clinical nurse specialist reveals that Mrs. James has generalized weakness, poor skin turgor, dark circles around the eyes, sticky mucous membranes, pale skin, a rectal temperature of 101° F, generalized abdominal tenderness, hyperactive bowel sounds, a thready but regular heart rate of 100, a blood pressure of 110/60, respirations of 24, and a weight of 110 pounds.

Following a complete physical examination the clinical nurse specialist orders a stool culture, electrolytes, and a complete blood cell count. After collaboration with the clinic physician the eldest son approves Mrs. James' admission to the hospital with her entire family in attendance. Mrs. James is crying as she enters the hospital. A diagnosis of dehydration and *Salmonella* poisioning is made. Arrangements are made for follow-up after discharge from the hospital.

CARE
PLAN

Nursing Diagnosis   Diarrhea related to inadequate refrigeration of food, resulting in six to seven watery brown stools per day.

Patient Outcome	*Nursing Interventions*
Patient will resume normal elimination and peristaltic action within the next 24 to 48 hours.	1 Measure daily weight. 2 Record amount, character, and volume of stools. 3 Obtain stool culture. 4 Assess pain status. 5 Explain specific reason for problem (i.e., lack of refrigeration of potato salad and other foods that need refrigeration). 6 Note results of CBC and electrolytes.

Nursing Diagnosis   Communication, impaired verbal, related to cultural differences, resulting in possible misinterpretation on the part of the nurse and other health care providers.

Patient Outcome	*Nursing Interventions*
Communication will be established between patient, nurse, and family to understand health condition and needs.	1 Determine meaning of verbal and nonverbal cues. 2 Establish rapport with patient and family. 3 Be aware of cultural factors such as avoiding eye contact. 4 Communicate with patient in an unhurried manner. 5 Communicate in specific terms. 6 Learn the form of language used by Appalachians. 7 Ask patient and family for their advice. 8 Avoid criticism and spend extra time with patient. 9 Communicate on a first-name basis.

Nursing Diagnosis   Home maintenance management, impaired, related to lack of refrigeration, resulting in inadequate food storage.

Patient Outcome	*Nursing Interventions*
Family will obtain proper refrigeration for patient prior to hospital discharge.	1 Determine beliefs related to assistance from government agencies. 2 Determine specific information family should learn and know. 3 Understand role reversal that takes place during illness. 4 Utilize Appalachians from patient's community. 5 Include family in decision making.

Nursing Diagnosis   Anxiety related to cultural belief that people go to the hospital to die, resulting in episodes of crying.

Patient Outcome	*Nursing Interventions*
Patient will show signs of decreased anxiety.	1 Utilize the clergy. 2 Exhibit a calm and unhurried manner. 3 Reassure patient. 4 Be flexible in visiting regulations. 5 Be accepting of patient's cultural differences. 6 Explain procedures to patient in specific terms. 7 Involve family in nursing care. 8 Provide arrangement for one family member to stay during the night.

Nursing Diagnosis   Fluid volume deficit related to six to seven watery stools per day, resulting in poor skin turgor, dark circles around the eyes, sticky mucous membranes, rapid thready pulse, and weakness.

Patient Outcome	*Nursing Interventions*
Patient will exhibit signs of adequate hydration within 24 hours.	1 Offer fluids such as tea from home when tolerated. 2 Maintain balanced intake and output. 3 Measure daily weight. 4 Specifically explain reason for and effect of IV therapy and medications. 5 Increase fluids as indicated. 6 Monitor for vital signs. 7 Keep items within reach to prevent accidents.

Nursing Diagnosis   Nutrition, altered: less than body requirements, related to frequent loose stools, resulting in absence of food intake for the past 48 hours and possible weight loss.

Patient Outcome	*Nursing Interventions*
Patient will consume a balanced diet for body size and maintain present weight prior to discharge.	1 Monitor weight. 2 Provide nutritionally balanced diet at times patient feels like eating. 3 Document food intake. 4 Explain necessity for proper diet in specific terms. 5 Determine what foods Appalachians like to eat. 6 Encourage rest.

STUDY QUESTIONS

1. List some strategies that may help the nurse communicate with an Appalachian family.
2. Describe the prevailing attitude of Appalachians toward hospitals and hospitalization.

3. Compare and contrast the differences in illness behaviors between persons in middle-class America and persons in Appalachia.
4. Describe the orientation and significance of the extended family and the relative role within the Appalachian family structure.
5. Describe the possible importance of folk medicine practices and folk healers to persons from Appalachian regions.
6. Describe ways in which the nurse and other health care professionals may develop sensitivity toward and acceptance of Appalachian folk medicine practices.
7. Indicate resources that health care providers can use to facilitate wellness.
8. List at least three major health problems that place many Appalachians at risk.

REFERENCES

Banziger, G., & Foos, D. (1983). The relationship of personal financial status to the utilization of community mental health centers in rural Appalachia. *American Journal of Community Psychology, 11*(5), 543-552.

Banziger, G, Smith, R.K., & Foos, D.T. (1982). Economic indicators of mental health service utilization in rural Appalachia. *American Journal of Community Psychology, 10*(6), 669-686.

Blondell, J.M. (1988). Urban-rural factors affecting cancer mortality in Kentucky. *Cancer Detection Preview, 11*(3-6), 209-223.

Chovan, M.J., & Chovan, W. (1985). Stressful events and coping responses among older adults in two sociocultural groups. *Journal of Psychology, 119*(3), 253-260.

Critchley, E.M., & Cantor, H.E. (1984). Charcot's hysteria renaissant. *British Medical Journal, 289*(6460), 1785-1788.

Culture of poverty revisited. (no date). A critique by the Mental Health Committee against Racism. New York: Mental Health Committee against Racism.

Dial, W. (1974). The dialect of the Appalachian people. In B. Maurer (Ed.), *Mountain heritage.* Morgantown, W.Va.: Morgantown Printing & Binding.

Durrance, J., & Shamblin, W. (1976). Appalachian ways: The Appalachian Regional Commission.

Ezell, J.M., Skinner, J.D., & Penfield, M.P. (1985). Appalachian adolescents' snack patterns: Morning, afternoon, and evening snacks. *Journal of American Dietetics Association, 85*(11), 1450-1454.

Finney, J. (1969). *Culture, change, mental health and poverty.* New York: Simon & Schuster.

Flaskerud, J. (1980). Perceptions of problematic behaviors by Appalachians, mental health professionals and lay non-Appalachians. *Nursing Research, 29*(3), 140-149.

Ford, T. (1967). The passing of provincialism. In T. Ford (Ed), *The southern Appalachian region.* Lexington: University of Kentucky Press.

Hicks, G. (1969). *Appalachian valley.* New York: Holt, Rinehart, & Winston.

Horton, C.F. (1984). Women have headaches, men have backaches: Patterns of illness in an Appalachian community. *Social Science Medicine, 19*(6), 647-654.

Jones, L. (1983). Appalachian values. In D. Whisnant (Ed.), *All that is native and fine: The politics of culture in an American region.* Chapel Hill: University of North Carolina Press.

Kluckhohn, F.R., & Strodtbeck, F.L. (1961). *Variations in value orientations.* Evanston, Ill.: Row, Peterson.

LaFargue, J. (1980). A survival strategy: Kinship networks. *American Journal of Nursing, 80*(9), 1636-1640.

Leaverton, P.E., Feinleib, M., & Thom, T. (1984). Coronary heart disease mortality rates in United States Blacks, 1968-1978: Interstate variation. *American Heart Journal, 108*(3, Pt. 2), 732-737.

Leichter, S.B., Hernandez, C., Fisher, A., Collins, P., & Courtney, A. (1982). Diabetes in Kentucky. *Diabetes Care, 5*(2), 126-134.

Lewis, S., Messner, R., & McDowell, W. (1985). An unchanging culture. *Journal of Gerontological Nursing, 11*(8), 20-26.

Messner, R., Lewis, S., & Webb., D.D. (1984). Unique problems and approaches in Appalachian patients with Crohn's disease. *The Society of Gastrointestinal Assistants Journal, 7,* 38-46.

Murdock, G. (1971). *Outline of cultural materials.* New Haven, Conn.: Human Relations Area Files.

Murray, R., & Huelskoetter, M. (1987). *Psychiatric/mental health nursing.* East Norwalk, Conn.: Appleton & Lange.

Nations, M.K., Camino, L.A., & Walker, F.B. (1985). "Hidden" popular illnesses in primary care: Resident's recognition and clinical implications. *Culture, Medicine, and Psychiatry, 9*(3), 223-240.

Rowles, G.D. (1983). Between worlds: A relocation dilemma for the Appalachian elderly. *International Journal of Aging Human Development, 17*(4), 301-314.

Schiller, P.L., & Levin, J.S. (1988). Is there a religious factor in health care utilization? A review. *Social Science and Medicine, 27*(12), 1369-1379.

Schwartz, J. (1973). Rural health problems of isolated Appalachian counties. In R. Nolan & J. Schwartz (Eds.), *Rural and Appalachian health*. Springfield, Ill.: Charles C Thomas.

Skinner, J.D., Salvetti, N.N., Ezell, J.M., Penfield, M.P., & Costello, C.A. (1985). Appalachian adolescents' eating patterns and nutrient intakes. *Journal of American Dietetics Association, 85*(9), 1093-1099.

Simpkins, O. (1979). Appalachian culture. In B. Mauerer (Ed.), *Mountain heritage*. Morgantown, W.Va.: Morgantown Printing & Binding.

Snow, L. (1976). High blood is not high blood pressure. *Urban Health, 5*, 4-55.

Spurlock, C.W., Moser, M., & Flynn, L.J. (1989). Regional differences in death rates among postneonatal infants in Kentucky, 1982-1985. *Kentucky Medical Association, 87*(3), 119.

Steinman, D. (1970). Health and rural poverty. *American Journal of Public Health, 60*, 1813-1823.

Stills, J. (1978). *River of earth*. Lexington: University of Kentucky Press.

Tripp-Reimer, T. (1982). Barriers to health care: Variations in interpretation of Appalachian client behavior by Appalachian and non-Appalachian health professionals. *Western Journal of Nursing Research, 4*(2), 179-191.

Tripp-Reimer, T., & Friedl, M.C. (1977). Appalachians: A neglected minority. *Nursing Clinics of North America, 12*(1), 41-54.

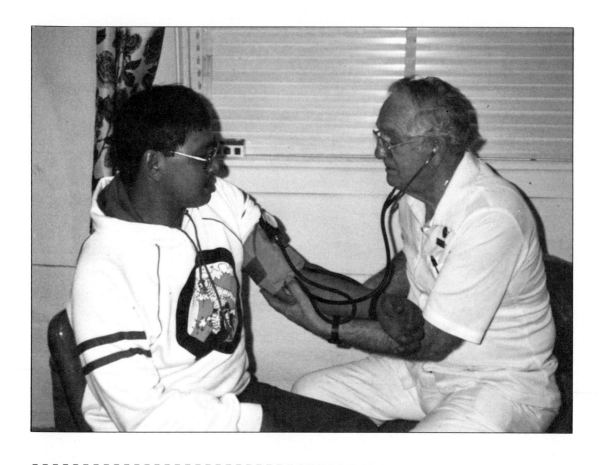

CHAPTER 12

■ ■

American Eskimos

Dolly Lefever and Ruth Elaine Davidhizar

BEHAVIORAL OBJECTIVES
After reading this chapter, the nurse will be able to:

1 Describe the stressful impact of acculturation of the Eskimo people into Western society, whether in Alaska or in the mainland United States.

2 Understand verbal and nonverbal communication barriers that may affect health care for the Eskimo people.

3 Describe attitudes and beliefs of the Eskimo people that relate to health and illness.

4 Identify the shift in health/illness patterns as the Eskimo people have adopted the Western diet and life-style.

5 Describe the problems related to providing health care to Eskimos residing in widely scattered and isolated villages in Alaska.

Settlements of Eskimos are found in diverse locations, including the northern territories of Canada, Alaska, Russia, and Greenland. While Eskimos may be found throughout the world, this chapter focuses on Alaskan Eskimos who have remained in their native land and those who have migrated to the mainland United States. However, comments are also made about Canadian Eskimos, whose health needs are very similar. To provide culturally appropriate nursing care, it is necessary for the nurse to understand the culture and heritage of the Eskimo people.

OVERVIEW OF ALASKA
The Land

Alaska is often described in superlatives. One fifth the size of the continental United States, Alaska has more coastline than the other 49 states combined and is by far the largest state in the continental United States; it is more than double the size of Texas, which by any standards is considered a large state. Furthermore, Alaska is larger than all but 16 of the nations in the world. Everything in Alaska appears to be on a grand scale. It is the home of the largest mountain in North America, Mount McKinley, which rises to a height of 20,320 feet and is joined by six other peaks that are over 14,500 feet high. Alaska also is the home of Malaspina, a great glacier that is larger than the state of Rhode Island. There are more than 100,000 glaciers in Alaska, and these generally cover more than 28,000 square feet each, providing Alaska with 125 times more glacier area than the rest of the United States combined (Kimble & Good, 1955). Alaska is a land where airplanes track icebergs the size of Cleveland and great black bears, polar bears, and other wild animals roam relatively undisturbed.

The chief influences on the climate in Alaska are its northernly latitude, its large land mass, and its coastal waters. Winters are long and bitterly cold, with the exception of the region along the southeast coast. Summers throughout the state are short and cool. The temperature varies by virtue of the season and geographic region; for example, the average temperature at Juneau, in the south of Alaska, is about 25° F in January and 55° F in July, whereas in Nome, in the north of Alaska, the average temperature is only about 4° F in January and 49° F in July. Because of its northernly latitude, an unusual feature of Alaska's terrain is permafrost, or permanently frozen ground. In the Arctic region continuous permafrost underlies surface dirt in depths of about 2000 feet. Some buildings and highways have been erected on permafrost. This has created some problems, because as the permafrost thaws, the structures may sink. In addition, in regions where there is permafrost, above-ground cemeteries are commonplace.

Parts of Alaska fall beyond the treeline. Thus in the far north only willows grow, and only in parts of the valleys protected from the wind. Lack of light, warmth, and water; the permafrost; and chilling winds cause the tundra in the far north to be covered with only a flat matting of short, ancient willows and birches (Lopez, 1986). Annual snowfall over most of the Arctic is light, often no more than 4 to 6 inches, and actual snowstorms are rare. Ground blizzards frequently occur in coastal areas, however, where most settlements are located. High winds and a furious swirling of dry snow already on the ground often persist for days and are commonly referred to as a "blizzard." When caught in a blizzard, an Eskimo can cut out a circle in the icy crust of snow covering the ground, dig a hole in the snow, crawl in, replace the icy lid, and remain there until the storm has passed (Holderman, 1989). Freezing temperatures, wind, and blizzards, which are experienced in some areas throughout the winter, have resulted in the wearing of native garb by both natives and nonnatives, including parkas and footgear (mukluks) made of animal skins (Lopez, 1986). Eskimos in the windy sea coast areas prefer seal skin, because this skin has no pores and is warmer (Holderman, 1989).

The People

Alaska is a land with many diverse populations. The native population is divided culturally into three distinct groups: Indians, Aleuts, and Eskimos. For centuries the native people of Alaska lived in isolated regions and were undisturbed by outside cultures. When outsiders discovered the wealth of Alaska's natural resources, the long-undisturbed culture at last came face to face with elements of the Western culture brought by Alaska's new occupants, the "outsiders." The gold rushes in the early 1900s brought miners and their families. In the 1940s and 1950s military personnel came to Alaska because of its strategic geographic location. Between 1941 and 1945 over 1 billion dollars was pumped into Alaska by the federal government to develop transportation systems: the railroad, highways, airfields, docks, and breakwaters. The most recent onset of Westerners arrived following 1969, when the largest auction in the history of mankind was held in Anchorage, Alaska. Some of the world's largest oil companies and consortiums gathered for the sale or lease of some 450,000 acres of the North Slope oil lands by the state of Alaska. In 1970 the population of Alaska was 302,173, which represented approximately a 33.6% increase in the population since the 1960s and made Alaska one of the largest growth areas in the United States. However, during the 1970s only 22% of the population was non-White.

Most of the non-Whites in Alaska in the 1970s were aborigines, including Indians, Aleuts, and Eskimos. In the 1970s almost 50% of the population and most of the aborigines lived in rural and isolated communities. Even natives in the rural areas, however, were not immune to the onslaught of Westerners and the concomitant cultural shock that continues today (Lopez, 1986).

There are approximately 401,851 people residing in Alaska (*Statistical Reports,* 1981). This includes approximately 21,869 American Indians, 8090 Aleuts, 34,144 Eskimos, 1595 Japanese, 522 Chinese, 3092 Filipinos, 1536 Koreans, 241 Asian Indians, 383 Vietnamese, 402 Hawaiians, 149 Guamians, 134 Samoans, and 6323 persons of other nationalities (*Statistical Reports,* 1981). Eskimos constitute 8.5% of the total population in Alaska.

OVERVIEW OF THE ABORIGINES

The Indian people who reside in Alaska and Canada are composed of several different tribes, including the Tsimshian, the Haida, the Tlingit, and seven small tribes belonging to the Athapascan language family. The Tsimshian's, the Haida's, and the Tlingit's ancestors migrated to Alaska from Canada in the eighteenth and nineteenth centuries. Many of the Tsimshiam Indians live along the Nass and Skeena rivers. The Haidas are located on the Prince of Wales Islands, and the Tlingits originally settled along the coastal region, which extended from Ketchikan to Katalla. The Haidas and the Tlingits are distantly related. Both tribes, but particularly the Haida, are noted for their totem pole carving. Today, many of the southeastern Indians are fishermen or work in fish canneries. For the most part these people have abandoned their former tribal customs. The Athapascan Indians are found along the wide, flat river valleys west of Fairbanks, Alaska. The mainstay of these tribes is hunting and trapping. Many Indians lived on the caribou herds and followed them as they roamed the northland.

The Aleuts inhabit the Aleutian Islands and the Alaskan peninsula. The Aleuts are closely related to the Eskimos, because both groups are descendants from Asian migrants who came to what is now known as Alaska about 10,000 to 15,000 years ago. The Aleuts have their own unique customs, traditions, and language. For survival the Aleuts engage in sealing, fishing, and farming (Brody, 1975).

The Eskimo people are found along the Bering Sea and the Arctic Ocean coasts, as well as along the lower Yukon and Kuskokwim river regions. Archaeologists believe that the ancestors of the Eskimos came across the Bering Strait from Asia about

10,000 to 15,000 years ago (Dunbar, 1968). Archaeologists have estimated that during the period 1750 to 1800, 48,000 Eskimos lived along the Arctic region of North America. Nearly one half (26,000) lived in the area now known as Alaska. Approximately two fifths of these early Alaskans spoke Yupik. These Eskimos lived in southwest Alaska, with the Yukon River as the natural dividing line between this group and the more northern coastal Inupiak (Milan, 1980).

While customs, traditions, and some heritage are shared among the aborigines, these groups have traditionally been enemies. Disputes over territorial rights to land or game resulted in the development of an animosity that has been carried on through the generations. For example, it has been reported that some Eskimo parents caution their children to stay near their village in order to avoid being "carried off by the Indians" (Holderman, 1989). These superstitions are kept alive through the retelling of tales, and when things are missing from an Eskimo village, "the Indians" are blamed (Brody, 1975; Damas, 1984; Hall, 1975; Holderman, 1960).

CULTURE AND HERITAGE OF THE ESKIMO PEOPLE

The word *Eskimo* is from the French *esquimaux,* possibly from *eskipot,* an Algonquian word meaning "eater of raw flesh." Some Eskimos feel this attribution puts them in a poor light with modern audiences and so use other terms for themselves. *Inuit,* the most widely used of these terms, refers specifically to Eskimos of the eastern Canadian Arctic. The Eskimos of the Bering Sea region prefer, instead, to be called *Yup'ik,* whereas North Slope Alaskan Eskimos prefer *Inupiat,* and Mackenzie Delta Eskimos prefer *Inuvialunit* (Damas, 1984).

Some people think the Eskimos once numbered about 100,000 and that this number dramatically decreased with contact with the White man in the nineteenth and twentieth centuries, which brought exposure to disease (Brody, 1975). Epidemics of smallpox, influenza, and measles have been credited with killing thousands. The Eskimo people, more than any other native Alaskans, have managed to preserve many interesting and unique native customs. Today, however, the traditional way of life is changing for the Eskimo as the Eskimo people become assimilated into the dominant culture, take on mechanical trades, and move away from reliance on the land. Young Eskimos are leaving the villages to go away to school and are returning with new knowledge of the outside world.

The Eskimo people have lived in harsh and frigid regions of the north. To survive in this frozen, non-crop-producing region, the Eskimos have hunted, fished, and trapped. Thus the dietary mainstay of the people traditionally consisted mainly of wild meat, such as reindeer, and seafood, such as seal, fish, and whale, which were supplemented by berries fermented in sealskin with fat, as well as wild greens, such as "sourdock."

Traditionally, whaling was an important component of the economy for most Eskimos who lived on the ocean (Lubbock, 1937; Stefansson, 1921). The popular Eskimo "blanket toss game" originated from the lofting of a member of the tribe as high as possible above flat terrain to look seaward to spot whales. When a whale was spotted, open sealskin boats called umiaks were outfitted with paddles, bailers, and harpoons and were launched from the shore. Great knowledge and skill were required to harpoon a whale and tow it back to shore, where the entire village participated in butchering the beast.

Eskimos traditionally have been noted for their honesty. For example, if a piece of driftwood were turned in a position in which it would not have washed ashore, others would know it had been claimed and would not take it (Holderman, 1989).

It is a popular misconception that most Eskimos live in dome-shaped ice block shelters called igloos. In fact, these shelters were used primarily as emergency bivouacs by the Canadian Eskimo. The early Alaskan Eskimos lived in dwellings that were partially underground and covered with sod. Both the ice igloo and the sod huts had long, dipped tunnels as entrances so that the cold air, which is heavier, was caught in a natural trap, thus permitting the interior of the hut to be heated more easily. Today, houses are constructed of wood frames in small modern villages that are scattered widely along the coast and major river systems. Permanent villages range in population from 20 persons to several thousand, with an average of 100 persons. Most of these villages share community water supplies, electricity, churches and stores, and irregular mail service by airplane.

Because of the remoteness of the villages, the U.S. Public Health Service Bureau sponsors clinics in each village, which are staffed by a community health nurse who travels to the villages by air or dogsled. Because of the shortage of field nurses, health care has been, and in some places continues to be, provided by White teachers and native, trained health aids (Holderman, 1962, 1989). Between visits by the public health nurse, teachers, often untrained in health care, have given antibiotics, pulled teeth, delivered babies, and handled both major and minor medical emergencies.

The following excerpts are from letters written by a teacher's assistant living in Deering, Alaska (Holderman, 1962):

The great variety of work and the fascinating Eskimo people make life in the Arctic very interesting for this farm girl from Johnstown, Pennsylvania. As special assistant to the teacher (my husband), I find my role also includes caring for the sick (there is no doctor within 100 miles) and my LPN training comes in very handy. I also help teach, prepare the school lunch, fill out applications for villagers who know little English for OAA and ADC checks from the Territory, help pull teeth and immunize the children, conduct women's meetings, write letters and reports for the Eskimo natives, and help the Eskimos place orders from the Sears Roebuck catalogue.

They caught me as I was coming out of church and told me about a sick baby with a temperature of 105.1. This baby is always sick and since the mother has had 8 that died I fear for the safety of this one. The mother was shaking her when I got to the sod hut where they live to try to get her to stop crying. Eskimos can't bear to hear their children cry. I told her to put her down and keep her very quiet and gave her a shot of penicillin. I wanted my husband to make this visit but when an Eskimo woman comes to the door and he answers it they just grunt and won't tell him. In the Eskimo culture women have their place and men have theirs. When I got home another mother came in with her two year old who had a temperature of 104.1. We are so lucky we haven't had a death this year. It is so depressing when we have to add another name to the death book. We are working very hard to help the Eskimos learn how to take better care of themselves and their babies and with constant teaching we can see less sickness. We are glad it will soon be winter because without the mosquitoes and flies and less spoiled food there will be less fevers, and sickness.

When we first came and I went through the dispensary supplies in the dispensary between our house and the school I came across this little black doctor's bag and thought "How quaint!" I wondered if there was any real occasion to use it. Now the little bag has lost its quaintness. There have been many occasions to carry it. When I start out at 20 below across town to see a patient I am always worried about what I'll find. I did a minor operation this week. This lady had a dreadful swollen shoulder and finally the mass came to a head the size of a fist and the doctor 100 miles away ordered me to lance it deep and wide. I went with my boiled instruments and went to work in the dimly lit cabin. One Eskimo held a flashlight and handed me what I needed. I was sure the blood would gush out but instead the pus poured forth, several cupfuls I am sure. Later, I stopped to redo the dressing and give her more penicillin and she is much better. She was very grateful and insisted I accept new fur mittens she had made out of reindeer skin as a token of her appreciation.

Last Saturday I was worried about Martha who had not been in to school for a few days. I had fixed her face up with salve on Monday but it had looked pretty bad. The old grandma she lives with had sent word on Friday she couldn't come to school because "The medicine never helped." The hut was terribly dirty and there was no one there to care for her and keep her clean. The bugs had apparently ate at her until the scabs spread all over. My husband and I both went and when we saw her knew we had to get her out of there if she was to get better. We sent for an interpreter and told the old grandma we would have to take her. The native pastor helped and the men just picked up the girl and carried her out to the infirmary on the porch of our house. We started with her head and gave her a general overhauling in our own portable tub. We spent hours soaking, bathing her face, and applying salve. Days later we got the scabs off and the healing process began. It had spread up her nose and smelled horrible. I think it was the first time in her whole life that she had to do anything she did not want to do. Eskimo children are rarely corrected. I'm sure she never had so much washing in her whole life. I made her a clean new dress and kept rewashing her clothes to get rid of the germs. Yesterday we sent her home after a week without a trace of illness or even a scar.

In addition to discussing the six cultural phenomena presented throughout this text as they relate to Eskimos and their impact on nursing care for these people, the remainder of this chapter emphasizes the impact created for the Eskimo people by the assimilation of cultural traits from Westerners who have moved into Alaska. Today, Eskimo leaders seek to create a modern Eskimo culture that combines the best of both the traditional Eskimo culture and the Western culture.

COMMUNICATION
Language

While some authorities have related the language of persons native to the Arctic to the Athapascan or Algonquian language groups (Szathmary, 1984), others have found the Eskimo language of Eskimauan to be a unique language of its own. Eskimauan is a difficult language because one word is often used to express a whole sentence. Originally the Eskimo language had no written forms; thus the recounting of events in story form and in dance provided the only record of Eskimo life. Today, a phonetically written form of the Eskimo language exists that was developed by linguists and Eskimo leaders. The early missionaries and educators demanded that the Eskimo people learn English, which has now become the primary language of the younger generation of Eskimos. A few school systems have initiated bilingual studies programs as a direct result of the desire of Eskimos to preserve the Eskimo heritage.

In the verbal language spoken by Eskimos, present-oriented actions are communicated with the Eskimos referring to themselves, as well as others, in the third person. For example, when referring to himself or herself, an Eskimo person would say, "Someone is going hunting," or "Someone is hungry." There is no terminology recognizing the future or vocabulary to discuss abstract concepts; language is used to describe action occurring in the present (Vaudrin, no date). In the past, each person in the Eskimo culture had a defined role in the group; therefore the anticipation of each person's action required little verbal communication. With the desire to be accepted by incoming Westerners, the Eskimo people learned to speak simple English. Idioms, abstract ideas, and double-meaning phrases were not understood in early acculturation (Vaudrin, no date). However, with English as a primary language of the young people and with the exposure to the world via satellite television and education, idioms and abstract ideas have begun to have meaning. Still, the nurse who cares for Eskimo patients from the bush or remote areas should avoid the extensive use of idioms, such as "a bull in a china shop," "out in left field," or "robbing Peter to pay Paul," since such idioms may lack meaning to these people who may have little or no background in urban living where such things as baseball fields are commonplace.

The language of the Eskimo people reflects their dominant concerns and interests. Certain words take on a more significant meaning than other words. Since Alaska for the most part is a land of snow and ice, these words take on a more significant meaning. For example, there are three different words for *snow* for which there are no single-word equivalents in the English language. Different words are used for falling snow, soft snow on the ground, and drifting snow. Another important word for the Eskimo is *ice*. Again, different words describe freshwater ice, saltwater ice, and icebergs, since ice also serves different and important purposes in this culture (Armstrong, 1973; Holderman, 1989).

For the older generation, English is the second language. Thus when one is speaking to an older person, comprehension can be facilitated by speaking slowly and in literal terms. Translators may be helpful, but it is important to remember that the Eskimo language has no translation for the future or for abstract ideas. When providing care to an Eskimo patient, the nurse should provide an explanation about specific therapeutic interventions both in English and, if a translator is available, in Eskimo (Glassetter, 1989).

Use of Silence

Eskimos tolerate periods of silence more easily than do people in Western society (Kleinfeld, 1971). In fact, it is considered rude to fill silences with chatter, since such chatter only prevents one from having the space to express viewpoints. The perceived Western intolerance of silence serves to increase the Eskimo's feelings of being dominated and inferior (Kleinfeld, 1971; Vaudrin, no date). Traditionally in Eskimo culture, each adult is given the opportunity to express a viewpoint without a time limit. For example, an Eskimo may go to see a White person for some reason and just sit in silence for many minutes before saying why he or she has come (Holderman, 1989). However, individuals in Western society may be insensitive to this mode of communication and interpret silence as nonparticipation or passive acceptance. Generally, Eskimos are a polite people and are unlikely to criticize other people's opinions and actions unless such actions cause a threat to the social group. In dealing with people in Western society, the younger generation of Eskimos have for the most part adapted to Western ways, which includes becoming more verbal.

Touch

There is a wide range of acceptable open demonstration of affection displayed in public among various subgroups in the Eskimo culture. However, the handshake is considered universally acceptable and a mandatory politeness. Hugging is an acceptable greeting between family members and between women friends. Eskimo men are more reserved in their expressions of affection, using handshakes as a common way to greet friends and family (Glassetter, 1989). Traditional Eskimos are very modest about exposing the body, and it is often difficult to persuade older Eskimo people to undergo complete physical examinations, particularly for diagnostic purposes. The nurse who cares for Eskimo patients needs to establish a trust relationship before diagnostic examinations will be allowed. In the presence of pain and illness, however, there is less resistance to physical examinations (Schaefer, 1973).

The late Eskimo healer Della Keats supposedly healed many people through the use of touch and love (Keats, 1985). According to Keats, she inherited the skill of her hands and learned the use of herbs for healing from her mother and other Eskimo elders. Through love, touch, and a combination of old and new medicines, Keats reportedly healed her people (Pender, 1987). The older Eskimo people give credence to the power of touch as a direct result of a shaman's healing powers (Glassetter, 1989). Shamanism, a belief that a person holds supernatural powers, is a doctrine held by some primitive societies and some Eskimos.

Kinesics

Eskimos use nonverbal communication extensively through body posture and facial expression (Albert, 1988; Boas, 1938). Years of watching animal behavior for survival needs have made the Eskimo people experts in the interpretation of nonverbal language. The nurse who understands the Eskimo culture will look for nonverbal clues, such as watching the face for raised eyebrows (indicating "yes") or a wrinkled nose (indicating "no"). Eskimos seldom disagree publicly with others. While smiles and head nods in the Western culture may indicate agreement, in the Eskimo culture they may simply acknowledge the other person's words. Among Eskimos actual agreement is determined by action. Insincerity and deceptiveness are quickly perceived through body talk and lead to distrust and eventually to social ostracism. Thus others are evaluated by body language, and this evaluation is nonverbally communicated back by inclusion or exclusion of the person in future activities. The nurse who lives and works among the Eskimo people over time will eventually understand the nonverbal language of the Eskimo people and its significance. The old adage is true for the Eskimo that one must listen with both the eyes and the heart to hear what the people have to say about themselves and others (Glassetter, 1989; Keats, 1985).

Implications for Nursing Care

For effective communication to occur, the nurse must develop a trust relationship with the patient that in time will give rise to acceptance of the nurse. When the nurse works in an Alaskan village, the villagers may appraise the nurse not on skills, but on the nurse's endorsement of the community. Some villagers may perceive acceptance in terms of the nurse's willingness to visit in homes, to take time to have a cup of coffee, and to participate in village activities. It is important for the nurse to recognize that some Eskimos have a need to know they are accepted as individuals and as a community. Thus insincerity and discrepancy between nonverbal and verbal language will cause mistrust and block communication. When dealing with Eskimo patients, whether in villages or in an integrated mainland U.S. society, the nurse should be assertive but not aggressive and use a suggestive rather than direct approach.

Some Eskimos respect the right of personal choice and self-determination so long as these actions do not impact on the welfare of the family or community. Above all, the nurse must avoid direct orders, because they tend to be viewed as being "bossy." When working with some Eskimo patients, it is best for the nurse to approach the situation in a roundabout way. For example, a public health nurse, while making a home visit, may notice a baby's bottle rolling around on a dirty floor. Later the nurse may see the toddler pick the bottle up, take a few sips, and throw it back on the floor. If the nurse corrects the mother about failure to protect the child from the dangers of unrefrigerated milk and bottle-mouth syndrome, that mother may not come to the clinic or allow the nurse in the house again. However the advice may be more readily accepted if the nurse waits until the mother brings the child in for health care, where teaching can be implemented and emphasis placed on the importance of refrigerated milk and the prevention of bottle-mouth syndrome.

SPACE

In the Eskimo culture individual space is often shared with family members (Roberts & Ross, 1979). What is perceived as crowded living conditions by individuals in the Western society may be viewed by the Eskimo as living in the warmth and security of the family group. The Western cultural need to be territorial, that is, to own private space, traditionally was not a value of the Eskimo people. Instead, the Eskimo people valued sharing and perceived it as an acceptable norm. Acculturation has weakened this particular value system, but family rights still take precedence over individual rights. For example, if a family member desires the privacy of a room for a few hours, this request may be accepted as a personal need. However, if this same individual demands such privacy continuously in a two-room house with five members, ridicule and accusations of selfishness may result. As the need for individual space arises, individual family members may go on hunting, fishing, or camping trips to meet privacy needs, as well as to return to nature.

A handshake distance between two people is considered the acceptable space for socialization on a daily basis. Closer approaches without permission are perceived as threatening, whereas greater distances are perceived as rude. An outsider who desires input from the Eskimos in a public meeting must recognize the decision-making process of the people and the impact that spatial requirements have on the decision-making process. The public zone for communication incorporates an intimate physical space where people sit in a circle, without a leader dominating the group. Some Eskimos view Westerners as masters of the savior attitude, which can serve to block communication with an impenetrable wall (Damas, 1984).

Implications for Nursing Care

The nurse who cares for Eskimo patients must remember that certain requirements for spatial distances must be observed. Requirements for space must take into account that the patient may have unique beliefs about space and may be disturbed when a nurse ventures into personal space to do such routine procedures as give a bed bath or provide oral care. The nurse must determine how much self-care can be implemented by the patient and how much must be implemented by the nurse. When self-care is threatened, patients who are protective of space may become withdrawn, overly aggressive, or overly passive. The nurse must be careful to allow the patient to make decisions about care, and thorough explanations should be given when the nurse must venture into the intimate or personal zone.

SOCIAL ORGANIZATION
Family

The extended family is the primary social unit; however, polyandry was common in traditional Eskimo society. Polyandry (the practice of a woman having more than one husband), while a cultural rarity, is thought to have existed in the Eskimo culture because of extensive female infanticide and because of the inability of some women to survive the long harsh winters (Carpenter, 1973; Holderman, 1989). The practice of female infanticide and the suicide of elderly people in Eskimo culture may be understood in light of the harsh and frigid geography (Seltzer, 1983; Travis, 1983). In many instances there simply was not enough food, and hence the killing of female babies (who were primarily consumers rather than procurers of food) was a kind of protection for the society as a whole. Similarly, when men got beyond the age when they were able to be active hunters and women were no longer able to chew the hides and thus prepare them, they were usually expected to commit suicide or to induce their friends or relatives to kill them. While this may seem inhumane, it was a purposeful way of preserving the culture (Nida, 1954; Seltzer, 1983). In a study of the attitudes toward the elderly in the Aleutian Islands today, Seefeldt (1984) reports that Eskimos sill place more value on youth.

Among some early Eskimos wife exchange had no negative connotations and was considered the mark of a good host (Holderman, 1989; Nida, 1954). Rules of hospitality suggested that a host should offer his wife to an unrelated visitor, with an understanding that the favor should be reciprocated.

The family unit, with its kinship ties, was paramount to survival in the harsh Arctic environment. The ideal Eskimo family group size has traditionally been considered to be four members (Holderman, 1989). While the Eskimo society has become a distinctively individualistic society, with primary reliance being on the individual and with the individual being relatively free to work out problems, the survival of the group traditionally was considered more important than the survival of the individual members. Several family units would band together in a migrating social group. These social groups were not permanent, because families could disband and join other groups during a lifetime. However, the roles for individuals and for families within a social group were clearly delineated, so that the groups were not weakened by the shifting of members (Nida, 1954). In fact, this shifting may have strengthened the culture by extending kinships. Extended families consisted of parents, their children (from a current or previous marriage or from adoption), grandparents, and single blood relatives. The husband was the head of the family, but the responsibility of bonding the family into a strong unit belonged to the mother. Thus if the family was not successful, the blame was placed on the woman.

Kinships were vital social relationships when Eskimos lived in isolated areas. Kinship boundaries extended beyond blood relations through such practices as wife sharing, hunting partnerships, and the adoption of children. The code of behavior between kin was as binding as that between blood relatives. These extensive kinship relationships were partially responsible for the cultural similarities in Eskimos that spread across the vast Arctic regions (Williamson, 1974). History has recorded incidences of lost Eskimo hunters who crossed paths with another Eskimo band and were subsequently killed if the lost person could not prove kinship to any member of the new group (Williamson, 1974).

In Eskimo culture today, the extended family plays a very important role. Survival no longer depends on kinships, but these relationships are far from dead. There still is a linking of families, which is evidenced by the sharing of native foods or the formation of business partnerships. These ties go beyond simple friendship considerations. The rapid entry of the Eskimo into the American cash economy and value system has led to the restructuring of the Eskimo social and economic system. The nurse who interacts with persons from this culture must recognize that partially accepted Western values may be superimposed over Eskimo values that may still be viable. The new elite class in Eskimo society is based on the ability to earn money without regard for old, established kinships and extended families, and a disregard for and severance of family and kinship ties underlie conflicts that may be found within villages today (Klausner & Foulks, 1982).

Individual freedom within the family or group

The culture maintains its respect for individual thought and personal freedom for behavior and decisions. Perhaps there is even more freedom for individual choices than in other traditional cultures, since survival of the group is less affected by personal preferences. At times, this individual freedom appears extreme, since others in the society take on a noninterference attitude. For instance, a husband may beat his wife without anyone lifting a finger to stop the beating, or a person may drink to oblivion day after day and no one will take the bottle away (Roberts & Ross, 1979). The value of individual choice of behavior is honored so long as the integrity of the group is not in jeopardy.

Social status within the family structure

Formerly, social status was attained by successful hunters who could provide food and skins not only to their own families, but also to others. Successful hunters soon were recognized as leaders in the social group by the members. The opinions of successful hunters were given precedence over the opinions of others. A woman's status was secondary to her husband's and was gained through her own skills in keeping her family well fed and clothed. Each family member had an expected role to play. Grandparents were the primary educators of the children and imparted knowledge and skills required for survival. Children learned skills through play activities that also contributed to family needs, such as finding bird's nests for the eggs or challenging a playmate in picking the most berries (Holderman, 1989).

Some Eskimo parents do not punish or even correct their small children because tradition says that the spirits of a deceased relative guides each youngster. In the Eskimo culture the spirit of the deceased relative is considered so paramount to the survival of the young child that while a women is in labor an old woman may be brought to the bedside to recite the names of the child's dead relatives. The name that is uttered at the time when the child becomes visible is regarded as the appropriate name, and thereafter this deceased ancestor becomes the guardian spirit of the young child (Holderman, 1989; Nida, 1954; Polk, 1987).

For the Eskimo child, praise from parents and grandparents provides a positive learning experience and a strong self-concept (Polk, 1987). In Eskimo culture undesirable behavior traditionally was ignored, and if the behavior continued, the child was shamed through teasing and ridicule. Social controls within the community followed a similar pattern. There were no rigid rules. If a social standard was broken, it was assumed that the individual had a valid reason for the breach of conduct. Behavior was kept in control through teasing, gossip, and ridicule; and if the behavior threatened group survival, the person was ostracized. To be isolated from the group meant certain death because an individual could not survive for long in the Arctic. The traditional Eskimo society is an example of a society that bases status on sharing and contributing to the well-being of the group and can thus establish a positive feedback system to control its members (Gove, 1982; Williamson, 1974).

Traditional Eskimos did not have any formal recognition of puberty (Polk, 1987). This was in marked contrast to other primitive societies wherein formal rituals frequently marked the coming of age.

For the nurse to give culturally appropriate nursing care to the patient whose cultural makeup encompasses traditional values regarding social status, it is necessary for the nurse to appreciate traditional family roles. In most cases it is necessary to involve both nuclear and extended family members in the planning, implementation, and evaluation of nursing care.

Political Structure

The political development of the Eskimo people has evolved out of the development of councils, native corporations, and health care corporations. The Native Land Claims Act of 1971 spurred a political development pattern similar to the political system in other states. Where once each community had an informal social structure that revolved around family and kin, now most villages have a decision-making council headed by an elected spokesman.

Implications for Nursing Care

Extended family ties can be used to pressure noncompliant patients into following recommended therapy. These ties can also be used to find reasons for noncompliance, since the patient may not feel free to contradict the nurse. In Eskimo culture it is not considered polite to openly disagree with others. The nurse may need to resolve a difficult situation by asking other family members for guidance. The traditional view of health as a way of life becomes cloudy with the squelching of shamanism and with the miracles that modern medicine provided during the devastating infectious disease era. Some Eskimos have become dependent on Western medicine. Thus the nurse must remember that some Eskimo patients may still put blind faith in the physician's decision regarding their treatment. The fatalistic acceptance of illness may also contribute to this dependency. With the increased educational levels of the younger people and with the help of the nurse as an advocate, some Eskimos are beginning to assume more autonomy to question medical therapy and social programs. It is essential that the nurse encourage the Eskimo patient to take personal responsibility for health or illness. The nurse should directly involve the patient in planning health care and in activities that pursue solutions to health needs.

There is a mixture of child-rearing practices in the Eskimo culture today. Eskimo parents tend to use more positive reinforcements, praising desired behavior and ignoring undesired actions. Children are considered individuals as soon as they learn to express themselves. What this means for the nurse is that a child is given the right to refuse or accept health-related care. Some parents will not force a child to do something that the child refuses to do. For example, a parent may make a statement such as, "I tell Sam to brush his teeth, but he won't do it" or "JoJo won't let me put drops in her ear." The parent may tease, shame, or ridicule the child in an attempt to persuade the child, but the parent will seldom demand the appropriate behavior. The nurse needs to emphasize that certain health care behaviors or techniques such as brushing teeth or using medications appropriately are important because they may prevent more overriding problems such as dental cavities and otitis media.

TIME

The Arctic Circle marks the point at which there is no sunrise on December 21, which is considered the winter solstice (or the shortest day of the year), and no sunset on June 21, the summer solstice (or the longest day of the year). This gives rise to a unique phenomenon that occurs in the northernmost part of North America. When the sun rises on May 10 in Barrow, Alaska, which is North America's northernmost city, it does not set again until August 2. As a result, there are 84 days of continuous sunlight; likewise, when the sun sets on November 18 in Barrow, it does not rise again until January 24. Therefore Barrow residents have 67 days of continuous darkness.

The extended periods of daylight and darkness give rise to seasonal, geographically related behavior. For example, it is not uncommon to see small children playing outside in the summer at 2 o'clock in the morning (Gottberg, 1988). Also during the summer months, the extended hours of daylight are used for fishing. Likewise, because of the extended periods of darkness in the winter, northerners tend to sleep late. While most northern people have rearranged their lives in recent times to synchronize themselves with the Western day/night rhythm, some Eskimos remain on "Eskimo time," which is a result of both the unusual daylight pattern and a present time orientation. Use of "Eskimo time" may prompt Eskimo families to keep their children out of school and in fish camp several weeks after school officially opens. Some Eskimos believe that fish camp, a present-oriented activity, is a time to be enjoyed, whereas school, a future-oriented activity, prepares children for future goals. Committing to year-round jobs on a 9-to-5 schedule is difficult for some Eskimos because of the strong urge to spend summer and fall in fish camps.

The present time orientation of this culture is sometimes reflected in the ways in which money is spent. There is an emphasis on consumable things that give immediate benefit. Budgeting and investing for the future may not be motivating concepts. Some Eskimos who have been away from the village and have earned a large sum of money during a season may come home and "blow" it in one spending spree for the family. This exemplifies two values: sharing what you have with others and living for today because tomorrow will take care of itself.

Use of "Eskimo time" requires readjustment by the nurse for such things as scheduling of appointments for health care, since some Eskimos prefer to come in when they feel like it. Consequently, a nurse who works in a remote area of Alaska should seldom schedule a clinic appointment before 9 or 10 AM and should be prepared to work late into the evening. A visiting nurse may be on a tight schedule and insist that the villagers accept a Western time frame. This insistence causes such comments as "you are always rushed," or "you must not like our village because you are always in a hurry to leave."

Implications for Nursing Care

It is important for the nurse to remember that a village may practice "Eskimo time," which is quite different from city time. For example, some people may stay up late and sleep late, which may cause stress for teachers because the children may come to school half asleep and without breakfast. In the summer, when it is daylight most of the time, villagers may sleep only when they are tired and children may stay up very late. This may present real challenges for the nurse, whether in a clinic or hospital setting, because the lack of a definitive schedule interferes with the nurse obtaining medical histories and the patient keeping appointments and taking medications on time and correctly. The public health nurse learns to take medical histories by village events and seasons. On the other hand, the hospital nurse must emphasize in simple terms the necessity for the medical history. In either case it is important to know a little about the patient's daily routine if nursing care is to be implemented and effective. Since schedules are flexible and time is relative, the nurse needs to inquire about daily schedules before requiring medication to be taken at a certain time. Many families do not eat meals together. Therefore telling a patient to take a pill at mealtime may have no meaning.

ENVIRONMENTAL CONTROL

The early Eskimos believed that the individual had three parts: body, soul, and name. All of these were considered of equal importance and combined to make the whole person. Early Eskimos also believed that everything, for example, earth, wind, flowers, animals, and birds, had a spirit. An extensive "taboo" system guided the Eskimo in harmonious living with the spirits (Holderman, 1960). Each family inherited a specific taboo system, and each person had a guiding spirit to help him or her during his or her lifetime. When a girl married, she had to abide by both families' taboos (Gove, 1982). The spiritual leader, called a shaman, had the vital role of keeping the group healthy by persuading the spiritual world to continue smiling on the people. When famine struck or illness occurred, the shaman communicated with the spiritual world during trances to learn what taboo had been broken and who needed to appease the spirits. Appeasement often meant that the guilty confessed to breaking the taboo and suffered humiliation. It is interesting to note that the shaman was not blamed if the shaman failed to find the cause for negative events. The people accepted their situation as a matter of fate (Blodgett, 1978; Lantis, 1960). Famine, bad luck, and failure in hunting meant the spirits were displeased with the Eskimo, whereas successful hunting and times of plenty meant the spirits were pleased. Consequently, the Eskimo perceived his or her relationship with nature as being in harmony or out of harmony with the spirital world. Today shamanism has been largely replaced by Christianity except for various remote areas of Alaska (Blodgett, 1978).

Illncss/Wellness Behaviors

Early Eskimos believed that each person had a spiritual healer, who could be offended by the person breaking a taboo. A broken taboo was manifested by the person becoming ill. Possession by harmful spirits was recognized as a cause of illness. For example, it was considered taboo to eat polar bear liver, and any Eskimo who offended the bear spirit in this manner became ill or died. Studies in the 1940s indicated that vitamin A toxicity, rather than the ill effects of the broken taboo, was the cause of illnesses associated with eating polar bear liver (Rodahl, 1964).

Written information on shamanism is limited because of the squelching of this religion by early missionaries. Folklore indicates that the shaman had predicted the coming of the strangers who would cause the death of the Eskimo; thus when nearly one half of the Eskimos died of diseases brought by the early traders, whalers, and missionaries, the prophecy was fulfilled. Unfortunately, while the Westerners brought medicine, they also brought new diseases to which the Eskimo people had not learned to adapt. With the influx of Westerners, the life-style of the Eskimos changed as they moved into permanent settlements to take advantage of schools, churches, and medical care. The spread of communicable disease became rampant among these people, who now lived in crowded, permanent houses. Prior to the influx of Westerners, the constant moving of living sites prevented the hygiene problems that were now incurred by permanent villages. Over the years the Eskimos have learned about the physical causes of illness and the appropriate techniques necessary to prevent the spread of disease. However, it has taken many years to increase their numbers.

Shamanism lost face with the people as they turned to the magic of medicine brought by the Westerners to cure the devastating infectious diseases. Many of the medical people were missionaries, who implied that illness was related to the people's sinfulness and that the cure depended partly on their confession and acceptance of Western religion. The early Eskimo did not oppose the switch to the new religion because it seemed similar to shamanism. Medical treatment by Westerners was often restricted to the Eskimos whose names appeared on the church roster.

In the Eskimo culture there is a generation gap in health and illness concepts. An older person may have a more holistic view of health in that the older person may believe a happy person is less likely to develop physical ills, whereas a younger person may assign illness to direct physical causes. For example, in the case of suicidal behavior, a young person may blame alcohol, stating that if the person did not drink, he or she would not commit suicide. Therefore the treatment for the prevention of suicide is to take the alcohol away. On the other hand, the older Eskimo person may see suicidal behavior as an illness of the spirit that creates a disharmony leading to the choice of drinking. The cure is to heal the spirit; then the need for alcohol will disappear.

Implications for Nursing Care

When giving culturally appropriate nursing care to Eskimo patients, whether in remote areas of Alaska or in the mainland United States, the nurse must realize that an individual's feelings of environmental control are an important factor in the nursing assessment of patient status. Illness and wellness behaviors among some Eskimo patients may be attributable to past belief systems and a belief in supernatural powers. The nurse may need to combat some superstitious beliefs, such as the belief that a pain in the head will be cured by wrapping a red yarn around the head (in this case the nurse must teach the patient that the continued wrapping of a red yarn to treat head pain may delay needed medical treatment).

Since some Eskimos tend to view nature as an entity that can be in equilibrium or disequilibrium, the nurse can build on this concept and teach the patient that certain conditions in the body can also be in equilibrium or disequilibrium. Coupling the theory of equilibrium or disequilibrium with supernatural beliefs, the nurse may explain that certain conditions such as edema of the lower extremities may be perceived as a disequilibrium in the body. Therefore the patient who attempts self-treatment with a red yarn around the leg to stop the rise of disequilibrium (edema) may actually be augmenting the chance for further disequilibrium in the body.

BIOLOGICAL VARIATIONS
Body Size and Structure

Ancestors of the Indians and Eskimos originated from the Mongolian race (Banks, 1956; Zegura, 1984). Anthropologists believe there was a land bridge between Asia and Alaska that was crossed by the early native people. Genetic studies have related the origin of Eskimos to a population of Asiatic Beringia (Szathmary, 1984). The Mongolian racial traits seen in the Eskimos include a short muscular body, large oblong skull with a definite occipital protuberance, well-developed lower jaw and maxillary bone, epicanthal folds, little or no body hair, dark-pigmented skin, and lumbar mongolian spots (Banks, 1956; Chance, 1966; Mann & Scott, 1962). The head shape and jaw structure have been attributed to the evolutionary process from prehistoric man and have little significance in the Eskimo culture today (Carpenter, 1973; Chance, 1966).

Early medical research noted the short stature and heavier weight per height of Eskimos, which was markedly different from that of europeans and other circumpolar people, such as Icelanders and Finns (Milan, 1980). Three theories were proposed to explain this difference: (1) genetic inheritance, (2) a combination of genetic and environmental adaptation, and (3) a condition of long-term nutritional deficiency. Part of this weight difference was attributed to the Eskimo's thicker bony skeleton and muscular chest and arms (Hrdlicka, 1930, 1941; Milan, 1980). Researchers demonstrated by the use of triceps and body skin-fold measurements that the extra weight was not due to an extra layer of fat, negating the adaptation theory that Eskimos carried extra fat to protect the body from the cold (Hrdlicka, 1941). Muscular development due to an active life-style and genetic inheritance contributed to the early Eskimo's body structure.

The birth weights and heights of present-day Eskimos are statistically similar to those of their White counterparts (Heller, 1947; Johnston et al., 1982; Mann & Scott, 1962). By the age of 11 months, Eskimo infants fall within the 5% range for height on Faulkner's growth charts, whereas their weight is in the 50% range. By 18 months of age, Eskimo children are consistently heavier than their White counterparts. This pattern of growth continues until the age of 6, when Eskimo children become lighter in terms of weight than White children. The average height of Eskimo children remains shorter throughout life. This pattern may be a genetic trait, although in the past three decades the Eskimos have had a growth (height) increase pattern of greater than 1 cm per decade (Milan, 1980). Some researchers believe that the growth increase is indirectly related to a decrease in hibernation. However, in 1972 Schaefer presented some convincing data directly linking the growth rate to sugar consumption. The pattern seen in Eskimos discredits the supposition that growth increase is due to a high-protein diet, since the Eskimo diet changed from an almost total protein intake to the present-day high-sugar, high-carbohydrate diet, yet their growth pattern has increased with this change (Bells, Draper, & Bergan, 1973). Unfortunately, obesity is now a problem.

When the Faulkner growth chart is used in health assessments of Eskimo children, it is important to remember that the chart is based on White averages. Sequential growth patterns are needed in health and nutrition assessment. For instance, it is easy to identify Eskimo children born with fetal alcohol syndrome by following the sequential growth pattern on the standard growth charts.

Skin Color

Eskimos have a "tanned" complexion that becomes deep brown to black with continuous exposure to the sun. This pigmentation is part of their Mongolian heritage. However, evolutionary selection may also explain this feature. Skin cancer research indicates that deeply pigmented skin has some natural protection from the ultraviolet rays of the sun. Therefore the evolutionary conclusion is that the Eskimo people are more protected from skin cancer because of their deep skin pigmentation (Young, 1986).

Other Visible Physical Characteristics

Mongolian heritage among Alaskan Eskimos is reflected in the lumbar pigmented spots and the epicanthal eye folds. However, neither of these characteristics gives rise to significant health problems. The nurse who gives care to Eskimo children needs to be able to distinguish between mongolian spots and those bruises that might be associated with child abuse. Child abuse may be reported to health care providers by well-meaning Westerners who notice "bruises" on an infant's arms and buttocks when these are only mongolian spots. However, it is important for the nurse to remember to document during physical assessment unusual placement of mongolian spots on areas such as the wrist, legs, and chest.

Enzymatic Variations

Enzyme deficiencies in lactase and sucrose have been documented in the Eskimo. When given a lactose load equivalent to 3 to 4 cups of milk, 80% of Eskimo adults and 70% of Eskimo children demonstrated intolerance symptoms of flatulence and diarrhea (Bells, Draper, & Bergan, 1973; Duncan and Scott, 1972). However, most of these people could tolerate a daily glass of milk without symptoms. In the past, Eskimos had no dietary source of milk after being weaned from the breast, and nutritional analysis of traditional foods indicates that the adult diet of Eskimos remains quite low in calcium. Research is needed to determine if there is a genetic protective factor for calcium metabolism or if this population is at risk for osteoporosis from calcium-deficient diets. It is essential that the nurse who works with Eskimo patients encourage the use of alternate forms of milk such as cheese, yogurt, and powdered milk. The nurse must also remember that another source of calcium that is readily available to Eskimos is found in fish bones that are canned with the flesh.

A small portion of Alaskan (approximately 5%) and Greenland Eskimos (approximately 10%) are intolerant of sucrose. Some classic research studies suggest that a can of soda pop or a piece of cake can cause debilitating diarrhea in some Eskimos (Bells, Draper, & Bergan, 1973; Shephard, 1974).

Friedrich and Ferrell (1985) found that the alpha-keto acid reductase locus is monomorphic in most cultural groups, despite earlier studies that suggested its existence as a genetic polymorphism. Thus the Eskimo population is no more prone to having an alpha-keto acid reductase locus than any other cultural group.

Susceptibility to Disease

The isolation of the Eskimo from outsiders caused these people to be more susceptible to the devastating effects of infection. Eskimos who lacked exposure to certain diseases failed to develop antibodies to these diseases. It has been documented that Eskimos do develop antibodies to antigens as well as their Western counterparts do. Thus the rapid spread of disease among Eskimos is thought to have occurred because of a lack of knowledge about hygiene techniques necessary to stop the spread of communicable disease, not because of failure to develop antibodies to antigens (Young, 1986).

Today, increased incidences of communicable diseases are still being reported among some populations of Eskimos. For example, in an epidemiological study of streptococcal disease that affected 706 Alaskan Eskimo children, throat cultures were obtained during a long-term surveillance program (Brant, Bender, & Marnell, 1982). In this study a binary variable, multiple-regression model was used to study the association between streptococcal colonization of the children and the following six potential risk factors: age, sex, number of children in the household, region, health aide rating, and colonization rate for the child from the previous year. According to the study's findings, the factors significantly associated with streptococcal colonization among the Eskimo children included age, past colonization, competence of the local health aide in providing care, and the region in which the care was provided. The study also found that the number of children in overcrowded homes and the child's sex were not apparently important to the incidence of streptococcal colonization (Brant, Bender, & Marnell, 1982).

There are still some remote villages in Alaska where hygiene techniques remain a nursing priority. When working with Eskimos, the nurse must implement teaching programs emphasizing hygienic practices and medical asepsis. Because some modern villages are extremely crowded, susceptibility to disease is augmented; thus the nurse must emphasize hygienic practices with these individuals as well. A study by Lum et al. (1986) reports the significant effect that improved immunization programs, prenatal care, and improved health care have had on infant mortality. Deaths from infectious diseases, measles, and pertussis were dramatically reduced as health care was improved among southwestern Alaskan Eskimos between 1960 and 1980.

Still another problem for Eskimo infants is increased exposure to *Haemophilus in-*

fluenzae type b disease (Hall et al., 1987). Alaskan Eskimos have the greatest known endemic risk for *Haemophilus influenzae* type b disease, which seems to have genetic factors that contribute to susceptibility (Petersen et al., 1987; Ward et al., 1986).

Tuberculosis

Tuberculosis used to be considered an illness for which natives in Alaska had inherited susceptibility (Stevenson, 1984). Today that is no longer considered true, but it is still an illness that is five times more prevalent among the natives in Alaska than in the general U.S. population. In the 1970s certain regions of Alaska experienced an incidence rate of 1200 per 100,000 population, in contrast to 14 per 100,000 in the rest of the U.S. population. However, rather than inherited susceptibility, this incidence is related to environmental and socioeconomic issues, such as very cramped houses because of the cold temperature and poor availability of clean water (Stevenson, 1984). Effective intervention includes both prevention and the curtailment of possible spread once a case is present. Health education is essential and needs to include not only direct information on tuberculosis, but also information on predisposing factors such as hygiene, overcrowding, alcohol abuse, and nutrition. Many rural health care providers have suggested that a general improvement in the standard of living is needed in order for this problem to be fully addressed (Stevenson, 1984).

Glaucoma

Eskimos are susceptible to primary narrow-angle glaucoma. Persons who have primary narrow-angle glaucoma have eyes that have a shallow chamber angle and a thicker lens, both of which are factors that contribute to glaucoma. It is thought that the sex and increasing age of the person, particularly in the case of women, are associated factors as well. Both genetic and environmental components appear to play a major role in the development of primary narrow-angle glaucoma (Schaefer, 1973; Van Rens et al., 1988).

Diabetes mellitus

While Alaskan Eskimos have been known to have low rates of diabetes mellitus, more recent studies have found that the incidence of diabetes mellitus appears to be increasing among these people (Schraer et al., 1988). Although some classic research studies suggest that a normal glucose response is found among Eskimos (Mouratoff, Carrol, & Scott, 1967; Scott & Griffin, 1956), with each passing decade there is an increasing number of glucose-intolerant Eskimos. There are many Eskimos of mixed heritage who are listed as being full-blooded Eskimos, and this could be a factor in the discrepancy.

The risk factors for diabetes are yet to be completely understood, but there is strong evidence that obesity and high sugar intake are contributory factors among Eskimos. Over the past decade, obesity among Eskimos has increased, and it is not uncommon for Eskimos (particularly women) to be as much as 50 to 100 pounds over their ideal weight. In Canada Schaefer (1972) noted that the incidence of diabetes was higher in the Arctic, where Eskimos have had a longer contact with a high-sugar diet. In this classic study, Schaefer concluded that the increase in known diabetes incidence among Alaskan Eskimos follows Campbell's rule, which states that diabetes morbidity generally trails 20 to 30 years behind the introduction of a Western diet.

Although Eskimos are not reported to have an increased incidence of glucose intolerance, it is essential for the nurse to keep in mind that some Eskimos have a prevalence for obesity and a high sugar intake, both of which can be contributory factors in the development of diabetes mellitus. In light of this fact, the nurse must implement teaching techniques that emphasize the importance of exercise and eating right. In addition, the nurse must bear in mind that if Campbell's rule is correct, an increase in glucose intolerance will be evident among the Eskimo people. The key to control of glucose intolerance is prevention. Thus the nurse needs to teach the Eskimo patient the necessity for prevention.

Cardiovascular disease

In Alaska the incidence of cardiovascular disease among Eskimos is low in comparison with the rest of the general population in the United States. It remains unclear whether genetic factors protect this population from a high incidence of cardiac disease. However, the nurse must keep in mind that the diet and life-style of the Eskimo people have changed dramatically in the last few decades, and that this will certainly have an impact on the cardiovascular health of the Eskimo people (Young, 1986). The Western world has done extensive research on arteriosclerosis and heart disease in a search for preventive clues. As a result, Americans are encouraged to eat a diet that is low in fat (less than 30% of daily caloric intake), limit their red meat and egg yoke intake, and do aerobic exercises. Traditionally the Eskimo people subsisted on a diet that was 44% protein (sea and land animals, fish, and birds), 47% fat (polyunsaturated), and 8% carbohydrates, which included berries, beach greens, and roots. In a recent analysis of the dietary intake of Eskimos, protein intake was 26%, fat intake was 37%, and carbohydrate intake was 37% (Mann & Scott, 1962). Although protein and fat intake decreased significantly, carbohydrate intake increased significantly. For some Eskimos the significant increase in carbohydrates is attributable to high intakes of sugar, and the implications for the nurse working with these people are that a focus on the prevention of cardiovascular problems is crucial.

In certain seasons the early Eskimos ate foods that were high in cholesterol. In other seasons their diet was devoid of cholesterol. Some studies suggest that the body uses stored cholesterol when there is no cholesterol intake (Feldman & Kang-ley, 1972). If this is correct, seasonal food variations among Eskimos have provided a protection against heart and blood vessel disease. Today, Eskimos continue to follow a seasonal pattern of dietary habits. Regardless of whether or not the body uses stored cholesterol, the nurse needs to caution against excessive cholesterol intake.

While medical knowledge regarding cardiovascular disease in the pre-Western-contact Eskimo is limited, arteriosclerotic plaquing was noted in the blood vessels of mummified bodies that were dated back to 1460. The oldest body had significantly greater evidence of vascular changes (Zimmerman & Aufderatrde, 1984).

In a study involving a Bering Strait Eskimo population, similar heart rates and heart rate rhythmicity and almost identical acrophases were found in the Eskimo, the Aymara Indian, and the French populations. The study also found that Alaskan Eskimos had heart rate means that varied by approximately 15 beats per minute (Rode & Shephard, 1984). This variation can have serious implications for the nurse who is monitoring the rhythmicity of the heart because of the variation in beats. When monitoring the pulse rate of an Eskimo patient, the nurse should, when possible, take an apical rather than a radial pulse and should count the heart rate for 1 full minute.

Anemia

Anemia, especially in infants and children, seems to be a direct result of a nutritional deficiency due to iron-poor food choices. Hereditary predisposition was eliminated as a possibility for anemia in one epidemiological study (Nobmann, 1984). For the Eskimos who live along the Kuskokwim and Yukon rivers, there is a tendency to have a diet high in fish and store items that are relatively iron poor. A typical meal for these people includes fish soup, "pilot" bread (so named because it was originally brought in by pilots) with shortening, and black, sugared tea. Even preschoolers drink black tea in these areas, and it is thought that the tannic acid in tea interferes with iron absorption (Nobmann, 1984). Thus the diet is considered to be iron poor and additionally has an agent (tannic acid) that prohibits absorption. Sea mammals are an excellent iron source, but with the decrease in subsistence living and the easy access to store-bought foods, even the coastal people succumb to anemia.

It is believed that anemia is one of the factors that contributes to morbidity in infants and children under 3 years of age (Nobmann, 1984). Lactating mothers should be taught nutritional education by the nurse who works in infant programs and in addition should be given vitamin and iron supplements. Infant iron-fortified formulas can now be found even in remote areas in Alaska and should be used instead of canned milk when a mother elects not to breast-feed. WIC (Women, Infants, and Children) and AFDC (Aid to Families with Dependent Children) programs have been established in areas throughout Alaska and provide money to purchase high-cost formula. Studies done by WIC suggest that its programs have effected a decrease in anemia (Nobmann, 1984).

Cancer

The incidence of cancer is not significantly different from that of the rest of the American population. However, the pattern of cancer is unique. Among Eskimo men, lung, colorectal, nasopharynx, stomach, and liver cancers are the most common. Among Eskimo women, colorectal, breast, lung, and gallbladder cancers are more common (Young, 1986). Data on 239 verified cases of malignant disease in the western and central Canadian Arctic were studied by Hildes and Schaefer (1984), who found Eskimos to be less prone to developing cancer of the skin, prostate, pancreas, and stomach. Cervical cancer is on the increase, but the cause for the rise is not clear (Toomey, Rafferty, & Stamm, 1987). Apart from risk factors such as smoking and diet, there is considerable interest in the role that infectious agents play as carcinogens. For example, hepatitis B virus (HBV) is the causative agent for hepatocellular carcinoma (McMahon et al., 1986). Children infected at an earlier age are at a greater risk for becoming HBV carriers, and once a carrier, a child has a 40% chance of developing liver cancer by the age of 40 (Lanier et al., 1980).

The Epstein-Barr virus has been implicated in the development of nasopharyngeal cancers. It has been reported that Greenland Eskimos have the highest documented Epstein-Barr virus titers in the world (Young, 1986). Other risk factors associated with this particular type of cancer development include the widespread life-style habits of smoking, alcohol, and chewing tobacco. Alaskan native hospitals have reported a significant rise in nasopharyngeal cancer among teenagers and young adults (Young, 1986), and epidemiologists have attributed this increase in nasopharyngeal cancer to tobacco habits (snuff and cigarettes) that begin in preschool-age groups rather than the Epstein-Barr virus.

Dietary habits such as the consumption of heavily smoked fish and fermented salted foods may also add some carcinogenic risks. There are insufficient data at the present time to determine whether or not genetic factors contribute to the cancer patterns of the Eskimo people.

Blood Variations

Eskimos as an ethnic group have a distinctive blood group variation; specifically, RH-negative blood is absent in Eskimos (Overfield, 1977, 1985).

Nutritional and Life-Style Preferences

Following the control of infectious diseases among Alaskan Eskimos, the health/illness pattern shifted to reflect an increase in chronic disease. This increase in chronic disease may be attributable to the fact that the Eskimo diet and life-style changed as these people assimilated many of the Western culture's bad habits, such as a sedentary life-style and a diet high in sugar, salt, and fat.

Instead of walking great distances, as in times past, modern Eskimos, even in the remote regions of Alaska, have adopted the Western habit of a more sedentary life-style. Some Eskimos now use some form of locomotion to get around villages that are less than a mile long or wide, minimizing needed exercise.

Clean water is sometimes a difficult commodity in Alaska. In some villages on the ocean, drinking water must be brought as ice from several miles up the river. In the process of being brought to the village, the chunks of ice may be handled by a number of people and must then be melted, boiled, and cooled.

Psychological Characteristics

"The suicide epidemic in Bush Alaska continues . . ." is a headline frequently seen in the Alaskan newspapers. The mental health status of Eskimos is complicated by the pressures created by traditional cultural demands, attempts at assimilation of Western values, and the harsh geographic region. Alcohol and drug abuse are the major causes of injury, accidents, and death among Alaskan Eskimos. Suicide is associated with alcohol abuse, which in turn is a symptom of a people attempting to assimilate in a rapidly changing society (Albert, 1988; Travis, 1983).

The suicidal behavior in Eskimo populations is thought to have changed in pattern and quantity over the last decade. The rate of attempted suicide among the Eskimos has more than quadrupled, and the incidence of completed suicides among young people has increased. In a study of Greenland Eskimos, it was found that almost 2/1000 of the adult population committed suicide yearly, and attempts at suicide were five times as frequent. The reasons for the suicides were found to be poor childhood home background and the effects of emotional conflicts with close contacts, alcohol affliction, criminality, and instability at work (Grove & Lynge, 1979). To understand the psychological makeup and characteristics of the Eskimo people, the nurse needs to have an awareness of their history and its relationship to self-destructive behavior as evidenced among some Eskimos, as well as an awareness of their present stress of acculturation.

For many Eskimos the rapid breakdown of organized traditional values, religion, and life-style, as well as social relationships, has led to an inability to find a meaningful role in the modern world (Albert, 1988). For example, a young Eskimo villager who is a student in a modern school and works on computers and studies about world events may become disillusioned at home when old roles are still present. In this situation the parents may feel inadequate because they are unable to relate to the child as a result of the knowledge that the child has acquired at school. On the other hand, the child may see little importance in subsistence living skills, such as fishing or hunting, which are areas where the parents excel. Following high school, the student may leave the village to attend college or trade school. However, the student may be unable to tolerate living away from the village or family and thus may return to the village after several months or years. This individual now has to be reaccepted into the village social life. Reestablishing satisfactory relationships in the village is difficult for many of these young people because they find that their own views and values have changed as a result of the outside experience, and thus village life becomes stifling. Also, the trade or occupation learned while away (for example, computer science) often is not useful in the remote village. The result of all of this is that the village now has a frustrated, angry individual who has not readapted to village life and does not have the emotional ability to survive away from home and family. These contributory factors may lead to depression and hence use of alcohol and drugs (Albert, 1988; Chance, 1966; Seltzer, 1980).

In a study that compared 567 native Alaskan criminal offenders referred to mental health professionals with 939 White offenders, it was found that alcohol abuse, which is the dominant social problem for some native Alaskans, is not clearly associated with the degree of sociocultural change. Residence in larger communities and higher educational achievement are associated with greater psychosocial maladjustment than is the incidence of alcohol abuse. The region of residence has a stronger influence on the rate and type of maladjustment than does the ethnic group (that is, Eskimo, Indian, or Aleut) or the ethnic density of the community of residence (that is, the proportion of native Alaskans in the population (Phillips & Inui, 1986).

For some Eskimos alcohol use has become an acceptable way to escape. Binge drinking has been related to the stress of acculturation (Mala, 1984) and is characteristic for some Alaskan natives (Albert, 1988). Since binge drinking is directly related to morbidity and mortality in Alaska, programs have been set up to deal with this problem. However, programs such as Alcoholics Anonymous have been relatively unsuccessful in Eskimo treatment, with effective treatment being related more frequently to successful resolution of the conflicts created by assimilation (Albert, 1988).

Some reports have identified the biological predisposition of some Canadian Eskimos to be more susceptible to the deleterious effects of alcohol (Seltzer & Langford, 1984). Canadian Eskimos are extremely rapid acetylators as tested with isoniazid (Schaefer, 1986). Eskimos also tend to clear phenytoin rapidly, as proved in Greenland Eskimos and supported by clinical observations in Canadian Eskimos. Schaefer (1986) also found that metabolism is significantly slower in Canadian Eskimos than in Whites. While the work with biological predisposition and alcoholism metabolism has been done with Canadian Eskimos, there is no reason why these data cannot be generalized to the Alaskan Eskimos in a more westerly area of the Arctic.

Implications for Nursing Care

Seltzer (1983) has reported three interesting cases of Eskimos who claimed to be possessed by spirits. The spirits appeared to represent culture-bound defense mechanisms and attempts at problem solving in Eskimos who had unresolved cultural conflicts. While reports of spiritual possession are not common among mental health professionals in Alaska, Seltzer's report does emphasize the importance of knowledge of myths and customs, as well as culturally significant methods of healing, on the part of health care providers.

As mentioned elsewhere in this text, an understanding of cultural differences will allow the nurse to relate in a positive way to persons from varied cultural backgrounds. If nursing interventions are to be successful, it is essential that they not oppose a particular cultural practice. On the other hand, if the cultural practice is detrimental to the health status of the people, the nurse must devise a teaching plan and alternative strategies to combat the negative practice. If the nurse is to use time and energy efficiently, it is important that the nursing care measures be planned and implemented cooperatively with the patient and family so that nursing care is perceived as being culturally relevant (Overfield, 1985).

The nurse who works with Eskimo patients needs to know certain biological concepts that are germane to the Eskimo people in order to give not only adequate care, but also nonharmful care. As the Western culture impacts on the Eskimo people, behaviors have changed. For example, Eskimos are consuming large quantities of carbohydrates, bottle-feeding instead of breast-feeding their infants, consuming large quantities of alcohol, increasing their tobacco use, and assuming a more sedentary lifestyle. As behaviors and health care needs of these individuals change, the nurse must modify approaches to patient care accordingly.

SUMMARY

Despite the apparent Americanization of the Eskimo people, these people have retained many of their traditional perceptions and responses to life situations. Whether a nurse works in an Alaskan village or in a clinic or hospital in the mainland United States and encounters an Eskimo patient, it is important for the nurse to incorporate a theoretical framework that encompasses knowledge of communication, spatial requirements, social organization, time, environmental control, and biological variations to enhance quality nursing care.

CASE STUDY	This case study focuses on a 6-year-old Eskimo girl with chronic otitis media, anemia, poor dietary habits, noncompliance with prescribed medication, and low self-esteem resulting in failure to adjust to school.

The mother brings the child to the village clinic for treatment. When taking the history from the mother, the nurse notes that the child has six siblings and comes from a home where the father is frequently absent and when present is often drunk. The nurse observes that the mother provides inconsistent direction and resorts to threats and ridicule when attempting to correct or change the child's behavior. For example, when the child does not sit still, the mother states, "You be good, or the nurse will give you a shot." The nurse notes that both ears have a gluelike discharge, which the mother states is being treated with ear drops given at the clinic 2 weeks earlier. However, the mother also states that the child refuses to allow the ear drops to be instilled because they "hurt" her ears. The nurse notes that only a small amount of the bottle has been used.

This is the second clinic visit. At the first visit, when asked about what the child ate, the mother responded that most food items came from hunting or fishing or the village store and that they usually had fish soup, pilot bread with shortening, and black, sugared tea. With a hemoglobinometer, the nurse now determines that the child's hemoglobin remains at the same low level as at the previous visit. The iron supplement tablets given at the last visit have not been taken. When questioned about whether she eats the school lunch provided by the public lunch program, the child replies that no one likes her and that the other children take her food, so she does not get much.

On examination of the child, the nurse finds a pale mucous membrane and poor muscle tone with decreased muscle activity. The child's temperature is 102° F, her pulse is 75, her blood pressure is 100/66, and respirations are 22. The nurse notes that the child complains of a sharp, constant pain in both ears and frequently pulls or tugs at both ears, seemingly in an attempt to gain relief. On examination of the ears, the nurse notes that the external canal is free of wax and that the mastoid process behind the ear is not tender to touch. However, the tympanic membrane appears inflamed.

CARE PLAN

Nursing Diagnosis   Nutrition, altered: less than body requirements.

Patient Outcomes	*Nursing Interventions*
1 Child will have increased iron level.	1 Educate mother and child about iron-rich foods.
2 Mother will understand safety measures.	2 Teach mother to recognize signs of pica as being iron related.
3 Parental knowledge of illness will be increased.	3 Do a 24-hour iron recall dietary history.
4 Patient will have adequate dietary intake.	4 Obtain height and weight measurements and plot on a standard chart that has been normed for Eskimo children.
	5 Assist mother in designing a medication reminder sheet.
	6 Reinforce with mother and child the need for taking appropriate dose of iron supplements.
	7 Teach mother and child about the need to eat a nutritionally balanced diet.
	8 Instruct mother to be certain to put iron supplements in a safe place so other children cannot take the medication indiscriminately, so as to avoid iron toxicity.

Nursing Diagnoses Body temperature, altered. Health maintenance, altered. Infection, potential for. Pain.

Patient Outcomes	*Nursing Interventions*
1 Child will have increased comfort.	1 Observe for symptoms of ear discomfort such as tugging or holding ears.
2 Levels of microorganisms will be reduced.	2 Assess for hearing impairment or loss.
3 Measures will be taken to prevent recurrence.	3 Examine external auditory canal for erythema.
4 Parental knowledge about condition will be increased.	4 Examine tympanic membrane for erythema, mobility, and bulging.
5 Measures will be taken to prevent the possibility of a tympanic membrane rupture.	5 Teach mother and child signs and symptoms of tympanic membrane rupture, which include sudden relief of pain.
	6 Teach mother and child the value of soft and liquid foods when chewing is extremely painful because of movement of the eustachian tube.

Nursing Diagnosis Nutrition, altered: less than body requirements.

Patient Outcomes	*Nursing Interventions*
1 Mother and child will describe causative factors related to inadequate nutrition.	1 Teach mother about importance of good nutrition for a child.
2 Child will experience adequate nutrition through oral intake.	2 Encourage a caloric intake of at least 80 calories/kg and 1.2 g protein/kg.
	3 Encourage mother to seek additional assistance for dietary supplements such as the WIC program.
	4 Encourage mother to talk with teachers about lunchtime intake.

Nursing Diagnoses Parental role conflict. Parenting, altered. Noncompliance with prescribed regimen.

Patient Outcomes	*Nursing Interventions*
1 Child will describe experiences that cause her to alter prescribed behavior.	1 Assess causative or contributing factors for noncompliance with prescribed therapy.
2 Mother will develop an appropriate alternative for previous plan for medication administration.	2 Assess child's rationale for noncompliance with medication.
	3 Initiate health teaching for mother and child.
	4 Teach mother and child importance of adhering to prescribed regimen.
	5 Teach mother and child what to expect from drug regimen, including side effects.

Nursing Diagnoses   Self-esteem disturbance.

Patient Outcomes	*Nursing Interventions*
1 Child will verbalize positive feelings about self.	1 Encourage child to express both positive and negative feelings.
2 Child will take part in activities with other children in a confident manner.	2 Encourage mother to set limits on problematic behavior, such as poor hygiene, noncompliance with medication, and other negative behaviors.
3 Child will achieve grade level objectives of school age.	3 Accept silence of child but let her know that the nurse is there for support.

Nursing Diagnosis   Infection, potential for.

Patient Outcomes	*Nursing Interventions*
1 Mother and child will learn value of washing hands and not placing foreign bodies into the ear.	1 Teach mother or child to take prescribed antibiotic.
2 Mother and child will learn value of taking prescribed antibiotic for the full amount of time.	2 Develop a medication reminder chart.
	3 Teach mother and child to seek early medical care for pharyngitis to prevent spread of infection through eustachian tube to middle ear.
	4 Teach parent and child to use ear plugs for swimming, showering, and hair washing if these are available.

STUDY QUESTIONS

1. Identify why otitis media may be a common illness among Eskimo children.
2. Identify cultural factors that affect the treatment of otitis media in Eskimo children.
3. List factors that predispose the Eskimo people to risk as a direct result of regular consumption of tea.
4. List factors that predispose the Eskimo people to risk as a result of consumption of large quantities of sugar.
5. Utilizing Campbell's rule, is this cultural group at risk for glucose intolerance?
6. List several contributing factors related to alcoholism among Alaskan Eskimos.
7. Formerly tuberculosis was a disease condition to which Eskimos were thought to have inherited susceptibility. Today, however, this is considered untrue. List two factors cited that do have contributing significance for this disease.

REFERENCES

Albert, D. (1988). *Impact of aculturation of Alaskan natives.* Paper presented at the Ob-Gyn Update 1988 Conference, Anchorage, Alaska.

Armstrong, T., et al. (Eds.). (1973). *Illustrated glossary of snow and ice.* Cambridge, U.K.: Scott Polar Research Institute.

Bank, T. (1956). *Birthplace of the wind.* New York: T.Y. Crowell.

Bells, R., Draper, H., & Bergan, J. (1973). Sucrose, lactose, and glucose tolerance in northern Alaskan Eskimos. *American Journal of Clinical Nutrition, 26,* 1185-1190.

Blodgett, J. (1978). *The coming and going of shaman: Eskimo shamanism and art.* Winnipeg, Canada: Winnipeg Art Gallery.

Boas, F. (1938). *The mind of primitive man.* New York: Macmillan.

Brant, L.J., Bender, T.R., & Marnell, R.W. (1982). Factors affecting streptococcal colonization among children in selected areas of Alaska. *Public Health Reports, 97*(5), 460-464.

Brody, H. (1975). *The people's land: Eskimos and Whites in the eastern Arctic.* Middlesex, U.K.: Penguin Books.

Carpenter, E. (1973). *Eskimo realities.* New York: Holt, Rinehart, & Winston.

Chance, N. (1966). *The Eskimo of north Alaska.* New York: Hoit, Rinehart, & Winston.

Damas, D. (1984). *Artic: Handbook of North American Indians* (Vol. 5). Washington, D.C.: Smithsonian Institute.

Dunbar, M. (1968). *Ecological development in polar regions: A study in evolution.* Englewood Cliffs, N.J. Prentice Hall.

Duncan, I., & Scott, E. (1972). Lactose intolerance in Alaska Indian and Eskimo. *American Journal of Clinical Nutrition, 25,* 867-868.

Feldman, S.A., & Kang-ley, H. (1972, July). Lipid and cholesterol metabolism in Alaskan Eskimos. *Artic Pathology, 94,* 42-58.

Friedrich, C.A., & Ferrell, R.E. (1985, May). A population study of alpha-keto acid reductase. *Annuals of Human Genetics, 49*(Pt. 2), 111-114.

Glassetter, M. (1989, Feb. 8). Personal interview with Dolly Leffever concerning Inupiak values.

Gottberg, J. (1988). *Frommer's dollarwise guide to Alaska.* Englewood Cliffs, N.J.: Prentice Hall.

Gove, C. (1982). *The conflict between cultural persistence and aculturation as it affects individual behavior of northwestern Alaskan Eskimo.* Dissertation presented to graduate faculty of the School of Human Behavior, U.S. International University, San Diego.

Grove, O., & Lynge, J. (1979). Suicide and attempted suicide in Greenland: A controlled study. *Acta Psychiatrica Scandinavica, 60*(4), 375-391.

Hall, D.B., Lum, M.K., Knutson, L.R., Heyward, W.L., & Ward, J.I. (1987). Pharyngeal carriage and acquisition of anticapsular antibody to *Haemophilus influenzae* type b in a high risk population in southwestern Alaska. *American Journal of Epidemiology, 126*(6), 1190-1197.

Hall, E. (1975). *The Eskimo storyteller: Folktales from Noatak, Alaska.* Knoxville: University of Tennessee Press.

Heller, C.A. (1947). *Alaska nutrition survey report.* Juneau, Alaska: Territorial Department of Health.

Hildes, J.A., & Schaefer, O. (1984). The changing picture of neoplastic disease in the western and central Canadian Arctic. *Canadian Medical Association Journal, 130*(1), 25-32.

Holderman, N. (1960, March). The little men. *Alaska Call,* p. 16.

Holderman, N. (1962). Personal correspondence about life as an Alaska Native Service teacher's wife.

Holderman, R. (1989, April 15). Personal correspondence regarding Alaska Native Service teaching experiences in the 1950s and 1960s in Deering and Shungnak, Alaska.

Hrdlicka, A. (1930). *Anthropological survey in Alaska.* 46th annual report. Washington D.C.: U.S. Department of Commerce, Bureau of Ethnology.

Hrdlicka, A. (1941). Height and weight of Eskimo children. *American Journal of Physical Anthropology, 28,* 331.

Johnston, F.E., Laughlin, W.S., Harper, A.B., & Ensroth, A.E. (1982). Physical growth of St. Lawrence Island Eskimos: Body size, proportion, and composition. *American Journal of Physical Anthropology, 58*(4), 397-401.

Keats, D. (1985). *Della Keats: Eskimo healer* (Video). Kotzebue, Alaska: Manillnaq.

Kimble, G., & Good, D. (1955). *Geography of the northlands* (Special Publication No. 32). New York: American Geographical Society.

Klausner, A., & Foulks, E.F. (1982). *Eskimo capitalists: Oil, politics, and alcohol.* New Jersey.

Kleinfeld, J.S. (1971). *Some instructional strategies for the cross-cultural classroom.* Juneau, Alaska: Alaska Department of Education.

Lanier, A., Bender, T., Talbert, M., et al. (1980). Nasopharyngeal carcinoma in Alaskan Eskimos, Indians, and Aleuts: A review of cases and study of Epstein-Barr virus, HLA, and environmental risk factors. *Cancer, 46*(9), 2100-2106.

Lantis, M. (1960). *Eskimo childhood and interpersonal relationships.* Seattle: University of Washington Press.

Lopez, B. (1986). *Artic dreams: Imagination and desire in a northern landscape.* New York: Charles Scribner's Sons.

Lubbock, B. (1937). *The Artic whalers.* Glasgow, U.K.: Brown, Son & Ferguson.

Lum, M.K., Knutson, L.R., Hall, D.B., Margolis, H.S., & Bender, T.R. (1986). Decline in infant mortality of Alaskan Yupik Eskimos from 1960 to 1980. *Public Health Reports, 101*(3), 309-314.

Mala, A. (1984). Circumpolar health, 1984: An Alaskan perspective. *Alaska Medicine, 26*(4), 108-111.

Mann, G.V., & Scott, E. (1962, July). The health and nutritional status of Alaskan Eskimos. *American Journal of Clinical Nutrition, 2,* 31-76.

McMahon, B.J., Heyward, W.K., Templin, D.W., Clement, D., & Lenier, A.P. (1989). Hepatitis B–associated polyarteritis nodosa in Alaska: Clinical and epidemiologic features and long-term follow-up. *Hepatology, 9*(1), 97-101.

Milan, F.A. (Ed.). (1980). *The human biology of circumpolar populations*. Cambridge, Mass.: Cambridge University Press.

Mouratoff, G., Carrol, N., & Scott, E. (1967). Diabetes mellitus in Eskimos. *JAMA, 199*(13), 107-122.

Nida, E. (1954). *Customs and cultures*. New York: Harper & Brothers.

Nobmann, E. (1984). *Dietary factors and iron deficiency*. Anchorage: Alaska Native Medical Center.

Overfield, T. (1977). Biological variations. *Nursing Clinics of North America, 12*(1), 19-27.

Overfield, T. (1985). *Biologic variation in health and illness*. Reading, Mass.: Addison-Wesley.

Pender, J. (1987, March). Little pinch: Memoir of a healer. *Anchorage Daily News Magazine*, p. 3.

Petersen, G.M., Silimperi, D.R., Rotter, J.I., Terasaki, P.I., Schanfield, M.S., Park, M.S., & Ward, J.I. (1987). Genetic factors in *Haemophilus influenzae* type b disease susceptibility and antibody acquisition. *Journal of Pediatrics, 110*(2), 228-233.

Phillips, M.R., & Inui, T.S. (1986). The interaction of mental illness, criminal behavior and culture: Native Alaskan mentally ill criminal offenders. *Culture, Medicine, and Psychiatry, 10*(2), 123-149.

Polk, S. (1987, Sept./Oct.). Helping our children. *Children Today*, pp. 19-20.

Roberts, L., & Ross, C. (1979). Nursing north of sixty. *Canadian Nurse, 75*(5), 26-29.

Rodahl, K. (1964). *Between two worlds*. London: Heinemann.

Rode, A., & Shephard, R.J. (1984). Ten years of "civilization": Fitness of Canadian Inuit. *Journal of Physiology, 56*(6), 1472-1477.

Schaefer, O. (1971). When the Eskimo comes to town. *Nutrition Today, 6*, 8-16.

Schaefer, O. (1972). Pre- and postnatal growth acceleration and increased sugar consumption in Canadian Eskimos.

Schaefer, O. (1973). The changing health picture in the Canadian north. *Canadian Journal of Ophthalmology, 8*, 196-204.

Schaefer, O. (1986). Adverse reactions to drugs and metabolic problems perceived in northern Canadian Indians and Eskimos. *Progress in Clinical and Biological Research, 214*, 77-83.

Schraer, C.D., Lanier, A.P., Boyko, E.J., Gohdes, D., & Murphy, N.J. (1988). Prevalence of diabetes mellitus in Alaskan Eskimos, Indians, and Aleuts. *Diabetes Care, 11*(9), 693-700.

Scott, E.M., & Griffin, I. (1956). *Diabetes mellitus in Eskimos*. Anchorage, Alaska: Artic Research Center.

Seefeldt, C. (1984). Children's attitude toward the elderly: A cross-cultural comparison. *International Journal of Aging and Human Development 19*(4), 319-329.

Seltzer, A. (1980). Acculturation and mental disorders in the Inuit. *Canadian Journal of Psychiatry 25*(2) 173-181.

Seltzer, A. (1983). Psychodynamics of spirit possession among the Inuit. *Canadian Journal of Psychiatry, 28*(1), 52-56.

Seltzer, A., & Langford, J.A. (1984). Forensic psychiatric assessments in the Northwest Territories. *Canadian Journal of Psychiatry, 29*(8), 665-668.

Sevenson, M. (1984). Tuberculosis in the North: A lifestyle issue. *Canadian Nurse, 80*(1), 41-43.

Shephard, R.J. (Ed.). (1974). *Circumpolar health: 3rd international symposium*. Yellow Knife, Northwest Territory, Canada.

Statistical reports. (1981). Washington, D.C.: U.S. Department of Commerce, Bureau of the Census.

Stefansson, V. (1921). *The friendly Artic*. New York: Macmillan.

Szathmary, E.J. (1984). Peopling of northern North America: Clues from genetic studies. *Acta Anthropologenet, 8*(102), 79-109.

Toomey, K.E., Rafferty, M.P., & Stamm, W.E. (1987). Unrecognized high prevalence of *Chlamydia trachomatis* cervical infection in an isolated Alaskan Eskimo population. *JAMA, 258*(1), 53-56.

Travis, R. (1983). Suicide in northwest Alaska. *White Cloud Journal, 3*(1), 23-30.

Van Rens, G.H., Arkell, S.M., Charlton, W., & Doesburg, W. (1988). Primary angle-closure glaucoma among Alaskan Eskimos. *Documenta Ophthalmologica, 70*(2-3), 265-276.

Vaudrin, B. (no date). *Native/nonnative communication.* Unpublished manuscript.

Ward, J.I., Lum, M.K., Hall, D.B., Similper, D.R., & Bender, T.R. (1986). Invasive *Haemophilus influenzae* type b disease in Alaska: Background epidemiology for a vaccine efficacy trial. *Journal of Infectious Diseases, 153*(1), 17-26.

Williamson, R. (1974). Eskimo underground social-cultural change in the Canadian Central Artic. *Occasional Papers* (Vol. 2). Uppsala, Sweden: The Institute for Allman Och Jamforande, Elnografi Vid Uppsala University.

Young, T.K. (1986). Epidemiology and control of chronic disease in circumpolar Eskimos/Inuit populations. *Artic Medical Research 42,* 25-47.

Zegura, S.L. (1985). The initial peopling of the Americas: An overview from the perspective of physical anthropology. *Acta Anthropogenet, 8*(1-2), 1-21.

Zimmerman, M.R., & Aufderatrde, A.C. (1984). Frozen family of Utqiaguiq: Autopsy findings. *Articantropology, 21*(1), 531-564.

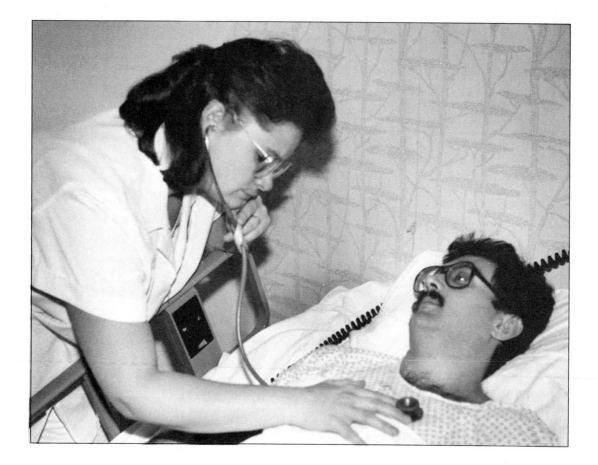

■ ■

CHAPTER 13

Italian Americans

Margaret Bowen

BEHAVIORAL OBJECTIVES

After reading this chapter, the nurse will be able to:

1 Explain the unique cultural background and heritage of Italians who have immigrated to the United States and Canada.

2 Describe factors that have led to discrimination against Italian individuals in the United States and Canada.

3 Explain the matriarchal family structure found in many Italian families.

4 Explain the conflicts Italian immigrants have felt between becoming assimilated into the dominant culture in the United States and Canada and retaining their own ethnic identity.

5 Describe culturally based customs that Italians in the United States and Canada may continue to practice today.

OVERVIEW OF ITALY

Italy, a republic in southern Europe, is bounded on the north by Switzerland and Austria, on the east by Yugoslavia and the Adriatic and Ionian seas, on the south by the Mediterranean Sea, on the southwest by the Tyrrhenian Sea, and on the north-west by the Ligurian Sea and France. The country is a boot-shaped peninsula measuring about 750 miles in length and averaging about 125 miles in width. Its territory includes two large islands— Sicily, lying just off the toe of the boot, and Sardinia, lying 130 miles off the southwest coast—as well as a number of smaller islands, including Elba, Capri, Ischia, Capraia, Giglio, and the Lipari Islands.

□ Special acknowledgment is given to Carol Pasquale, R.Ph., Director of Pharmacy, Logansport State Hospital, Logansport, Indiana, for reviewing this chapter.

Bordered on the north by the Alps, with the Apennines extending down through the peninsula, much of Italy is hilly and mountainous, with limited amounts of land available for agriculture. The only sizable plain is the valley of the Po River, in the north. Italy is also crossed by rivers, including the Po, the Adige, the Arno, and the Tiber, and shorter streams originating in the mountains.

The climate in Italy is varied, with the north having warm summers and cold winters. The south, on the other hand, has a typically Mediterranean climate, with hot, dry summers and mild, rainy winters.

Traces of Paleolithic and Neolithic culture found throughout the peninsula indicate that Italy has been inhabited since early times. However, the history of Italy has not been peaceful. With constant warfare among city-states, Italy became prey to powerful neighbors, including Spain, Poland, Austria, and the French. Influences from invading armies made their impact on the Italian culture, resulting in diverse ethnic practices throughout the country. In 1814 the Napoleonic Empire collapsed, and Italy was reorganized at the Congress of Vienna. During this time, the goal of a unified Italian nation captured the imagination of increasing numbers of Italians (McKay, Hill, & Buckler, 1988), and many looked hopefully toward the autocratic kingdom of Sardinia-Piedmont. When Sardinia's monarch, Victor Emmanual, appeared to come to power in 1848, many Italians believed that the goal of unification was close to being realized. In 1861 the provinces were united under one agreement, and Italy became a nation at last. However, while the country became united politically, internal divisions remained, with a great social and cultural gap existing between the progressive, industrialized north and the more stagnant and agrarian south. During these years many Italians left in search of democracy and a more stable government. Politically, before World War I, Italy was a liberal state moving gradually toward democracy. However, the wars worsened the political situation as Italy suffered first from Mussolini's dictatorship and then from Hitler's. Today, while the Italian government continues to change frequently, the economy continues to expand, and Italy's place in the United Nations and the European Economic Community has resulted in more stability. The earlier trend for Italians to migrate has significantly diminished.

The economy of Italy over the centuries has primarily revolved around agriculture, fishing, and tourism. Despite the scarcity of farmland, in the 1800s as many as 75% of Italians depended on agriculture for a livelihood. The influx of cheap North American wheat accentuated the long-standing economic problems of the Italian villagers and prompted migration by many poor Italian farmers in order to survive. Since the 1950s rapid industrial growth has resulted from Italy's participation in the European Economic Community and the government's encouragement of industrial development (McKay, Hill, & Buckler, 1988). Today, only one fourth of the labor force is employed in agriculture, and Italy can boast of trade throughout the world.

Italy is densely populated and for many years had the highest birthrate of any European country. The crowded countryside may also account for the way many Italians drive. (Many Italians appear to drive as though they are race car drivers in ordinary traffic. In fact, Italy has produced a number of famous car racers, including Michael Andretti, Mario Andretti, and Enzo Ferrari.) The Italian temperament is also commonly demonstrated in driving situations where it is not uncommon to see an Italian driver emerge from a car at a stoplight to wave a fist at a fellow driver who appears to be taking too much of the road. Italy is traditionally urban, with over half the people living in cities, including the large and world-famous metropolitan areas of Rome, Milan, Turin, and Naples. While the present population increase, taking emigration into account, is less than 1% a year, overpopulation has long plagued Italy, resulting in migration to other parts of the world, including large settlements in Argentina, Brazil, France, and North America (Simons, 1976).

Today, travelers in Italy, particularly in Rome, can still view the remains of a civilization that once ruled the world. The outline of the forum designed by Julius Caesar as the heart of the city of Rome, the villas and country houses both in and outside the city that were occupied by the rich, the Roman Colosseum where gladiators once fought, and the ruins of cities destroyed by volcanoes still provide visitors to Italy with fascinating ventures into history.

IMMIGRATION TO THE UNITED STATES AND CANADA

Italian immigrants can be divided into four groups: (1) the elderly living in Italian enclaves; (2) a second generation living both within the neighborhoods and in the suburbs; (3) a younger, well-educated group living mainly in the suburbs, and (4) the new immigrants (Ragucci, 1981).

For the most part, Italian immigrants to the United States and Canada have been landowning peasants from villages and towns who fled the country because of rural overpopulation, agricultural depression, lack of opportunity, and political oppression. In addition, some Italians came as cheap labor for profiteering steamship companies (Gioseffi, 1987). The number of Italian immigrants began to rise in the late 1800s, reaching an annual rate of 10,000 by 1880 and rising to 100,000 by 1900. This trend continued until World War I, when the number of Italian immigrants fell sharply. However, this number was increased by 200,000 by 1921. During the years between 1820 and 1975 Italians composed 11.1% of persons immigrating to the United States and were exceeded only by the Germans, with their 14.8% (Bernardo, 1981). Today, some 30,000 Italians immigrate to the United States from Italy annually (McKay, Hill, & Buckler, 1988), bringing the population of Italian persons in the United States to 6 million (U.S. Department of Commerce, Bureau of the Census, 1983). However, the number of persons who claim Italian descent by having at least one Italian parent is approximately 12 million (Giordano, 1986; U.S. Department of Commerce, Bureau of the Census, 1983).

The Italian American community has immigrants from mainland Italy, from Sicily and Sardinia, and from other Mediterranean islands that are part of Italy (Spector, 1985). Many persons who left Italy came from the south, where they were known as Neapolitans, Syracusans, or Clabrians. On arriving in the United States, however, they became known at Italians.

The ties of family and friends, as well as regionalization, have played a crucial role in the migration process. People from villages and provinces often settled together in rural enclaves or tightly knit urban neighborhoods with their families and friends. Often direction for this relocation was given by a strong individual—a businessman or religious leader—who migrated first and paved the way for families and even whole communities of Italian people to follow. Thus clusters of family groups and persons from Sicily often could be found living on the same street, whereas Neapolitans could be found in another area. Erie, Pennsylvania; Cleveland, Ohio; and Buffalo, New York, which are all located near Ellis Island and the northwest Canadian border, soon had large Italian communities (Smeal, 1988). Today, New York, New Jersey, Pennsylvania, California, and Massachusetts are the states with the largest settlements of Italians, with these states each having over 1 million persons with Italian ancestry (U.S. Department of Commerce, Bureau of the Census, 1983). The highest concentration of Italian descendants in cities can be found in New York, Philadelphia, Chicago, Boston, and Newark (Bernardo, 1981).

Italian Americans have a proud heritage in the United States, which started with the founding of America by the Italian explorer Christopher Columbus. In fact, America was named after an Italian, Amerigo Vespucci, and was initially explored by Italians, namely Verrazano, Cabot, and Tonti (Bernardo, 1981). By and large, first-generation immigrants found vast opportunities and prospered in America. These early Italian immigrants seemingly managed to prosper despite the many difficulties encountered. In spite of these difficulties, the Italian immigrants chose to remain in America and considered the problems encountered less austere than the poverty and lack of opportunity that most left behind in their native land.

A philosophy of "if you are going to make it, you must make it for yourself" prompted many Italians to "make it good" in America in spite of discrimination in relation to job opportunities, place of residence, and racial stereotyping of Italians as gangsters, dirty, or lazy (Cateura, 1987). Discrimination in schools included giving children harder assignments, more homework, and placement in the back of the classroom (M.D. Pasquale, 1989). Unlike some other minority groups in America, many of the Italian immigrants were educated, had a history of civilization, and a tradition of culture that gave them strength and confidence as they struggled to adjust to their new surroundings (Smeal, 1987).

Most of the early Italian immigrants settled in large cities. Only a small minority of the early settlers followed agricultural trades, and by the latter part of the nineteenth century, nearly half of all Italian immigrants were laborers. While the cliche "Italians are idle" may have applied to some Italians who lost their ambition when hard work did not result in a satisfying job, this stereotype was certainly not generally true (Venturi, 1987). The stereotype of laziness would also seem to have some association with the Italian custom of taking a siesta in the afternoon (many Italian shops close for a few hours after lunch). However, rather than being regarded as a sign of laziness, this custom may be explained as demonstrating the importance of leisure to productivity. The stigma against Italians as members of the Mafia is decreasing today as the Italian government is being more aggressive in combating the Mafia in Italy. Giuliani (1987) has suggested that the power of the Mafia is also decreasing because the Mafia no longer has the ability to recruit large numbers, since persons who formerly might have been recruited are now attending American colleges, law schools, and medical schools and are no longer in isolated Italian communities.

Today, second-generation Italian Americans, or those born to Italians living in the United States, continue to enjoy prosperity in America. Cateura (1987), in a book describing 24 Italian Americans, emphasizes that second-generation Italian Americans combine two very opposite cultures—the Italian and the Anglo-Saxon, and thus vary greatly from their forefathers, who primarily maintained their Italian culture. As Italian Americans are becoming assimilated into the mainstream dominant culture, discriminatory practices are decreasing. However, in spite of the merging of many cultural beliefs and the assimilation of Italians into the mainstream of life in the United States, many Italian American families still maintain significant portions of their cultural heritage. Italian Americans seem to have a heightened and mature appreciation for the arts of all kinds, including music, art, and clothes. Giuliani (1987) attributes this appreciation to an enjoyment of being alive that has been related to the Renaissance and to the present reemergence of Italy as one of the cultural centers of the world.

The ethnic consciousness movement in the 1970s in the United States prompted many Italian Americans to perceive their ethnic heritage in a more positive light and to be less eager to discard it for the customs of those they encountered (Auletta, 1988). Many Italian Americans still keep their roots alive in Italy by returning time and again to renew acquaintances and to keep the heritage alive (Cateura, 1987).

COMMUNICATION

Italian is the nearly universal language spoken in Italy. However, in addition, dialects indigenous to particular regions of Italy cause some Italians to have difficulty understanding persons from another locality. In a study by Bates et al. (1984), sentence interpretation in American and Italian children between the ages of 2 and 5 were compared. The Italians were found to rely primarily on semantic cues, whereas American children relied on word order. An earlier study reported by Bates et al. (1984) indicated that abstract semantic strategies may be a core strategy for phrasing in Italian. In addition to Italian as the spoken language in Italy, there are a few linguistic minority groups, the largest being the German-speaking population in the northern area of South Tyrol. The English that is spoken in the United States and Canada today contains some words that have been borrowed from the Italian language, for example, *spaghetti* and *bologna* (Nida, 1954).

Nonverbal Communication

Many persons with an Italian background relate to others—strangers, as well as friends and family—in a warm and affectionate manner. Italians are "full of gusto and have great joy for living life" (Venturi, 1987). Many Italians appear to have a relaxed manner and therefore are able to present themselves in a less defensive manner (Cateura, 1987). Warmth can be expressed by loud and expressive verbal communication but is also expressed nonverbally. In other words, Italians traditionally express warmth to others not just through words, but also through body language, such as outreaching hands and raised arms, hugging, kissing, and a pleasant facial expression. Italians are perceived as being physically very expressive, and this perception has resulted in some Italian Americans working very hard at avoiding overexaggerated nonverbal expression in order to try to fit in with the dominant culture (M.D. Pasquale, 1989).

Another important means of nonverbal communication for Italians is found in the practice of sharing food with friends and family. The practice of sharing special ethnic dishes has contributed to the preservation among many Italian Americans of this important aspect of cultural heritage (Burtis, Davis, & Martin, 1988). Mealtime is a leisurely affair associated with warmth and fellowship.

Implications for Nursing Care

Having an understanding of the communication patterns of persons of Italian descent is important if the nurse is to give culturally appropriate nursing care to such individuals (Rozendal, 1987). The nurse needs to understand that the warmth and friendly manner of Italian Americans is part of the Italian culture and may have a different meaning than the same behavior patterns encountered in other persons. For example, what may appear to be seductive language and touching on the part of a male Italian American patient may simply be this person's manner of relating and should not be taken personally by the nurse.

The nurse needs to be aware that newly immigrated or elderly Italian patients may hesitate to describe symptoms to the nurse or interpreter or to answer questions because of modesty. Information that can be obtained from relatives who do not have these inhibitions may assist the nurse in making a diagnosis and planning treatment.

In a study comparing similarities and differences in pain experiences among Black, Irish, Italian, Jewish, and Puerto Rican patients, Lipton and Marbach (1984) found that the pain experiences reported by the Black, Italian, and Jewish patients were the most similar and that interethnic differences could be identified concerning issues such as stoicism and expressiveness in response to pain, as well as daily functioning affected by pain. Duration of pain was a significant variable for Italian patients. It is important for the nurse to appreciate that Italian Americans may be unusually expressive and describe physical complaints in a dramatic manner (Koopman, Eisenthal, & Stoeckle, 1984). It is also important for the nurse to evaluate complaints carefully and to assess the patient thoroughly to determine the exact nature of the symptoms that are present. The nurse should also be aware that the patient's concern for symptoms should be treated with as much concern as the actual physical symptoms that may be present, and that it is important to listen carefully to the patient for both verbal and nonverbal messages that may be communicated. This information could assist the medical team in avoiding the misdiagnosis of an Italian American patient as having both pain and a hysterical emotional problem, which has sometimes occurred because the symptoms were reported so dramatically (Rotunno & McGoldrick, 1982).

SPACE

Some individuals who have immigrated from southern Italy, where parlors were uncommon and homes were often small, are unaccustomed to use of a living room. Today in America, some Southern Italians still use living rooms infrequently and may keep the living room furniture covered with plastic (Cateura, 1987).

Houses in some communities in Italy were joined by common walls, resulting in a physical "closeness" between families. This geographic closeness for many continued in America when Italian immigrants settled in urban areas close to other Italian immigrants.

Implications for Nursing Care

It is important for the nurse to appreciate that Italian American patients may have the need for physical closeness to others, especially their family. When the nurse relates to Italian American patients during hospitalization or even during outpatient treatment, this possible need for closeness should be considered as the patient is assessed and nursing care is delivered. Relaxed visitation policies may be demanded by the patient, family, and friends and may be in the best interests of meeting the intense patient's needs for closeness during this time of stress.

SOCIAL ORGANIZATION

Italians have a great appreciation for cultural heritage, including allegiance to other Italians. This appreciation was actualized by the settlement of Italian immigrants into clusters forming Italian neighborhoods with strong feelings of support, loyalty, and camaraderie. While the strong appreciation for kinship is changing, for many years Italian American professionals who could have left the Italian neighborhood to advance in their profession chose instead to stay.

Family

Strong family ties are extremely important for Italian Americans with nuclear and extended families (for example, uncles, aunts, cousins, and in laws), all keeping in close proximity or at least close contact with one another. Family traditions are strong in regard to holidays, weddings, and deaths. For example, Christmas calls for a *presepio* (a manger) and Christmas Eve for a meal with many different types of fish (as many as 13 or more) and frittole, or little fruit cakes made with yeast and fried. Easter for many Italian individuals requires Easter pizza made with two crusts filled with sausage, ricotta cheese, fennel seed, parsley, sweet basil, red pepper, and rice; a round and sweet Easter bread; and a confectionary dish called cruist (ribbons) (M.D. Pasquale, 1989). Thanksgiving for many persons of Italian descent is celebrated with lasagna or ravioli. A wedding calls for a "velvet bag" placed in front of the bride and groom at the reception for monetary gifts; a wedding meal, including wedding soup with spinach and meat balls in chicken broth; pasta; meat; dozens of varieties of cookies; and for some Italian individuals a special dish of toast with sugar and wine.

Different areas of Italy have special feast days, including the town of Civitella/Alfendene's Feast of St. Lucia (M.D. Pasquale, 1989) and the Feast of St. Anthony (DeLuise, 1988). These feast days are associated not only with food, but also with dancing. St. Joseph's Feast Day, celebrated in some areas in March, is uniquely celebrated with cream puffs. Other special foods such as scrupel, fried beaten dough made with egg (Italian donuts); pannetoni, a cake sprinkled with powdered sugar; and pizzellas, a special pastry desert, are often associated with certain holidays by individual families (Bohm, 1989). Traditionally birthdays have been less of a special holiday and may be celebrated merely with a sponge cake (Bohm, 1989).

Many Italian families today continue the tradition of Sunday being a day for family visiting, eating a marathon meal, drinking, women cooking, talking, gathering around the piano singing, exchanging jokes, political arguing, storytelling, and card games. In some families the meal goes on all day, starting with an antipasto tray of anchovies, salami, cheeses, olives, and blistered peppers; soup; pastas, including homemade macaroni, mostaccioli, spaghetti, and rigatoni; and meatballs. Sunday dinner in many families has traditionally been served at 3 PM, with time after the meal for the men to take an afternoon nap while the women visit with the cousins and aunts (Auletta, 1987). These meals have contributed to strong feelings of togetherness among families, so much so that some people from Italy have strong antipathy for those who choose to leave the Italian community. In other words, for some Italians, leaving the community is seen as leaving the family.

Roles of men and women

Roles of men and women are clearly defined in the Italian culture, with men having a role outside the home whereas the woman's role is in the home. Traditionally, Italian men were unlikely to assist in household work, considering chores such as grocery shopping, carrying out the garbage, cleaning, and child care to be woman's work (M.D. Pasquale, 1989). While popular stereotypes hold Italian men to be "sexist, macho types" who hold their wives subservient, the traditional Italian family is matriarchal (Sirey, 1987). While the role of the Italian American woman has been primarily in the home, the woman has a tremendous, innate sense of power that is actualized by her influence on her children. Unlike some other cultural groups where the woman's role is in the home, Italian women have not tended to feel oppressed but have maximized the importance of this role. Some have described the relationship of Italian couples by saying the father is the head of the Italian household whereas the mother is the heart of the household (Rotunno & McGoldrick, 1982).

Traditionally, the role of females in the Italian culture was very protected. Italian girls were prohibited from unlady-like activities such as tennis, swimming, and bike riding. Dating was often prohibited, with marriages arranged. Thus some Italian women did not spend any time alone with their husbands until they were married (M.D. Pasquale, 1989). While the Italian family might have been impoverished even after immigration, this protection of the woman continued as a characteristic; women were not to work outside of the home and definitely were not to be someone else's servant (M.D. Pasquale, 1989). Interestingly, Talese (1987) has noted that very few prostitutes in America are Italian.

Children

Children growing up in Italian families frequently have been taught to value relationships with people and the importance of caring and loving members of the family, as well as family friends. Children are used to affectionate hugs and kisses. Italian parents generally are self-sacrificing for their children; for example, an Italian mother would be unlikely to buy something for herself if her child were in need.

Despite the value placed on the role of women by Italian people, many Italians traditionally have rejoiced more over the birth of a boy than over the birth of a girl, even though Italian immigrant children of both sexes worked very hard to help support families that had recently immigrated (Venturi, 1987). It has been only recently that children have been able to change roles from that of wage earner to that of student.

In the past, some Italian immigrants to the United States appeared to view education as a threat to the values of the family. In addition, education was considered costly, because children lost the opportunity for work. Education was not considered as valuable as practical knowledge. The value of formal education seems to be increasing, however, and the earlier high rates for truancy, the tendency for children to work after school, and the pattern of children withdrawing from school well before the legal age are decreasing. In 1972 statistical data indicated that young Italian Americans

(23 to 34) had finally reached the national average in regard to schooling. Despite the delay in gaining education, census studies revealed that the average income level of Italian American families was already above the national average in 1968 and has remained above normal (*Statistical Reports,* 1981).

Relationship of mothers to sons

The bond between Italian mothers and sons traditionally has been even stronger than the bond between mothers and daughters. Italian mothers frequently have communicated a strong message to their sons: "You can't live without me." Italian sons have often appeared to be "waited on hand and foot" by their mothers and are "defended to the death." An Italian son can "do no wrong" (M.D. Pasquale, 1989).

The elderly

Italians hold the elderly in positions of respect. Even today, Italian families tend to care for their elderly at home rather than place them in nursing homes. When an elderly person is hospitalized, the nurse should anticipate that the patient is likely to be surrounded by family and should incorporate this phenomenon into the plan of care (Cacciola, 1982).

Marriage

As persons from Italy settled in the United States, marriage was almost invariably to other Italians. This tendency has continued through the second generation, although it is decreasing as time goes on. Weddings today remain large family events. In earlier years it was not uncommon for the mother to miss the wedding ceremony because she was supervising the preparation and cooking of the wedding meal (M.D. Pasquale, 1989).

Divorce

Traditionally, Italians did not divorce. This practice is changing today, although to many it still carries a strong negative stigma. To these persons the attitude is, "If we don't get along, we just put up with each other" (M.D. Pasquale, 1989).

Names and the significance to family structure

Italian surnames are very distinctive, such as Bernardin, Talese, Gian-Carlo, Sofia, Roman, Scorcese, and Coppola. Some Italians seek to preserve their heritage by giving their children distinctively Italian names. Some Italian surnames were accidentally changed during immigration by errors made by immigration officers. Other names were intentionally changed by immigrants in an effort to Americanize the name to make it less noticeably Italian.

Some names can be related to certain locations in Italy. For example, many of the family names in northern Italy end in a consonant rather than a vowel. On the other hand, Italian names ending in vowels may be found in other parts of the country.

Some Italian individuals follow a tradition found in some parts of Italy in which the first girl is named after the father's mother, the second girl is named after the mother's mother, the first boy is named after the father's father, and the second boy is named after the mother's father.

Religion

While many Italians are members of the Catholic church, the assumption cannot be made that all Italians are Catholic. Today, Rome, while predominantly Catholic, also has Protestant churches, including some Methodist churches.

The Church is an important focus for life for many Italians, and many Italians in the United States and Italy continue to celebrate the many church festivals and observances of saints' days. For example, weekend celebrations of a saint's special day can be found in cities in the United States with large Italian settlements. On the other hand, the Catholic church has not always appeared to have a strong hold philosophically on persons of Italian origin, either in Italy or in the United States (Rotunno & McGoldrick, 1982). Religion seems to be more of a personal issue. Some Italian individuals raised in the Catholic church can recall restrictions that limited their activities. Catholic schools were associated with discipline, and many children objected to the lack of permissiveness, such as restrictions in associating with non-Catholics. Even today, some Italians leave the church during their youth and return when they are older (Cateura, 1987). Previously, many persons of Italian origin viewed the church as a kind of family rather than a bureaucratic structure. Today, this is changing and the church is being seen as more bureaucratic (Bohm, 1989). Still, some Italian Catholic churches seem more informal than other Catholic churches, with more apparent freedom of spirit, more moving around, and more talking. Italian churches in America are more likely to have children in the church and to have a more relaxed atmosphere.

Traditionally, few Italian individuals were bishops in the Catholic church. Dating back to the historic controversy between the Irish Catholics and Italian Catholics, this is gradually changing as the strife between the two groups is decreasing; today, bishops can be found from both groups.

Implications for Nursing Care

It is important for the nurse to be aware that Italian Americans tend to be a proud people. Early immigrants, who did not have Social Security, health insurance, or unemployment insurance, often did not seek assistance outside the family. Many immigrants preferred to starve rather than ask anyone other than a relative for money. The nurse should be alert for possible financial need and should try to assist the patient in making arrangements that are compatible with personal values.

The nurse should also be cognizant of the practice by some Italian Americans of observing numerous religious traditions surrounding the illness and death of a family member. Both funeral masses and anniversary masses may be observed if the family is Catholic. Traditionally, Italian woman have worn black when a family member dies.

Families of Italian American patients may be uncomfortable discussing the impending death of a relative. It is important for the nurse to be aware that family members may take great measures to avoid discussing death and may appear to be ignoring the obvious.

Because of the importance of family, family therapy is an appropriate form of intervention with Italian Americans. On the other hand, gaining entrance to and developing the trust and acceptance of the family may be difficult, and the nurse must be careful to convey that the health care professionals do not consider anyone to blame for the patient's illness. Rotunno and McGoldrick (1982) suggest that one of the most essential tasks in working with Italian American families is developing the ability to view the family in its basic healing context and to mobilize and capitalize on this helping system.

Because of the importance placed on food in many Italian American families, the nurse should be aware that family members may bring the patient food in the hospital. Also, compliance with a prescribed diet may be difficult because of the importance food plays in the social organization of the Italian family.

TIME

Persons who have immigrated from Italy are often labeled as being fatalistic and thus present time oriented (Migliore, 1989; Rotunno & McGoldrick, 1982). There are behaviors found in persons from southern Italy that support this classification, for example, arriving late for appointments, seeking immediate relief from pain, and generally displaying a high degree of emotion and expression about symptoms of illness. It is important, however, to avoid labeling all Italians as being present time oriented, since these behaviors can also be explained by Sicilian conceptions of punctuality and the communicative dimension of the pain experience.

Some Italian Americans seem to have a past orientation, since they return to Italy to visit and reminisce with friends about relatives who have died (Bohm, 1989). This may be based on the history of Italians, in which they appeared to have little to look forward to and learned to appreciate what was and what had been.

Implications for Nursing Care

Italian Americans who are present oriented tend to present symptoms to their fullest and expect immediate treatment for the illness presented (Spector, 1985). On the other hand, some Italian Americans have a fatalistic sense about death and believe that terminal illness and death are part of God's will.

ENVIRONMENTAL CONTROL

Italian Americans tend to be individualistic and at the same time tend to blend forces from both their cultural heritage and the culture of the dominant society. Historically, Italians reported folk beliefs that generally indicated a belief in an external locus of control. While most Italians use Western medicine today, the belief in the ability to influence those around one can currently be evidenced by the involvement of Italian Americans in politics. Italian power in politics in America has been significant, although political success for Italian Americans was late in coming. The first Italian American senator was not elected until 1950; the first Italian American cabinet member was not appointed until 1962. As a rule, Democrats fare better than Republicans among Italian American voters. However, extremely liberal candidates tend to do poorly with Italian American voters. Black versus Italian political confrontations have been long-standing, and anti–civil rights candidates have tended to fare well among Italian American voters (Spector, 1985).

Beliefs about Health and Illness

Illness traditionally was viewed as being caused by (1) winds and currents that bore diseases, (2) contagion or contamination, (3) heredity, (4) supernatural or human causes, and (5) psychosomatic explanations (see box on p. 304).

BELIEFS ABOUT ILLNESS AND TREATMENTS

Moving air, such as a draft, was a way to explain illnesses such as pneumonia. Moving air may be the reason why an elderly Italian American patient refuses to have surgery for cancer, since this individual may feel that when the inside of the body is exposed to moving air, the illness will spread more rapidly.

Beliefs about contamination may cause an individual with Italian heritage to avoid persons who are ill; the hesitancy of Italian women to discuss sex and menstruation may also be related to these beliefs.

Traditionally, some Italians believed that the blood was responsible for illness. Blood could be "high" or "low" and "good" or "bad."

Superstitions have also been used by Italians to explain illness. Some superstitious beliefs reported by Italians include (Spector, 1985):

1. Congenital anomalies can be attributed to the unsatisfied desire for food during pregnancy.
2. If a woman is not given food that she smells, the fetus will move inside and a miscarriage will result.
3. If a pregnant woman bends, turns, or moves in a certain way, the fetus may not develop normally.
4. A woman must not reach during pregnancy, because reaching can harm the fetus.

Italians also report a traditional belief in the "evil eye," or *mal ochio*. It was thought that if another individual admired a good-looking child or adult, the look could cause the child or adult to receive evil spirits. Various remedies were available for ridding the individual of the evil spirits, including placement of a bowl of olive oil on the head of the person who had been given the evil eye, accompanied by prayers. Both evil people and God were thought to be the cause of curses. A curse from God could be a punishment for bad behavior (Ragucci, 1981).

Folk remedies practiced by Italians in the past and to a limited extent today also indicate belief in an internal locus of control. For example, in the folk medicine tradition, warm spirit of camphor rubbed on the chest followed by a warm cloth placed on the chest is a cure for a cold; leeches are a cure for backache, pain in the kidney area, and pneumonia; *abbaiare* (water boiled with bay leaves) is a cure for colicky babies; castor oil is a treatment for a variety of childhood illness (Bohm, 1989; M.D. Pasquale, 1989); and mineral waters taken as tonics are used to cleanse the blood (Spector, 1985). Chicken soup is used in some Italian families to cure a cold and to speed recovery after delivery. Often the care of the ill person in an Italian family is shared by family members.

Finally, Italians have recognized the relationship of emotions to illness, and many believe that emotions should not be bottled up, since suppressed emotions can lead to harm (Ragucci, 1981).

Illness prevention

Many health maintenance practices among the Italian people are related to food; for example, eating is known as a way to solve both emotional and physical problems. It is further thought that fruit at the end of a meal will clean the teeth and thus decrease decay. Hard bread is also thought to be good for the teeth. A hearty intake of pasta, wine (even for children), homegrown vegetables, salads, fruit, and cheese have been related by Italians to staying healthy.

Illness prevention has been related by some Italians to practices such as placing garlic cloves on a string around the neck of infants and children to prevent colds and "stares" by other people. Keeping warm and dry, staying out of drafts, avoiding washing hair before going out or during a menstrual period, and placing a pair of scissors under the mattress of the newborn to prevent "evil" from occurring are health-seeking traditions that many Italians brought with them to the United States (Spector, 1985).

Implications for Nursing Care

It is important for the nurse to assess the patient's locus of control and to provide education about control. Since Italians are perceived as having an external locus of control and a somewhat fatalistic outlook on life, it is essential for the nurse to emphasize the importance of illness prevention techniques. Because some Italians may also attribute the cause of illness to external forces in the environment, such as the "evil eye," curses, or mystical thought, it is important for the nurse to assess whether such health care practices have neutral, beneficial, or harmful effects on the patient's health care status, as well as assessing health-seeking attitudes and behaviors. Since some Italians believe that illness can also be caused by the suppression of emotions, as well as by stress, fear, grief, or anxiety, it is important for the nurse to assist the Italian American patient in finding healthy emotional outlets to prevent illness and/or disease. Since illness prevention techniques may not be part of the patient's way of looking at disease and illness, the nurse should carefully provide information on medication and should assess the patient for noncompliance. The nurse may find the Italian American patient generally reluctant to take medications, and special intervention may be required before the patient agrees to participate in the recommended therapy (C. Pasquale, 1989).

BIOLOGICAL VARIATIONS
Enzymatic and Genetic Variations and Susceptiblity to Disease

Not all Italians fit the stereotype of having dark hair and eyes; there are also Italians with blue eyes and blond hair. There is some research suggesting that favism, a severe hemolytic anemia produced by the eating of fava beans and the deficiency of an X-linked enzyme, and thalassemia syndromes, including Cooley's anemia and alpha thalassemia, are genetic illnesses affecting Italians (Crowley et al., 1987; Marinucci, 1982; Thain et al., 1987; Zago, Costa, & Bottura, 1982). Other possible genetic links have been suggested; for example, studies of blood samples indicate significant differences in HLA alleles in individuals throughout Italy (Santolamazza, Benincasa, & Scozzari, 1986). HLA gene frequencies place continental Italy and Sicily in a position similar to that of other Mediterranean populations, whereas the genetic isolation of Saradinia is quite evident. A study by Olivetti et al. (1986) found that the most significant linkage disequilibrium values observed in the Italian population were in agreement with those found in other White populations. The differences between northern and southern Italy and between continental Italy and Sardinia were emphasized by the linkage disequilibrium values and the principal component analysis. This adds further weight to the sociological evidence of family stability in certain areas of Italy.

Differences were also found in the etiology of chronic nonalcoholic liver disease between residents of Naples and residents of Copenhagen (Del Vecchio-Blanco et al., 1984). There were more hepatitis B virus (HBV)–induced cases among Italians (38.8% versus 15.5% in the Danish), but the sex ratio and biochemical activity in the Italians were not different from those in the Danish. Autoimmune markers were much more frequent and in higher titers in Danish HBV–negative patients than in Italian ones. Thus Italians fit the theory of autoimmune disease, but their chronic liver disease seemed to be caused by hepatitis viruses other than B.

Some studies have been done indicating significant variations in the incidence of certain illnesses in different European populations. For example, Allen and Phelan (1985) found that the incidence of cystic fibrosis among the Australian-born children of parents born in Italy was 1 per 3625 live births, and among Australian-born children of parents born in Greece, the incidence was 1 per 3726 live births. Studies have also compared mortality rates among persons of different countries. In a study comparing mortality amenable to medical intervention from 1959 to 1980 in six countries—the United Kingdom, the United States, France, Japan, Italy, and Sweden—Italy was found to have the least favorable infant and maternal mortality rates in the European Economic Community (Charlton & Valez, 1986). Mortality from heterogeneous "avoidable" causes declined faster than mortality from all other causes in each of the countries. England, Wales, and Italy experienced the smallest decline in stroke mortality.

As mentioned elsewhere in this text, racial differences have been noted in terms of physical development. For example, menarche occurring at about 12.5 years of age has been found in girls in rural Naples and other specific localities, whereas menarche occurring at a later age than 15 has been found in some areas of Africa and Egypt (Eveleth & Tanner, 1976; Overfield, 1985).

Sickle cell disease occurs at a much higher incidence among Blacks. However, occasional cases have appeared in children of Greek, Italian, Turkish, and Arabian ancestry (Campbell & Oski, 1977).

Lactose malabsorption and intolerance

Some Italians have a problem with lactose malabsorption and intolerance (Bozzani, Penagini, & Velio, 1986; Ceriani et al., 1988). In a study of 40 Italian patients with irritable bowel syndrome, malabsorption was frequent in the "low milk consumers" group (P less than 0.05). During a 4-month period in which a lactose-free diet was the only treatment, 7.5% of patients were symptom-free and remained so for the duration of the 8-month period of the diet, during which time 52.5% improved and 40% showed no change.

Nutritional Preferences

The kitchen is the center of many Italian homes. Food consumption studies in Italy in the 1960s revealed a high consumption of cereals (grains and wheat), meat, vegetables, fruit, and wine (Kromhout, Keys, & Aravanis, 1989). Many dishes prepared in the homes of Italian individuals involve days of preparation, and there is enjoyment not only in eating the food created, but also in the preparation process.

The Italian culture is famous for its cuisine, including dishes made from cheeses, pasta, ham, and sausages. Commonly used spices include sweet basil, garlic, and parsley. Wine, tomato puree, and olive oil are also used to season food. Many delicious Italian dishes were developed years ago by creative imaginations when little meat was available and the pastas were a way to stretch small meat portions in a large family. Special recipes have been passed down through the generations. Polenta is a dish made of cornmeal that is very popular in northern Italy. While Polenta itself is rather bland, it is served with a sauce containing sausage or other meat, as well as with different kinds of cheese. Another special Italian delight is cappelletti, which requires hours of preparation. The word *cappelletti* means "little hats." Small ravioli are made in the shape of hats, filled with different kinds of meats and seasonings, and served with chicken broth or sauce. Other Italian dishes include strufoli, a fried dough sprinkled with candy, and frittata, an omlet made with leftovers, including potatoes, zucchini, or meat. Gnocchi is another special Italian dish made with dough containing mashed potatoes and served with a sauce. Types of sauces vary with the geographic origin of the family. In the northern segment of Italy a thick meat sauce that requires 6 to 8 hours of cooking is served, whereas southern Italy is known for its sauce and meatballs.

Food is used by many Italians to improve physical and psychological well-being. DeLuise (1988) reported situations where the Italian mother responded to depression or heartache with "Eat this; it will make you feel better" and also responded to complaints of being too full after a gigantic meal with "Eat this; it will make you feel better."

A healthy Italian habit is the eating of many greens. Salads are common at lunch and dinner, and popular vegetables include artichokes, broccoli, escarole, asparagus, cauliflower, and mushrooms. Heavy deserts are not desired, and meals are commonly finished off with fresh fruit and cheese. Milk is generally avoided in Italy because of milk-borne epidemics that were common in the past. Some Italians believe it is healthy to drink wine with meals (Burtis, Davis, & Martin, 1988).

Psychological Characteristics
Mental health

Many Italian people feel that if the family is not able to help the individual, going to outsiders is inappropriate (C. Pasquale, 1989). Sirey (1987) has reported that more and more Italians are going into counseling. The upward mobility that is promoted by the American people comes into conflict with the strong ties that many Italian Americans feel for the family. As Italian Americans leave their Italian communities and extended families, the way in which the family is viewed must also change. This conflict between the present demands of society and the cultural heritage is also felt by Italian women who no longer have the strong extended family network available for support. The National Organization of Italian American Women (NOIAW) addresses this issue by promoting sharing among Italian American women with common cultural values.

While there are contrasting approaches for treating schizophrenia in Italy and in the United States (during acute phases of schizophrenia in Italy patients are admitted to general hospital psychiatric wards for an average duration of 1 month and then discharged into the community), in a study comparing symptoms of positive and negative schizophrenia, the results of assessment scales were very similar in spite of different languages and different cultures (Moscarelli, Maffei, & Cesana, 1987).

Alcoholism

People living in Italy have traditionally had a high consumption of wine and have been the focus of a considerable amount of research in this area (Heien & Pompelli, 1987; Kromhout, Keys, & Aravanis, 1989; Muhlin, 1985; Trevisan et al., 1987). Many Italian American individuals make their own wine with recipes brought from Italy. However, research on drinking patterns indicates low abstention and low problem rates among Italians as compared with Irish individuals, who have high prevalence rates of heavy drinking with problems, and with British and German individuals, who have intermediate rates (Bales, 1962; Blane, 1987; Clark & Midanik, 1982). The low rate of alcoholism among Italian American individuals has caused these persons to be viewed by employers as dependable on the job.

Suicide

Catholic dogma proclaims that suicide is a sin. Members of Italian families who are practicing Catholics may feel dishonored by a suicide in the family, may find themselves barred from certain occupations, and may find they cannot bury the body in consecrated ground. This attitude is so strong among some Italian individuals that physicians and members of the clergy may falsify death certificates, listing mental illness, which is more acceptable to the Catholic church (Pasquali, Arnold, & DeBasio, 1989). According to Farberow (1975), it is important for the nurse to assist the family members in understanding the dynamics of suicidal behavior. Since the family may serve as a primary source of support, the family should be assisted in providing love, help, and protection to the potentially suicidal individual or to the person who has already attempted suicide. Many Italian Americans believe that each individual is accountable for the welfare of others. Although the family can be a vital support system, this belief may place great demands on family members and subsequent guilt if they feel they cannot meet the needs for nurturance that are requested. Family members may attach strings to nurturing behavior and increase the conflict experienced by the individual already in emotional distress. It is important for the nurse to understand that while the patient and family may be members of third, fourth, and successive generations of Italian Americans and may not appear to be strongly attached to the Catholic church, the concern and value for life may remain strong. Ambivalence experienced by an Italian American individual considering suicide may result from the inability to escape the intricately woven net of doctrine laid by the family and the church (Pasquali, Arnold, & DeBasio, 1989).

Implications for Nursing Care

It may be useful for the nurse caring for Italian American patients to know that systematic mandatory immunization of children against tetanus began in Italy in 1968. This is an important fact, because in a national sample of Italian young men born between 1958 and 1963, about one third were not protected. The prevalence of nonimmune subjects was greater in the southern regions, in the island rural areas, among the unemployed, and among older individuals (Rosmini, Gentili, & Wirz, 1987). For a patient who has not been immunized for tetanus, a booster will not be appropriate.

Since milk is seldom used as a beverage by Italian individuals, the nurse should evaluate whether or not calcium intake is adequate, particularly when assessing the dietary intake of children in Italian American families. When doing a family assessment, it may be important for the nurse to assess not only the calcium intake of the children in the family, but that of the adults as well. Use of whole grains and enriched breads should be encouraged, since some Italian breads may not be enriched and may not contain milk. For a family concerned with the cost of food, the nurse might suggest that domestic oils, such as soybean, cottonseed, and corn, are less expensive for cooking and seasoning foods than olive oil and may be an acceptable substitute (Burtis, Davis, & Martin, 1988).

As Italian Americans are becoming more accepting of outside help for physical and mental illness, the number of Italian Americans hospitalized is gradually rising (C. Pasquale, 1989). As this number rises, nurses will increasingly be called on to provide support for these patients. Nurses are in a unique position in caring for Italian Americans, since nurses tend to be viewed as more nurturing and nonjudgmental than physicians (Rozendal, 1987). However, nurses must devote a substantial amount of time to assessment of Italian American patients, since trust does not come easily (Rotunno & McGoldrick, 1982).

SUMMARY

Cultural diversity is a great strength in America. When Italians first settled in the United States, they were fearful of people outside the cultural group, and an intense desire to preserve the cultural heritage emerged. Today, as Italian Americans become more assimilated into the mainstream of the dominant American culture, more selective behaviors based on personal preference are being used.

CASE STUDY

Maria Mamolenti, a 22-year-old Italian American married woman, comes to the clinic because she is pregnant. With Mrs. Mamolenti are her husband, her mother, two sisters, and a cousin. This is her first pregnancy. Mrs. Mamolenti, who is approximately 3 months pregnant, relates to the nurse that she fears the baby has been harmed because it was necessary for her to do considerable reaching above her head to put things away in her new apartment. In the interview Mrs. Mamolenti relates to the nurse practitioner that she has had the following symptoms: (1) bloating, (2) flatulence, (3) cramps, (4) abdominal distention, and (5) diarrhea.

The nurse examines Mrs. Mamolenti and finds that her vital signs are as follows: pulse 72; respirations 18; blood pressure ll0/80. Further examination reveals that there is some abdominal distention; however, the abdomen is not tender to touch. On further questioning, Mrs. Mamolenti reveals that she has been drinking at least six to eight glasses of milk as instructed by the nurse at her last visit. She states that before her pregnancy she rarely drank milk and in fact drank wine with most meals, particularly with dinner. However, when she did drink milk, she experienced no difficulty.

After a lactose loading dose of 50 g (approximately the same amount of lactose found in 4 cups of milk), Mrs. Mamolenti exhibits similar symptoms and therefore is diagnosed as lactose intolerant. In addition, after a breath-hydrogen assay, she is found to have a very low level of lactose tolerance.

At her next clinic visit Mrs. Mamolenti, accompanied by the same family members, is given an explanation for her illness. While she verbalizes an understanding of the nature of the condition, the nurse notes that both Mrs. Mamolenti and her family verbalize a need to have the problem corrected immediately to prevent harm from occurring to the unborn baby.

CARE
PLAN

Nursing Diagnosis   Nutrition, altered: less than body requirements of calcium and riboflavin for a pregnant woman.

Patient Outcome

Patient will reduce or eliminate causative factors related to lactose intolerance from diet.

Nursing Interventions

1   Instruct patient to do a 24-hour recall to determine calcium deficiency.
2   Reduce or eliminate causative factors by instructing patient to drink only small amounts of whole milk at breakfast.
3   Instruct patient to substitute whole milk with low-lactose milk treated with Lactaid or Lacterase if discomfort is experienced from milk ingested at breakfast.
4   Instruct patient to substitute whole milk with one cup of yogurt as midmorning snack.
5   Instruct patient to eat at least two slices of cheese as midafternoon snack.
6   Instruct patient to drink at least one glass of buttermilk as an h.s. snack.
7   Instruct patient to increase intake of meat, fish, poultry, eggs, breads, and cereals.
8   Instruct patient to increase caloric intake of high-carbohydrate foods such as fruit to the diet.

Nursing Diagnosis   Coping, family: potential for growth.

Patient Outcome

Family will verbalize an understanding of the need for adequate nutrition.

Nursing Intervention

Instruct patient and family about the need for adequate nutrition throughout life and particularly during pregnancy.

Nursing Diagnosis   Health maintenance, altered, related to cultural folk beliefs.

Patient Outcome

Patient and family will verbalize an understanding of beneficial, neutral, and harmful cultural health practices.

Nursing Interventions

Instruct patient and family about differentiation between beneficial, neutral, and harmful cultural health practices.

Nursing Diagnosis   Health-seeking behaviors related to culture and cultural beliefs.

Patient Outcomes

1   Patient will consume a high-protein diet with at least 1200 g of calcium per day.
2   Patient and family will verbalize an understanding about beneficial, neutral, and harmful cultural health practices.

Nursing Interventions

1   Assess each family member for knowledge and skill needed to monitor health.
2   Utilize audiovisual aids such as pamphlets and pictures to teach this family about pregnancy, as well as lactose intolerance.

STUDY
QUESTIONS

1. List some strategies that may help a nurse communicate with an Italian American family.
2. Describe the matriarchal family structure and the influence this may have on the way a nurse should approach an Italian American family for health teaching.
3. Identify nutritional preferences that may be found in persons of Italian descent.
4. Explain how dietary intake needs can be maintained by a patient who is lactose intolerant.
5. Explain the folk beliefs and practices that may influence how an Italian individual approaches a health problem.
6. Identify communication problems a nurse may encounter when interacting with an Italian American family.

REFERENCES

Allen, J.L., & Phelan, P.D. (1985). Incidence of cystic fibrosis in ethnic Italians and Greeks and in Australians of predominantly British origin. *Acta Paediatrica Scandinavica 74*(2), 286-289.

Auletta, K. (1987). Ken Auletta. In L. Cateura (Ed.), *Growing up Italian.* New York: William Morrow.

Bales, R.F. (1962). Attitudes toward drinking in the Irish culture. In Pittman, D.H., & Snyder, G.R. (Eds), *Society, culture, and drinking patterns.* New York: John Wiley & Sons.

Bates, E., MacWhinney, B., Caselli, C., Devescovi, A., Natale, F., & Venza, V. (1984). A cross-linguistic study of the development of sentence interpretation strategies. *Child Development, 55*(2), 341-354.

Bernardo, S. (1981). *The ethnic almanac.* New York: Doubleday.

Blane, H.T. (1987). Acculturation and drinking in an Italian American community. *Journal of Studies in Alcohol, 38*(7), 1324-1346.

Bohm, C.G. (1989, Sept. 26). Personal communication.

Bozzani, A., Penagini, R., & Velio, P. (1986). Lactose malabsorption and intolerance in Italians. *Digestive Diseases and Sciences, 31*(12), 1313-1316.

Burtis, G., Davis, J., & Martin, S. (1988). *Applied nutrition and diet therapy.* Philadelphia: W.B. Saunders.

Cacciola, E.J. (1982). Ethnic and cultural variations in the care of the aged: Some aspects of working with the Italian elderly. *Journal of Geriatric Psychiatry, 15*(2), 197-208.

Campbell, J.J., & Oski, F.A. (1977). Sickle cell anemia in an American White boy of Greek ancestry. *American Journal of Diseases in Children, 131,* 186-188.

Cateura, L. (Ed.). (1987). *Growing up Italian.* New York: William Morrow.

Ceriani, R., Succato, E., Fontana, M., Zuin, G., Ferrari, L., Principi, N., Paccagnini, S., & Mussini, E. (1988). Lactose malabsorption and recurrent abdominal pain in Italian children. *Clinical Pediatrica, 7*(6), 852-857.

Charlton, J., & Valez, R. (1986). Some international comparisons of mortality amenable to medical intervention. *British Medical Journal, 292,* 295-301.

Clark, W.B., & Midanik, L. (1982). Alcohol use and alcohol problems among U.S. adults: Results of the 1979 national survey. In National Institute of Alcohol Abuse and Alcoholism: Alcohol consumption and related problems. *Alcohol and Health Monograph, 1*(DHHS Pub. No. ADM 82-1190), 3-52.

Crowley, J.P., Sheth, S., Capone, R.J., & Schilling R.F. (1987). A paucity of thalassemia trait in Italian men with myocardial infarction. *Acta Haematology, 78*(4), 249-251.

Del Vecchio-Blanco, C., Caparaso, N., Tage-Jensen, U., Di Sapio, M., & Schlichting, P. (1984). *Scandinavian Journal of Gastroenterology, 19*(8), 1081-1085.

DeLuise, D. (1988). *Eat this: It'll make you feel better.* New York: Simon & Schuster.

Eveleth, P., & Tanner, J. (1976). *Worldwide variation in human growth.* New York: Cambridge University Press.

Farberow, N. (1975). *Suicide in different cultures.* Baltimore: University Park Press.

Giordano, J. (Ed.). (1986). *The Italian American catalog.* New York: Doubleday.

Gioseffi, D. (1987). Daniela Gioseffi. In L. Cateura (Ed.), *Growing up Italian.* New York: William Morrow.

Giuliani, R. (1987). Rudolph Giuliani. In L. Cateura (Ed.), *Growing up Italian.* New York: William Morrow.

Heien, D., & Pompelli, G. (1987). Stress, ethnic and distribution factors in a dichotomous response model of alcohol abuse. *Journal of Studies in Alcohol, 48*(5), 450-455.

Koopman, E., Eisenthal, S., & Stoeckle, J. (1984). Ethnicity in the reported pain, emotional distress and requests of medical outpatients. *Social Science and Medicine, 189*(8), 487-490.

Kromhout, D., Keys, A., & Aravanis, C. (1989). Food consumption patterns in the 1960's in seven countries. *American Journal of Clinical Nutrition, 49*, 889-894.

Lipton, J.A., & Marbach, J.J. (1984). Ethnicity and the pain experience. *Social Science Medicine, 19*(12), 1279-1298.

Marinucci, M., Massa, A., Care, A., Cianetti, L., Tenturi, L., & Sauli, S. (1982). Occurrence of Hb Riverdale-Bronx (beta 24 [b6] Gly replaced by Arg) in an Italian carrier. *Hemoglobin 6*(4), 423-425.

McKay, J., Hill, B., & Buckler, J. (1988). *A history of world societies.* Boston: Houghton Mifflin.

Migliore, S. (1989). Punctuality, pain, and time-orientation among Sicilian-Canadians. *Social Science and Medicine, 28*(8), 851-859.

Moscarelli, M., Maffei, C., & Cesana, B. (1987). An international perspective on assessment of negative and positive symptoms of schizophrenia. *American Journal of Psychiatry, 144*(12), 1595-1598.

Muhlin, G.L. (1985). Ethnic differences in alcohol misuse: A striking reaffirmation. *Journal of Studies in Alcohol, 46*(2), 172-178.

Nida, E. (1954). *Customs and cultures.* New York: Harper & Brothers.

Olivetti, E., Rendine, S., Cappello, N., Curtoni, E.S., & Piazza, A. (1986). The HLA system in Italy. *Human Heredity, 36*(6), 357-372.

Overfield, T. (1985). *Biological variation in health and illness.* Reading, Mass.: Addison-Wesley.

Pasquale C. (1989, Oct. 12). Personal communication.

Pasquale, M.D. (1989, Sep. 26). Personal communication.

Pasquali, E.A., Arnold, H.M., & Debasio, N. (1989). *Mental health nursing: A holistic approach.* St. Louis: C.V. Mosby.

Ragucci, A. (1981). Italian Americans. In A. Harwood (Ed.), *Ethnicity and medical care.* Cambridge, Mass.: Harvard University Press.

Rosmini, R., Gentili, G., & Wirz, M. (1987). Immunity to tetanus among Italians born between 1956 and 1963. *European Journal of Epidemiology and Biostatistics, 3*(3), 302-307.

Rotunno, M., & McGoldrick, M. (1982). Italian families. In M. McGoldrick, J.K. Pearce, & J. Giordano (Eds), *Ethnicity and family therapy.* New York: Guilford Press.

Rozendal, N. (1987). Understanding Italian American cultural norms. *Journal of Psychosocial Nursing and Mental Health Services, 25*(2), 29-33.

Santolamazza, D., Benincasa, A., & Scozzari, R. (1986). *Human Heredity, 36*(5), 281-285.

Simons, B. (Ed) (1976). Italy. In *The volume library.* Nashville, Tenn.: Southwestern Company.

Sirey, A. (1987). Aileen Riotto Sirey. In L. Cateura (Ed.), *Growing up Italian.* New York: William Morrow.

Smeal, E. (1987). Eleanor Cutri Smeal. In L. Cateura (Ed.), *Growing up Italian.* New York: William Morrow.

Spector, R. (1985). *Cultural diversity in health and illness.* East Norwalk, Conn.: Appleton-Century-Crofts.

Statistical reports. (1981). Washington, D.C.: U.S. Department of Commerce, Bureau of the Census.

Talese, G. (1987). Gay Talese. In L. Cateura (Ed.), *Growing up Italian.* New York: William Morrow.

Thain, S.L., Wainscoat, J.S., Sampietro, M, Old, J.M., Cappellini, D., Fiorelli, G., Modell, B., & Weatherall, D.J. (1987). Association of thalassaemia intermedia with a beta-globin gene haplotype. *British Journal of Haematology, 65*(3), 367-373.

Trevisan, M., Krogh, V., Farinaro, E., Panico, S., & Mancini, M. (1987, Dec.). Alcohol consumption, drinking pattern and blood pressure: Analysis of data from the Italian National Research Council Study. *International Journal of Epidemiology, 16*(4), 520-527.

U.S. Department of Commerce, Bureau of the Census. (1983). *1980 census of population—Ancestry of the population by state: 1980.* Washington, D.C.: U.S. Government Printing Office.

Venturi, R. (1987). Robert Venturi. In L. Cateura (Ed.), *Growing up Italian.* New York: William Morrow.

Zago, M.A., Costa, F.F., & Bottura, C. (1982). Thalassaemia intermedia in a family with beta o-thalassaemia and Hb hasharon. *Journal of Medical Genetics, 19*(6), 437-440.

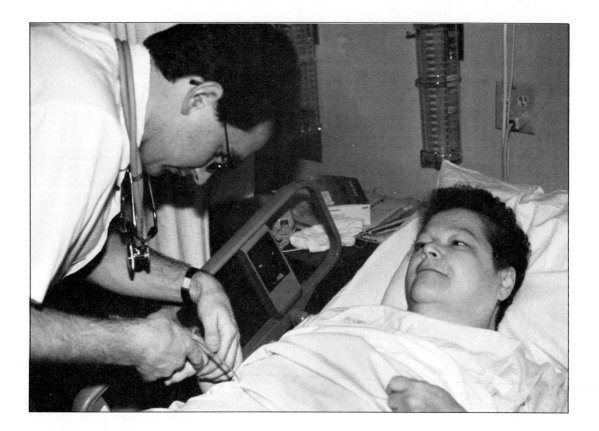

CHAPTER 14

■■

Irish Americans

Cheryl Martin

BEHAVIORAL OBJECTIVES
After reading this chapter, the nurse will be able to:

1 Recognize cultural factors that affect the health-seeking behaviors of Irish Americans.

2 Identify specific communication approaches for Irish Americans that influence health and wellness behaviors

3 Explain the distance and intimacy behaviors of Irish Americans and how health and wellness behaviors are influenced.

4 Identify the Irish American orientation to time and its influence on social and psychological behavior.

5 Recognize physical and biological variances that exist within and across Irish American groups in order to provide culturally appropriate nursing care.

OVERVIEW OF IRELAND

The Republic of Ireland covers approximately 85% of the island that bears its name. The Republic of Ireland comprises 26 counties that became the Irish Free State in 1921. The capital of Ireland is Dublin. In 1937 the Irish Free State was given the Gaelic name *Erie* by the constitution. Ireland is bordered on the northeast by Northern Ireland, which today remains a part of the United Kingdom, and is washed by the Atlantic Ocean to the west and south. St. George's Channel, the Irish Sea, and the North Channel separate Ireland from Great Britain by distances averaging at least 50 miles, or 80 kilometers.

The Republic of Ireland is primarily an agricultural country and is noted for the Irish potato. Industry is flourishing, and mining has become increasingly important because of recent discoveries of lead, silver, zinc, and copper deposits. Most of the countryside in Ireland is low land, is situated less than 500 feet above sea level, and is underlain by limestone rock. Most of the surface is covered by glacial drifts that are a legacy of the Pleistocene Ice Age. In some places in Ireland the drifts have been shaped into distinctive landforms that form a continuous belt across the island.

Most of Ireland has a cool, maritime climate. For example, in July temperatures vary from 61° F in the south to 57° F in the north. Winters are extremely mild, with January temperatures varying from 44° F in the Valentia to to 40° F in the northeast.

Ireland was colonized from Europe. For at least 5000 years there were successive waves of settlers who arrived from the island of Great Britain. Each group of settlers contributed to the heritage of the modern Irish nation. Even today, the Celtic influence remains dominant in Ireland. However, the eastern portion of Ireland has been particularly influenced by the Anglo-Normans, whose initial invasion of 1170 was followed by the subsequent immigration of settlers from England, Wales, and Scotland. The population of Ireland rapidly expanded during the eighteenth and early nineteenth centuries and reached a peak of 8.1 million people in 1841. However, the great potato famine, which began in 1845, brought a reversal of the population trend as a result of the many deaths and massive migration to the United States and Great Britain. This exodus continued over the next 100 years, and by 1930 the population of Ireland numbered little more than half of the original 1845 figure. Today, the population is approximately 3,368,217 (*Statistical Reports,* 1981) and is of mixed origin (McKay, Hall, & Buckler, 1989).

Nursing is less institutionalized in Ireland because of the rural society with "country" traditions. Even in Dublin, which contains more than one third of the population, many of the people have relatives who live in the country, and therefore there is a mass exodus on weekends to the countryside. Nursing is considered a desirable career, and families are proud to claim a nurse "in the family" (Slack, 1982).

IMMIGRATION TO THE UNITED STATES

The large number of Catholic Irish immigrants of the famine years were not the first Irish people to have immigrated to the United States. The famine immigrants were preceded by their Irish countrymen in the seventeenth and eighteenth centuries, although in smaller numbers (Fallows, 1979). Many of the earlier immigrants, particularly during the seventeenth and eighteenth centuries, were Protestants from the northern county of Ulster and thus came to the United States under less dramatic circumstances than the population that came later. The early Ulster immigrants arrived in the United States just in time to help the Americans win independence from England. At that time many Irish American immigrants regarded themselves as members of the Anglo-American society. This distinction was not made to deny their Irish origin, but to embrace their new heritage. By the mid-1800s Irish organizations were established in the major cities of America, but even today, Irish descendants note their Irish extraction more as a point of historical interest than as an identification with social relevance for their lives. According to Greeley and McCready (1975), Irish Americans, in the process of adapting to American life, began to think and behave like their American counterparts.

There are approximately 16 million people of Irish descent who reside in the United States, or approximately 8% of the U.S. population (*Statistical Reports,* 1981). Irish Americans have become so assimilated into the mainstream of American society that today they are more likely to be professionals or managers and less likely to be laborers, service workers, or factory hands (Blessing, 1980).

COMMUNICATION

The official language of Ireland is Irish. However, English is recognized as the second official language. English is universally spoken throughout Ireland, and approximately 27% of the population know both Irish and English. Irish is more widely used in the west and is the first language of people in remote areas of Ireland.

To understand the development of language in Ireland, it is essential to understand the historical significance of the Celtic language. Because the Celtics developed a written language quite late, the people were forced to rely heavily on the oral transmission of laws, customs, religions, and philosophy; and poetry became a useful mnemonic device for transmitting tradition. According to legend, the ancient heroes of the mythological cycle, which included Finn MacCool and Cuchulain, were clearly in love with the sound of their own voices. Modern-day Irish people are much like the ancient Celtics; the Irish politician and the Irish priest have the same love for using many words (Greeley, 1981). Greeley (1981) suggested that for Irish people, playing with the language was not only a means of communication, but also provided a portion of their enjoyment and pleasure. It should be noted that languages throughout the world that have survived from an earlier period have not only elaborate language structures, but also more extensive vocabularies. It has been suggested that the reason for this is that spoken language needs to be more flexible and descriptive than written language.

For people in the western part of Ireland, the vocabulary is about one half as extensive as the vocabulary of the well-educated English speaker of London. It has also been noted that people who live in the Gaeltacht, or the Irish-speaking regions in the west, tend to have an extensive English-speaking vocabulary. According to Greeley (1981), modern-day Irish people delight in ridicule, scatology (elaborate obscenity), limericks, puns, and riddles. Although a modern-day Irish language exists, the Irish language for all practical purposes was almost destroyed during the second half of the nineteenth century with the onslaught of the English language.

Since many Irish persons arrived in the United States with knowledge of English, assimilation into the predominant culture was enhanced. However, in spite of the use of English words, some words have different meanings for the Irish. For example, the word *homely,* which is commonly used in the United States to describe someone who is plain and not attractive, is used by some Irish people as an endearing word to describe hospitality. An Irish guest after a dinner may hug the host or hostess and say, "Thank you for being so homely."

Implications for Nursing Care

It is important for the nurse to understand that some Irish Americans who may be encountered in the health care system may not have an extensive vocabulary, but the words they use may be used with exaggeration. Since for some Irish people language is a form of entertainment and power, the patient may attempt to communicate needs through flowery and sometimes exaggerated words. For example, the nurse should be careful to evaluate physical signs and symptoms of pain in addition to verbal descriptions to assist in an accurate assessment of the need for nursing intervention.

Zola (1966) compared Italian Americans and Irish Americans and their descriptive methods of presenting complaints. The findings of the study indicated that when Italian Americans and Irish Americans were asked, "Where does it hurt?" the Irish American respondents were more likely to locate chief problems in the eyes, ears, nose, or throat. In a similar question the respondents were asked to identify the most important areas of the body. Again, for the Irish American respondents, the emphasis was on the eyes, ears, nose, and throat. Another finding of the study was that the Irish Americans more often than the Italian Americans denied that pain was a part of their illness. When Irish American respondents were asked about the presence of pain, some of them hedged their replies with qualifications such as "It is more a throbbing than a pain," "It is not really a pain; it feels more like sand in my eye," or " It feels more like a pinprick than a pain." The conclusion of the study was that the Irish Americans, through such comments, were reflecting something more than an objective reaction to their physical condition. The Irish Americans were found to describe their chief problems in terms of specific dysfunctions, and what appeared to emerge from the study was that Irish persons limit and understate their physical difficulties, whereas Italians spread and generalize theirs.

The importance of culture in the way Irish persons respond to questions regarding pain is further substantiated by the work of Zborowski (1952), who noted that Irish people pretend they have no pain (Spector, 1985). The astute nurse must keep in mind that the Irish American patient may tend to be overly verbose in descriptions of conditions, but this does not imply that the patient is being objective or accurately descriptive about the nature of the condition. The nurse should use a combination of open-ended and closed questions to solicit specific information from which culturally appropriate nursing care can be planned.

SPACE

Space is an essential component in a cultural framework of nursing, since from the beginning of modern time, philosophers, mathematicians, psychologists, and ethnologists have studied the phenomenon of space. *Territoriality, proximity,* and *personal space* are all terms that have been used to describe space. The word *territoriality* was initially used to describe the physical area that animals claim as their own and defend from predators, but in modern times the term has been extended to describe human behavior as well (Hall, 1959). Hall (1963) coined the term "proxemics" to describe the use of space as an elaboration of a culture. According to Hall (1966), individuals by virtue of their culture have four ways of perceiving distance: as intimate distance (from 6 to 8 inches), as personal distance (from 6 inches to 4 feet), as social distance (from 4 to 12 feet), or as public distance (from 12 to 25 feet). Hall (1966) concluded that the use of space explains communication in various cultures.

Space is a cultural phenomenon that is infrequently noted in the literature about the Irish. Greeley (1981) has noted, however, that Irish American students often require more time to become articulate and self-confident in a high-powered academic environment, and that this can be seen in the student's spatial relationships with others. The Irish American student is more likely to sit off in a corner for several semesters, only to be "discovered" later as having produced brilliant work, for the most part in solitude (Greeley, 1981). Some authors (Fallows, 1979; Greeley, 1981) have also noted that Irish individuals are less likely to be physically affectionate in both their interpersonal and their family relationships.

Implications for Nursing Care

The use of space, in its simplest terms, is a means of nonverbal communication (Stillman, 1978). How individuals feel about their own personal space determines how much intrusion by others is considered acceptable. Since health care often occurs in what is described as an intimate zone, spatial issues have important implications for the nurse.

Since Irish Americans are perceived as having a past-oriented culture that relies heavily on extended family ties, the personal space of some Irish Americans is extremely limited (Fallows, 1979). In other words, since some Irish American patients may be accustomed to having family members close by, they may have a need for close proximity of family members during illness; however, according to Greeley (1981), despite the closeness of the family unit, Irish American families have a tendency to collapse the personal space inward, more so than in other cultures.

One difficulty that has been noted in Irish American families is difficulty expressing love and affection. Some have more difficulty in expression with close family members than with more distant persons, creating an isolated and greatly expanded personal space. Others express feelings somewhat readily with a close group of intimates but not with persons more distant. The nurse should be cognizant of the possible effects of attitudes and values about space that may affect individuals from different cultures. By assessing the patient on an individual basis, the nurse can provide culturally appropriate care. One major objective for the nurse may be to assist the family in recognizing the need to convey warmth, feelings, and attitudes in order to create a supportive and nurturing spatial environment for the patient that will promote recovery.

SOCIAL ORGANIZATION
Family

The famine years had a significant impact on the structure of the Irish American family. As the famine progressed, the resulting experiences dramatically altered the family system in Ireland. The immigrants brought this altered family structure to America and formed their own ethnic societies. Most of those who immigrated to the United States from Ireland were between the ages of 15 and 35, since it was these able-bodied individuals who were most able to leave (Kennedy, 1973; McKay, Hill, & Buckler, 1989).

Ireland stands alone in losing such a large proportion of its population to emigration. Even in modern times, more Irish people live outside Ireland than in it, and most Irish families have at least some members living in the United States (Fallows, 1979). A wide range of disparity has been noted regarding the link between Irish Americans and the family in the homeland. For some Irish Americans there appears to be an almost mystical link between the family in America and the roots in Ireland. These roots often lead to a particular farm that may still be inhabited by a remnant of that particular clan. For other Irish Americans there is almost no link remaining except the knowledge that an ancestor originated in Ireland. The family values and ethnic traits are often transmitted to the next generation unconsciously by imitation of the parental model.

Prior to the famine years, families in the southern and western parts of Ireland were traditionally Irish speaking, Catholic, and subsistence farmers. The typical couple married early, had many children, and on the father's death subdivided the land among the sons. The agricultural pattern of the prefamine years no doubt was instrumental in creating the almost total reliance of the Irish on the potato crop. However, this pattern of continuous subdividing of the land among family members also contributed to the close family bonds, which were evidenced by parental demands for respectful attention and by obedience to marriages arranged by the parents to ensure appropriate bonds between families and clans. These family bonds continued even after immigration to America, as evidenced by the fact that it was the responsibility of many immigrants to send back money to pay the passage for another family member to come to America (Kennedy, 1973).

Marriage

In the past there was intense social pressure among Irish Americans regarding mate selection; marriage within the Irish Catholic community was considered preferable. Therefore the Irish neighborhoods in the United States often served as the social context for the meeting and pairing off of the young immigrants (Wessel, 1931). For the early Irish settlers, marriage with non-Irish Catholics was a permissive alternative. However, these marriages generally followed a preferential hierarchy in which the early-arriving English or German Catholics were considered more suitable than the later-arriving Irish Catholics (Abramson, 1973; Alba, 1976). By the time of the third generation of immigrants, a tendency was noted for the socially aspiring Irish Catholic to marry a Protestant or even convert to Protestantism. These practices were generally disapproved of by other Irish American Catholics. Even today in stable communities in the United States, intermarriage between Irish families remains one of the clearest distinctions of social acceptance and social equality in the Irish American community.

A number of studies have portrayed marriage among the Irish as an uneasy practical alliance that provided little affection or intimacy between partners. Sex and procreation were reported to be duties rather than joys or expressive activities in some of the marriages reported in the studies by Albon and Cunningham (1981)

Bachelorhood and spinsterhood are infrequent among Irish Americans, with only 14% of men and 12% of women not married according to a study by Greeley (1981). The typical Irish American Catholic woman marries at 22 years of age, and the typical Irish American Catholic man marries at 24.5 years of age. Although this is a bit older than the American average, the practice in ancient Ireland was to delay marriage until the early 30s. Greeley (1977) has noted that Irish American Catholics are less likely than Irish American Protestants to marry before the age of 21. Greeley (1977) has also noted that Irish American Catholics are less likely to become divorced and are more likely to have three or more children. The mean number of children for Irish American families is 2.6, as compared with the national mean of 2.4. As family planning becomes more progressive among Irish American Catholics, the number of children is decreasing.

Role of women

One traditional view of Irish women was that they were controlling matriarchs on whom sons and husbands were dependent (Messenger, 1969). A contrasting view held that male dominance began as a pattern in Ireland following the mass emigrations. According to Fallows (1979), the women were expected to be subservient in every way and assist their husbands with what was considered "men's work" in addition to completing their own, traditionally female tasks.

Greeley (1972) has noted that some Irish women find it hard to resist the temptation to become stiff, if not frigid, when sexual advances are made by a mate. According to Greeley (1972), sexual relations have been viewed as a matter of duty by some Irish women, whereas others are able to be warm and loving with their mate. Also, according to Greeley (1972), some Irish American Catholic women have reported feeling obligated to admit any failures regarding sexual performance at the next confession, and some Irish American women have felt such an obligation to the "duty" of marital sexual relations that this obligation has continued for periods of 20 or 30 years of marriage even if no pleasure is experienced.

A representative study of female college graduates by Greeley and McCready (1975) found that Irish American women are more likely than their Anglo-American counterparts to view the wife-mother role as the dominant one in marriage. The findings also suggest that Irish-American women view the mother's working as detrimental to children and see the role of the wife as a helpmate to the husband. The data further suggest that Irish American women are less likely to stress the importance of security or of keeping up family contacts or relationships with parents or in-laws, or to view their daughters' independence as important. A final conclusion of the study was that Irish American women are less likely to report tense relationships with their mothers; however, they are more likely to report tense relationships with their fathers.

Role of men

Greeley (1972) has noted that while Irish men, particularly when intoxicated, may spin tall tales and recite romantic poetry about their true love, in intimate relationships they often become awkward and tongue-tied, and may become clumsy, if not rough, in any attempts at intimacy. The male dominance that began in Ireland as a result of the change in family structure between 1840 and 1940 is paralleled even today among Irish Americans (Fallows, 1979).

Adolescent Irish Americans

Porteous (1985) conducted a study of adolescents in England and Ireland to determine if problems experienced by adolescents varied systematically with age, sex, and culture. The data from this study suggest that in both countries boys are less mature than girls in problem experience and at the same time are more concerned with authority, self-image, and behavioral problems, whereas girls appear to have more worries in personal and emotional areas. The data also suggest that in both countries boys, as well as girls, are more concerned with feelings of self-inadequacy, which increase with age, whereas the concerns expressed by both boys and girls in other areas seemingly decrease with age. The data further suggest that Irish adolescents have a less mature problem pattern than their English counterparts; however, Irish adolescents in the study admitted to having more worries. The conclusion of the study was that cultural differences are specifically reflected in adolescent problem experiences.

Religion

The church of Ireland is an independent Anglican church found in both the Republic of Ireland and Northern Ireland. The church traces its Episcopal succession from the pre-Reformation church in Ireland. Christianity is thought to have existed in Ireland before the missionary activities of Patrick, the Patron Saint of Ireland, in the late fifth century. The early church in Ireland was monastic, without parochial or diocesan divisions or central government. If there was authority within the structure of the church, it rested with the abbot and the bishops.

As church members in the United States, both Irish American Protestants and Irish American Catholics have had a significant impact on the development of hospitals, schools, colleges, and churches, not only in the growing cities on the East Coast, but in towns and cities across the country (Shannon, 1981).

In Ireland the Catholic church has been faced with a dilemma because of the desire to preserve the Catholic moral tone. In this regard the Catholic church has found it necessary to relegate the prevention of AIDS through the promotion of condoms and safe sexual practices to the government as its official responsibility. Most Catholic churches advocate abstinence before marriage and avoidance of sexual behavior by some high-risk groups, such as homosexuals.

Political Influences

Immigrants from Ireland have significantly contributed to the development of the United States from its inception (Griffin, 1981). In fact, eight Irish individuals signed the Declaration of Independence, and five died in the Boston Massacre. About one third of the people in the United States can trace all or part of their lineage to Irish ancestry. It has been reported that three presidents, including Andrew Jackson, James Buchanan, and Chester Arthur, were sons of Irish immigrants. Irish individuals have been active in all walks of American life, including the formation and growth of trade unions and active service on police forces across the country, and have served admirably in the army and in the navy (Griffin, 1981).

Irish Americans have enjoyed a significant and spectacular rise in the political arena in this country, in part because of the block voting of these individuals in large cities, where they generally were the largest single group. The fact that this voting practice assured the Irish of political influence was evident by the 1800s, particularly in Boston, where the first Irish American mayors were elected. During this same period in New York, the Irish controlled many political machines. Among the most noted Irish American political bosses were John F. Fitzgerald, Richard J. Daley, "Big Tim" Sullivan, and James Michael Curley. The success of the Irish was due in part to their strong sense of group solidarity, to their fluency with the spoken word, and to personal charm. Historically the Irish were known as the most successful enhancers of corrupt politics. Today, the voting patterns for Irish Americans remain about the same as for other Americans. In addition, with the election of the first Irish Catholic president in 1960, the issue of an Irish Catholic president became obsolete.

Implications for Nursing Care

The nurse must keep in mind that the one reemerging theme among Irish Americans is the significance of the family and family structure. It is difficult for people from other cultures to perceive the importance of the family structure to some cultural groups such as the Irish Americans. Since Irish Americans are viewed as having a relational orientation that is lineal in nature, nursing interventions are likely to be successful only if family involvement in the care and treatment of the patient is maximized.

Kluckhohn and Strodtbeck (1961) viewed relational orientation in families as having three subdivisions: lateral (collateral), lineal, and individualistic. For families with a lateral (collateral) mode of orientation, the goals and welfare of laterally extended groups, including siblings and peers, take on paramount importance. This type of family assumes responsibility for all of its members. Therefore the goals of the individual family members become subordinate to those of the family group. When the lineal mode is present as the major focus in family groups, the goals and welfare of the group may also have primary importance, because the family members view culture and kinship bounds as the primary basis for maintaining lineage.

A contrasting mode that is held by some families is the individualistic mode of orientation. For families with this orientation, individual goals are viewed as being more important than specific lateral or lineal goals. In this type of family each individual member is held responsible for personal behavior and is therefore judged according to personal accomplishments (Haber et al., 1987).

Since Irish Americans are perceived as having a lineal relationship, it is important for the nurse to seek the family's advice and opinions on treatment for the patient. In addition, since the family is perceived as being a source of anxiety and tension because of restricted family roles, it is important for the nurse to assist the family in identifying the boundaries of each role and the characteristics of the roles. If the family determines that the boundaries are restricted and do not overlap, the nurse must accept this fact and recognize and appreciate that such families function with a hierarchical ranking of family roles. Therefore lack of recognition on the part of a nurse may foster feelings of anxiety and tension on the part of those persons who are considered to be at the top of the hierarchical ranking, such as the father or the mother.

Since Irish Americans tend to delineate roles and behaviors within the family structure by virtue of sexual orientation (female or male), it is important for the nurse not to minimize the significance of ranked ordering of behavior. For example, some Irish American women may view their role as primary caretaker of the family, and therefore when this person is ill, her role function is greatly compromised. In this case the patient must be assisted in developing strategies to help the family meet its needs in the absence of the primary caretaker.

It is also important for the nurse to remember that for some Irish Americans religion and religious views take on paramount importance in maintaining the social integrity of the individual. The astute nurse should solicit information on religious practices that are deemed essential to the optimal functioning of the Irish American patient. Lack of recognition of the significance of religious beliefs may serve to augment problems and difficulties encountered with illness.

TIME

According to Kluckhohn and Strodtbeck (1961), the cultural interpretation of time has a three-point range of variability that includes past, present, and future orientations. In this model Irish Americans are viewed as having a past-oriented culture.

Kluckhohn and Strodtbeck have noted that all cultures must deal with all three time orientations. Where cultures differ regarding time perspective is in the preferential ordering of the orientations, and a great deal about a society can be learned and predicted from this preferential ordering. For example, Irish Americans are perceived as members of a first-ordered past-oriented society, since some Irish Americans have a strong allegiance to the past, worship their ancestors, and have a strong family tradition. In addition, persons from cultures with past-oriented time perspectives may have the attitude that nothing new ever happens in the present or will ever happen in the future because it all happened in the far-distant past. For example, an Irish American who is shown a new invention may remark, "Our ancestors were making something similar to this 100 years ago." Persons in the dominant culture may find it difficult to understand the respect that Irish Americans have for tradition, and at the same time some Irish Americans do not appreciate the typical American disregard for tradition.

Implications for Nursing Care

Since some past-oriented people are perceived as lacking an understanding of rhythmicity and periodicity, it is likely that they may also be perceived as being noncompliant regarding scheduled medical and therapeutic interventions. Because some individuals with a past time orientation view man as being subjugated to nature, there may be a tendency for a fatalistic orientation that affects the time orientation. In other words, some people with a past time orientation believe that time and nature will alleviate the problem and tend to wait until the last possible moment to seek medical intervention for acute or chronic medical problems.

The astute nurse must recognize that noncompliance is not necessarily an inherent quality of the personality but may be related to a lack of understanding regarding the time perspective. For example, individuals with a past-oriented perspective view time as being elastic, and therefore a moment in time has the possibility of being recaptured (Mbiti, 1970). The nurse must plan activities with the patient that encourage the patient to adhere to the necessary aspects of the time perspective, as in the case of time-released insulin or heart medication. The patient should be advised or encouraged to arrive at least 30 or 45 minutes early for other activities that require adherence to a fixed schedule.

ENVIRONMENTAL CONTROL
Locus of Control

Kluckhohn and Strodtbeck (1961) developed a five-concept value orientation framework that includes (1) perceptions of human nature, (2) the relationship of man with nature, (3) time orientation, (4) activity orientation, and (5) relational orientation. In this model Irish Americans are viewed as being a past-oriented culture because some Irish Americans hold the view that man is basically evil and subjugated to nature, and they have family and social relationships that are lineal in nature. Also, they tend to cling to a past-oriented value orientation in regard to the family and family relationships and tend to consider past values and traditions to be of paramount importance to future growth and development. Greeley and McCready (1975) found in a national sample of Anglo-American Protestant males and Irish American Catholic males that the Irish Americans in the study were more fatalistic, less authoritarian, less anxious, and more trusting than their Anglo-American counterparts. Because Irish Americans hold a value orientation that views man as being subjugated to nature, some Irish Americans are viewed as having an external locus of control.

Perception of Illness

According to Zola (1966), every individual has an orientation to problems that corresponds with the way this person handles problems. For Irish Americans the world view of life is expressed through fasts, which are symbolic of prior deprivations in their lives. Some Irish Americans have life patterns that have alternated between overindulgence and self-deprivation (Zola, 1966). Many psychologists believe that the expected and limited nature of these irregular, extreme cycles is correlated with alcohol use, and that for some Irish Americans continued use of defense mechanisms to ignore or dispel previous conditions or symptoms is the norm rather than the exception. Some Irish Americans have a view of life that states, "Life is black and long suffering and therefore the less said about life the better" (Zola, 1966). It is this statement that best reflects the way in which some Irish Americans handle the concept of illness.

While in some cultural groups the ignoring of bodily complaints is not normative, for some Irish Americans this appears to be a culturally prescribed and supported defense mechanism. For some Irish Americans the use of defense mechanisms (ignoring and denying) appears to be the typical way of coping with psychological and physiological needs. An example of this is that some Irish Americans will state regarding an illness, "I ignore it as I do most other things." This point reemphasizes the fact that for some Irish Americans there is a tendency to understand the implications of the illness but, at the same time, to refrain from expressing illness-related complaints.

Illness/Wellness Behaviors

It can be said that the consistency of the Irish illness behavior can also be perceived in two other contexts. First, for some Irish Americans illness or the perception of illness helps perpetuate a self-fulfilling prophecy. It has been said that the way in which some Irish Americans have communicated complaints, and at the same time done very little to make treatment easy, for the most part has assured these individuals of continued suffering (Zola, 1966). In addition, for some Irish Americans illness behavior can be linked to sin and guilt ideology, which seems to pervade a major portion of Irish American society even today. This is evidenced by the fact that in the Irish American culture there is great restraint, which opens the door for constant temptation, which must be denied. The perception held by some Irish Americans is that the flesh is weak and the individual is very likely to sin. This theme is reinforced even in the way in which symptoms are localized. According to Zola (1966), Irish Americans localize complaints in the eyes, ears, or throat, which might be a symbolic reflection of the more immediate source of sin and guilt. For example, it might be said that these three localizing areas of complaints are congruent with what should have been seen, what should have been heard, or what should have been said.

Folk Medicine

Some Irish Americans subscribe to folk medicine beliefs that can be perceived as neutral health practices (neither having benefit nor producing harm), such as the "blessing of the throat" and the wearing of holy medals to prevent illnesses. Additional folk medicine beliefs that are considered neutral include the practices of tying a bag of camphor around the neck to prevent flu during the flu season, never looking in a mirror at night and closing closet doors to prevent evil spirits from entering the body, and finally, above all, maintaining a strong family with lots of love to prevent illnesses.

Other folk medicine beliefs practiced by some Irish Americans may be perceived as harmful, such as the practices of eating lots of oily foods, cleansing the bowels every 8 days with senna, and seeing a doctor only in an emergency. For some Irish Americans the first level of intervention is often home treatment because of the belief that a doctor should be seen only in an emergency, and this practice may create a reactive rather than a preventive model of treatment. For example, for the treatment of a throat condition, the first level of intervention may be home treatment with such things as iodine or kerosene to paint the throat or honey and lemon to soothe the throat. Another example of a practice that might be perceived as harmful is the home treatment of nausea and other stomach ailments that might have serious implications with such remedies as hot tea, castor oil, or eating potatoes or gruel.

Some Irish Americans subscribe to folk medicine practices that may be perceived as beneficial, such as the practices of getting lots of rest and going to bed early, enjoying fresh air and sunshine and exercising outdoors, dressing warmly, and keeping the feet warm. Many also believe that one must eat good food, take vitamins, and balance the diet. In addition, there seems to be an overriding belief that in order to stay healthy, one must be goal oriented and nurture a strong religious faith. The combination of positive thinking along with healthy practices such as exercise and adequate rest can contribute to optimal wellness (Spector, 1985).

Implications for Nursing Care

Since some Irish Americans are perceived as having an external locus of control, the astute nurse must devise a teaching plan that emphasizes the importance of preventive techniques to maintain optimal wellness and prevent illness. The nurse should recognize the importance of assisting the patient in developing a sensitivity and an understanding about wellness that will alleviate fatalistic beliefs about life in general and illness in particular. It is important for the nurse to understand that compliance with a health regimen is much more complex than the mere recognition and prescription of such a plan. The nurse must keep in mind that philosophical beliefs and attitudes play a major role not only in the perception of health and wellness, but also in compliance behavior.

Since the first level of treatment for an illness for some Irish Americans may be home treatment, it is important for the nurse to ascertain for the patient which of these practices are neutral or beneficial and thus may be retained and incorporated into the plan of care, and which of these practices are harmful. The nurse must devise teaching strategies that assist the patient in developing an understanding about harmful folk medical practices in order for such practices to be eliminated from the typical health care regimen of the patient. The nurse must realize that complete avoidance of harmful practices is initially difficult and that a reduction in such behaviors should be considered significant.

BIOLOGICAL VARIATIONS

Lipton and Marbach (1984) conducted a study to examine interethnic differences and similarities in reported pain experiences among Blacks, Irish persons, Italians, Jewish persons, and Puerto Ricans and found that responses, attitudes, and descriptions of pain were relatively similar after controlling for variables shown by previous studies to influence reported pain experiences. These variables included symptom history; signs elicited on physical, radiographic, and laboratory examination; and social, cultural, and psychological data. No significant intraethnic differences were noted regarding the patients' emotionality (that is, stoicism versus expressiveness) in regard to pain and the overall interference in daily functioning attributed to pain. The data suggest that the pain experiences reported by Black, Italian, and Jewish patients were almost identical, whereas the pain experiences of Irish and Puerto Rican patients appeared to be relatively distinctive from those of the other groups and from those of each other. The variable that most influenced differences for Irish patients was social assimilation. The conclusion of the study was that intraethnic homogeneity is present for most aspects of the pain experience; however intraethnic heterogeneity also exists for factors that influence the experience of pain.

AIDS Risk

Of the number of reported cases of acquired immunodeficiency syndrome (AIDS) in the United States among Irish Americans, there is a low incidence reported for homosexuals (Lewis, 1988). The number of reported cases of AIDS among Irish Americans appears to be predominantly related to intravenous drug use. This has been further substantiated in a study by Walsh (1987), in which 11,640 persons in Ireland were tested for antibodies to the AIDS (human immunodeficiency) virus. Of this number, 626 were found to have antibodies to the virus, and 412 of these were identified as being intravenous drug users, including 28 infants born to mothers who were intravenous drug users (Lewis, 1988). The data would suggest that Irish people subscribe, in part or in full, to the doctrines of the Catholic Church, which include monogamous relationships, no premarital relationships, and no homosexual relationships. On the other hand, lack of sexual enhancement, failure to relieve aggressive tendencies, and the characteristics of a dominant family life-style may be related to the incidence of AIDS among Irish persons who are intravenous drug users (Lewis, 1988).

Psychological Characteristics
Alcoholism

Among American ethnic groups, Irish Americans have been ranked the highest or near highest in terms of heavy alcohol intake, loss of control, and untoward social consequences (Estes & Heinemann, 1986; Walsh, 1968, 1969; Walsh & Walsh, 1973). The Irish in Ireland have ranked among the highest groups internationally for the prevalence of alcohol-related problems (Walsh, 1969). Stivers (1976) concluded that heavy drinking among Irish men is directly related to the patterns and characteristics of the family, social, and economic systems. It has been further suggested that membership in the hard Irish drinking peer group was traditionally legitimized because of the status of the sons who did not inherit land (Ablon & Cunningham, 1981).

Greeley (1972) concluded that the Irish often drink for reassurance, to escape from intolerable psychological burdens, and to repress sexuality and aggressiveness. Greeley (1972) has further characterized the domination of the Irish American mother as a causative factor in male alcoholism because she rules her family by strong will or by subtly manipulating the sympathies of her husband and children. Ablon and Cunningham (1981) have substantiated the possibility of female domination as an etiological factor in the development of alcoholism among Irish men. They found in their study that problem drinking was positively linked most closely to the Irish and that in cases where a man's parents were both Irish, a serious alcohol problem was likely to be present. They also found that in cases where a man had an Irish mother but a father from another ethnic group, if that father was characterized as a heavy drinker, even if not an alcoholic, the subject was likely to have a drinking problem.

Adolescents and drinking behavior

O'Conner (1978) noted that an expectation for enhanced sociability was directly related to drinking among Irish young adults. The respondents in this study had a prominent wish for a reduction in anxiety. Very little information is available regarding the drinking behavior of Irish adolescents. More information about adolescent Irish drinking would be helpful in addressing Irish adult drinking behavior.

Christiansen and Teahan (1987) conducted a study that examined the drinking behavior of Irish adolescents in two stages. The first stage compared the drinking behavior of Irish adolescents with the drinking behavior of American adolescents. During the second stage the adolescents' expectations regarding the effects of alcohol were measured. In the study it was thought that adolescent expectancies might initially arise from social learning processes, including acculturation from parents who drink or are alcoholics. However, the data from the study suggest that Irish adolescents drink less and experience fewer alcohol-related problems than their American counterparts across all ethnic adolescent groups, including Irish Americans. The findings of Christiansen and Teahan are not surprising, since approximately 95% of the population in Ireland are reported to be Roman Catholic, and adolescents are prohibited from drinking as a religious decree at the time of confirmation and are expected to pledge abstinence until age 21. However, although Irish adolescents did not report as many alcohol-related problems as their American counterparts, when social drinking occurred among these adolescents, drinking-related problems were noted. A conclusion was that Irish adolescents had a lower expectation for sexual enhancement; however, they believed that alcohol would result in increased arousal and release of aggression.

The problems identified in Irish adolescents, such as lack of sexual enhancement and lack of ability to release aggression, have also been noted among adult Irish alcoholics. Although Irish adolescents are noted to drink less and experience fewer alcohol-related problems, Ireland has one of the highest rates of alcoholism among the adult population.

Implications for Nursing Care

The nurse should keep in mind that for Irish Americans the problem of alcoholism is one that is influenced by a variety of factors, including patterns and characteristics of the family, social and economic conditions, and psychological orientation, rather than a biological variation per se. Since some Irish American adults and adolescents drink for reassurance and to escape what is perceived as an intolerable burden, the nurse must develop strategies to teach such individuals more positive ways to alleviate stress and tension. Such individuals should be taught to verbally communicate feelings and anxiety rather than repressing or denying such feelings. The patient must be taught the value of verbal expression to communicate needs. In addition, it is important to assist these patients in developing positive outlooks on life that may be perceived as positive coping strategies. The nurse also must remember the value of working not only with the patient, but also with the family, since some Irish Americans perceive family relationships as being paramount to a healthy existence.

The nurse might devise a family systems strategy that identifies perceived and actual roles within the family structure. After the roles are delineated, the nurse should assist the family in identifying undesirable behaviors manifested by persons in the particular roles. Changing behaviors that negatively impact on the entire family system cannot be accomplished overnight. Such interventions are likely to need repeated reinforcement over a period of time. However, the nurse must keep in mind that since some Irish Americans report that their drinking behavior is a result of their situation in life, it is important to consider the family's social and economic variables as a realistic beginning point in the initial intervention and treatment of such patients.

SUMMARY

Irish Americans have enjoyed extraordinary success in the United States. Although once faced with religious bigotry and economic hardship, Irish Americans nevertheless managed to cope with these problems and frequently turned them to their advantage.

Nurses should develop a sensitivity and understanding of individuals from a transcultural perspective in order to provide culturally appropriate nursing care. Nursing schools throughout the United States should incorporate transcultural courses and transcultural concepts into the nursing curriculum to foster the development of a transcultural understanding. One such institution that has developed a course to facilitate transcultural understanding is Vanderbilt University, which has a course entitled "International Perspectives of Nursing and Health Care." This course was designed to offer graduate and undergraduate students an experiential learning opportunity for the development of a theoretical base in nursing and health care in countries other than the United States. During this experience students spend time in Dublin, Edinburgh, and London. Macy and Morgan (1988) described the experiences of students in this course; for example, while in Dublin students noted that 90% of the deliveries were attended by midwives, who were usually assisted by student midwives. During this experience students were able to compare the differences in nursing and medical techniques found in other countries and to assess the need to modify care based on transcultural concepts.

CASE
STUDY

Mr. Jonathon McMartin, a 46-year-old Irish Catholic American, is admitted to an in-house alcoholic treatment center at a local hospital. Mr. McMartin came to the United States 10 years ago with his wife and his five children, who now range in age from 11 to 23. Of the five children, four still live at home. In addition, Mr. McMartin's mother and father live within five blocks of him. Mr. McMartin also has seven siblings; three of these siblings still reside in Ireland, and four live in the same city as Mr. McMartin. Mr. McMartin reports to the nurse therapist who admits him to the unit that his problem occurred because he feels isolated from his immediate family. He states that his wife is very cold and unaffectionate and appears to mobilize the children to her way of thinking. Mr. McMartin says his children appear very distant from him and closer to their mother. He also reports that as a child growing up, he felt the same way about his mother and father: he felt close to his mother and very distant from his father. Mr. McMartin reveals to the nurse that he believes he can stop drinking any time he desires.

CARE
PLAN

Nursing Diagnosis   Health maintenance, altered, related to use and abuse of alcohol.

Patient Outcomes	***Nursing Interventions***
1 Patient and family will verbalize a desire to learn more about alcoholism and appropriate techniques to reduce symptomatology.	1 Identify with patient and family sociocultural factors that influence health-seeking behaviors.
2 Patient and family will verbalize a willingness to comply with psychiatric therapeutic regimen.	2 Determine with patient and family their knowledge level about alcoholism and the severity of this illness.
3 Patient and family will verbalize an understanding of the need to comply with routine, scheduled follow-up visits to maintain an alcohol-free environment.	3 Determine with patient and family their willingness to adapt to an alternate lifestyle free of alcohol.

Nursing Diagnosis   Parenting, altered, potential, related to perceived emotional distance in family.

Patient Outcomes	***Nursing Interventions***
1 Parents will develop an adequate base for effective parenting.	1 Assist parents in identifying present expectations of self, spouse, and children within the family system.
2 Parents will develop realistic expectations of self, spouse, and children within the family system.	2 Assist family in developing and creating a positive learning environment for family growth.
	3 Identify with family perceived areas of failure to meet expectations.
	4 Provide family with opportunities to express feelings about unmet expectations.
	5 Assist family in identifying major components within role identity that may create conflict within family system.
	6 Encourage family to engage in closeness-related behavior such as touching in order to develop a more cohesive family system.

Nursing Diagnosis Communication, impaired, related to sociocultural variables creating interpersonal distance in family.

Patient Outcomes	*Nursing Interventions*
1 Family will be able to communicate with health care personel, personal and family-related needs. 2 Family will be able to communicate feelings about interpersonal relationships and effects of alcohol on the family system. 3 Each family member will be able to send precise, understandable messages to one another through appropriate verbal and nonverbal communication.	1 Assist family in developing adequate communication techniques to communicate feelings and anxieties to one another. 2 Assist family in developing the ability to determine discrepancies in communicated verbal and nonverbal behavior. 3 Assist family in developing appropriate language skills and nonverbal perception to decrease the possibility of faulty perception.

Nursing Diagnosis Family processes, altered, related to an alcoholic family member.

Patient Outcomes	*Nursing Interventions*
1 Family will participate in care and maintenance of the alcoholic family member. 2 Family will assist nurse in assisting patient to return to a high level of wellness. 3 Family will verbalize difficulties encountered in seeking appropriate external resources.	1 Determine family's understanding of patient's condition. 2 Determine support systems available to family from external resources. 3 Determine with family supportive networks of friends and extended family members. 4 Involve family in care and management of patient. 5 Encourage family to verbalize fears and anxieties.

Nursing Diagnosis Self-esteem disturbance related to emotional distancing of significant others.

Patient Outcomes	*Nursing Interventions*
1 Patient and family will verbalize positive and realistic feelings about self and the family system. 2 Patient and family will make positive statements about self and the family system and display appropriate behavior accordingly. 3 Patient and family will set realistic goals for self and the family system and implement a plan to follow through on activities to achieve these goals. 4 Patient and family will perceive self and family in a positive manner.	1 Design and implement patient and family education to clarify values and beliefs that are perceived as negative influences. 2 Encourage patient and family to engage in family therapy. 3 Assist family in developing an understanding about the need for the patient to engage in psychotherapy, whether individual or group. 4 Encourage family to seek and attend appropriate self-help groups.

STUDY
QUESTIONS

1. List appropriate nursing interventions that can be implemented to facilitate communication within this family system.
2. Describe the family structure of some Irish American families and the effect the family organization may have on health-seeking behaviors, and explain how this may affect nursing interventions when providing care for Mr. McMartin.
3. Identify how Mr. McMartin's behavior may be affected by time and space variables.
4. List at least two etiological reasons for the development of alcoholism within an Irish American family.
5. Identify sociocultural variables within an Irish American family that may facilitate perceived emotional distance.

REFERENCES

Ablon, J., & Cunningham, W. (1981). Implications of cultural patterning for the delivery of alcoholism services. *Journal of Studies on Alcohol 42*(Suppl. 9), 185-206.

Abramson, H. (1973). *Ethnic diversity in Catholic America*. New York: John Wiley & Sons.

Alba, R. (1976). Social assimilation among American Catholic national-origin groups. *American Sociological Review, 41,* 1030-1046.

Blessing, P. (1980). Irish. In S. Thernstrom (Ed.), *Harvard encyclopedia of American ethnic groups*. Cambridge, Mass.: Belknap Press.

Christiansen, B., & Teahan, J. (1987). Cross-cultural comparisons of Irish and American adolescent drinking practices and beliefs. *Journal of Studies on Alcohol, 48*(6), 558-562.

Estes, N., & Heinemann, M.E. (1986). *Alcoholism*. St. Louis: C.V. Mosby.

Fallows, M. (1979). *Irish Americans*. Englewood Cliffs, N.J.: Prentice Hall.

Greeley, A. (1972). *That most distressful nation: The taming of the American Irish*. Chicago: Quadrangle Books.

Greeley, A. (1977). *The American Catholic: A social portrait*. New York: Basic Books.

Greeley, A. (1981). *The Irish Americans*. New York: Harper & Row.

Greeley, A., & McCready, W. (1975). The transmission of cultural heritages: The case of the Irish and Italians. In N. Glazer & D.P. Moynihan (Ed.), *Ethnicity: Theory and experience*. Cambridge, Mass.: Harvard University Press.

Griffin, W. (1981). *A portrait of the Irish in America*. New York: Charles Scribner's Sons.

Haber, J., Hoskins, P., Leach, A., & Sideleau, B. (1987). *Comprehensive psychiatric nursing*. New York: McGraw-Hill.

Hall, E.T. (1959). *The silent language*. New York: Fawcett.

Hall, E.T. (1963). A system for the notation of proxemic behavior. *American Anthropologist, 65*(5), 1003-1026.

Hall, E.T. (1966). *The hidden dimension*. New York: Doubleday.

Kennedy, R. (1973). *The Irish: Emmigration, marriage, and fertility*. Berkley: University of California Press.

Kluckhohn, F., & Strodtbeck, F. (1961). *Variations in value orientation*. Evanston, Ill.: Row, Peterson.

Lewis, C. (1988). AIDS in Ireland. *Canadian Medical Association Journal, 138,* 553-555.

Lipton, J.A., & Marbach, J.J. (1984). Ethnicity and the pain experience. *Social Science and Medicine, 19*(12), 1279-1298.

Macey, J., & Morgan, S. (1988). Learning on the road: Nursing in the British Isles and Ireland. *Nursing Outlook, 36*(1), 40-41.

Mbiti, K. (1970). *African religions and philosophies*. New York: Anchor Books.

McKay, J., Hall, B., & Buckler, J. (1989). *A history of world societies*. Boston: Houghton Mifflin Co.

Messenger, J. (1969). *Inis Beag: Isle of Ireland*. New York: Holt, Rinehard & Winston.

O'Conner, J. (1978). *The young drinkers: A cross-national study of social and cultural influences*. London: Tavistock Publications.

Porteous, M.A. (1985). Developmental aspects of adolescent problem disclosure in England and Ireland. *Journal of Child Psychology and Psychiatary, 26*(3), 465-478.

Shannon, W. (1981). Foreward. In W.D. Griffin, *A portrait of the Irish in America*. New York: Charles Scribner's Sons.

Slack, P. (1982). Nursing in Southern Ireland. *Nursing Times, 78*(4), 138-141.

Spector, R. (1985). *Cultural diversity in health and illness.* East Norwalk, Conn.: Appleton-Century-Crofts.

Statistical reports. (1981). U.S. Department of Commerce, Bureau of the Census.

Stillman, M. (1978). Territoriality and personal space. *American Journal of Nursing, 78,* 1671-1672.

Stivers, R. (1976). *A hair of the dog: Irish drinking and American stereotype.* University Park: Pennsylvania State University Press.

Walsh, B.M., & Walsh, D. (1973). Validity of indices of alcoholism: A comment from Irish experience. *British Journal of Preventive Social Medicine, 27,* 18-26.

Walsh, D. (1968). Alcoholism in Dublin. *Journal of the Irish Medical Association, 61*(371), 153-156.

Walsh, D. (1969). Alcoholism in the Republic of Ireland. *British Journal of Psychiatry, 115,* 1021-1025.

Walsh, J. (1987, Sept. 8). AIDS. *The Irish Times.*

Wessel, B. (1931). *An ethnic survey of Woonsocket, Rhode Island.* Chicago: University of Chicago Press.

Zborowski, M. (1952). Cultural components in response to pain. *Journal of Social Issues, 8,* 16-30.

Zola, I. (1966). Culture and symptoms: An analysis of patients' presenting complaints. *American Sociological Review, 31,* 615-930.

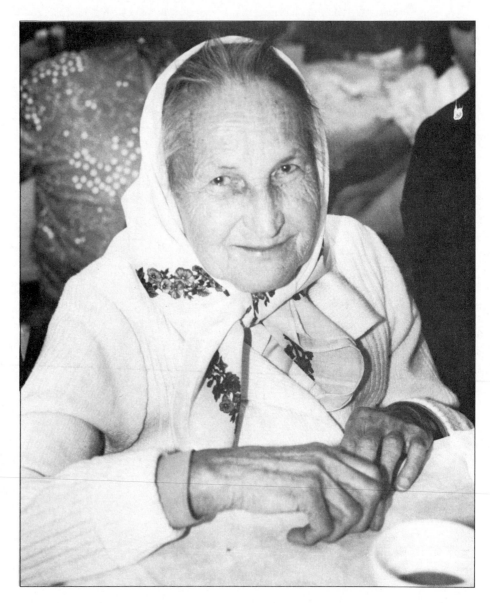

CHAPTER 15

. . . .

Soviet Americans

Linda S. Smith*

BEHAVIORAL OBJECTIVES
After reading this chapter, the nurse will be able to:

1 Identify the importance of spiritual beliefs to Soviet Americans.

2 List at least two future-oriented values for Soviet Americans.

3 Describe specific characteristics of the Russian language

4 Explain how Soviet people use gestures as a part of communication.

5 Identify at least two health problems unique to Soviet Americans.

6 Describe how health care practices in the Soviet Union have impacted on the health of Soviet Americans.

OVERVIEW OF THE USSR

The Union of Soviet Socialist Republics (USSR) is the largest sovereign state in the world. In the USSR there are 15 separate republics, each of which has its own cultural traditions, foods, language, national heritage, and economic climate. While each of these republics is unique, they are united by one political structure. Each republic is made up of states.

The USSR is bound on the north by the Arctic Ocean; on the east by the Pacific Ocean; on the south by North Korea, China, Afghanistan, Iran, the Caspian Sea, Turkey, and the Black Sea; and on the west by Romania, Hungary, Czechoslovakia, Poland, the Baltic Sea, Finland, and Norway. The USSR is divided into five major land regions: the European–West Siberian Plain, the Central Siberian Plateau, Eastern Siberia, and the Soviet Far East and Central East. Depending on the region, the

*First nurse-author/editor to enter into a collaborative agreement (in 1989) with officials of the USSR to write and distribute nursing literature with and for Soviet nurses.

physical terrain of the USSR differs. In the European–West Siberian Plain the physical region consists of rolling plains, wide river valleys, and coastal lowlands.

The Siberian region consists of level plains that stretch unbroken for approximately 1200 miles east from the Ural to the Yenisey River. The Central Siberian Plateau is sparsely settled and extends to the Lena River. Because the region is covered entirely by forest, those that inhabit it are mostly miners, hunters, and trappers.

Eastern Siberia is found beyond the Lena River and stretches eastward to the Pacific Ocean and the Bering Straits. The terrain of this region is comparable in length to the Appalachians. The mountains and valleys of Eastern Siberia are thought to be the most remote and least inhabited in the world. Even today, Eastern Siberia remains the least known region of the USSR.

The Soviet Far East is separated from the Central Siberian Plateau and Eastern Siberia by the Stanovoi and Yablonovy mountains. This region is the USSR's link with China, Japan, and the Pacific Ocean. The major waterway found in this area is the Amur River. Some of the most populated areas in the USSR are found in the Far East. Soviet Central Asia is east of the Caspian Sea and south of Siberia. In the northern region the terrain consists of plateaus, whereas in the central and southern regions there are mostly lowlands. There are very few rivers that cross this region, and those that do drain into salty, brackish lakes such as the Aral Sea and Blakhash Lake. Some of the rivers disappear altogether into the desert sands.

The Soviet Union and its territories are thought to be too distant from the sea or facing too cold of a sea to enjoy the moderating effects that large bodies of water have on the climate. With the exception of the coastal areas of the Black Sea and the Caspian Sea, the majority of territory in the Soviet Union has a continental climate. The climate in the Soviet Union is characterized by extremes in temperature and rainfall. Throughout most of the USSR, winter temperatures are generally well below freezing, and the coldest regions are in the northeast. Siberia, for example, is the coldest part of the country, with an average January temperature of −20° F. Even more extreme temperatures are found in the northern part of Eastern Siberia, where average January temperatures are as low as −50° or −60° F. Summers throughout the USSR are likely to be warm, with the exception of the far northern regions. In fact, some of the highest summer temperatures on Earth have been recorded in Soviet Central Asia. Approximately 40% of the Soviet Union is covered with permafrost, a permanent frozen soil, varying in depth from 1 foot to several hundred feet and thawing only a few inches in the summer months. Because of the extensiveness of the permafrost, agriculture, railroad building, and road building can be carried out only with extreme difficulty.

The Soviet Union is a multinational state, with at least 108 separate groups residing in it. Nearly three fourths of the population are from the East Slavic language group, consisting of Russians, Ukrainians, and the Belorussians (White Russians). Within the Slavic group, the Russian population numbers more than 114 million, making this group the largest ethnic group found within the USSR (Simons, 1976). Because Russians are found in every region of the Soviet Union, Russian is the official language of the Soviet Union. The second largest population group in the Soviet Union is the Ukrainians, who number more than 37 million. Ukrainians reside in the southern European region of the Soviet Union and maintain a separate cultural and historical tradition.

The Belorussians number more than 7 million and live north of the Ukrainians. Along the shores of the Baltic Sea are found the Baltic people, which include the Estonians (more than 1 million), Latvians (more than 1.3 million), and Lithuanians (more than 2.3 million). The Latvians and Lithuanians speak languages that are common to the Indo-European group found in the Soviet Union. The Estonians, on the other hand, inhabit the northern part of the country and speak a language that is closely related to Finnish.

The Moldavians number more than 2.3 million and primarily reside along the southwestern boundary of the Soviet Union. The Moldavians are closely related to Romanians and thus speak Romanian. The Chuvash, who number more than 1.5 million, reside in the middle Volga region and speak a Turkic language. The Tatars, who number more than 5 million, speak Asian languages. Also found in the Soviet Union are the Bashkirs, who number more than 1 million and also speak a Turkic language.

The most diverse people within the Soviet Union are the peoples of the Caucasus. There are three major groups found in this area: the Georgians (more than 2.7 million), the Armenians (more than 2.8 million), and the Azerbaidzhans (more than 2.9 million). Within the Caucasus and central Asia, there are also about 25 other minority groups, which range in size from 4000 to 300,000.

In Soviet Central Asia the people are for the most part Turkic and fall into four major subgroups. Residing in the central part of this region are the Uzbeks, who number more than 6 million and live in the central part of the region. In the northern part of this region are the Kazakhs, who number more than 3.6 million. The people who live in the mountains and the valleys of the east are called Turkmenians (more than 1 million). The last major group found in Soviet Central Asia are the Tadzhiks people, who number more than 1.4 million and reside along the Afghanistan border, speaking a language related to Persian.

In the eastern region there are small but diverse native populations. With the exception of the Yakuts (more than 250,000), a Turkic-speaking people of the Lena Valley of Eastern Siberia, none of the surviving native groups of Siberia has a population of over 25,000, and some of these groups have populations of less than a 1000. There are Koreans found in the Soviet Far East, as well as Buryats found in southern part of Siberia, who are related to the Mongols of the neighboring Mongolia.

While there are at least 108 diverse cultural groups found throughout the USSR with populations of significant numbers, the Jewish population has greatly diminished since World War II because of the persecution of Jews in German-occupied parts of the Soviet Union.

Today in the USSR, 13% of the population are reported to live below the official Soviet poverty level ($1920 a year). When the Soviet poverty level is computed at the black market rate, this figure is similar to $300 a year in the United States. Since poverty is so widespread in the USSR, the use of commodities such as meat and dairy products is on the decline (down 30% since 1970). It has also been reported that at least 30 million Soviets drink water that is not considered potable (Auster, 1989; Doerner, 1989). There has been a decline in the life expectancy of Soviet men because of increasing alcohol consumption. In the USSR 65% of the rural hospitals have no hot water, and 27% lack sewage systems. Common items found in the U.S. health care system, such as disposable syringes, are considered a luxury in the Soviet Union; needles are routinely reused after being cleansed with steel wool. It has also been reported that about 30% of USSR hospitals have no indoor toilets (Dentzer, Trimble, & Auster, 1989).

IMMIGRATION TO THE UNITED STATES

There are approximately 406,022 persons in the United States who are reported to be Russian immigrants. Of this number, 112,725 reside in New York City and 58,642 reside in California (U.S. Department of Commerce, Bureau of the Census, 1988). For the most part, those who have immigrated to the United States are well-educated, courageous people who are voracious readers and passionately devoted to the arts. Because poverty is so widespread in the USSR, most Soviet immigrants have survived years of hardship. In spite of this hardship, the Soviet immigrants generally appear to be a proud people. Soviet immigrants to the United States come to a specific location because they have relatives or contacts in that location. Although this is a requirement for resettling, it means that pocket populations of Soviet Americans have emerged in various regions of the United States.

There are also differences related to dates or times of immigration. More recently, Soviet immigrants have been younger and less often Jewish. Recent immigrants have not endured the long delays and confusion that their counterparts had to endure in the past. They can be often processed and arrive in the United States within a year or less. Of course, some resentment has surfaced among the earlier immigrants, who often endured 10 years or more of waiting and turmoil.

Interestingly, for the past 20 years the United States encouraged the Soviet Union to allow free immigration, particularly for the 2 million Soviet Jews still residing in the country. A wave of Soviet Jews immigrated to the United States in 1973 as a direct result of a law passed by Congress to facilitate Jewish immigration. As a result of this new law, more than 66,480 Soviet Jews immigrated to the United States during the period of 1975 to 1980 (Schiff, 1979). Of this number of Soviet Jewish immigrants, approximately 50% settled in New York City and most of the rest settled in Chicago, Los Angeles, and Philadelphia (Wenger, 1985).

Until recently, however, Soviet officials have very carefully regulated the flow of immigrants. Washington has responded to these strict controls by placing restrictions on Soviet trade. Chairman Gorbachev of the USSR initiated efforts to improve the Soviet Union's public relations status in the hope that Washington would lift expensive trade restrictions. In August of 1989, 18,000 Soviets applied for U.S. visas. Of this number, one third of the applicants were Jewish, and one third were from the Soviet Republic of Armenia. This was a dramatic increase from 1988, when 13,458 visas were issued for the entire year ("Give Us Your Masses", 1989). In the 1970s total immigration per year was approximately only 1000. It was predicted that in 1990 Soviet immigrants would number over 100,000. With this influx of Soviet immigrants, health care workers are beginning to see larger numbers of Soviet American patients enter into the health care system.

While the United States has urged the Soviet Union to loosen immigration restrictions, the United States has also held limited slots open to refugees. In October of 1989, Roberts and Auster noted that of the 125,000 refugee slots available over the next 12 months, 50,000 were reserved for immigrants, primarily Jewish, from the

Soviet Union. Also in October of 1989, the State Department of the United States indicated that 47,000 Soviets already had been approved for admission to the United States. Even with this phenomenal number, it was predicted that after the quota was filled, 300,000 Soviet Jews would still be waiting to come to America. The U.S. Senate Appropriations Committee report in September of 1989 indicated that the response to the refugee need has been entirely inadequate and that quota restrictions need to be adjusted to respond to the changes in emigration practices from the Soviet Union (Roberts & Auster, 1989).

To facilitate an understanding of the Soviet immigrant, it is necessary to know that in the Soviet Union preventive care and medical treatment are free. Education, including postsecondary university and professional studies, is also free (Smith, 1989). Therefore many of the the Soviet immigrants have had some form of technical training or advanced education. Nevertheless, among Soviet immigrants, the concepts of insurance, private pay, diagnostic related groups (DRGs), malpractice, etc., are new and difficult to understand.

COMMUNICATION
Dialect, Style, and Volume

The official language of the Soviet Union is Russian. Approximately one sixth of the people in the world speak Russian. Russian is composed of a 33-character Cyrillic alphabet named after the ninth-century apostle for the Slavs, St. Cyril. It was St. Cyril who created the alphabet so that the Bible could be translated and therefore used for liturgy in the Slavic countries (Moore, 1988).

Soviet people from the Republics of Armenia and Georgia (as well as some of the other Baltic regions) will often initially speak only their native language. The Georgians and Armenians have kept their old Japhetic alphabets (from Aramaic and Greek), whereas the Latvians, Lithuanians, Estonians, and Karelians have continued with a Latin-based language (Moore, 1988). Younger people from these areas recognize the need to be bilingual in order to advance professionally and therefore have learned Russian in addition to their native language.

For most Soviets English is considered to be the most popular language of all of the Western languages. This newfound popularity of English on the part of the Soviet people is related to the fact that the Voice of America (VOA) and the British Broadcasting Corporation (BBC) are transmitted now without interference in the Soviet Union. In addition, professional literature (including health and medicine) is often English based (Moore, 1988).

Russian is one of the three most important languages of the world. It is not possible to fully understand a culture until the language of that culture is also understood (Kinsey, 1989). Great Russian writers such as Tolstoy, Pasternak, Dostoyevski, Gogal, etc., have written not only about places and events, but also about human emotions and the spiritual nature of human existence.

Russian is sometimes referred to as a "house green" language because articles (for example, *the*) and verbs (for example, *is*) are often not needed. The Russian language is a flexible, beautifully rich language. Paralanguage qualities such as tone, inflection, speed, verbal pauses, etc., contribute to the variety and meaning of Russian words and sounds. Russians freely use paralanguage and other nonverbal indicators to denote the value being placed on what is said. The spirit of the Soviet people, their warmth and love, comes through clearly in this unusually exciting dialect (Binyon, 1983; Black, 1989).

Although most of the well-educated Soviets have taken English at some point in their education, English proficiency is not easy for the older Soviet immigrants. However, younger immigrants have made the adjustment to English with less difficulty. For younger Soviet immigrants the first priority on arrival in the United States is to learn conversational English; the second priority is to enroll children in school; and the third priority is to find employment. Many Jewish elderly immigrants speak Yiddish. For these people the practice of speaking Yiddish has been greatly discouraged by the Soviet authorities as being an "anti-state" activity. Younger Jewish immigrants seldom speak Yiddish (Gennis, 1989; Smith, 1989).

Touch

Soviets often use touch freely. It is not unusual to see Soviet women embracing and kissing other women and Soviet men embracing and kissing other men. Friends who have been separated often greet each other, in public or in private, in this fashion. The technique of kissing each cheek three times seems to be a cultural trait adopted from the Middle East. The gentle kiss on the hand is a gesture—male to female—of respect and admiration. Also, a handshake has great meaning and significance for the Soviet people; the handshake of agreement from a Soviet is often more binding than a signed document (Kinsey, 1989).

Emotions are also freely expressed. Soviets have a quick appreciation for jokes and satire—often venting their feelings in this form of expression. It has been said that Russian people can cry and laugh easily. In the Soviet Union it is permissible and socially acceptable for men to cry at funerals.

Context

The Soviet people are commonly perceived as being kind, caring, and generous. When trust has been established, they express these feelings willingly and publicly. They are by nature and experience, however, cautious; some Soviets evaluate situations and people with great care. Many Americans have been led to believe that Soviets are not trustworthy, because their affect is flat and their communication style may be described as dull. One possible reason for these faulty assumptions may be found in the language barrier; because of their language difficulties, some Soviet Americans speak carefully, slowly, and cautiously.

An additional language difficulty is the very nature of the English language. Although many Soviets take English in Soviet schools, they rarely learn English from a native speaker, but from native Soviets. Tourists traveling in the Soviet Union are often approached by native Soviets who are eager to practice conversational English. However, for most new Soviet immigrants, conversational English is likely to be completely unrecognizable and thus difficult to comprehend. This is particularly true for immigrants who relocate in eastern and southern parts of the United States, where variations in dialects are noted.

Kinesics

Until trust and comfort have been established, Soviet Americans will use few gestures. They do, however, feel free to maintain eye contact. Older Soviet Americans who have recently immigrated are more entrenched in social amenities, often preferring to express themselves verbally. "Please" and "thank you" are integral to their speech, and they use these words at every possible opportunity. The nod of the head is a gesture of approval; the outstretched hand is a gesture of salute. When compliments are given, they are sincere, and flowers are presented during important meetings as a gesture of tribute.

The person seated first in a room is the one with the most authority or prestige. Children are not permitted to mingle with distinguished guests and are required to eat in the kitchen rather than in the dining area when the family entertains.

Implications for Nursing Care

Soviet Americans expect the nurse to be warm and caring, to "feel" for them and to help them cope with physical and emotional problems. Some Soviet Americans will not appreciate a light, "chatty" approach to health care. In most instances Soviet Americans will comply with medical directives and teachings if they believe that the nurse is trustworthy, sincere, and competent. Nurses will not be believed and trusted by Soviet Americans if they are perceived to be masklike, robotic, or phony in their caring behaviors. The Soviet American will be critical of caregivers who say they care but whose behavior is not reflective of a caring attitude. Once language is no longer an issue or problem, the nurse will find warmth and "humanness" within easy reach.

The nurse should address Soviet adults as "Mr." or "Mrs.," followed by the surname. In so doing, the nurse will convey to the patient an attitude of respect.

It is important for the nurse to be aware that while the younger Soviet immigrant adapts well to English, older Soviet immigrants may not. Often, elderly Soviet immigrants choose to associate only with Russian-speaking friends and relatives, failing to assimilate the American culture and language. This presents a difficult problem if an interpreter is unavailable. To add to this difficulty, Soviet American households may impose a "Russian-only" rule on their children (allowing only Russian to be spoken at home).

Because many Soviet Americans are multilingual (Yiddish, German, French, Polish, Czechoslovakian, Latin, etc.), it is an advantage if the nurse is able to understand Russian or another language familiar to the patient. One way to convey respect and an understanding of the culture is to provide avenues for patient teaching through Russian literature. Health literature written in Russian may be better patient teaching aids than video films.

SPACE

The Soviet culture exists on two very different levels. To strangers and new acquaintances, a Soviet person will remain aloof, preferring to speak and work in the social or public zone. However, once friendship and familiarity have been established, the Soviet people are comfortable within a personal zone. The intimate zone is reserved for spouse or children except for health care workers performing within a professional capacity. It appears that a Soviet person when hospitalized tolerates the loss of privacy well.

Individuals are perceived according to the boundaries they maintain, which include the degree of permeability and flexibility. *Permeability* is generally defined as the degree to which a boundary is open or closed; for the most part, permeability varies from closed to open. When an individual has closed boundaries, there tends to be very little exchange between this person's internal and external environments, and the person may be perceived as being quiet, withdrawn, and set in his or her ways. On the other hand, if the boundaries are open, there appears to be much exchange between the person's internal and external environments, and this individual may be perceived as being talkative, social, and one who enjoys taking risks.

The definition for *flexibility* is the ability of a person to move along a permeability continuum. An individual who is sometimes closed and sometimes open, and who thereby uses the entire permeability continuum, is considered flexible. On the other hand, an individual who always gravitates toward the closed end of the continuum, which is indicative of a low degree of flexibility, will be described as a rigid, closed person. An individual who is always open and never closed will be described as an open individual. People who are perceived as being rigid and closed may be quiet and withdrawn, and seldom if ever share intimate secrets, dreams, or thoughts, even with best friends or a spouse (Scott, 1988).

Some Soviet individuals are perceived as being rigid and closed because they prefer to remain aloof and distant. However, the word *friend* is not a casual term to people from the Soviet Union. It appears that friendship is taken more seriously by Soviet Americans than by many others in the United States. Close Soviet friends may embrace, but mere acquaintances are likely to not even shake hands. Soviets may prefer to greet and meet acquaintances on a verbal level only.

It is not proper to call an adult Soviet American by his or her first name. In the Soviet Union it is standard to address adults by their first name and then by their father's name (for example, Lyudamilla Victorana—Victor being Lyudamilla's father's name). For Soviet Americans the accepted, preferred method of addressing adults is by "Mr." or "Mrs." plus the last name. To address a Soviet person by his or her first name only is improper and presents a grave social error. Soviets also strongly object to terms of endearment when used by health care workers. Terms such as "dear" "hon" and "hi-guy" are abhorred.

Implications for Nursing Care

The nurse caring for a Soviet American patient will generally find that health assessment procedures done in the intimate zone are accepted without argument or problem provided that the nurse has given adequate information and justification before the procured, and permission from the patient has been requested and provided. For the most part, the nurse should be aware that Soviet people prefer to remain at a social distance rather than an intimate distance with caregivers. If personal distance must be invaded to provide therapeutic assistance, the nurse should provide careful explanation before the intervention to alleviate stress and anxiety created by the violation of space. As with all aspects of care, it is important for the nurse to modify approaches based on an evaluation of the individual patient and family.

SOCIAL ORGANIZATION
Family

Family relations and family roles exert a significant influence on the Soviet people. Both in the Soviet Union and in the United States, extended families often live together, relying on each other for support, child care, and the completion of household tasks. Children learn that if a parent says "no," they can always ask one of their grandparents (Gioiella, 1983).

The Soviet people are very family oriented. For the Soviet immigrant, who may have left children, siblings, and parents to come to America, the family that is here become even more significant. Therefore Soviet Americans are a very closely knit group. Within a few years after immigrating to the United States, however, the children become assimilated into the American culture, leave home, and may even leave the geographic area. The remaining family members are often elderly and without job or language skills. They tend to isolate themselves from American contacts.

It appears that the father has the greatest influence within the Soviet family structure. Children, especially male children, look up to this figure and absorb his values and beliefs. One particular story exemplifies the Soviet people's love and respect for family. A young Soviet, born on a Lithuanian peasant farm, was one of several children in the family. He stated that he grew up loving and respecting his father and having a good, balanced, accepting attitude toward life. However, the only occupation available to any of the children was farming, and there was no more land available. Therefore the family was forced to divide the small family plot among all the children. Rather than fight over this land with his brothers, this man left his country and has not seen his family since. "My family was so important to me," he explained, "that I knew I had to leave in order not to hurt them."

Education and cultural activities are family values that begin when children are still infants. To educate their children, fathers will walk arm and arm with them through art museums in an effort to instill an appreciation of history and culture. Both girls and boys are encouraged to do well in school, achieve good grades, and go to college.

Nuclear and extended families

Soviet American families, just as Soviet families in the USSR, are small. The average number of children is two or less. In the Russian Republic, the largest Republic in the Soviet Union, 56% of all couples have only one child (Binyon, 1983).

Individualism

Soviet people are hard working and have very little tolerance for people who do not have jobs. They are self-reliant and independent. Soviet Americans who become ill will use home care and/or hospitalization as much as possible rather than become a burden to their family. They have a strong desire to stay in their own homes and will remain independent, not wanting to move in with their children, until the last possible moment.

This strong individualism seems to contradict the Soviet social structure, wherein individual achievements are seen in terms of their value to the group as a whole. This "collective" idea instills a sense of self-esteem based on how well the group has accepted one's work (Hess, 1971).

Position of Women in the Family and in Society

Soviet women, who are almost completely liberated on the job and in professional circles, are not liberated at home. Although husband and wife both have full-time jobs outside the home, most Soviet men prefer to have their wives do all the cooking, shopping, and housework. Without the modern conveniences of time- saving electric appliances (microwave ovens, washers, dryers, vacuum cleaners, etc.), the Soviet woman spends at least an additional 40 hours per week on household chores (Binyon, 1983).

Jobs for women are considered equal, but salary is not. Soviet women on an average earn 30% less than their male counterparts. Soviet women now account for 67% of Soviet physicians, 87% of economists, 58% of engineers, and 89% of bookkeepers (Koval, 1989). Ninety two percent of all working-age women either work or study, and one out of three marriages fail (Binyon, 1983).

Spirituality and Religious Beliefs

The Soviet people take religion very seriously. Although religious expression in the Soviet Union has had major social roadblocks since the 1917 Bolshevik Revolution, recent *perestroika* and *glasnost* changes have witnessed a resurgence of religious freedoms. The Christian church has had a remarkable revival. As one of the largest and most influential divisions of Christianity, the Russian Orthodox Church celebrated the one-thousandth anniversary (in 1988) of the decision by Prince Vladimir of Kiev to embrace that religion (Binyon, 1983).

The Russian Orthodox Church requires followers to observe fast days as well as a "no meat" rule on Wednesdays and Fridays. During Lent all animal products, including dairy products and butter, are forbidden. Food is fried in linseed oil. Toward the end of Lent, pregnant women have reported alopecia and night blindness. Fasting also takes place during Advent. It is believed that God is served in a more powerful way during periods of fasting. However, even if fasting is strictly observed, special allowances are made for illness and pregnancy.

There are 5000 Baptists in the Soviet Union, and this number is growing rapidly. Most Soviet Baptists live in the Republic of Ukraine. There are a few Soviet Catholics (especially in Lithuania and the Ukraine) and Lutherans in the Baltic republics. A high concentration of Christians exists in Georgia and Armenia. However, many churches lie rotting and unattended as a result of repressive actions by the Communist Party.

The Soviet Union is the fifth largest Muslim country in the world (Binyon, 1983). Tartar Muslims have lived in the central part of Russia and the Crimean area. Their religious beliefs allow several wives, and Tartars do not eat pork.

Traditionally in the Soviet Union, Jews could not own property or land, which perhaps explains why many Soviet Jews became merchants. As a result of this new role, other Soviet people developed resentment and anti-Semitic feelings. With the relaxation of censorship and a new emphasis on Soviet nationalism, there has been a resurgence of this anti-Semitism.

Soviet Jews immigrate to the United States and other countries in a greater percentage than non-Jewish Soviet people. The more Jewish oppression and anti-Semitism in the Soviet Union, the greater the rate of immigration, and this leads to further discrimination. New freedoms of speech and expression have brought out old, otherwise buried, prejudices. In this newfound climate, Soviet Jews feel persecuted and fear greatly for their children.

Implications for Nursing Care

Despite persecution and hardships, the Soviet people have maintained a significant degree of individualism. Soviet parents have taught their children an appreciation for land and country. In all human societies the things that are done for survival, such as eating, elimination, sex, and health practices, though physical, take on cultural and social regulations. These cultural functions and norms dictate behavior patterns in a profound way. It is essential for nurses to understand the role culture plays in order to provide safe, compassionate, and effective nursing care. Although some Soviet immigrants have maintained feelings of nationalism for the motherland, it is important for the nurse to understand that strong feelings of nationality (national pride) may not be experienced by all Soviet Jewish immigrants. This lack of national pride is individual, however, and cannot be assumed. Many Soviet immigrants are very proud of their homeland and do not reject their roots. One Soviet immigrant explained, "Whether good or bad, it is still mine. I still love my homeland."

Because Soviet Americans value family orientation, the nurse must remember to involve the entire family, including extended family members, in the planning and intervention of care. Since the father is perceived as having a paramount role and function in the Soviet family, the astute nurse will solicit the opinions and advice of the father before presenting a treatment and intervention plan to the rest of the family. In this instance if the father's opinions and advice are solicited prior to the presentation to the rest of the family, the father may be of particular assistance in getting the family's cooperation and assistance.

Some Soviet Americans hold particular beliefs in regard to religion, as well as death and dying. Therefore it is important for the nurse to respect these beliefs and practices and to incorporate them into a therapeutic plan of care to assist the patient in returning to a high level of wellness.

TIME

Some Soviet Americans hold a perspective of time that is past, present, and future oriented. For these people there is no future without the present and no present without the past. On the other hand, some Soviet Americans hold only a future orientation. This ideology represents the thinking of the well-educated Soviet American, because a future-oriented perception may be equated with position and power. One example of this cultural attitude is seen in the very nature of immigration. Regardless of orientation, the Soviet people have endured hardships and pain, loneliness, and isolation in order to achieve greater freedom and a better quality of life for themselves and their families.

Another important example of future orientation is seen in the Soviet people's almost universal belief in education for themselves and their children. Education begins early and is reinforced in the home. Children as young as 5 years old learn to read classic literature and attend the ballet, the opera, and concerts.

For Soviet Americans who espouse a belief in future orientation, education is viewed as an awakening or a light, whereas a lack of education is viewed as a void or darkness. Self-learning and lifelong learning are valued and practiced. To help Soviet children cope with problems they will encounter, educational institutions are encouraging a spirit of inquiry. Under Gorbachev, Soviet schools are transforming children into self-starters with the goal of moving toward free thought and expression (Traver, 1989).

On immigration to the United States, Soviet children are encouraged to attend school immediately, even before they have any knowledge of English. In fact, Soviet children learn English very readily. It is obvious, then, that for Soviet immigrants present efforts are vehicles for future achievements.

Implications for Nursing Care

For some Soviet immigrants who hold a time orientation that is a combination of past, present, and future beliefs, it is important for the nurse to remember that such an individual may be reluctant to seek preventive therapeutic interventions because of a fatalistic orientation. The nurse must design and implement teaching strategies that will assist the patient in developing an understanding about the implications of past and present behavior on future wellness behavior.

On the other hand, some Soviet immigrants hold only a future orientation and as such value preventive therapeutic techniques that have long-range future benefits on wellness and wellness behavior. Because these individuals hold a future orientation, the nurse will find it less difficult to encourage preventive screening techniques such as cholesterol screenings, mammograms, and blood pressure screening than with past-oriented individuals. In fact, the patient may even request information on preventive techniques and their benefits.

ENVIRONMENTAL CONTROL
Locus of Control and Impact on Wellness/Illness Behaviors

The Soviet culture instills in its members a belief that man does have some control over nature (but this is not absolute). This control is especially apparent in health care activities. Spiritually, however, those Soviet Americans with Russian Orthodox beliefs may have difficulty with current self-help practices. These beliefs center around ideas of Christ's teachings. It is believed that Christ will give as much help as is deserved in relation to the strength of the beliefs, which means that an ill person who is not recovering must somehow not have had enough faith. Illness in this sense is perceived as a punishment. For those Soviet Americans who espouse these beliefs, this is perceived as an external locus of control because of a fatalistic orientation.

In contrast, some Soviet Americans hold the belief that one can control both internal and external forces in the environment, thereby creating opportunities for high-level wellness. This perception is regarded as an internal locus of control. When individuals have an internal locus-of-control orientation, they are likely to have a unique self-care approach to illness and hospitalization. Soviet health care efforts are now being focused on disease prevention as a paramount trend in their health care system ("Health Care," 1988). With an increased concern about diet, obesity, and blood pressure levels, the Soviet people are demonstrating an interest in aerobic exercise, calorie counting, and lower salt and fat intake; they are also becoming more conscious of how they look. Soviet television carries daily exercise shows, and joggers can be seen lining the streets and parks. Joggers are more often men, and fitness clinic attendees are more often women (Black, 1989).

Alternative Methods of Treatment

In the Soviet Union feldshers deliver a great deal of primary health care. The feldsher is a medical aide with 3 years of training (Vlassov, 1989). After 3 years of medical school, the feldsher is trained in basic preventive medicine, with special focus on mothers and preschool children. The feldsher is also trained in suturing and emergency care techniques. Feldsher centers generally serve collective farms and therefore are in the center of each village. Because of their proximity to the population, Feldsher centers become the first point of referral for patients. Feldsher centers are organized by regions, with approximately four feldsher centers to every hospital (Brown, 1979). When Soviet people are ill, they are expected to stay in bed and call the clinic. The physician or feldsher will make a house call that same day, determine the severity of the problem, and make a recommendation (Maloof, 1970). Twice each year, all women of childbearing age and all preschool children are screened.

Other health care alternatives sometimes used have been charm men and barber shops. In the past, barber shops were equipped to do a procedure called "cupping," which was done primarily for the treatment of respiratory tract disorders and may still be practiced today in some heavier Jewish Soviet American populations. In this procedure, approximately 15 cups are heated, placed up and down the back, and left in place for about 10 minutes. Believed to extract evil humors from the body, these cups leave ecchymotic-like marks for days (Carr, 1983).

The Soviet Health Care System

It has been estimated by some that the Soviet health care system lags about 40 years behind that of the United States (Allen, 1983; Anthony-Tkach, 1985; Brown, 1984; Cox, 1983; Kershbaum, 1983; Kinsey, 1989; Latinis-Bridges & Clancy, 1988; Latinis-Bridges & Dayani, 1984; Myco, 1984; Wells & Starpe, 1985); however, other sources suggest that this statement may be empirically unfounded (Smith, 1989). The suggestion that the Soviet health care system lags behind that of the United States is supported by the observation that high-tech equipment and disposable items are conspicuously absent from Soviet hospitals (Kinsey, 1989). Although routine abdominal surgery in the Soviet Union for appendectomies and gallbladder procedures is comparable to that in the United States, Soviet people have far fewer hysterectomies. Labor and delivery are traditional, without Lamaze techniques. Birth control rests with an almost total reliance on abortion. It is not unusual for a 37-year-old Soviet woman to have had as many as 10 abortions. Contraceptives are of poor quality and difficult to obtain, and all types of hormones, taken for any reason, are unpopular. Therefore more abortions are done in the Soviet Union than in any other country in the world, and the average Soviet woman has six to eight abortions in her lifetime. Abortions, using the suction method, are usually performed during the eighth to twelfth week of pregnancy (Binyon, 1983).

In addition, Soviets with advanced coronary artery disease have not had access to cardiac surgical interventions such as bypass surgery. In a recent case involving a 14-year-old Lithuanian boy, a heart valve needed to save his life was unavailable to his physicians in the Soviet Union. Plans to send the valve to Lithuania were abandoned when it was learned that the valve would probably end up on the black market, and the boy was flown to Milwaukee, Wisconsin, where a new valve was implanted (thanks to private donations and free medical services) (Manning, 1989).

While the health care system may in some respects lag behind that of the United States, there is some indication that preventive health care is practiced. Physical screening is believed by the Soviet people to be the answer to good health care ("Health Care," 1988) and is widely accepted among younger Soviet immigrants. Female Soviet Americans are quite familiar with frequent and routine pelvic and Pap screenings, gastric acid tests, sedimentation rates, and prothrombin times. They are neither familiar with nor accepting of mammograms, routine breast examinations, or cholesterol screenings.

Folk Medicine

Soviet immigrants, especially the elderly, may still practice some homeopathic or folk medicine. For example, one patient had an amber necklace from Riga and refused to allow treatment for a thyroid condition, explaining, "Those pills make me sick. My necklace will cure everything with my thyroid except cancer." When laboratory work proved to her that the condition was worsening, she accepted medication (Ruby, 1989). Ground into a powder and added to hot water, amber is also used as a kind of tea.

Other home remedies include herbs, which are prepared as drinks or enemas, and charcoal in water, which is ingested for the treatment of stomach acidity. Hot steam baths are considered medicinal for pneumonia and upper respiratory tract infections. Mineral water and plasters are also used. Because of their belief in the healing qualities of mineral water, emerging Soviet health centers are said to use products that are rich in curative properties.

Soviet Americans have a very strong belief in the usefulness of massage. This philosophy seems to stem from a kind of chiropractic idealism related to the spine and back. In addition, orthopedic shoes for foot or leg pain are commonly asked for and used.

Practices at the Time of Death

Soviet families with members who have recently died often keep vigil over the coffin for hours. The deceased is washed, dressed, and placed in the coffin prior to the wake and funeral. A black wreath is placed on the door of the deceased person's home. At the funeral a priest (if the family is Catholic or Russian Orthodox) places holy oil on the forehead while making the sign of the cross. A paper band is placed on the forehead with this prayer: "Oh God, Father, be merciful to thy servant (name), accept into thy fold (name)." A piece of paper is placed on the dead person's chest, symbolic of a ticket into heaven. Each grieving member of the family symbolically places a few grains of soil onto the coffin.

Implications for Nursing Care

It is important for the nurse to be aware that in Soviet hospitals patients take care of each other. Giving bedpans, feeding patients, performing patient teaching functions, and even bathing patients are tasks that are more often performed by other patients than by nursing staff. Patients assume a major role in their own care and are discharged after lengthy hospital stays (Dennis, 1989). Soviet Union patients report their love and admiration for the wonderful, dedicated nurses who care for them. "I couldn't have made it without my nurses," one cardiac patient explained (Smith, 1989). The role of nursing in the Soviet Union seems to be changing. While previously nursing was held in low esteem as a profession, literature today indicates that nursing is gaining in stature as an essential component of the health care system (Kinsey, 1989).

Soviet immigrants are generally surprised by the accessibility of American hospitals, which differs from the complicated referral process that is encountered in the Soviet Union (Kinsey, 1989). Soviet immigrants are generally impressed not only with accessibility, but also with the thoroughness of American health care. The nurse should be aware that the Soviet American patient will find the way in which health professionals relate somewhat different from that to which they are accustomed. Traditionally, American physicians and nurses have been taught to have a nondirective, listening approach to patient interactions. This approach is unsatisfactory for many Soviet immigrants, who seem to need almost immediate information and answers. Subjective symptoms may be difficult to assess in relation to descriptions of severity and because of a dearth of presented information.

Soviet Americans are nearly 100% compliant with follow-up medical appointments. Generally, Soviet Americans are respectful and patient, and admire their physicans and nurses. They ask appropriate questions and accept what is told to them. Soviet Americans do not, however, often use walk-in or emergency department services. Usually the Soviet American will call the physician and wait until he or she is available. This most likely is due to their past medical experiences in the Soviet Union.

Soviet Americans will comply with most medical directives, doing whatever is necessary to get well and stay independent. However, these individuals may stop taking medications with any sign of a side effect, even if the side effect is unrelated. This is particularly noted with the psychotropic drug groups. The nurse may also notice that there seems to be a kind of cancer phobia among elderly Soviet immigrants. These people seem to have an "if it isn't broke, don't fix it" philosophy in relation to screenings for stool guaiac tests, sigmoidoscopy, and mammograms. Diagnostic tests such as these are often refused, causing later stages of discovery and less favorable prognoses (Ruby, 1989). Soviet families may also forbid health care professionals from disclosing a cancer diagnosis to elderly parents, which further complicates care. The concept of DNR ("do not resuscitate") may be a problem for the Jewish family that is unable to understand not doing everything possible for a loved one.

BIOLOGICAL VARIATIONS
Body Size

Obesity is common among female Soviet individuals, especially the elderly. This problem is attributable to the virtual unavailability of fresh fruits and vegetables in the Soviet Union. Many culturally preferred foods are high in saturated fats and salts. Because Soviet immigrants retain their traditional dietary preferences in the United States, the problem continues. Soviet physicians estimate that as many as 50% of their population are overweight (Black, 1989). Stature among Soviet Americans is quite similar to that of other patients seen by the health care provider.

Enzymatic Variations

Soviet Americans do not have problems with hypervitaminosis or hypovitaminosis, and biochemically, laboratory parameters are the same (Gennis, 1989). The one exception is that the cholesterol levels of Soviet Americans are generally well above normal.

Susceptibility to Disease

Hypertension

Blood pressure screening is routine in the Soviet Union; however, antihypertensive pharmacological treatment is not. Soviet Americans are keenly aware of the causes and effects of hypertension and will identify themselves as hypertensive or borderline hypertensive, as the case may be. However, although Soviet Americans are often very hypertensive, they may not have been treated for the disorder. One reason for this is the lack of available antihypertensive drugs ("Health Care," 1988). Diet is likely to be a contributing factor to hypertension.

Tuberculosis

Tuberculosis exposure has also been noted in greater incidence among Soviet immigrants. The population in the Soviet Union is routinely immunized 2 days after birth with bacillus Calmette-Guérin (BCG). This is an effective treatment when a high prevalence of tuberculosis exists. The problem, however, is that it causes tuberculin reactions to read positive and makes purified protein derivative (PPD) readings unclear. BCG immunization cannot be assumed, however, following positive PPD readings; many radiographs show signs of old cases of tuberculosis (Gennis, 1989).

Dental Needs

Previous dental care for Soviet immigrants has been noted to be adequate. Rarely are gaps caused by missing teeth seen in Soviet men and women. Soviets have easy access to qualified dental care and often come to the United States with bridges and removable plates.

Eye Care Needs

Soviets also have access to good eye care in the Societ Union. Eye care and eye surgery receive a great deal of Soviet money and attention.

Nutritional Preferences and Deficiencies

Recent efforts toward a national fitness movement in the Soviet Union have been slowed because of the Soviet Union's chronic shortage of fresh fruits and vegetables. Sausage, potatoes, and bread are standard foods for breakfast, lunch, and supper. The Soviet immigrant who has come from a rural district (two thirds of the Soviet population live in urban areas) will prefer to eat cabbage, buckwheat, millet, barley, and bread (Russian bread is a kind of heavy rye bread and can weigh as much as 12 pounds per loaf), along with sour milk and salted pork (if the person is non-Jewish). Usually salted meats are kept in a barrel and stored all winter in a kind of fruit cellar. Meat, as a delicacy, may be planned out and rationed. Chicken may be served during celebrations and illness. Most Soviet immigrants thus respect food and handle it with great care. Not a single morsel of food, especially meat, is to be wasted.

Psychological Characteristics

Mental health

For many years in the Soviet Union, Soviet citizens who tried to evangelize others or to organize labor unions have been labeled as insane and hospitalized in prisonlike psychiatric hospitals. This practice has been scorned by the rest of the world's psychiatric community, who have found the diagnosis of "sluggish schizophrenia" used in the Soviet Union to describe these persons very objectionable. Such practices have additionally been scorned within the Soviet Union. For example, the Nov. 23, 1987, edition of *Health Week* included an item that appeared in *Komsomolskaya Pravda,* the Communist youth newspaper, which reported that some individuals who resist arrest are labeled as schizophrenics and placed in psychiatric hospitals by police ("Soviets under Fire," 1987). Hospitalization is said to occur in spite of Soviet law, which states that citizens can be forcibly hospitalized only if they display signs of deep depression, are suicidal, or threaten the lives of others.

There are indications that such psychiatric practices are changing. In 1987 the May 1 issue of *Psychiatric News* carried a report of a change in policy in the USSR relevant to aspects of psychiatric treatment and the homeless, which were discussed at a meeting between the chairman of the American Psychological Association (APA) Council on International Affairs, Harold Visotsky, M.D., and the Soviet Deputy Ambassador, Yevstafiev ("APA Representatives," 1987). In the meeting with the APA delegation, Yevstafiev identified a change to "maximum humanization." It would appear that Soviet psychiatrists are trying to improve their tarnished image by releasing these political prisoners and placing psychiatry under the governance of the Ministry of Health, rather than the Ministry of Internal Affairs (police) (DeWitt, 1989). Today, psychiatric therapies include hydrotherapy, physiotherapy, insulin therapy, inhalation therapy, work therapy, and drug therapy. Work therapy is considered of great importance, even for children (Hess, 1971).

One of the most common mental health problems seen in Soviet Americans is depression. This is seen primarily in elderly immigrants who have traveled with children to the United States. They are unfamiliar with the language and customs, have left home and family, and often can get only minimum-wage jobs because of their age. Yet they are especially reluctant to maintain compliance with antidepressant drugs because of side effects.

Posttraumatic Stress Disorder

Another mental health problem seen in Soviet World War II veterans is a kind of posttraumatic stress disorder (PTSD). Memories of the traumatic war experiences cannot easily be erased. The Soviets lost over 20 million people during World War II. It has been said that not a single family was left untouched by this tragedy. When one speaks to Soviets about "The Great War," it becomes apparent that memories are as strong as if it had taken place yesterday.

Alcoholism

In the Soviet Union, alcoholism is a major and growing national health problem. However, under the direction of *glasnost,* the first Alcoholics Anonymous (AA) groups are emerging in Moscow. In 1985 Gorbachev launched an all-out antidrinking campaign by increasing the drinking age and the tax needed to be paid for all liquor purchases. Despite these efforts, alcoholism in the Soviet Union continues to increase (Garelik, 1989).

Alcoholism is seldom seen, however, among Soviet immigrants. Neither do Soviet immigrants smoke, use drugs, or become sexually permissive. Perhaps the lack of these self-abuse problems is attributable to the attitudes and values, high levels of education, and cohesiveness of this skewed Soviet population.

Radiation Accidents

Many new Soviet immigrants are arriving from cities and towns in the Republic of Ukraine (Trimble, 1989). Two important Ukrainian cities are Kiev (its capital), with 2.4 million people, and Chernobyl. At 1:23 AM Saturday, April 26, 1986, a catastrophic accident occurred at the Chernobyl Nuclear Power Station. Although, 26,000 Chernobyl-area residents were evacuated, this evacuation did not take place until 36 hours after the explosion (Raloff & Silberner, 1986). The evacuation occurred long after lethal radiation was absorbed. Experts consider the region surrounding the plant to be dangerous, with the extent of the danger unknown.

Kiev lies 80 miles south of the Chernobyl reactor site, downwind and downstream from the accident. Scientific studies have been able to estimate Chernobyl's effects on human health at no greater than a 0.02% risk for cancer (Knox, 1988; Serrill, 1986); however, recent Soviet immigrants strongly distrust the Soviet government's claims of safety, believing that the government has been less than truthful. Among the immigrants from this geographic area, nonspecific health symptoms are generally blamed on Chernobyl. Thus far, radiation has not been specifically identified as a cause.

Implications for Nursing Care

American nurses quickly recognize that Soviet Americans are very friendly, interesting, likable, and generally well educated. Soviet immigrants do not tend to overuse or abuse health care services. On the other hand, the nurse should be aware that Soviet immigrants may be skeptical of psychiatric services, since psychiatric treatment has often appeared in the Soviet Union to be associated with persecution. Education about psychiatric symptoms and the modalities of treatment available in the United States are an essential part of a psychiatric intervention strategy. The patient and family should be made to feel that they are participants in treatment selection and should be invited to choose treatment strategies.

It is important for the nurse caring for a Soviet immigrant to be aware of possible nutritional implications for nursing care. Since very recent immigrants may not be able to tolerate the richer American foods, the nurse would be wise to introduce new foods slowly. Religious dietary restrictions may also be a concern.

While alcoholism is not reported to be a problem among Soviet Americans, residual effects of alcoholism, whether physiological or psychological, must be looked for in individuals and families. In addition, the nurse must assist the Soviet American patient in identifying coping strategies that will reduce anxiety and tension, thereby reducing the potential for alcohol abuse.

Since hypertension is reported to have a high incidence among Soviets and Soviet Americans, the nurse should devise teaching strategies that emphasize the benefits of dietary restraints, weight control, and adequate exercise. In addition, the Soviet American patient who is hospitalized for hypertension must learn to develop an appreciation of the need to take prescribed medication for hypertension in a timely manner and to report unusual symptoms to health care professionals.

SUMMARY

As nurses transcend their care beyond their own cultural mind-set, they learn to accept and use cultural uniqueness as an indicator for nursing interventions. Among experiences that are assisting nurses in gaining a transcultural perspective are transcultural educational experiences, including those described by MacAvoy (1988), in which 20 registered nurses visited several USSR health care facilities as part of an educational tour. In the experience described by MacAvoy (1988), 35 continuing education hours were acquired through reading assignments and listening to educational lectures given by persons in the Soviet Union. In addition to gaining an understanding of persons in other cultures, the nurse must increase knowledge in order to provide culturally appropriate care to immigrants to the United States. Certainly, complexity, variety, and cultural diversity contribute to the nurse's challenge and responsibility for Soviet Americans.

CASE
STUDY

Victor and Slava have immigrated to Milwaukee, Wisconsin, from Kiev, the capital of the Ukraine, in the USSR. They are Jewish and believed that the strong anti-Semitism they felt in the USSR had become unbearable and that their only alternative was to leave the country and join relatives in Milwaukee. Mt. Sinai Samaritan Hospital offered 1 year of free health care to them when they first arrived. Now, 3 years later, Victor and Slava continue to seek services at this large teaching hospital and clinic. Victor and Slava are both 58 years old, and Slava speaks very little English. Victor has found a new peer group at the brewery, his place of employment. However, Slava has been unable to find work and prefers to stay near family and friends. The Milwaukee Jewish Family Services has been minimally successful in involving Slava in social activities. Slava reads and sits in her chair most of the day. Recently, she has become more withdrawn, with an overwhelming feeling of sadness and loneliness for her native land. She regrets coming to the United States and has focused her bitter feelings inward.

A painful venous occlusion brings Slava to the health clinic, where the nurse examines her lower extremities and finds swelling, tenderness, edema, and a positive Homans' sign on Slava's left leg. A health history is difficult because of the language barrier, but with the help of Victor and an interpreter, the nurse learns about Slava's sedentary life-style, high fat and high cholesterol intake, and recent episodes of sadness. Victor is supportive but impatient for his wife to "get back on her feet again." Slava says very little.

On laboratory examination, Slava's plasma low-density lipoprotein (LDL) level is 240 mg/100 ml. Left ventricular hypertrophy is noted on the electrocardiogram. Slava is obese and has a blood pressure of 200/120. Hemorrhages of the retinas are also noted.

Slava is presented with two medical diagnoses: symptomatic hypertension and depression. The nurse realizes that Slava's dietary instructions need to be presented with great care and attention given to cultural habits and beliefs. The nurse shows Slava an extensive list of "good" foods and asks her to identify her favorites. With Slava's help and the help of the dietitian, the nurse works out a weekly menu. The nurse must also teach Slava specific techniques for controlling her hypertension. Slava is instructed to take her own weight and blood pressure every morning, record them on a graph, and bring the graphs with her for her every-other-week clinic visits. It is explained to Slava that she will need to diligently follow medication, dietary, and exercise regimens in order to decrease her risk for further disability. Slava is especially motivated to help herself because of her fear of losing her eyesight and thus being unable to read (her favorite pastime). Walking is encouraged after Slava's leg becomes asymptomatic.

After these instructions are repeated carefully several times, Slava is escorted into a private office. The nurse, who has known Slava for 3 years, asks her about her sadness and isolating behaviors. Slava adamantly rejects the nurse's suggestion that she see a psychiatric consultant.

CARE
PLAN

Nursing Diagnosis   Nutrition altered: more than body requirements (fat, salt), related to cultural food preferences and sedentary life-style.

Patient Outcomes	*Nursing Interventions*
1 Patient will maintain a 1500-calorie/day low-cholesterol diet.	1 Teach patient about importance of exercise.
2 Patient will decrease her weight by 4 pounds per month.	2 Teach patient about menu planning in relation to avoidance of high-salt, high-fat foods.
3 Patient will walk 2 miles per day (after leg has healed).	3 Encourage and support compliance with medications, exercise, diet, and follow-up care.
4 Patient will learn to swim and will swim twice weekly at the Jewish Activity Center.	

Nursing Diagnosis   Coping, ineffective individual, related to chronic feelings of loneliness and isolation.

Patient Outcomes	*Nursing Interventions*
1 Patient will attend activities at Jewish Family Services twice a week.	1 Encourage and support social networking.
2 Patient will join a social group at the local synagogue.	2 Introduce patient to Jewish Services and involve patient's family in relation to compliance.
3 Patient will enroll in English at the Milwaukee Area Technical College (MATC).	3 Arrange for patient to visit the library of Russian books and journals located at Jewish Family Services.
	4 Help patient make initial contacts for English-as-a-second-language (ESL) classes held at MATC.
	5 Arrange transportation for patient for all activities and clinic visits.

Nursing Diagnosis   Coping, ineffective individual, related to lowered self-esteem and separation from previous contacts.

Patient Outcome	*Nursing Interventions*
Patient will network with other Soviet immigrants.	1 Show respect for patient's cultural preferences.
	2 Provide reading materials for patient.
	3 Introduce patient to other Soviet immigrants outside of her family and follow up with kindness, caring, and honest concern.

STUDY
QUESTIONS

1. Why is it important that Slava's own list of foods be used when making out a weekly menu?
2. How will the nurse keep Slava motivated toward self-care?
3. What role will Slava's family play in her recovery?
4. During patient teaching, how much space should be between the nurse and Slava?

5. How may the nurse use Slava's spiritual values and beliefs to the best advantage?
6. Why is Slava likely to be compliant?
7. What role does language play in this nurse-patient relationship?
8. In addition to what is listed in the care plan, how else might the nurse increase Slava's self-esteem and decision-making potential?
9. When talking with Slava, what should the nurse be careful *not* to do?
10. How may Slava's attitudes toward self-learning and lifelong learning enhance nursing care strategies?
11. Why did Slava adamantly refuse psychiatric consultation? What should the nurse do now?

REFERENCES

Allen, M. (1983, Jan.). A Soviet study trip. *Nursing Mirror, 156,* 17-20.

Anthony-Tkach, C. (1985). Nursing and health care in the Soviet Union. *Nursing Forum, 22*(2), 45-52.

APA representatives meet with Soviets to discuss abuse of psychiatry in USSR. (1987, May 1). *Psychiatric News*, p. 37.

Auster, B.A. (1989, April 3). When high hopes meet harsh realities. *U.S. News and World Report*, pp. 43-44.

Binyon, M. (1983). *Life in Russia*. New York: Berkley Publishing.

Black, A. (1989, April 10). Here come the trainers. *Time Magazine*, p. 102.

Brown, L. (1979). At the centre of things. *Nursing Mirror, 148*(10), 20-21.

Brown, M.S. (1984). Health care in the Soviet Union. *Nursing Practitioner, 9,* 50-52.

Carr, M. (1983). Kindness and consideration. *Nursing Mirror, 157*(2), 26-28.

Cox, M. (1983, April). A peek at nursing in the Soviet Union. *Weather Vane, 52,* 6-7.

Dennis, L.I. (1989). Soviet hospital nursing: A model for self-care. *Journal of Nursing Education, 28*(2), 76-77.

Dentzer, S., Trimble, J., & Auster, B. (1989, Nov. 20). The Soviet economy in shambles. *U.S. News and World Report*, pp. 25-44.

DeWitt, P.E. (1989, April 10). A profession under stress. *Time Magazine*, pp. 94-95.

Doerner, W.R. (1989, June 19). Soviet Union: Hard lessons and unhappy citizens. *Time Magazine*, pp. 28-29.

Garelik, G. (1989, April 10). Where Slava starts over again. *Time Magazine*, pp. 32-34.

Gennis, M. (1989, Sept.). Personal communication (Assistant Professor of Medicine and Program Director of Internal Medicine, Sinai Samaritan Medical Center/University of Wisconsin; in charge of health care for all Soviet immigrants).

Gioiella, E.C. (1983). Russia: The Soviet health care system for the aged. *Journal of Gerontological Nursing, 9*(11), 582-585.

Give us your masses—up to a point. (1989, Sept. 18). *US News and World Report*, p. 12.

Health care in communion with Hippocrates. (1988, June). *Soviet Life*, pp. 30-31.

Hess, G. (1971). Impressions of mental health service delivery systems in Finland, Poland, Soviet Russia and Czechoslovakia. *International Journal of Nursing Studies, 8*(4), 223-235.

Kershbaum, L. (1983). The PNA visit to the Soviet Union. *Pennsylvania Nurse, 38,* 13.

Kinsey, D. (1989). Nursing and health care in the U.S.S.R. *Nursing Outlook, 37*(3), 120-122.

Knox, C. (1988). Chernobyl health effects may never be seen. *Science News, 134*(25), 391.

Koval, V. (1989, March). Working women: Common problems. *Soviet Life*, pp. 24-25.

Latinis-Bridges, B., & Clancy, B.J. (1988, March). An American perception of Soviet health care. *Kansas Nurse, 63,* 1-2

Latinis-Bridges, B., & Dayani, E. (1984, March). Perspectives on Soviet nursing and health care. *Kansas Nurse, 59,* 2-4.

MacAvoy, S. (1988). A cross-cultural learning opportunity: USSR, 1985. *The Journal of Continuing Education in Nursing, 19*(5), 196-200.

Maloof, E.C. (1970, May). A firsthand report of health facilities in the USSR. *Dental Economics*, pp. 27-30.

Manning, J. (1989, Sept. 28). Boy will have a story with heart to tell. *Milwaukee Sentinel*.

Moore, R. (Ed.). (1988). *Fodor's 89 Soviet Union*. New York: Fodor's Travel Publications.

Myco, F. (1984, Feb. 1-7). Health care in the Soviet Union. *Nursing Times, 80,* 40-43.

Raloff, J., and Silberner, J. (1986). Chernobyl: Emerging data on accident. *Science News, 129*(19), 292-293.

Roberts, S., & Auster, B. (1989, Oct. 23). The new refugees. *U.S. News and World Report,* pp. 34-37.

Ruby, M. (1989, March 3). Sinai Samaritan to double free care for Soviets. *Wisconsin Jewish Chronicle,* p. 8.

Schiff, A. (1979). Language, culture and Jewish acculturation of Soviet Jewish emigres. *Journal of Jewish Communal Service,* 44-49, 56-57.

Scott, A. (1988). Human interaction and personal boundaries. *Journal of Psychosocial Nursing, 26*(8), 23-27.

Serrill, M.S. (1986). Anatomy of a catastrophe. *Time Magazine, 128*(9), 26-29.

Simons, B. (1976). *The volume library*. Nashville, Tenn.: Southwestern Company.

Smith, L.S. (1989). Soviet nursing and health care. *Advancing Clinical Care, 4*(5), 41-44.

Soviets under fire for committing sane people. (1987, Nov. 23). *Health Week,* p. 5.

Traver, N. (1989, April 10). Restructuring the 3 R's. *Time Magazine,* pp. 96-97.

Trimble, J. (1989, April 3). The Ukraine: The critical republic. *US News & World Report,* pp. 45-47.

U.S. Department of Commerce, Bureau of the Census. (1988). *Current population reports, divisions and states*. Washington, D.C.: Superintendant of Documents.

Vlassov, P.V. (1989). History of paramedical training in Russia. *Advancing Clinical Care, 4*(5), 27-31.

Wells, J.M., & Starpe, D.C. (1985, Aug.). Nursing administrator's perspective on the USSR health care system. *ANNA Journal, 12,* 255-288.

Wenger, A. (1985). Learning to do a mini ethnonursing research study: A doctoral student's experience. In M. Leininger (Ed.), *Qualitative research methods in nursing*. Orlando, Fla.: Grune & Stratton.

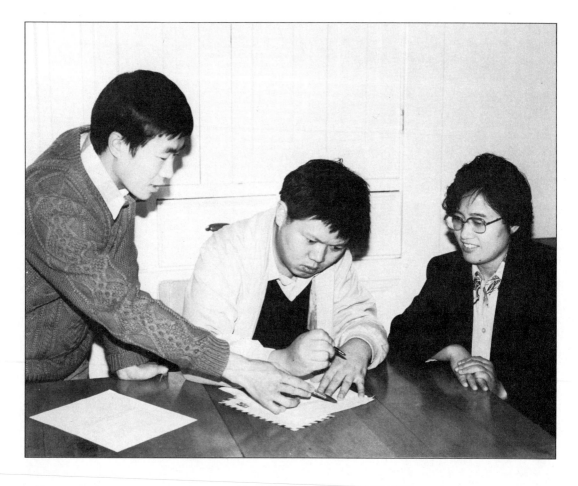

··

CHAPTER 16

Chinese Americans

Karen Chang

BEHAVIORAL OBJECTIVES
After reading this chapter, the nurse will be able to:

1 Describe the impact of Chinese philosophy and values on Chinese Americans.

2 Explain the ways that Chinese Americans communicate.

3 Describe the influences of the family system on Chinese Americans.

4 Explain the time concept of Chinese Americans.

5 Describe the illness behaviors of Chinese Americans.

6 Identify the biological variations of Chinese Americans.

7 Articulate the implications for providing effective nursing care to Chinese Americans.

OVERVIEW OF CHINESE AMERICANS

The majority of Chinese Americans are immigrants from Taiwan, Hong Kong, and mainland China. Chinese Americans have the largest population among Asian immigrants. According to the 1980 census, the United States has 812,000 Chinese Americans, and it was estimated that by 1990 the number would be 1.25 million. It is estimated that by the year 2000, there will be 1.7 million Chinese immigrants living in the United States (*Statistical Abstracts,* 1988).

Before 1965 most Chinese immigrants had little or no education, and many were alone because their families were not allowed to come with them. They were forced to immigrate for political, social, or economic reasons. The majority of them came from Canton and took up occupations such as mining, railroad construction, and farming. After 1965 immigration laws eased in the United States, and better-educated professionals and specialists began to immigrate. Now families were allowed to immigrate together. These immigrants came from Taiwan, mainland China, and Hong Kong. As a result, a wide cultural and linguistic diversity exists among Chinese Americans.

A wide range of educational levels exists among Chinese Americans. There are many college-educated professionals, yet there is a larger number of barely literate individuals working in low-paying occupations (Mangiafico, 1988; Wong, 1982; Yeun & Schwartz, 1986).

Chinese culture is dominated by Confucius' teachings, which encourage individuals to pursue love, righteousness, decorum, and wisdom. A harmonious relationship with nature and other people is stressed, and a person is expected to accommodate rather than confront. If private interest conflicts with community interest, a person is expected to submit to the interest of the group rather than advocate personal concerns. Public debating of conflicting views is not acceptable. A person is expected to be sensitive to what people think, and to be gracious toward others so as not to make them "lose face." Self-expression and individualism are discouraged, whereas showing filial piety to parents and loyalty to family, friends, and government is highly praised. Modesty, self-control, self-reliance, self-restraint, and face-saving are frequently taught to Chinese people. When they fail to follow these cultural practices, they feel shame or guilt. Consequently, Chinese people appear to be quiet, polite, pleasant, and nonassertive and often suppress feelings such as anger or pain.

Reciprocation or treating others as one would wish to be treated is often used in interpersonal relationships. Interpersonal interactions have a hierarchical structure, so that older or higher-status people have authority over younger or lower-status people. A person's status is always referred to during interactions. For example, brothers address each other as "older brother" and "younger brother" in addition to the first name. Educational achievement and professional success are highly valued because pride and honor are brought to the family and the community as a result. Therefore Chinese parents willingly provide support for children to pursue higher education.

The sharp contrasts between the Chinese and American cultures cause a high level of stress among Chinese Americans during the acculturation process. Some may hold on to traditional Chinese culture, observe holidays according to the lunar calendar, and maintain Chinese customs; some may reject all their traditional heritage; and some may assimilate both the Chinese culture and the American culture. Ill-adjusted individuals may not be able to perform tasks productively, may have low self-esteem, and may exhibit some lawless behaviors. Second- and third-generation Chinese Americans, who are already well assimilated into the Western culture, may not be influenced much by traditional Chinese culture. However, they may experience an identity problem: culturally and linguistically they are Americans, yet others may perceive them as Chinese (Albert & Triandis, 1985; Becker, 1986; Chang, 1981; Chen & Yang, 1986; *Encyclopedia Americana,* 1983; Louie, 1985; Orque, Bloch, & Monrroy, 1983).

COMMUNICATION
Dialect

Linguistic diversity causes communication problems among Chinese people. Although the official Chinese language is Mandarin, there are many dialects spoken that are not understood by other groups of Chinese people. All the languages have the same written characters, however, which have not been changed for 3000 years. This stability in the language permits all literate Chinese persons to be able to communicate in writing. Each Chinese word consists of only one syllable. Each word has its own meaning, but if a word is combined with another word, the meaning of the combined words could be changed. There are four tones, and changes of tone could also change the meaning of the word. The Chinese language has no copulas, plurals, or tenses (Becker, 1986; *Encyclopedia Americana,* 1983; Hall, 1976).

Style, Volume, and Touch

The Chinese value silence more than Americans and avoid disagreeing or criticizing. Disagreements are not verbalized, so that harmonious relationships will be maintained, at least outwardly. To raise one's voice to make a point, a common behavior for some Americans, is viewed by some Chinese people as being associated with anger and as a sign of loss of control. To avoid confrontation, the word "no" is rarely used; furthermore, the word "yes" can mean "no" or "perhaps." A direct "no" is avoided because it may cause the same individual to lose face. Hesitance, ambiguity, subtlety, and implicity are dominant in Chinese speech. Understanding nonverbal cues and contextual meanings is also necessary during communication. For example, serving a banana with tea indicates an unacceptable marriage arrangement. To communicate effectively, all parties involved must participate (Argyle, 1982).

Chinese people do not ordinarily touch each other during conversation. Touching someone's head indicates a serious breach of etiquette. Touching during an argument indicates shameful loss of self-control. In the same respect, putting one's feet on a desk, table, or chair is regarded as impolite and disrespectful. On the other hand, public displays of affection toward a person of the same sex are quite permissible. Public displays between the opposite sex, however, are not considered acceptable, and as a result, Chinese people are often viewed as shy, cold, polite, unassertive, or uninterested (Chen & Yang, 1986; Watson, 1970).

Context

Communication among the Chinese is high-context communication, which is the opposite of communication among mainstream Americans in many ways.

A high-context communication is one in which most of the information is either in the physical context or internalized in the person, while very little is in the coded, explicit, transmitted part of the message. A low-context communication is just the opposite, i.e., the mass of the information is vested in the explicit code. (Hall, 1976)

Chinese people perceive and value more nonverbal and contextual cues than do Americans. For example, facial expressions, tensions, movements, the speed of interactions, and the location of interactions are perceived during interactions and have some meaning (Anderson, 1986). Chinese people have a tendency to view what is immediately perceptible, especially visually perceptible, and seek intuitive understanding through direct perception. Intuitive understanding is valued more than logical reasoning (Gudykunst, Stewart, & Toomey, 1985).

Kinesics

Chinese people greet others by bowing. When they nod their heads, this may indicate "yes," whereas shaking the head may indicate "no." To answer a question such as "Haven't you had anything to eat?" is problematic for many Chinese Americans.

They may be confused about whether to answer affirmatively or negatively: "Yes, I haven't had anything," or "No, I would like something." Many Chinese Americans experience feelings of shame and embarrassment when they cannot communicate well. Some apologize frequently for their linguistic inabilities because they think they are inconveniencing others. Even though most Chinese people do not express their emotions, some may narrow their eyes to express anger and disgust (Argyle, 1982). Chinese people have less eye contact than Americans because in their culture excessive eye contact may indicate rudeness (Watson, 1970).

Chinese Americans experience a great amount of stress when they are in health care facilities. The language barrier and different cultural background often cause these people to experience confusion, depression, frustration, helplessness, and powerlessness. However, they feel that they would inconvenience the health care worker and thus are often embarrassed to ask questions when no health care workers speak their language (Smith & Ryan, 1987). These emotional experiences are often not verbally expressed but may be indicated by nonverbal cues. Frequently, observing nonverbal behaviors and encouraging patients to verbalize will help identify these psychological problems.

Implications for Nursing Care

It is important for the nurse to remember that there are diversified Chinese dialects that are not comprehensible to other Chinese groups. If the patient needs a translator in the health care setting, the nurse should find out whether this patient speaks Mandarin or not. If not, the nurse needs to find a translator who can speak the same dialect as the patient.

Since the Chinese language is quite different from English, the nurse needs to keep in mind that when Chinese Americans communicate with their second language, they often experience a great amount of stress. The nurse may observe these symptoms of stress and can help the patient relax to lower the stress level. Since Chinese Americans tend to be quiet, polite, and unassertive and tend to suppress feelings such as anxiety, fear, depression, or pain, it is important for the nurse to recognize nonverbal cues and their cultural meanings in order to develop culturally appropriate nursing care plans.

Some Chinese Americans hesitate to ask questions when they do not understand; therefore after rapport has been established, the nurse should elicit and encourage Chinese Americans to verbalize their feelings and ask questions. The nurse should avoid using negative questions to elicit responses, because negative questions are comprehended differently in the Chinese language.

In addition, since some Chinese Americans do not ordinarily touch another individual during conversation, it is important for the nurse to explain the necessity of touching, particularly when therapeutic assistance is needed. Showing respect, demonstrating empathy, and being nonjudgmental can help establish rapport with Chinese American patients. The nurse can communicate better with Chinese Americans by understanding cultural practices, as well as differing communication styles. Therapeutic communication techniques can be used to promote conversations to help Chinese American patients express thoughts and feelings, and to ensure mutual understanding, especially when the nurse thinks the patient is experiencing anxiety, fear, depression, or pain.

SPACE

In studying human spatial relationships, Hall (1976) divided humans into two groups: contact and noncontact. People from a contact group interact with each other by facing each other more directly, being closer, touching more, employing more eye contact, and speaking more loudly than members of a noncontact group. People from a contact group may perceive people from a noncontact group as being shy, uninterested, cold, and impolite. Conversely, people from a noncontact group may view people from a contact group as being pushy, aggressive, obnoxious, and impolite (Hall, 1963). Both Chinese Americans and most middle-class mainstream Americans are categorized as being in noncontact groups. However, from the Asian's point of view, Americans face each other more, touch more, and have more visual contact than Asians. Chinese people feel more comfortable in a side-by-side or right-angle arrangement and may feel uncomfortable when placed in a face-to-face situation. Americans prefer to sit face-to-face or at right angles to each other. In the Asian culture the person of higher status has the prerogative of sitting as proximally as desired; thus the burden of correct behavior is on the person of lesser status (Porter & Samovar, 1988; Watson, 1970).

Implications for Nursing Care

Since Chinese Americans are categorized as a noncontact group, it is important for the nurse to remember that some Chinese Americans may be erroneously perceived as being extremely shy or withdrawn. It is equally important for the nurse to remember that some Chinese Americans may view tasks that are associated with closeness, increased eye contact, and touch as being offensive or impolite. The nurse can reduce these misunderstandings by providing explanations when performing these tasks. Since some Chinese Americans feel uncomfortable with face-to-face arrangements, the nurse may seek the patient's input in terms of comfortable seating arrangements.

SOCIAL ORGANIZATION
Impact of Immigration on Social Organization

Many early Chinese immigrants came to this country as contract laborers or with money that was borrowed from various Chinese American organizations. These organizations assumed a supervisory role for these early immigrants once they arrived in the United States. The Chinese immigrants were very similar to other immigrants from other ethnic and cultural groups in that most of them were unfamiliar with the language and the culture of the United States. Therefore many of the early Chinese immigrants worked as laborers in gangs. Although many of these individuals were physically smaller than those in other ethnic or cultural groups in the United States, they nevertheless were hard workers. Historically Chinese Americans helped forge and build the United States in such areas as railroad building and other equally taxing jobs. Early Chinese immigrants worked very cheaply and saved money by living very frugally. These virtues made many of the early Chinese immigrants employable, but they were feared and hated as competitors by other American workers (Lyman, 1974).

By 1851 there were 25,000 Chinese Americans living in California alone (Sung, 1967). By 1870 the number of Chinese immigrants in the United States had increased to 63,000. In 1880 approximately 6000 Chinese persons entered the United States. Nearly twice as many entered the United States in 1881, and nearly five times as many entered in 1882 (Sung, 1967). However, in 1882 an exclusionary immigration law reduced the inflow of Chinese immigrants to less than 1000 until the year 1890. It is because of this law that the initial Chinese immigration was almost exclusively male. It is thought that the immigration of Chinese men to the United States was a tentative rather than a permanent move, and during the 1880s the number of Chinese persons leaving the United States was greater than the number coming in.

In addition to the Chinese exclusion act of 1882, other laws were enacted in the United States that severely curtailed not only immigration, but also the possibility of a Chinese person becoming a naturalized citizen. Furthermore, some of these laws were specific enough to require citizenship as a prerequisite for entering many occupations and for owning land (Sowell, 1981). Also, during the period from 1854 to 1874, there were laws that prevented Chinese people from testifying in court against White men (Lyman, 1974). Some historians believe that such laws in effect made it possible to declare "open season" on Chinese Americans because many of these individuals had no legal recourse when robbed, vandalized, or assaulted. The almost total exclusion of Chinese immigration from 1882 to 1890 had devastating long-range effects on Chinese Americans that are evident even today. Since the early Chinese immigrants were almost exclusively male, there was very little hope for a normal social or family life. Many of these early male immigrants had wives and children in China whom they would not see for many years if at all; because of the severe restrictions on economic opportunities, it was not possible to earn enough money to book passage back to China.

Over the years the few Chinese women who had managed to immigrate to the United States were able to produce a small number of second-generation children. When these children grew up, there was a slight ease in the serious shortage of women that remained characteristic of Chinese Americans from the early immigration period until World War II. In addition, an unknown number of Chinese women were smuggled into the United States for the specific purpose of prostitution (Lyman, 1974). As recently as the 1960s a number of illegal aliens also entered the country to pursue a better life. As a result, many Chinese residents deliberately avoid census takers.

Despite the fact that economic opportunities for early Chinese immigrants were highly restricted, many Chinatown communities took care of their own indigents. It is perhaps for this reason that even during such disasters such as the San Francisco earthquake in 1906 and the Great Depression of the 1930s, many Chinese Americans did not seek or receive federal aid.

In 1943 there was a repeal of the Chinese exclusion act of 1882, which did help ease the imbalance of the male/female ratio and permitted a more normal family life to develop among a very family-oriented people. After the repeal of the Chinese exclusion act of 1882, the bulk of the new Chinese immigrants were female (Sung, 1967). The labor shortages of World War II opened many new job opportunities that were not previously available to Chinese Americans. Thus many Chinese Americans abandoned traditional Chinatown occupations to move into these new jobs (Sowell, 1981).

In 1940 only 3% of Chinese Americans in California had jobs that were considered "professional," as compared with 8% of the White population. By 1950 the percentage of Chinese Americans in professional fields had doubled to 6%, and over the next decade the percentage of Chinese Americans working in professional fields tripled and for the first time passed the percentage of Whites working in professional fields. In 1970 it was reported that Chinese Americans in general had a higher income or higher occupational status than most other Americans. In 1970 at least one fourth of all employed Chinese Americans were working in scientific or professional fields (Sowell, 1981).

Today, approximately 63% of Chinese Americans are foreign born. States with the largest percentages of Chinese Americans are California (40.1%), Hawaii (6.9%), New York (18.1%), Illinois (3.6%), and Texas (3.3%). The median age for Chinese Americans is reported to be 29.6 years as compared with 30 years for the rest of the nation. Today, 49% of Chinese Americans are women as compared with 51% in the rest of the population. Seemingly, the disparity between males and females that existed during the earlier immigration of Chinese people has been resolved. The number of married-couple families among Chinese Americans is 87% as compared with 83% for the rest of the population. Chinese Americans are reported to have an average of 3.7 persons per family. In 1980 approximately 75% of the male Chinese American population and 67% of the female Chinese American population had at least a high school education. In addition, in 1980 44% of Chinese American men and 30% of Chinese American women had completed college. Approximately 66% of Chinese Americans are in the work force. Chinese Americans own or operate 26% of the number of businesses in the United States, with gross receipts exceeding 6 billion dollars. These gross receipts represent approximately 39% of the gross receipts received throughout the United States. The average income per family for Chinese Americans is $22,600 as compared with $19,900 for the rest of the population (*Statistical Abstracts,* 1988). However, while more than 60% of Chinese families have more than one wage earner, there still are many low-income Chinese families in the United States; approximately 13.5% of Chinese Americans live below the poverty level as compared with 12% for the entire United States (Orque, Bloch, & Monrroy, 1983).

Family

The Chinese culture emphasizes loyalty to family and devotion to tradition, and deemphasizes individual feelings (Chen & Yang, 1986). Chinese individuals are willing to submit their own interests to those of the family, which maintains a strong and cohesive bond. The family is expected to take care of its members, both immediate and extended. Doing so brings honor to the family; not doing so brings shame (Kim, 1988; Louie, 1985).

The Chinese family generally has a hierarchical structure. The older children have authority over younger children, and the younger children must show respect and deference to authority figures. Failure to do so causes shame for the family. The authority figures have more influence on decision making, and these decisions are made on the basis on consensus rather than majority. The individual learns to submit to the prevailing opinion rather than disagree (Anderson, 1986; Gudykunst, Stewart, & Toomey, 1985). However, the values of the Chinese American family are eroding in the acculturation process; many youngsters do not show respect to the elderly, and many elderly persons cannot count on their children or relatives for help. Many older Chinese Americans thus suffer mental illnesses, and some commit suicide (Tien-Hyatt, 1987).

Marital status

Because of the early exclusion act in the United States, there was a disproportionately large number of Chinese men as compared with Chinese women. Many of the early unmarried Chinese men who came to the United States had virtually no opportunity to marry; thus in 1890 only 26.1% of the total number of Chinese men in the United States were married. The percentage of married Chinese women from 1890 to 1950 ranged from 57.4% to 69.1%. During this time period there appeared to be a lower percentage of single Chinese women who immigrated, which was partially accounted for by the Chinese tradition of females marrying at a younger age. Chinese Americans divorce less frequently than their American counterparts (Sung, 1967).

Religion

The four primary religions of China are Taoism, Buddhism, Islam, and Christianity. Of these four primary religions, Taoism has the least number of professed followers. Among the Chinese and Chinese Americans, Christianity is regarded as a newcomer; nevertheless, its effects are pronounced. Christianity is viewed as being partially responsible for the introduction of the Western culture into China as well as to Chinese persons living in the United States. Today the number of Chinese Roman Catholics is increasing rapidly, particularly among foreign-born Chinese Americans (Sowell, 1981).

Implications for Nursing Care

It is important for the nurse to remember that Chinese Americans are a family-oriented people who normally put family loyalties before personal interests. In addition, the Chinese American family has traditionally had a hierarchical structure. Chinese Americans perceive that they have a major responsibility in taking care of family members and relatives. Therefore family members may view the hospitalization or health care needs of a family member as a personal concern. The nurse needs to understand this sense of responsibility on the part of the family and be sensitive to their needs. Opinions and ideas of the family members should be incorporated into the plan of care. Also, it is important to provide health care education to all family members, not just the patient, when procedures are to be done.

Chinese Americans vary widely in educational background and socioeconomic status, have varied cultural and religious values and practices, and have different rates of acculturation. For example, some Chinese Americans speak English very poorly, whereas some can communicate in English without any problem. Some have medical insurance, whereas some do not. Some use herbal medicine, whereas some do not. If the patient has a language barrier, a translator is needed and can usually be found in the local Chinese community. Visual displays, flip charts, or exhibits can be used to facilitate the patient's understanding.

Most Chinese Americans have strong family ties. By assessing the patient's kinship relationship and identifying authoritative family members, the nurse can effectively use the influential family members to achieve the therapeutic goals. The nurse should help Chinese Americans with few support systems to seek community resources.

Chinese women are very uncomfortable and uneasy when examined by male health professionals. The nurse should be present and assist in the examination to ease the Chinese American woman's tension.

TIME

The Chinese have a different perception and experience regarding time; it is not past, present, or future oriented. Some Chinese Americans perceive time as a dynamic wheel with circular movements and the present as a reflection of the eternal. This metaphoric wheel continually turns in an unforeseeable direction, and individuals are expected to adjust to the present, which surrounds the rotating wheel, and seek a harmonious relationship with their surroundings (Kim, 1988; Yeun, 1987).

Hall (1963) has described the time concept of the Asian as "polychronic" and that of the Westerner as "monochronic." An individual with a polychronic time orientation adheres less rigidly to time as a distinct and linear entity, focuses on the completion of the present, and often implements more than one activity simultaneously. On the other hand, an individual with a monochronic orientation to time emphasizes schedules, promptness, standardization of activities, and synchronization with clocks.

When making decisions regarding current and future events, some Chinese people may be affected by traditions and customs. They may seek symbols, correlations, and intuitive understanding, as well as consider significances, consequences, future situations, and present factors before making decisions. They do not make decisions according to an individual's own benefit (Gudykunst, Stewart, & Toomey, 1985).

Implications for Nursing Care

Since Chinese Americans are perceived as being polychronic, which more or less implies that they are present time oriented, it is important for the nurse to remember that some Chinese Americans may not adhere to fixed schedules. Polychronic individuals may arrive late for appointments; may insist on completing a task before moving on to a new task, even though the new task may be time related; and may implement more than one task at a time. It is important for the nurse to recognize that when some Chinese Americans make decisions related to current events, they may appear hesitant because of the need to consider as many variables as possible.

ENVIRONMENTAL CONTROL

Many Chinese Americans may not believe that they have control over nature, since some Chinese people subscribe to a belief in fatalism and may view people as adjusting to the physical world, not controlling or changing the environment (Gudykunst, Stewart, & Toomey, 1985). In traditional Chinese teaching, a harmonious relationship with nature is stressed. The concepts of yin and yang represent the power that regulates the universe and that exists also within the body, as well as food.

Yang represents the positive, active, or "male" force, and *yin* represents the negative, inactive, or "female" force. Body systems are categorized into yin and yang groups. For example, the liver, heart, spleen, lungs, and kidneys are yin, whereas the gallbladder, stomach, large intestine, small intestine, bladder, and lymphatic system are yang. The yin forces store the strength of life, and the yang forces protect the body from outside invasions. Some Chinese people believe that an imbalance between yin and yang will result in illnesses, whereas a balance between yin and yang can enhance health.

Food is also grouped into yin/"cold" and yang/"hot" groups and is considered to be either the cause or the treatment of illnesses. A person with leukemia may believe that too many cold foods have been consumed. Diseases or conditions with excessive yin forces, such as cancer, postpartum psychoses, menstruation, or lactation, are treated with foods with yang quality, such as beef, chicken, eggs, fried foods, spicy foods, hot foods, vinegar, and wine. Diseases or conditions with excessive yang forces, such as infections, fever, hypertension, sore throat, or toothache, require the intake of foods with yin quality, such as bean curds, honey, carrots, turnips, green vegetables, fruits, cold foods, and duck (Ludman & Newman, 1984). In addition, the Chinese often use vegetables (for example, bok choy), tea, honey, or prunes to treat constipation; they use chrysanthemum, crystal, ginseng, or other teas to treat indigestion (Hess, 1986).

Illness/Wellness Behaviors

The cultural differences and language barriers play a major role in the utilization of health services among Chinese Americans. Many Chinese Americans use both Western medical services and Chinese medical services (predominantly herbal medicine) in the case of illness. Typically, a Chinese American will treat minor or chronic illnesses with Chinese medical services and acute or serious problems with Western medical services (Liu, 1986). Traditionally, the Chinese believe in preventive health practices. Some Chinese Americans will first seek Chinese medicines and try to manage on their own. When physiological signs indicate that conditions are getting worse, they will then seek Western medicines. This is especially common among Chinese American psychiatric patients because of the emphasis the Chinese culture puts on self-control and self-sufficiency.

Many Chinese Americans tend to underutilize medical services because of their low socioeconomic status. Although unemployment rates for Chinese Americans are lower than those for the general population, underemployment among Chinese Americans is much higher. Underemployment problems include a shorter working week, a mismatch between education and employment, and longer working hours for the same pay. In addition, at least 13% of Chinese Americans live at or below the poverty level. Many elderly male Chinese Americans live alone with a low income as a result of early immigration laws. Immigrant families may have no medical insurance because they may not be familiar with medical insurance, they may not believe in insuring health, or they may not be able to afford it (Liu, 1986).

Some Chinese Americans fear medical institutions because of language barriers and unfamiliarity with medical institutions, or because of an inadequate understanding of illnesses and treatment modalities. As a result, some Chinese Americans may not comply with medical treatments. Many diagnostic tests, such as amniocentesis, glucose tolerance testing, ultrasonography, or drawing blood, are often perceived as being dangerous and unnecessary (Minkler, 1983).

Some Chinese Americans have a tendency to self-medicate with over-the-counter drugs, herbal remedies, tranquilizers, and antibiotics (Campbell & Chang, 1973; Gallo, Edwards, & Vessey, 1980; Hess, 1986; Louie, 1985; McLaughlin et al., 1987). In addition, some Chinese Americans may save part of a prescribed medicine and take it at their own discretion at a later time (Campbell & Chang, 1973). Some Chinese people respond to pain stoically because of a fear of addiction and because of the value the culture puts on self-control (Thiederman, 1989). For some Chinese people the predominant pain preparations are topical ointments and balms (Hess, 1986).

Some Chinese Americans use both herbal medicines and Western medicines at the same time to treat illnesses, and since some herbal and Western medicines have similar effects, using both can create problems. For example, ginseng is a tonic stimulant and an antihypertensive medicine. The patient may overmedicate by taking antihypertensive drugs and ginseng at the same time.

Chinese herbal medicines are boiled in a specified amount of water over low heat until the desired concentration is reached. The medicines are then taken as a single dose. If the patient does not feel better after the initial dose, the patient may need to return to the herbalist. Because of this tradition, some Chinese Americans are not familiar with the practice of taking drugs when feeling well. In addition, the practice of taking multiple drugs in tablet or capsule form at various times and over several days or weeks can be confusing (Hess, 1986; Liu, 1986; Louie, 1985).

Folklore and Folk Practices

Restoring the balance of yin and yang is the fundamental concept of Chinese medical practice and includes acupuncture, herbal medicines, massage, skin scraping, and cupping. Acupuncture involves the insertion of metal needles through specific body points to treat or cure illnesses with excessive yang forces, such as pain, stroke, or asthma. Herbal medicines are categorized according to the properties of yin or yang and their therapeutic functions and are prescribed on the basis of the yin-yang nature of the particular illness.

"Moxibustion" is another folk practice that involves heat treatment of illnesses such as mumps or convulsions. When moxibustion is used as a treatment, the ignited moxa plants are placed near specific areas of the body. After moxibustion, tiny craters about 1 cm in diameter can be observed on the skin.

Massage is used to stimulate the circulation, to increase the flexibility of the joints, and to improve the body's resistance to illnesses.

Skin scraping is a method of applying special oil to the symptomatic area and rubbing the area with the edge of a coin in a firm, downward motion. This treatment is used to treat colds, heatstroke, headache, and indigestion. Linear multiple bruises may be observed on the skin as a result of this process.

Cupping is used to treat headaches, arthritis, and abdominal pain. A vacuum is created inside a cup by burning a special material, and the cup is then placed immediately on the selected area and kept there until it is easily removed. Circular, ecchymotic, painful burn marks 2 inches in diameter can be observed on the skin after this treatment (Boyle & Andrews, 1989; Louie, 1985; Spector, 1985).

Implications for Nursing Care

Since Chinese Americans often believe that they do not have control over nature and maintain a fatalistic outlook on life, they may be hesitant about seeking health care treatment. In addition, since some Chinese Americans subscribe to the theory of yin and yang, which attempts to restore balance to the body, such individuals are more likely to engage in self-treatment. Therefore the nurse must be able to distinguish between practices that could be harmful, neutral, or beneficial to the patient's particular medical problem. For example, some Chinese Americans from Southeast Asia or urban areas in China may practice native healing processes wherein they may tie a string around the wrist, burn incense, or make food offerings to the spirits. As long as these practices are not harmful, the nurse should respect them and allow them to continue (Gallo et al., 1980). The nurse who observes that a Chinese American patient is taking herbal medicine in addition to the prescribed medicine should caution the patient about the possibility of overmedicating.

Some Chinese Americans who subscribe to the theory of yin and yang believe that food has yin and yang qualities. Therefore the nurse must help the patient select the appropriate foods according to these beliefs. Also, hospital food could be foreign to some Chinese Americans. If the patient wishes, the nurse may encourage the family to bring in some native foods.

BIOLOGICAL VARIATIONS

People are the product of both genetic factors and environmental influences. For example, it has been theorized that the epicanthic fold that gives the Chinese a slant-eyed look may have evolved as a protection against blinding blizzards of snow or sand (Bleibtreu & Downs, 1971). The "yellow" color of the Chinese skin is thought to be due to a smaller amount of melanin in the skin than is in the skin of Black people (*Time*, 1967). Others have theorized that Chinese people may have a thickened corneum, creating the yellowish skin color (Molnar, 1983). Most Chinese people have thick straight hair. Chinese men tend to lack facial hair.

Body Size and Structure

Chinese Americans tend to be shorter at all ages and tend to complete their growth earlier than other Americans (Molnar, 1983). On the standard growth charts, the mean height and weight of Chinese American children fall in the tenth percentile, whereas the mean height and weight of mainstream American children fall in the fiftieth percentile (Boyle & Andrews, 1989). Asians on the average have longer trunks and shorter limbs than Whites. Some Chinese Americans have wider hips and narrower shoulders than other Americans. The children of Chinese immigrants are generally taller than native Chinese children, but their sitting/standing height ratio does not change. Asians have smaller chest volumes than Whites. The average forced expiratory volume (FEV) for Chinese Americans is 2.53 liters versus 3.22 liters for White Americans. The average forced vital capacity (FVC) is 3.27 liters for Chinese Americans versus 4.30 liters for White Americans (Overfield, 1985).

Skin Color

The majority of Chinese infants have mongolian spots (irregular areas of deep blue pigmentation observed primarily in the sacral and gluteal regions and occasionally in other parts of the body). Neonatal jaundice is seen in 50% of Chinese infants. The bilirubin level peaks on the fifth and sixth days of life, as compared with the second and third days for other races. Twenty-five to forty percent of Chinese infants have bilirubin levels higher than 12 mg/dl, and 15% to 23% of Chinese infants have blood levels higher than 15 mg/dl. Breast-feeding enhances the bilirubin level. The physician may suggest that the mother stop breast-feeding until the baby's bilirubin levels return to normal (Boyle & Andrews, 1989; Overfield, 1985).

Enzymatic and Genetic Variations

A majority of Chinese Americans have a lactase deficiency and are thus unable to tolerate fresh milk. Lactase splits milk sugar, lactose, into the simple glucose and galactose. A lack of lactase may cause a person who drinks fresh milk to have flatus, abdominal cramps, diarrhea, or vomiting. However, the person can often eat cheese because bacteria does the work of lactase. This enzyme also may be induced by long-term consumption of fresh milk.

The Chinese have relatively high incidences of thalassemia and glucose-6-phosphate dehydrogenase (G-6-PD) deficiency. Thalassemia is a type of hemoglobin abnormality characterized by a high rate of red blood cell destruction, necessitating frequent blood transfusions. G-6-PD deficiency is another red blood cell defect causing fragility of the red blood cells. People with G-6-PD deficiency are prone to anemia when exposed to certain drugs such as analgesics (aspirin, phenacetin), sulfonamides and sulfones, antimalarials (primaquine, quinacrine), antibacterials (nitrofurantoin, chloramphenicol, para-aminosalicylic acid), vitamin K, probenecid, and quinidine (Molnar, 1983; Overfield, 1985).

Another genetic difference is that Chinese people usually experience marked facial flushing and vasomotor symptoms after drinking alcohol. This may explain the low alcoholism rate among the Chinese (Overfield, 1985).

Susceptibility to Disease

Immigrants from Indochina and mainland China have common health problems, such as tuberculosis, intestinal parasites, malaria, malnutrition, anemia, and hepatitis. Most Southeast Asians received vaccinations (bacillus Camette-Guérin [BCG]) against tuberculosis in their childhood (Gallo et al., 1980).

Cancer

Chinese people are known to be at risk for cancers of the nasopharynx, esophagus, stomach, liver, and cervix. The intake of fermented and moldy foods, as well as nitrosamines contained in corn, bran, millet, and pickled vegetables, is thought to be a possible contributing factor for esophageal and liver cancers. Recent studies have revealed a downward trend for these cancers among Chinese Americans. On the other hand, the low-risk cancers for Chinese people (colon/rectum, lung, female breast, and leukemia) are gradually increasing among Chinese Americans (King & Locke, 1988; Yu, 1986). Further investigations are needed regarding the causes of these changes.

Mortality and Leading Causes of Death among Chinese Americans

In 1980, mortality data revealed the four leading causes of death for Chinese Americans to be identical to those for White Americans: first, heart disease; second, cancer; third, cerebrovascular disease; and fourth, accidents. The proportional mortality rates are different. Chinese Americans have a lower mortality from heart disease (32%) than White Americans (39%) and a higher mortality from cancer (27%) than White Americans (21%). The fifth leading cause of death for Chinese Americans is pneumonia and influenza. Suicide ranks seventh as a cause of death for Chinese Americans as compared with ranking tenth for White Americans. Chinese women have a higher suicide rate than White women. The causes of the higher suicide rate need further investigation (Yu, 1986).

Psychological Characteristics

Many Chinese Americans believe that psychiatric illnesses indicate an inability to solve problems or are manifested by behavior that is out of control, bringing shame to the individual and the family. Because of this, the family will often attempt to manage the sick person on their own until they can no longer handle the situation. As a result, hospitalized Chinese psychiatric patients appear more disturbed than other patients (Binder, 1983).

Chinese Americans experience multiple psychosocial stresses while adapting to the new culture and environment, including cultural conflicts, language difficulties, poverty, and discrimination. Many Chinese Americans experience depression and social loneliness, but few seek help until psychosomatic discomfort is experienced. Chinese Americans tend to seek help from physicians rather then psychiatrists or other mental health professionals for psychosomatic complaints (Hsu, Hailey, & Range, 1987; Kuo, 1984; Yeun & Schwartz, 1986).

Recent empirical studies have revealed that Asians require lower dosages than Whites for several psychotropic medications such as lithium, antidepressants, and neuroleptics. Asians require lower oral dosages and blood levels of lithium. The plasma levels of desipramine (an antidepressant) are higher and peak earlier for Asians than for Whites. Asians experience extrapyramidal effects at lower neuroleptic doses than do Whites. The plasma levels of diazepam at a given oral dose are higher in Asians than in Whites. Asians are reported to tolerate better the sedating effects of diphenhydramine. The causes for such differences are considered to be both genetic and environmental, suggesting that further investigation is needed (Lawson, 1986; Pi, Simpson & Cooper, 1986).

Implications for Nursing Care

It is important for the nurse to know that growth and development norms for Chinese Americans are different from White American standards. A standard growth chart for healthy Chinese children and adolescents is available (Whaley & Wong, 1987). However, the nurse should not rely on the growth chart alone. An assessment of general health status is necessary to identify malnutrition, anemia, or growth retardation (Gallo et al., 1980).

The nurse should reassure the Chinese American mother that it is normal for her newborn to exhibit more jaundice than other American babies. Otherwise, the mother may feel guilty and think the jaundice is due to something she ate. The observed mongolian spots on Chinese American infants should not be interpreted as lesions.

When working with a Chinese American family that has a family member with a physical or mental problem, the astute nurse will make using general or mental health facilities easier by providing information regarding the services, encouraging the family to seek help early, and arranging for follow-up care. Rather than waiting until the symptoms are advanced, the family should be assisted in getting appropriate care for their family member as soon as possible.

A case report illustrates the impact of the Chinese culture on a patient with a medical problem and psychotic symptoms. An 83-year-old Chinese woman exhibited psychotic symptoms at home for 15 months until the family could not handle the situation any longer and admitted her to a hospital. The family members felt guilty and ashamed because they could not take care of their mother. After admission, a health history revealed that the patient had had a gastrectomy about 13 years earlier, and her blood level of vitamin B_{12} was 91/dl (normal is 180 to 900/dl). She was treated with vitamin B_{12}, and the psychotic symptoms disappeared. If the family had brought the patient to the hospital earlier, they could have avoided 15 months of agony (Binder, 1983).

Patient and family teaching are important in providing care for the Chinese American patient and family. Lack of knowledge related to illnesses and treatment is a common problem and causes fear and anxiety. The nurse can assess the family's understanding of illnesses and treatment and provide education accordingly. If the patient takes herbal medicines, the nurse should provide education to increase the patient and family's awareness of the synergistic and antagonistic effects of Western and herbal medicines taken together. Since Asians are known to require lower dosages of psychotropic medications, the nurse should provide education about these medications and observe their effects and side effects. The nurse should also emphasize the importance of taking medicines as prescribed and discourage the practice of taking medicines only when symptoms of the illness are present. In addition, the nurse should keep in mind that Chinese Americans have a relatively high incidence of G-6-PD deficiency and alert the patient to seek help early when any side effects of medication are experienced.

The need for teaching about medication is illustrated by the following example. A Chinese American man took captopril at home as prescribed for 1 week and developed severe thirst and hyponatremia, leading to irreversible neurological damage (Al-Mufti & Arieff, 1985). He was polydipsic and drank about 7 liters daily. If he had been taught the side effects of captopril and had been encouraged to seek help when he experienced this side effect, his death could have been avoided.

Although many Chinese women breast-feed their babies, recently many Chinese American women have changed to bottle-feeding in adapting to the Western culture. The nurse should provide information regarding the benefits of breast-feeding and encourage mothers to breast-feed for at least 6 weeks (Minkler, 1983). If the mother has to stop breast-feeding because of jaundice, the nurse can teach the mother to express milk in order to continue breast-feeding when the baby is ready to be breast-fed again.

Dietary education is also very important in providing care for the Chinese American patient and family (Kolonel, 1988). Some Chinese Americans believe in the theory of yin and yang and eat foods accordingly when they are sick. For example, postpartum and following surgery, some Chinese Americans will not drink or eat anything with a yin nature, such as cold drinks, vegetables, salad, or cold meat; they will eat only chicken, beef, or fried foods. The nurse should help the patient select foods and drinks and encourage the family to bring the desired foods from home.

Chinese foods usually are cooked with soy sauce and monosodium glutamate (MSG). The nurse must remember that many preserved foods are also high in salt content. Therefore the nurse should inform patients who require a salt-restricted diet to reduce their sodium intake gradually by reducing the use of soy sauce, MSG, and preserved foods, and should discourage the high intake of fermented and moldy foods, which is considered to contribute to the high incidence of esophageal and liver cancer. The nurse should also encourage patients to reduce their intake of foods that have no nutritional value. Since many Chinese Americans may not be able to tolerate fresh milk because of a lactase deficiency, the nurse should encourage the use of tofu (bean curd) or other protein and calcium-rich foods to replace the need for fresh milk.

SUMMARY

The number of Chinese Americans is steadily increasing in the United States. As immigration of the Chinese continues, the nurse will encounter more Chinese Americans in health care facilities. Because of the complex cultural values and beliefs, diversified acculturation, and various educational levels among Chinese Americans, the nurse needs to work with individuals to assess their unique values, communication styles, social organization, time concepts, illness behaviors, and biological variations to provide effective and individualized nursing care. The nurse should convey respect to the patient, encourage pride in the Chinese culture, reduce feelings of shame, and facilitate adaptation to the Western culture.

CASE STUDY

A 40-year-old Chinese woman is admitted to a local hospital with the diagnosis of uremia. Her blood urea nitrogen (BUN) level is 168 mg/dl (normal is 8 to 18 mg/dl). She has a history of hypertension and was previously given a prescription for hydrochlorothiazide (HCTZ), which she stopped taking because of increasing dizziness, dry mouth, and weakness. She is single, lives alone, has no immediate family nearby, has a temporary job, and has no medical insurance. Her physician prescribes peritoneal dialysis and HCTZ. The following are noted by the nurse on assessment: blood pressure 180/100; respirations 20 per minute; pulse 110 per minute; height 5 feet 1 inch; weight 100 pounds; dry skin with multiple scratching marks; no urine output; and complaints of blurred vision, itchiness, weakness, and insomnia. Her gait is slightly unsteady. She talks with a soft and low voice and speaks English slowly but not fluently. She sometimes asks questions that have already been discussed. Although she smiles frequently during conversation, she appears tense and restless. The nurse notices some hand tremors, a shaky voice, and twisting fingers. Although she has limited information about peritoneal dialysis, the woman changes the subject as the nurse explains the procedure.

CARE PLAN

Nursing Diagnosis Pain related to pruritis.

Patient Outcome	***Nursing Interventions***
Patient will verbalize discomfort to others when it exists and will relate relief with therapeutic measures.	1 Explain pruritis will be decreased when patient's BUN level is down.
	2 Keep patient's room cool and avoid excessive warmth from clothes or blankets because warmth will increase itchiness.
	3 Apply cool lotions to dry and itchy areas.
	4 Apply cool wet soaks to reduce itchiness if patient desires this.
	5 Ask patient's doctor if any medicines can be used to decrease itchiness.
	6 Encourage patient to engage in diversional activities.
	7 Advise patient to keep her fingernails short to avoid injury to her skin when she scratches.

Nursing Diagnosis   Anxiety related to peritoneal dialysis.

Patient Outcome	*Nursing Interventions*
Patient will verbalize her understanding of peritoneal dialysis and will experience less anxiety after teaching.	1 Assess patient's understanding of peritoneal dialysis. 2 Present information to patient related to peritoneal dialysis by using pamphlets and drawings. 3 Explain rationale for peritoneal dialysis. 4 Describe feelings the patient may have during dialysis. 5 Contact dialysis nurse to obtain some audiovisual aids to help patient understand.

Nursing Diagnosis   Noncompliance related to side effects of HCTZ.

Patient Outcome	*Nursing Interventions*
Patient will describe the experience that caused her to stop taking HCTZ, describe appropriate treatment of side effects, and demonstrate appropriate alternatives to the previous plan.	1 Assess any other contributing factors for stopping HCTZ (e.g., cost; refer to social worker to seek any financial help). 2 Identify current effects and side effects of HCTZ on patient. 3 Teach effects and side effects of HCTZ. 4 Assist patient in reducing discomfort (e.g., dizziness—change positions slowly; dry mouth—ice chips, hard candy; weakness—get plenty of sleep and ask for help for what she is limited in doing). 5 Explain patient's dizziness; weakness could be improved when her BUN level is down. 6 Ask patient to verbalize what she understands.

Nursing Diagnosis   Communication, impaired verbal, related to foreign language barrier.

Patient Outcome	*Nursing Interventions*
Patient will be able to communicate basic needs and relate feelings of acceptance.	1 Talk slowly and clearly to patient. 2 Write down important information. 3 Use gestures, actions, pictures, and drawings to facilitate patient's understanding. 4 Encourage patient to teach others some Chinese words. 5 Seek a translator to discuss important matters.

STUDY
QUESTIONS

1. List at least three contributing factors for hypertension among Chinese Americans.
2. Delineate at least two things that the nurse can do to facilitate the communication process between the nurse and the Chinese American patient.
3. Identify at least two factors about lack of family structure and its significance to the Chinese culture that may contribute to the difficulties of hospitalization for this patient.
4. Describe factors in regard to the time concept that may hinder health care services where a Chinese American patient is concerned.
5. Describe health/illness practices that may augment problems associated with the treatment of hypertension for patients of Chinese descent.

REFERENCES

Albert, R.D., & Triandis, M.C. (1985). Intercultural education for multicultural societies: Critical issues. In L.A. Samovar & R.E. Porter (Eds.), *Intercultural communication: A reader* (5th ed., pp. 373-385). Belmont, Calif: Wadsworth.

Al-Mufti, H.I., & Arieff, A.I. (1985). Captoril-induced hyponatremia with irreversible neurologic damage. *The American Journal of Medicine, 79,* 769-770.

Anderson, J.M. (1986). Ethnicity and illness experience: Ideological structures and the health care delivery system. *Social Science Medicine 22*(11), 1277-1283.

Argyle, M. (1982). Intercultural communication. In L.A. Samovar & R.E. Porter (Eds.), *Intercultural communication: A reader* (5th ed., pp. 31-44). Belmont, Calif.: Wadsworth.

Becker, C.B. (1986). Reasons for the lack of argumentation and debate in the Far East. In L.A. Samorar & R.E. Porter (Eds.), *Intercultural communication: A reader* (5th ed., pp. 243-252). Belmont, Calif.: Wadsworth.

Binder, R.L. (1983). Cultural factors complicating the treatment of psychosis caused by B_{12} deficiency. *Hospital and Community Psychiatry, 34*(1), 67-69.

Bleibtreu, H.K., & Downs, J.F. (1971). *Human variations: Readings in physical anthropology.* Beverly Hills, Calif.: Glencoe Press.

Boyle, J.S., & Andrews, M.M. (1989). *Transcultural concepts on nursing care.* Glenview, Ill.: Scott, Foresman.

Campbell, T., & Chang, B. (1973). Health care of the Chinese in America. *Nursing Outlook, 21*(4), 245-249.

Chang, B. (1981). Asian-American patient care. In G. Henderson & M. Primeaux (Eds.), *Transcultural health care* (pp. 225-278). Reading, Mass.: Addison-Wesley.

Chen, C.L., & Yang, D.C.V. (1986, winter). The self image of Chinese-American adolescents: A cross-cultural comparison. *International Journal of Social Psychiatry, 32*(4), 19-26.

Encyclopedia Americana. (1983). (International ed., Vol. 6). Danbury, Conn.: Grolier.

Gallo, A.M., Edwards, J., & Vessey, J. (1980). Indochina moves to main street: Little refugees with big needs (Part 4). *RN, 43,* 45-48.

Gudykunst, W.B., Stewart, L.P., & Toomey, S.T. (1985). *Communication, culture, & organizational process.* Newbury Park, Calif.: Sage.

Hall, E.T. (1963). A system for the notation of proxemic behavior. *American Anthropologist, 65,* 1003-1026.

Hall, E.T. (1976). *Beyond culture.* New York: Anchor Press/Doubleday.

Hess, P. (1986). Chinese and Hispanic elders and OTC drugs. *Geriatric Nursing, 7*(6), 314-318.

Hsu, L.R., Hailey, B.J., & Range, L.M. (1987). Cultural and emotional components of loneliness and depression. *The Journal of Psychology, 121*(1), 61-70.

Kim, Y.Y. (1988). Intercultural personhood: An integration of Eastern and Western perspectives. In L.A. Samovar & R.E. Porter (Eds.), *Intercultural communication: A reader* (5th ed., pp. 344-351). Belmont, Calif.: Wadsworth.

King, H., & Locke, F.B. (1988). The national mortality survey of China: Implications for cancer control and prevention. *Cancer Detection and Prevention, 13*(3-4), 157-166.

Kolonel, L.N. (1988). Variability in diet and its relation to risk in ethnic and migrant groups. *Basic Life Science, 43,* 129-135.

Kuo, W.H. (1984). Prevalence of depression among Asian-Americans. *Journal of Nervous and Mental Disease, 172*(8), 449-457.

Lawson, W.B. (1986). Racial and ethnic factors in psychiatric research. *Hospital and Community Psychiatry, 37*(1), 50-54.

Liu, W.T. (1986). Health services for Asian elderly. *Research on Aging, 8*(1), 156-175.

Louie, K.B. (1985). Providing health care to Chinese clients. *Topics in Clinical Nursing, 7*(3), 18-25.

Ludman, E.K., & Newman, J.M. (1984). The health-related food practices of three Chinese groups. *Journal of Nutrition Education, 16,* 4.

Lyman, S. (1974). *Chinese Americans.* New York: Random House.

Mangiafico, L. (1988). *Contemporary American immigrants.* New York: Praeger.

McLaughlin, D.G., Raymond, J.S., Murakami, S.R., & Goebert, D. (1987). Drug use among Asian-Americans in Hawaii. *Journal of Psychoactive Drugs, 19*(1), 85-94.

Minkler, D.H. (1983). The role of community-based satellite clinics in the perinatal care of non-English speaking immigrants. *The Western Journal of Medicine, 139*(6), 905-909.

Molnar, S.C. (1983). *Human variation: Races, types, and ethnic groups* (2nd ed.). Englewood Cliffs, N.J.: Prentice Hall.

Orque, M.S., Bloch, B., & Monrroy, L.S.A. (1983). *Ethnics in nursing care: A multicultural approach.* St. Louis: C.V. Mosby.

Overfield, T. (1985). *Biological variations in health and illness.* Reading, Mass.: Addison-Wesley.

Pi, E.H., Simpson, G.H., & Cooper, T.B. (1986). Pharmacokinetics of desipramine in Caucasian and Asian volunteers. *American Journal of Psychiatry, 143*(9), 1174-1175.

Porter, R.E., & Samovar, L.A. (1988). *Intercultural communication: A reader* (5th ed.). Belmont, Calif.: Wadsworth.

Smith, M.J., & Ryan, A.S. (1987). Chinese-American families of children with developmental disabilities: An exploratory study of reactions to service providers. *Mental Retardation, 25*(6), 345-350.

Sowell, T. (1981). *Ethnic America.* New York: Basic Books.

Spector, R.E. (1985). *Cultural diversity in health and illness* (2nd ed.). East Norwalk, Conn.: Appleton-Century-Crofts.

Statistical abstracts of the United States. (1988). Washington D.C.: U.S. Department of Commerce, Bureau of the Census.

Sung, B. (1967). *A story of Chinese in America.* New York: Collier.

Thiederman, S. (1989). Stoic or shouter, the pain is real. *RN, 52*(6), 49-51.

Tien-Hyatt, J.L. (1987). Self-perceptions of aging across cultures: Myth or reality? *International Journal of Aging and Human Development, 24*(2), 129-148.

Time Magazine. (1967, Sept. 29, pp. 46-47).

Watson, O.M. (1970). *Proxemic behavior: A cross-cultural study.* The Hague, Netherlands: Mouton.

Whaley, L.F., & Wong, D.L. (1987). *Nursing care of infants and children* (3rd ed.). St. Louis: C.V. Mosby.

Wong, B.P. (1982). *Chinatown: Economic adaptation and ethnic identity of the Chinese.* New York: Holt, Rinehart, & Winston.

Yeun, J. (1987). Asian Americans. *Birth Defects Original Article Series, 23*(6), 164-170.

Yeun, W.H., & Schwartz, M.A. (1986). Emotional disturbance in Chinese obstetrical patients: A pilot study, *General Hospital Psychiatry, 8,* 258-262.

Yu, E.S.H. (1986). Health of the Chinese elderly in America. *Research on Aging, 8*(1), 84-109.

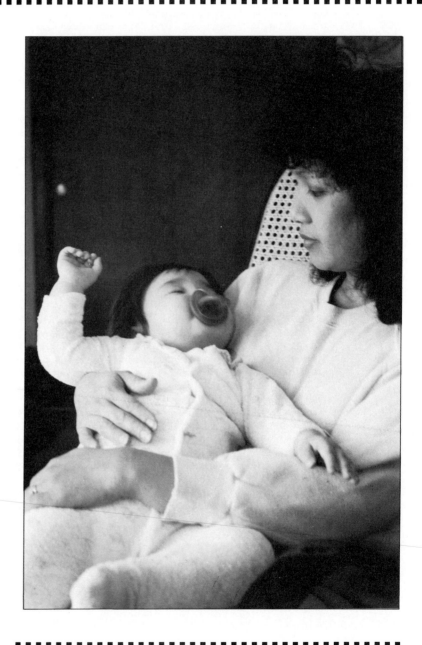

CHAPTER 17

∎∎

Filipino Americans

Anna Rambharose Vance

BEHAVIORAL OBJECTIVES

After reading this chapter, the nurse will be able to:

1 Describe the problems encountered in regard to communication when giving culturally appropriate nursing care to Filipino American patients.

2 Explain the Filipino American orientation to time and space and the relevance to culturally appropriate nursing care.

3 Describe how health care beliefs, values, behaviors, medical and folk practices, and attitudes affect health-seeking behaviors of Filipino American patients.

4 Identify how beliefs of Filipino Americans affect the internal locus of control and subsequently the environmental control variable.

5 Develop a culturally sensitive care plan for persons of Filipino descent.

OVERVIEW OF THE PHILIPPINES

The Philippine islands constitute an independent nation located in the Pacific Ocean approximately 450 miles off the southeastern coast of China. Taiwan is the nearest neighbor and is approximately 65 miles to the north; Indonesia is 150 miles to the south.

More than 7000 islands compose the Philippine Archipelago; however, the largest islands account for 94% of the country's total land area. The largest islands are Luzon (40,420 square miles) and Mindanao (36,537 square miles). All of the remaining islands are less than 6000 square miles in area. Most of the Philippine islands are hilly and mountainous, with very little level land. The principal island, Luzon, has several mountains that run from the north to the south of the island. The range,

□ This chapter is lovingly dedicated to the memory of my husband, Ronald Vance, Nov. 23, 1989.

known as the Sierra Madre, runs parallel to the northeastern coast, with the central Cordillera combining to form the spine of the Philippines.

The Philippine islands enjoy warm, even temperatures throughout the year. The average monthly temperature in the Philippines ranges from 76° to 84° F. Cooler temperatures are found at higher altitudes; however, temperatures below 60° F are a rare occurrence. Typhoons are known for striking the Philippines at least once a year. The average rainfall for most of the islands is at least 60 inches of rain a year, with some areas receiving up to 125 inches of rain. Most of the people found in the Philippines are of Malaysian descent. However, there are also people of Chinese, American, and Spanish origin who are native to the Philippines. The population is unevenly distributed, with Luzon, Cebu, Negros, Bohol, Leyte, and Panay being the most heavily populated islands.

The economy of the Philippines is based on agriculture; approximately 60% of the labor force is dependent on agriculture for its livelihood. One of the principal crops is rice, which occupies about half of the cropped land in the Philippines. Corn and coconut are also very important crops. Other crops of some significance include root crops, fruits, nuts, sugar cane, abaca, tobacco, ramie, kapok, and rubber. Although agriculture is the principal industry, the yields per crop per acre are among the lowest in Asia (Ennis & Inaba, 1977). It is thought that the causes of low productivity of agriculture in the Philippines are poor farm management, inadequate use of fertilizers, poor seeds, and lack of incentive on the part of the farmers because many are tenant farmers (Ennis & Inaba, 1977).

Fishing is also a major industry in the Philippines, with the number of persons engaged in fishing being second only to those in agriculture. Because fishing is a major industry, it is one of the primary dietary mainstays, second only to rice.

More than 40% of the country is covered by forest. Resources found in the forest include Philippine mahogany and pine. Minerals mined in the Philippines include gold and copper ore and chromite. The country continues to lack adequate supplies of mineral fuels, although coal is mined on the islands of Cebu and Mindanao.

The Philippine islands suffered enormous destruction during World War II (McKay, Hill, & Buckler, 1988). During the war the United States extended economic aid to the Philippines because it maintained large military bases on the islands. Following through on its promise to grant independence, which was made during the war, the United States granted independence to the Philippines in 1946. From 1946 to 1965 the Philippines pursued an American-style, two-party government. However, in 1965 President Ferdinand Marcos subverted the constitution and ruled as a lifetime dictator. Marcos abolished marshal law in 1981 but retained most of his own power. From 1981 to 1986 there was a growing resistance to Marcos' rule. In 1986 Corazon Aquino, whose politically involved husband was assassinated, possibly by Marcos' supporters, won a spectacular electoral victory over Marcos and forced him to flee the country (McKay, Hill, & Buckler, 1988).

IMMIGRATION TO THE UNITED STATES

Three different waves of Filipino immigrants have come to the United States: the first-wave or pioneer group, the second-wave group, and the third-wave or new immigrant group (Orque, Bloch, & Monrroy, 1983).

First-Wave Immigrants

The first-wave or pioneer group is diverse particularly because of the diverse times of arrival of its members in the United States and their reasons for immigrating. The first-wave Filipino immigrants were originally drafted to work on trade ships that were traveling from China to the United States (Bartlett, 1977). Between the years 1565 and 1815 hundreds of Filipinos escaped from the trading ships and went first to Mexico and finally to Louisiana and other regions throughout the United States. In 1907 with the passage of the gentleman's agreement that restricted Japanese immigration, Filipinos were recruited to work in Hawaii on sugar plantations (Daniels & Kitano, 1970; Laskar, 1969). Many of the first-wave Filipino immigrants worked on California farms or in Alaskan canneries, and still others worked as cooks or domestic helpers. Filipinos from 1907 to 1930 provided inexpensive and unskilled labor as housekeepers, janitors, farmhands, cooks, and so forth. Most of the first-wave immigrants were men who came from the Ilocos region, whereas others did come from the Bisayan and Manila areas of the Philippines (Hart, 1981; Melendy, 1977). In 1934 the United States passed what was known at the Tydings-McDuffie Act, which held Filipino immigration to an annual quota of no more than 50 persons. It was the Tydings-McDuffie Act that established a Philippine commonwealth and changed the legal status of Filipinos from "nationals" to "aliens" in the United States. When Filipinos were labeled "nationals," they had the rights of citizenship except the rights to vote, own property, or marry. However, with the new alien status the technical rights of limited citizenship were abolished (Parreno, 1977).

Second-Wave Immigrants

The second wave of immigration began after the Philippine islands won independence from the United States in 1946, when the annual quota was raised to 100 persons. Many Filipinos who served in the U.S. armed forces immigrated to the United States with their families after World War II. Lott (1976) noted that during this period many of the Filipino men were physically separated from their immediate kin and denied full participation in the larger American society. Therefore many of the second-wave group, particularly the men, relied on communal arrangements as their social group.

Third-Wave Immigrants

The new immigration group, or the third wave of immigrants, is composed of those Filipinos who have immigrated to the United States since 1965 as a result of the liberalization of the immigration quota. In 1974 Urban Associates, Inc., reported that in the 10-year period from 1960 to 1970, the Filipino population doubled, with 343,000 Filipinos residing in the United States.

Since 1965 the population of Filipinos has almost doubled again, and according to the 1980 census there are 781,894 Filipinos in the United States. Approximately 46% (350,378) of Filipinos reside in California, with another 16.9% residing in Hawaii, 4.6% in New York, 5.7% in Illinois, and 2% in Texas (*Statistical Abstracts,* 1988). Today in the United States, Filipino Americans constitute the third largest group of Asians and are only outnumbered in terms of population by the Chinese and Japanese.

COMMUNICATION
Dialect

One of the greatest difficulties that faced Filipinos during the 1960s was the task of forming a more integrated national community. This task was made even more difficult because of sociological diversity and because more than 80 dialects were spoken in the Philippines at the time. Although 86% of Filipinos spoke one of eight major dialects as their mother tongue, the fact remained that many diverse dialects were spoken across the country. Filipinos have long recognized the problem with dialect and language, and in 1930 a policy was adopted by the government to develop a national language based on Tagalog. In addition to Tagalog, English and Spanish were also adopted as the official languages of the Philippines. However, adoption of a national language by the people was slow, and by 1960 only 44.5% of Filipinos spoke Tagalog; 39.5% spoke English and 2% spoke Spanish (Corpuz, 1965). At this time more than 80 Filipino dialects were still being spoken in the country, with 86% of the total population speaking one of the eight major dialects as their mother tongue (Melendy, 1977). Today, although the most widely used dialect is Tagalog (Orque, Bloch, & Monrroy, 1983), 85% of young and middle-aged Filipinos do speak English. While Tagalog is the official national language, English appears to be the universal language of the Philipines. In fact, the Philippine islands make up one of the largest English-speaking nations (Zabilka, 1967).

In the United States Filipino immigrants have been willing to undergo discomfort and cultural alienation with the hope that the children might improve the economic status of the people through education. However, one tragic flaw in this scheme is the language barrier encountered by the children in the public school systems in the United States (Melendy, 1977). Even today, the public schools are not able to cope with the problem of bilingual education in languages other than Spanish and English.

Style

Shimamoto (1977) noted that the elderly Filipino man is generally concrete in thinking and pragmatic in problem solving. Shimamoto also noted that when a Filipino man acknowledges emotions in a verbal manner, this may be interpreted as a sign of unmanliness or weakness.

Context

There is a tendency for Filipinos to avoid direct expression of disagreement. This protects them from losing face or respect. For example, it was noted in a regional psychiatric hospital that a Filipino male physician, who was a family practitioner, would not disagree directly with a female psychiatrist. In this case the physician, in areas of disagreement, would communicate information to the psychiatrist by telling the nursing staff to relay the message. In this scenario the difficulties were encountered because Filipinos are a polite people who do not like to disagree, particularly with people in authority, and because some Filipino men experience discomfort with women as authority figures.

Some Filipino people experience difficulties when discussing topics that are considered personal, including sex, tuberculosis, and socioeconomic status. The issues of sex and sex education are considered so sensitive that Filipino parents generally do not openly or deliberately discuss them with their children (Guthrie & Jacobs, 1976). Because tuberculosis is a dreaded and feared disease among Filipino people (in the Philippines the morbidity and mortality rates for this disease remain high as a result of unsanitary living conditions), discussion about tuberculosis may also be avoided by some Filipino people (Hooper, 1958; Orque, Bloch, & Monrroy, 1983; Wooley, 1972).

Some Filipinos have an expressed need for modesty, privacy, and confidentiality. Therefore it is often difficult for the nurse to immediately begin interventions without a period of "small talk," which includes topics considered safe conversation, such as the weather, the condition of family members, or sports events. It is also important for the nurse to remember that Filipino American patients may be hesitant to express feelings and emotions in a group setting.

Kinesics

Nonverbal language is important for Filipino persons. For example, direct eye contact in the Filipino culture between an older man and a younger woman may be indicative of either seduction or anger. Another situation in which a nurse may encounter nonverbal communication on the part of a Filipino American patient is in a group setting. Because some Filipino people fear losing face in public situations, the Filipino American patient may be very hesitant to express personal feelings in a group setting and may resort to remaining silent.

Some Filipinos tend to behave agreeably even to the extent of personal inconvenience. The term for this form of agreement is *pakikisama,* which means getting along with others at all costs. Another trait for which some Filipinos are known is *amor propio,* which is really a Spanish word adapted to the Filipino language, meaning self-esteem. Therefore when a Filipino's *amor propia* is wounded, there is a tendency to preserve personal dignity by silence or aloofness in order to demonstrate self-pride. Filipinos will tend to agree even when they mistrust the physician or nurse because they do not want to risk hurting the other person's feelings. Therefore for some Filipinos a hesitant "yes" could be indicative of a positive "no," because they wish to avoid a direct, blunt "no." In the Filipino language there are hierarchial terms for "yes" and "no." The term used depends on whether one is speaking to a person of lower, equal, or superior status. When uncertain as to the status of the person with whom they are conversing, some Filipino Americans will use a silent nod to avoid giving possible offense. Also, a Filipino American patient will commonly address a physician or nurse as "doctor" or "Mrs"; however, if the name is not known, this same individual may only nod (DeGracia, 1979).

Implications for Nursing Care

It is important for the nurse to remember that since a large majority of first-wave Filipino immigrants came to this country with little or no education, it may be extremely difficult for such a person to comprehend English, especially English spoken in medical jargon. Therefore the nurse should use interpretive aids such as pictures and interpreters. It is also important for the nurse to remember that if an interpreter is used, the interpreter should speak the same language, as well as the same dialect, as the patient.

Regardless of immigration wave status, the Filipino American patient may view the nurse as an authority figure and therefore may relate to the nurse with formality and modesty. Since gender and age differences also have particular significance in the Filipino culture, it would be wise for the nurse to consider both gender and age when communicating with the patient. For example, since an elderly person is highly revered in the Filipino culture, it would be inappropriate, as well as disrespectful, for the nurse to address the elderly Filipino American patient by the first name. The nurse might try using such Tagalog designations as *"opo"* or *"oho,"* which are used to show respect and honor to the person being addressed (Orque, Bloch, & Monrroy, 1983). The Tagalog designation *"po"* should be inserted when an elderly Filipino American is addressed, because it conveys respect and is similar to designations in the English language such as "madam"or "sir" (Guthrie & Jacobs, 1976).

Since direct eye contact for Filipinos has various connotations, it is important for the nurse to remember that eye contact may be viewed in a variety of ways. A young female nurse who is assigned an elderly Filipino American male patient may encounter difficulties when communicating with this patient because the patient may remain aloof and reserved, and may avoid eye contact altogether (Bush & Babich, 1978).

Since Filipino men, regardless of age, have a great deal of difficulty verbally acknowledging emotions, Shimamoto (1977) recommended that the nurse assume an authority figure role during the development of the nurse-patient relationship. Because of the Filipino trait of deference toward authority figures, Filipino American men, regardless of age, are likely to respect the nurse's position and to listen and adhere to the nurse's suggestions because of the position. It is important for the nurse to appear knowledgeable and competent when communicating with a Filipino American patient and at the same time avoid talking down to the patient. It is also important for the nurse to remember that since some Filipino men experience discomfort with women as authority figures, difficulties may arise even in nurse-physician relationships. For example, when a female nurse is communicating with a Filipino American male doctor, the nurse should use sensitivity in offering suggestions or criticism. Some Filipino Americans encounter difficulties in group settings, particularly in situations where both men and women are present. Therefore one-to-one encounters may be best, so that the patient or professional the nurse is talking with feels free to express true feelings and emotions (Orque, Bloch, & Monrroy, 1983).

SPACE

Some Filipino Americans tend to collapse their space inward and to limit the amount of personal space available. This is due in part to the fact that Filipinos have a strong feeling for family, which is manifested by old-fashioned patterns imposed by the family patriarch. On immigration to the United States the personal space of Filipino Americans was also collapsed inward because some of the people lived in urban ghettos that were vastly overpopulated, so much in fact that these areas became known as "little Manilas" (Burma, 1954).

Implications for Nursing Care

Filipino Americans are perceived as a family-oriented cultural group. Therefore it is not uncommon for a Filipino patient to have the entire family, which includes nuclear and extended family members, hovering at the bedside. Even an adult who is unmarried with no relatives in the vicinity is likely to have swarms of Filipino American visitors because these people are sensitive to the loneliness that illness can provoke. The astute nurse will use family members to the advantage of the patient. Rather than viewing their presence as an overcrowding of space in the hospital for both the health care professionals and the patient, the nurse should capitalize on these customs and traditions by involving family members in educational training programs that will assist the patient in returning to an optimal level of functioning. In addition, it is important to solicit family, as well as patient, input in order to develop shared goals.

It is also important for the nurse to remember that Filipino Americans are familiar with a limited personal space, since it is always shared with other family members. Therefore the space provided in a hospital setting may appear to be overextended, thus necessitating the need for the patient to collapse personal space inward even more so. Filipino Americans, while hospitalized, may be reluctant to venture out of the personal space that is allocated and may be reluctant to leave their room for any reason (DeGracia, 1979).

SOCIAL ORGANIZATION
Family

Among the first-wave immigrants were young men with little or no education. Most of the first-wave immigrants who came to the United States were not allowed to immigrate with their wives; therefore most of the early male immigrants were single. This immigration pattern was responsible for a disproportional ratio of males to females. The male/female ratio in 1930 for Filipinos residing in the United States was 14 to 1 as compared with 1.1 to 1 for the rest of the population (Melendy, 1977). Lott (1976) noted that because Filipino men were separated from their families, these men tended to rely on communal arrangements with other Filipino immigrants who often came from the same island in the Philippines. Most of the first-wave immigrants came with little or no education and because of discriminatory practices that existed throughout the United States did not receive a better education or job. Of the first-wave immigrants, elderly men continue to live alone. According to Urban Associates, Inc. (1974), approximately 63% of Filipinos residing in the United States are poor, elderly men who live alone.

After World War II, when the immigration policies became more relaxed in the United States, more Filipino women began to enter the country and a more normal family pattern ensued. Despite the fact that more women were able to immigrate during the second and third waves, it has been noted that the age of Filipino American husbands continues to exceed that of their wives. It is because of the disproportional age of Filipino American women and men that many young women have been widowed early, thus leading to the establishment of the Filipino matriarchal system. In 1974 it was reported that a total of 69% of Filipino American families were matriarchal with young children and that at least 23% of all Filipino American families were extended (Urban Associates, 1974). Wagner (1973) noted that the ratio of extended families to nuclear families was at least twice that of the rest of the U.S. population. Today, however, married couples represent approximately 83.6% of all Filipino

American households, whereas female-headed households (matriarchal) make up only 11.8% of Filipino American families (U.S. Department of Commerce, Bureau of the Census, 1988).

In 1974 it was reported that 38% of all Filipino American families had five or more members (Urban Associates, 1974). Today, this number is decreasing somewhat, and the average Filipino American family has 4.2 persons as compared with the national average of 3.3 (U.S. Department of Commerce, Bureau of the Census, 1988).

It is probably because of the matriarchal system that the family has taken on paramount importance for Filipino Americans. This is evidenced even during times of illness. When a member of a Filipino American family becomes ill, the role of the family is emphasized and evidenced by the continuous presence of family members at the bedside and by their desire to be actively involved in patient care.

Third-wave immigrants appear to be better educated than members of the first or second group; however, some of these people still experience discrimination. The income level of Filipino Americans has not kept pace with educational attainment. In 1974 in the 25- to 34-year-old age-group for men, the ratio of persons not attending college but earning $10,000 was 0.9% as compared with 2.4% for the rest of the population. For persons over 25 years of age, 73% and 75% of all Filipino men and women, respectively, complete high school; 32% and 41% of Filipino men and women, respectively, complete college. The median age for Filipino Americans is 28.5 as compared with 30 for the rest of the population. Filipino Americans enjoy one of the lowest poverty levels among Asians and other Pacific islanders living in the United States. The poverty rate for Filipino Americans is 7.1% as compared with 35.5% for Vietnamese Americans, 29.5% for Samoans, 15.8% for Hawaiians, and 13.5% for Chinese Americans. However, it should be noted that Filipino Americans have a higher median family income ($23,700) than the national mean ($19,900) because at least three or more family members work. The percentage of family members working per family in Filipino American households is 17%, which is considerably higher than the national average of 13% (U.S. Department of Commerce, Bureau of the Census, 1988).

Family systems and the relationship to culture

The Filipino culture is a blend of various heritages, although there are some basic traits that most Filipino people manifest. Individualization is a key to understanding the Filipino culture and an individual of Filipino descent. As a result of the Chinese influence on family solidarity, Filipinos on the Philippine islands tend to socialize with people from the same region. This same clannishness is evident in the United States among the many organizations in the Filipino communities. Persons in the younger generations may have values that are in direct opposition to the traditional values held by older persons. In the Philippine islands today, many youths resemble their Western counterparts, particularly in areas of social values, dress, and music (De-Gracia, 1979). Although these same similarities exist among adolescents in the mainstream United States and Filipino American adolescents, many Filipino American youths still observe such traditional values as respect for elders, love of family, and preservation of self-esteem.

In the Filipino culture there is a strong feeling for family, which is a result of the Chinese influence. Today, these strong feelings for family continue and may be manifested by old-fashioned patterns imposed by the family patriarch or the equally authoritarian matriarch. The Filipino child is taught always to give deference to an elder and never to question the decision of an elder. In return for such obedience, the Filipino child receives solicitous protection from elders. In the absence of both parents, the eldest Filipino child becomes the ruling authority and must be obeyed. A study by Lantican and Corona (1989) comparing Mexican American primigravidas in El Paso, Texas, with Filipino primigravidas in Manila found that both groups had adequate social support. The network size for the Filipinos was 5.74 as compared with 5.78 for the Mexican Americans. In the case of 78% of the Filipinos studied, immediate family members provided the most support; however, Filipinos also reported that sisters were most likely to have been the first to receive information about the pregnancy, with husbands listed third. This was in contrast to the Mexican Americans studied, who reported first discussing the pregnancy with their husbands.

Religion

Filipinos are predominantly Roman Catholic, which has been attributed to the influence of the Spanish missionaries in the Philippines as early as 1520. In 1965 82.9% of the Filipino population were Roman Catholic, 7.6% were Aglipayan, 4.1% were Mohammedan, 2.3% were Protestant, 0.5% were *Iglesia ni Kristo*, 0.2% were Buddhist, 0.5% were other religions, and 1.8% had no religion (Zabilka, 1967).

Implications for Nursing Care

In the Philippine islands the family unit is the basic unit of social organization. Several generations of Filipinos are linked by descent and marriage. For some Filipinos family relationships are so important that many of the kinfolk live under the same roof or as close to each other as possible. Furthermore, membership in a family union is perceived by some Filipinos as being more important than membership in a trade union (Caringer, 1977). Therefore many of the nursing implications that arise are based on family structure and organization. Since Filipino American patients are very family oriented, it is important to remember that these patients may always have their families hovering about them. The sick Filipino child may feel lost without the mother constantly at the bedside, and when grandparents are ill, the entire family may keep vigil at the bedside out of respect for the elderly.

It is important for the nurse to remember that the family structure of first- and second-wave immigrants may be significantly different from that of third-wave immigrants in that more matriarchal family structures may be found in the earlier generations. Thus the varying family structures may present the need for unique and varying approaches to health care needs. Another implication for nursing care is associated with the fact that some first- and second-wave immigrants had a limited education as compared with third-wave immigrants, who came to this country better educated. When a Filipino American patient from the first- or second-wave group is hospitalized, it is important that the nurse not only involve families but also recognize the need to modify educational approaches to the family and patient's level of understanding.

TIME

Filipino Americans appear to have both a past and a present time orientation. According to Kluckhohn and Strodtbeck (1961), human nature has a postulated range of variations, including evil, good and evil, and good. People react to these value orientations by virtue of a time frame of reference. For example, past-oriented people view human nature as being basically evil, so that control and discipline of the self are continuously required if any real good is to be achieved. On the other hand, present-oriented people view human nature as a mixture of good and evil, so that although control and effort are needed, lapses in control and effort can be understood and need not always be severely condemned. For some Filipino Americans there is a prevailing attitude that one should unquestionably accept what life and death bring because irrespective of human effort, supernatural forces are mitigating and do control the world. It is this attitude that influences some Filipino Americans' time orientation.

Since Filipino Americans have both a past- and present-oriented time frame of reference, they distinguish between social and business time in the sense that they tend not to become too aggravated when social functions do not start on time. This is perhaps due in part to the fact that some Filipino Americans are perceived as past-oriented people who value human relationships and human nature over current events. However, Filipino Americans do equate success in business in Western society with a prompt observation of business time, which is perceived as being both present and future oriented (Orque, Bloch, & Monrroy, 1983). Nevertheless, for some Filipino Americans there is a prevailing attitude that time and providence will solve all (Corpuz, 1965).

Implications for Nursing Care

Since Filipino Americans are both past and present time oriented, it is important for the nurse to remember that often a Filipino American patient may ignore health-related issues, preferring to leave these things in the hands of God (*bahala na*). Some Filipino Americans may use the term *talaga,* which means destined or inevitable. When some Filipino Americans are ill, past time orientation become obvious because of a tendency to attribute conditions to the will of God and to cope with illness by praying and hoping that whatever God's will is, it is best for the individual.

Because of their past time orientation, there is a tendency among some Filipino Americans toward noncompliance in regard to medical regimens. In addition, these same individuals may not adhere to appointments or scheduled deadlines for health-related matters.

ENVIRONMENTAL CONTROL

As indicated in the preceding section, Filipino Americans are perceived as being both past and present time oriented and have a tendency to believe that events, particularly illnesses, are related to supernatural forces. As a result of this belief, some Filipino Americans have a value orientation that is perceived as fatalistic. Thus some Filipino Americans have an external locus of control that is evidenced by a belief in supernatural forces and by the methods of treatment of illness.

Folk Medicine

Filipinos and Filipino Americans support at least two, often competing, medical systems. A Filipino individual who becomes ill might consult both a folk healer and a Western-trained physician. Filipino Americans are like other ethnic groups in that they continue to practice folk medicine simply because it works (McKenzie & Chrisman, 1977). In some situations folk remedies may be the only treatments available for Filipino Americans, whereas in other situations some Filipino Americans will combine folk remedies with the therapy prescribed by Western health professionals. It is important for the nurse to remember that folk beliefs are an important part of some Filipino Americans' lives and therefore may significantly influence health practices.

Folk medicine has enjoyed a long history; in fact, folk medicine is thought to be older than contemporary scientific medicine. Some anthropologists believe that folk beliefs have persisted through the generations because they are so closely interwoven with other aspects of culture. Moreover, the therapeutic value of many of the health practices has been verified scientifically (McKenzie & Chrisman, 1977). The Filipino folk medicine system is based primarily on the Malaysian culture but may also be based on the Bisayan culture. Throughout the generations the Filipino heritage has been influenced by Indian, Chinese, Arabian, Spanish, Mexican, and American belief systems. It is thought that many of the elements of the health practices found in the Philippines may actually have been borrowed from these cultures. In the Filipino culture certain illnesses may be assigned to natural causes such as overeating, poor diet, or excessive drinking. In these cases these illnesses would normally be treated with home remedies. Home remedies could include such things as herbal preparations, teas, massage, sleep, and exercise.

Another category of illnesses is believed to be caused by supernatural agents. Some Filipino people associate disease with the total life situation, with the result that disease can have both natural and supernatural causes. Some Filipinos believe that there are invisible spirits that replicate the life of the individual and possess supernatural powers that are generally denied to most humans (Hart, 1966; McNall, 1989).

Individuals who subscribe to supernatural causation of disease may feel protected from harmful supernatural influences by such things as talismans, amulets, prayer, and seeking advice from a folk healer. Sickness and death are thought by some Filipinos to be the result of actions of angry ancestral spirits or witches, evil eyes, or the lethal bite or power of a supernatural animal. In such cases, if the patient does not recover or if the illness worsens, the patient will generally seek the advice of various folk medicine specialists. If the patient has the resources, it is not uncommon for this individual also to seek the advice of a conventional medical practitioner. In the Philippine islands it is not uncommon for a physician to incorporate certain aspects of the folk medicine belief system, such as the theory of hot and cold, when implementing the treatment plan (Hart, Rajadhon, & Coughlin, 1965).

A variety of folk medicine healers are found in the Filipino culture, including shamans and curers. A shaman is a priest or priestess who practices folk remedies. A curer diagnoses illness by palpating the pulse; many Filipino curers believe that the pulse is the best place to detect an illness because the pulse is an outlet, or a substation, of the heart. It is believed that if the pulse lies, then the heart lies (Lieban, 1967). An ill person's pulse may be either "hot" or "cold," depending on the type of illness. Some Filipinos believe that a healthy person has a balance in regard to hot and cold and air elements in the body. However, it is thought that if the body becomes too hot or subsequently too cold, the circulation of the blood will be increased or decreased, and the person will experience a loss of appetite and fatigue that will ultimately lower the body's natural defenses against the illness. It is thought by some Filipinos that both metaphysical and real hot and cold temperatures, if absorbed by the body in excessive amounts, will cause an illness.

Many Filipino individuals also subscribe to the theory of the four humors. The body humors include phlegm or mucus, air or vapors, bile, and blood. Filipinos who subscribe to this theory accept one overriding theme that includes health in relationship to air or wind (mal aire). For these Filipinos there are two ways in which one can get an illness. One of these ways is related to air and includes exposure to a normal draft or breeze that results in an illness such as a cold. The other way in which one can get an illness is by absorbing excessive amounts of hot or cold air, which ultimately will cause an imbalance of these principles in the body. A Filipino mother may wrap the navel of her baby with a cloth to prevent air from entering the body through the navel cord. Some Filipinos use coconut oil to soak or rub the skin in order to prevent wind from entering the pores. Some Filipinos believe that air circulates in the veins and that if hot air is absorbed through the pores, it will be carried to the brain by the blood, resulting in mental illness (Hart, 1981). Another mal aire illness includes the means by which the spirits penetrate the body by magically propelling thorns, pebbles, bones, and other foreign objects into the body.

Illness/Wellness Behaviors

Three concepts underlie Filipino health beliefs and practices: flushing, heating, and protection. Flushing is thought to keep the body free from debris; heating is thought to maintain a balanced internal temperature; and protection is thought to guard the body from outside influences. Flushing is based on the premise that if the body is a container, it can collect impurities. Heating involves the belief that hot and cold qualities must be in balance in the body. Protection involves safeguarding the natural boundaries of the body from supernatural, as well as natural, forces. Among Filipinos who subscribe to the theory of flushing, there is a complex system of beliefs based on the theory that flushing is a complex system of stimulating perspiration, vomiting, flatulence, or menstrual bleeding for the sole purpose of removing evil forces from the body. A common home remedy used to promote flushing is vinegar. Vinegar may be used to flush the body to cure an ailment such as a fever or a chest cold. In such cases the vinegar, when mixed with such items as water, salt, or hot pepper, may stimulate the individual to perspire and subsequently remove all of the evil or bad things from the body. It must be remembered that such practices are not all that unorthodox when compared with the Western medical system (McKinzie & Chrisman, 1977).

Since Filipinos are deeply religious and God-fearing people, they believe that many diseases and illnesses are the will of God. When a Filipino patient is given a poor prognosis, this patient may keep on hoping for a cure despite the severity of the problem. This attitude may help to explain why some Filipino patients are uncomplaining and frequently suffer in silence.

Implications for Nursing Care

It is important for the nurse to remember that Filipino folk- related health practices may be beneficial, neutral, or harmful. Folk practices that are beneficial or neutral should be incorporated into the plan of care. However the nurse should develop educational training programs that will help the patient and family to identify and eliminate folk practices that are harmful.

Some Filipino Americans have an external locus of control that is based on the belief that illness may be caused by external forces, which may be either natural or supernatural. Therefore it is important for the nurse to remember that the patient's noncompliance with medical regimens may be based on a fatalistic based system. It is important for the nurse to ascertain whether the patient's noncompliance is based on fatalistic beliefs or a lack of understanding.

BIOLOGICAL VARIATIONS
Body Size and Structure

In the United States prematurity is defined as a birth weight of less than 2500 g (5 pounds 8 ounces). When controls for income, maternal age, parity, and smoking were done, Filipino Americans tended to have a lower mean birth weight than their White counterparts (Morton, 1977). Morton suggested that the birth weight requirement for maturity should be lowered for some ethnic groups, including Filipino Americans, and in fact recommended that prematurity be redefined as less than 2200 g (4 pounds 14 ounces) for Filipino Americans and Blacks.

Filipinos are short in stature and tend to have very small frames. Some Filipinos have short limbs in comparison with the trunk size. At age 3 the mean standing height is 85.7 cm (33.7 inches) for Filipino boys and 84.8 cm (33.4 inches) for Filipino girls. Thus Filipino children are considerably shorter than White children, in whom the mean standing height is 95 cm (37.4 inches) for American White boys and 93.9 cm (37 inches) for American White girls (Meredith, 1978). However, the average height and weight of Filipinos is quite similar to that of Thais and Vietnamese persons. Filipinos tend to lag behind Japanese persons in both height and weight. The height of Japanese boys and girls from birth to 1 year of age exceeds the height of Filipinos (Matawaran, 1966). It is thought, however, that Filipinos overcome this difference by age 21 and that their growth increments are quite similar to those of Japanese persons.

In a classic 1958 study, Jose and Salcedo observed that Filipino women tended to be leaner and slimmer than their American White counterparts. Anchacosa-Angala and Marquez-Sumabat (1964) noted that body weight for Filipino Americans increased significantly when an increase in skin-fold thickness occurred. Based on this data, they concluded that skin-fold thickness could be used as an index of leanness and fatness for Filipino Americans.

Skin Color

Mongolian spots are commonly found at birth on Filipino infants. Normal pigmentation among Filipinos ranges from brown to peach brown, and it is extremely difficult to detect conditions such as cyanosis in darker-pigmented skin. In addition, some darker-skinned Filipinos may also have heavy deposits of subconjunctival fat, which contains high levels of carotene in sufficient quantities to mimic conditions similar to jaundice. If the nurse is to distinguish between carotenemia and jaundice, it is necessary for the nurse to inspect the posterior portions of the hard palate of the patient in an extremely good light or in bright daylight (Roach, 1977).

Other Visible Physical Characteristics

Filipinos are classified as members of the Asiatic race because of very common racial characteristics, including the brown skin color mentioned above, almond-shaped inner eye folds, and extremely sparse body hair, particularly in men, in whom chest hair is often absent. Hair on the head is typically coarse but also tends to be either straight or wavy (Garn, 1965). In addition, male pattern baldness appears to be a rarity among Filipino Americans (Garn, 1965).

Chung and Kau (1985) noted that the tendency for cleft lip or cleft palate was highest for the Japanese, Chinese, and Filipinos as compared with Whites and Hawaiians. These researchers also noted that the high-risk groups had smaller dimensions than Whites and Hawaiians in regard to cranial base measurement, facial height, palatal length, and mandibular length, which might be contributing factors to the higher incidence of cleft lip and cleft palate.

Enzymatic and Genetic Variations

Motulsky et al. (1964) found a high prevalence of glucose-6-phosphate dehydrogenase (G-6-PD) deficiency among Filipinos. It would appear that G-6-PD deficiency affects Filipinos as severely and as quanitatively as it affects persons found in the Mediterranean group. In addition, alpha-thalassemia, which is known as the hemoglobin H disease, is prevalent in Filipinos, Chinese persons, Thais, and Greeks (Wallerstein, 1976).

Susceptibility to Disease

Cardiovascular disease

Diseases of the heart remain the leading cause of death in the United States. In this category are coronary artery and hypertensive heart diseases. Both of these diseases vary in frequency by racial group. Weisse, Abiuso, and Thind (1977) and Gorden (1976) noted that Whites and Blacks in the United States have similar age-adjusted mortality rates for coronary artery disease. Gerber (1980) noted that White mortality rates for coronary artery disease are higher than those of either Japanese Americans or Filipino Americans. Gerber's study also suggested that mortality rates for coronary artery disease are higher in urban areas than in rural areas and that differences in mortality noted among races are probably not attributable to genetic factors but to environmental ones. This conclusion was based on the fact that when Japanese Americans or Filipino Americans moved from rural to urban areas, the mortality rate for coronary artery disease rose, which was thought to be directly related to changes in living styles, changes in diets, and changes in work patterns.

Other research studies have demonstrated a connection between a high rate of coronary artery disease and sedentary living patterns. It is thought by some researchers that the effect of sedentary life-styles is to increase total cholesterol blood levels and, in particular, low-density lipoproteins. These conditions are thought to be conducive to the development of coronary artery disease across races (Clarkson et al., 1981; Hartung, et al., 1980).

Frerichs, Chapman, and Maes (1984) conducted a study of mortality rates of seven ethnic groups in Los Angeles county during 1980. The study found that for all causes of death, age- and sex-adjusted rates were highest among Blacks, intermediate among Whites and Hispanics, and substantially lower among Asians and Pacific Islanders. The study also found that for cerebrovascular diseases the mortality rate among Blacks was again the highest, with Whites and Japanese being intermediate, and Hispanics, Filipinos, Chinese, and Koreans being the lowest.

Gerber (1983) noted that the life expectancy at birth for both males and females is greatest for Japanese persons, followed by Filipinos and then Whites. The findings of this study suggest that Filipino Americans would benefit more from the elimination of variables and/or stressors that predispose them to coronary heart disease and cerebrovascular accidents than would other ethnic groups excluding Japanese persons because of this higher predicted life expectancy at birth.

Hypertension

Stavig, Igra, and Leonard (1988) found that the prevalence of controlled and uncontrolled hypertension in the United States is lower for persons of Asian descent with the exception of Filipinos. In fact, the California Department of Health Services Hypertension study found that Filipino Americans have one of the highest prevalence rates for hypertension, second only to Blacks (Requiro, 1981). The analysis of the data from the study by Stavig, Igra, and Leonard suggested that Asians and Pacific Islanders with hypertension are less likely to be aware of the condition, to seek treatment or take medication for the condition, or to control the condition through diet. In addition, these ethnic groups recorded lower frequencies of hospital stays for the condition, fewer days of bed disability, and fewer days of not feeling well as a result of hypertension than all other ethnic groups. The study concluded that because of their high levels of poverty and lack of education, and the relationship of these factors to health-seeking behavior for hypertension, additional study is needed to help improve health care for Filipino Americans.

Young et al. (1987) noted a high positive relationship between sodium intake and the prevalence of hypertensive disease. This study examined the relationship between ethnicity and blood pressure in young adults of six ethnic groups residing in Hawaii. The findings suggested that body weights and heights of Whites and Hawaiians tended to exceed those of Chinese, Filipinos, Japanese, and Koreans. The study noted that both systolic and diastolic pressures were significantly higher in men than in women across all races. The study also found no significant differences between sexes or across races in regard to urinary excretion of sodium and potassium.

Stavig et al. (1986) conducted a study to determine the death rates in California for hypertension-related diseases for the periods 1969 to 1971 and 1979 to 1981. The data suggested that during both periods, age-standardized rates for composite hypertension-related mortality were highest for Blacks, followed by Whites, and lowest for Asians and Pacific Islanders. Filipinos, who were noted to have high prevalence rates of hypertension, tended to have a lower rate of hypertension-related mortality. The study concluded that the possible reasons for the decline in hypertension-related mortality may include population awareness, level of treatment, control of hypertension, knowledge of cardiovascular risk factors, improved medical technology, and modification of behavior.

Diabetes mellitus

There is an increased incidence of diabetes mellitus among Filipino Americans. Sloan (1963) concluded that diabetes mellitus occurs three times more often among Filipino Americans than it does among White Americans.

Cancer

Kolonel (1985) conducted a study comparing the cancer incidence rates for Filipinos in Hawaii. In the study it was noted that the significant increases in the incidence of thyroid cancer among Filipino women in Hawaii caused this group to have the highest incidence of thyroid cancer among all ethnic groups in Hawaii. In addition, the data suggested a lack of increase in female breast cancer rates among Filipinos in Hawaii and a lower than expected increase in colon cancer rates. In contrast to this study, Goodman, Yoshizawa, and Kolonel (1988) noted that the incidence rates for thyroid cancer remained relatively stable during the 25-year period from 1960 to 1984. However, this study also concluded that when Filipinos in Hawaii were compared with other ethnic groups in Hawaii, Filipinos were found to have the highest reported incidence rates for thyroid cancer. The conclusion of this study was that environmental influences may be responsible for the unusually high rate of thyroid cancer among Filipinos in Hawaii.

Young, Ries, and Pollach (1984) found that the rates of gallbladder and urinary bladder cancer for women exceeded those for men among the Filipino population. The primary site of cancer having the highest survival rate for both Filipino men and women was found to be the thyroid gland. The 5-year relative survival rate for cancer of the thyroid gland was found to be 91%, whereas the survival rate for other primary sites of cancer, including cancer of the esophagus, cancer of the liver, and cancer of the pancreas, were found to be uniformly low .

Gallbladder disease

Yamase and McNamara (1977) examined the hospital admission rates for gallbladder disease in Chinese, Japanese, Koreans, Filipinos, Hawaiians, Portuguese, Puerto Ricans, and Whites. This study found that while differences in admission rates among races were statistically significant, they were not clinically significant.

Amyotrophic lateral sclerosis

Studies have suggested that there is a prevalence for amyotrophic lateral sclerosis among Filipino Hawaiians that exceeds that found among Whites and Japanese Hawaiians (Matsumoto, 1972). However, the findings from other studies suggest that the excess in regard to amyotrophic lateral sclerosis found among Filipinos in Hawaii is more or less a function of population and age distribution rather than a true racial or ethnic difference (Kurtzke, 1982).

AIDS

Research by Woo et al. (1988) in San Francisco indicates that the number of AIDS cases has disproportionately increased among persons of Asian and Pacific Island descent (177%) as compared with increases among Blacks, Whites, Latinos, American Indians, and Alaskan natives (54%). The incidence of AIDS among Filipinos was reported to be 92 per 100,000.

Nutritional Preferences

Some Filipino Americans reflect their culture through the preparation and consumption of specific foods. Since some Filipino Americans subscribe to a theory of hot and cold, foods with these properties are incorporated into their dietary regimen.

For example, it is customary to include both "hot" and "cold" foods in cooking, such as mixing beans, which are considered hot foods, with green vegetables, which are considered cold foods regardless of how they are prepared (Orque, Bloch, & Monrroy, 1983). In addition, Filipino Americans who practice imitative magic may incorporate the concept of magic into the preparation and consumption of foods. For example, a pregnant Filipino women may believe that eating dark foods such as prunes will produce a dark-complected baby (Affonso, 1978; Pimentel, 1968).

For some Filipino Americans religious or family customs also dictate foods that are prepared and consumed. For example, Filipino Catholics may abstain from eating meat during Lent, particularly on Ash Wednesday and Good Friday. Zaide (1961) concluded that Filipino beliefs and customs are so entrenched in the culture that some Filipinos may even refrain from eating meat during the burial of a relative.

The traditional foods for Filipinos include rice, fish, and vegetables. For Filipino Americans typical dishes include adobo, pancit, and lumpia. Adobo is a method of preparation that includes cooking certain meats, such as pork, chicken, or beef, that have been marinated in vinegar, garlic, and other typical Filipino condiments. The meat is simmered slowly until it becomes tender and brown (Day, 1974). Pancit is a pasta made of rice or wheat noodles and is cooked with chicken, ham, shrimp, or pork in a soy and garlic–flavored sauce. Lupia is similar to the Chinese egg roll and is either deep fried or prepared fresh with selected vegetables (Day, 1974). Although Filipino Americans have changed their diets to reflect customs traditionally found in the United States, they also tend to retain ethnic food habits (Lewis & Glasby, 1975).

Psychological Characteristics

Flaskerud (1984) conducted a study to determine whether there was a difference in perspective placed on problematic behaviors exhibited by six minority groups: Black Americans, Native Americans, Chinese Americans, Mexican Americans, Filipino Americans, and Appalachians. The findings of the study suggested that there are differences in perceptions of problematic behavior and its management between mental health professionals and minority groups and concluded that while these differences are related to different levels of education and expertise, they are more than likely also to be related to cultural influences on conceptual explanations of problematic behavior and appropriate management. Cultural groups that were considered to be predominant viewed problematic behavior as mental illness and recommended psychiatric treatment, whereas cultural groups that were considered minority groups (including Filipino Americans, Chinese Americans, Mexican Americans, Black Americans, Native Americans, and Appalachians) viewed the behavior from a broader perspective that encompassed spiritual, moral, social, economic, vocational, recreational, personal, physical, and psychological assessment.

Alcohol use

A study by Danko et al. (1988) found that while Filipinos and Hawaiians have substantial alcohol usage if they drink, a large proportion of Filipino Americans continue to be abstainers. Lubben, Chi, and Kitano (1988) found that approximately 50% of the women in a population sample of 298 Filipinos were abstainers, whereas approximately 80% of the men in the sample were drinkers, suggesting that heavy drinking is almost exclusively a male activity among Filipinos. The study concluded that the only significant variable found among Filipino men and women in regard to drinking was regular participation in religious services.

Implications for Nursing Care

It is important for the nurse to remember that since Filipino Americans tend to have darker-pigmented skin than White Americans, it is essential to be able to distinguish between the norm and carotenemia, jaundice, or cyanosis. When inspecting the skin of a Filipino American, it is important that the nurse inspect the buccal mucosa for petechiae. When looking for evidence of carotenemia, the nurse can substantiate this finding if a yellow tint is absent in the palate when the scleras are yellow (Roach, 1977). If the nurse is unable to determine the presence of carotenemia, the patient's stool may be observed to determine if it is light or clay colored and the urine may be examined to determine if it is a dark golden color.

Since some Filipino Americans have a prevalence for enzymatic conditions such as G-6-PD deficiency, lactose intolerance, or thalassemia, it is important for the nurse to encourage the patient to eat meals that are high in protein and to replace whole milk with high-calcium substitutes such as buttermilk, yogurt, and sharp cheese, or by adding lactic aids to foods or other dairy products.

Filipino Americans are essentially very gentle and mild and have passive temperaments. It is thought that the reason for the passive temperament is the desire of Filipinos to maintain a harmonious balance between man and nature. These people generally are neither assertive nor aggressive and may often appear guarded or reticent. The nurse may often misunderstand this need for passivity and may misconstrue and mislabel this behavior as an inferiority complex. Very often Filipino Americans are erroneously labeled as passive-aggressive and as having a personality disorder with anger as the underlying cause. When angry, Filipino Americans do have a temperament that is passive-aggressive, and this anger often produces anxiety, which is usually handled through covert and passive means. Behavioral manifestations of passive-aggressive behavior are evidenced through such behavior traits as procrastination, stubbornness, intense craving for acceptance, and varying demands for attention (DeGracia, 1979).

The nurse should be cognizant that some Filipino foods are high in purine, such as dinu-guan, which is a food prepared from the small intestines, liver, heart, kidney, and blood of pork. Because dinu-guan is extremely high in purine, a patient who is on a purine-restricted diet should be instructed to modify the diet with leaner meats instead of pork organs. Since Filipinos, particularly Filipino men, have been reported to be hypertensive, the nurse should instruct the patient to modify traditional high-sodium Filipino diets. Foods that are considered high in sodium include traditional Filipino condiments such as soy sauce. For the patient on a diet moderately restricted in sodium, the nurse may suggest brands of soy sauce that have a lower or reduced sodium content. The patient who is on a diet totally restricted in sodium can be taught to prepare certain dishes such as adobo by marinating the meat overnight in a mixture of lemon juice, onions, garlic, sugar, and crushed peppercorns (Orque, Bloch, & Monrroy, 1983).

SUMMARY

The literature dealing with Filipino Americans has sometimes been confusing because Filipino individuals have been lumped together in the literature with Asians,

Spanish-speaking people, and "other" categories (Orque, Bloch, & Monrroy, 1983). Thus it is important for the nurse to apply data carefully from the literature to Filipino American patients who are cared for. In addition, the nurse should be careful to notice the dates on research studies of Filipino Americans, since many studies in the literature are old and may not reflect current needs. It is important for the nurse to assess the Filipino American patient carefully and to keep in mind what is known about the patient's cultural background so that culturally appropriate care can be provided.

CASE *STUDY*	Mr. Rom Recio, a 46-year-old Filipino American, is admitted to the hospital with a diagnosis of hypertension. Mr. Recio has lived in an urban area in Los Angeles, coming from the Philippines 2 years earlier. This is Mr. Recio's third admission to the hospital because his hypertension has not been controlled. Mr. Recio has repeatedly refused to comply and take the aldomet the physician prescribed for him during the initial diagnostic hospitalization. The nurse notes on examination that Mr. Recio's blood pressure is 140/104; his pulse is 88; his respirations are 16; and his temperature is 98.6° F. Although Mr. Recio speaks English, occasionally he has difficulty understanding what is being communicated in English terminology. Mr. Recio has a wife and three children ages 10, 12, and 15. Mr. Recio's wife speaks very little English; however, all of the children are proficient in the use of English. When the nurse examines Mr. Recio, he states that he thinks the problem with his blood has occurred because of disfavor with God.

CARE *PLAN*	*Nursing Diagnosis* Health maintenance, altered, related to hypertension.

Patient Outcomes

1 Patient and family will verbalize desire to learn more about condition and preventive techniques to reduce symptomatology.
2 Patient and family will verbalize a willingness to comply with prescribed medical regimen.
3 Patient will verbalize an understanding of the need to comply with routine schedule for antihypertensive drugs.

Nursing Interventions

1 Identify with patient and family socio-cultural factors that influence health-seeking behavior.
2 Determine with patient and family knowledge of hypertension and severity of illness.
3 Determine with patient and family knowledge and level of adaptation to news about condition of hypertension.
4 Identify with patient and family the necessity for adherence to prescribed time limits for taking antihypertensive drugs.

Nursing Diagnosis Communication, impaired verbal, related to recent immigration and the use of English as a second language.

Patient Outcomes

1 Patient and family will be able to communicate basic needs to health personnel.
2 Patient will be able to communicate feelings and anxieties about present diagnosis.

Nursing Interventions

1 Use visual aids that will aid patient in understanding the condition.
2 Use gestures or actions that communicate various tasks and procedures to be done.
3 Write down messages to provide visual stimulation about procedures to be accomplished.

Nursing Diagnosis   Family processes, altered, related to an ill family member.

Patient Outcomes	*Nursing Interventions*
1 Family will participate in care of the ill family member.	1 Determine family's understanding of patient's condition.
2 Family will assist nurse in assisting patient in returning to a high level of wellness.	2 Determine support systems available to family from external resources.
3 Family will verbalize difficulties encountered when seeking appropriate internal and external resources related to care and management of a family member with hypertension.	3 Determine with family a supportive network with friends available.
	4 Involve family in care and scheduling of patient-centered activities (e.g., taking Aldomet on time).
	5 Encourage family to verbalize difficulties.

Nursing Diagnosis   Noncompliance related to anxiety as manifested by ideology that the present condition is a result of God's disfavor.

Patient Outcomes	*Nursing Interventions*
1 Patient will verbalize fears related to health needs.	1 Identify with patient and family negative experiences with present conditions or delivery of services of the health care system.
2 Patient will verbalize factors that contribute to feelings of anxiety.	2 Correct any misconceptions about illness and/or medication regimen.
3 Patient will identify alternatives to present coping patterns necessary to reduce feelings of anxiety.	3 Identify health care practices that are beneficial, neutral, or harmful.
4 Patient will verbalize understanding for compliance with taking Aldomet when scheduled.	4 Give patient simple and precise instructions about medication regimen.
	5 Determine whether noncompliance in taking medication is a result of side effects or anxiety.

STUDY QUESTIONS

1. What factors related to culture are most likely to influence the noncompliance exhibited by Mr. Recio?
2. Explain how the Filipino American orientation to time may influence Mr. Recio's health-seeking behavior and his adherence to specific schedules.
3. Describe the locus-of-control variable that some Filipino Americans have that may influence health-seeking behavior.
4. Describe at least three other nursing interventions that can be implemented to facilitate communication between Mr. Recio, his family, and the health care team.
5. Describe the structure of some Filipino American families and the relationship the family may have on health- seeking behavior.

REFERENCES

Affonso, D. (1978). The Filipino American. In A. Clark (Ed.), *Culture, childbearing, health professionals* (pp. 128-153). Philadelphia: F.A. Davis Co.

Anchacosa-Angala, S., & Marquez-Sumabat, L. (1964). Skinfold thickness as indication of leanness-fatness in some female college students. *Philippine Journal of Nutrition, 17,* 176-197.

Bartlett, L. (1977). The Filipino "Cajuns." *Dixie,* p. 9.

Burma, J. (1954). *Spanish-speaking groups in the United States.* London: Duke University Press.

Bush, M., & Babich, K. (1978). Cultural variation. In D. Longo & R. Williams (Eds.), *Clinical practice in psychosocial nursing: Assessment and intervention.* East Norwalk, Conn.: Appleton-Century-Crofts.

Caringer, B. (1977). Caring for the institutionalized Filipino. *Journal of Gerontological Nursing, 3*(5), 33-37.

Clarkson, P., et al. (1981). High density lipoprotein cholesterol in young adult weight lifters, runners, and untrained subjects. *Human Biology, 53*(2), 251-257.

Chung, C.S., & Kau, M.C. (1985). Racial differences in cephalometric measurements and incidence of cleft lip with or without cleft palate. *Journal of Craniofacial Genetic Development and Biology, 5*(4), 341-349.

Corpuz, O. (1965). *The Philippines.* Englewood Cliffs, N.J.: Prentice Hall.

Daniels, R., & Kitano, H. (1970). *American racism: Exploration of the nature of prejudice.* Englewood Cliffs, N.J.: Prentice Hall.

Danko, G.P., Johnson, R.C., Nogoshi, C.T., Yeun, S.H., Gidley, J.E., & Ahn, M. (1988). Judgments of "normal" and "problem" alcohol use as related to reported alcohol consumption. *Alcoholism, 12*(6), 760-768.

Day, B. (1974). Philippine fare. *Gourmet,* p. 25.

DeGracia, R.T. (1979, Aug.). Cultural influences on Filipino patients. *American Journal of Nursing,* pp. 1412-1414.

Ennis, T., & Inaba, M. (1977). Philippines. In *The volume library.* Nashville, Tenn.: Southwestern Company.

Flaskerud, J. (1984). A comparison of perceptions of problematic behavior by six minority groups and mental health professionals. *Nursing Research, 33*(4), 190-197.

Frerichs, R.R., Chapman, J.M., & Maes, E.F. (1984). Mortality due to all causes and to cardiovascular diseases among seven face-ethnic populations in Los Angeles Country, 1980. *International Journal of Epidemiology, 13*(3), 291-298.

Garn, S. (1965). *Human races* (2nd ed.). Springfield, Ill.: Charles C Thomas.

Gerber, L.M. (1980). The influence of environmental factors on mortality from coronary heart disease among Filipinos in Hawaii. *Human Biology, 52*(2), 269-278.

Gerber, L.M. (1983). Gains in life expectancies if heart disease and stroke were eliminated among Caucasians, Filipinos and Japanese in Hawaii. *Social Science and Medicine, 17*(6), 349-353.

Goodman, M.T., Yoshizawa, C.N., & Kolonel, L.N. (1988). Descriptive epidemiology of thyroid cancer in Hawaii. *Cancer, 61*(6), 1272-1281.

Gordon, T. (1976). Heart disease in adults. *Vital Health Statistics, 11*(6), 1-43.

Guthrie, G., & Jacobs, P. (1976). *Childbearing and personality development in the Philippines.* University Park: Pennsylvania State University Press.

Hart, D.V. (1966). The Filipino villager and his spirits. *Solidarity, 1,* 66.

Hart, D.V. (1981). Bisayan Filipino and Malayan folk medicine. In G. Henderson & M. Primeaux (Eds.), *Transcultural health care.* Reading, Mass.: Addison-Wesley.

Hart, D.V., Rajadhon, P.A., & Coughlin, R.J. (1965). *Southeast Asian birth customs: Three studies in human reproduction.* New Haven, Conn.: Human Relations Area Files.

Hartung, G., et al. (1980). Relation of diet to high-density-lipoprotein cholesterol in middle-aged marathon runners, joggers, and inactive men. *New England Journal of Medicine, 302*(7), 357-361.

Hooper, H. (1958). A Filipino in California copes with anxiety. In G. Seward (Ed.), *Clinical studies in cultural conflict.* New York: Ronald Press.

Jose, F., & Salcedo, J. (1958). Subcutaneous fat distribution and body form of Filipino women. *Acta Medica Philippina, 14,* 161.

Kluckhohn, F., & Strodtbeck, F. (1961). *Variations in value orientations.* Evanston, Ill.: Row, Peterson.

Kolonel, L.N. (1985, Dec.). Cancer incidence among Filipinos in Hawaii and the Philippines. *National Cancer Institute Monogram, 69,* 93-98.

Kurtzke, J.F. (1982). Epidemiology of amyotrophic lateral sclerosis. *Advances in Neurology, 36,* 281-302.

Lasker, B. (1969). *Filipino immigration.* New York: Arno Press.

Lantican, L., & Corona, D. (1989, Nov. 14). *A comparison of the social support networks of Filipino and Mexican-American primigravidas.* Sigma Theta Tau International Conference, Indianapolis.

Lewis, J., & Glasby, M. (1975). Food habits and nutrient intakes of Filipino women in Los Angeles. *Journal of American Dietetic Association, 67,* 122-125.

Lieban, R.W. (1967). *Cebuano sorcery: Malign magic in the Philippines*. Berkeley: University of California Press.

Lott, J. (1976). Migration of a mentality: The Filipino community. *Social Casework, 57,* 165-172.

Lubben, J.E., Chi, I., & Kitano, H.H. (1988). Exploring Filipino American drinking behavior. *Journal of Studies of Alcohol, 49*(1), 26-29.

Matawaran, A., et al. (1966). Preliminary report on the average heights and weights of some Filipinos. *Philippine Journal of Nutrition, 19,* 318-332.

Matsumoto, N., et al. (1972). Epidemiology study of amyotropic lateral sclerosis in Hawaii: Identification of high incidence among Filipino men. *Neurology, 22,* 934-940.

McKay, J., Hill, B., & Buckler, J. (1988). *A history of world societies*. Boston: Houghton Mifflin.

McKenzie, J., & Chrisman, N. (1977). Healing herbs, gods, and magics. *Nursing Outlook, 25,* 326-328.

McNall, C. (1989). Healing we cannot explain. *American Journal of Nursing, 89*(9), 1162-1164.

Melendy, H. (1977). *Asians in America: Filipinos, Koreans, and East Indians*. Boston: Twayne.

Meredith, H. (1978). Research between 1960 and 1970 on the standing heights of young children in different parts of the world. In H. Reese & L. Lipsitt (Eds.), *Advances in child development and behavior* (pp. 1-59). New York:; Academic Press.

Morton, N.E. (1977). Genetic aspects of prematurity. In D.M. Reed & F.J. Stanley (Eds.), *The epidemiology of prematurity*. Baltimore: Urban & Schwartzenberg.

Motulsky, A., et al. (1964). Glucose-6-phosphate dehydrogenase (G6PD) deficiency, thalassaemia, and abnormal haemoglobins in the Philippines. *Journal of Medical Genetics, 1,* 102-106.

Orque, M.S, Bloch, B., & Monrroy, L.S.A. (1983). *Ethnics in nursing care: A multicultural approach*. St. Louis: C.V. Mosby.

Parreno, H. (1977). How Filipinos deal with stress. *Washington State Journal of Nursing, 49,* 3-6.

Pimentel, L. (1968). *The perception of illness among the immigrant Filipinos in Sacramento Valley*. Master's thesis, Sacramento State College, Sacramento, Calif.

Requiro, R. (1981). Filipino hypertension rate leads Asian-Pacific group. *Philippine News, 20,* 12.

Roach, L. (1977). Color changes in dark skin. *Nursing '77, 7,* 48-51.

Shimamoto, Y. (1977). Health care to the elderly Filipino in Hawaii: Its cultural aspects. In M. Leininger & K. Carbol (Eds.), *Transcultural nursing care of the elderly: Proceedings from the Second National Transcultural Nursing Conference*. Salt Lake City: University of Utah College of Nursing.

Sloan, N. (1963). Ethnic distribution of diabetes mellitus in Hawaii. *Journal of the American Medical Association, 183,* 419-424.

Statistical abstracts of the United States. (1988). Washington, D.C.: U.S. Department of Commerce, Bureau of the Census.

Stavig, G.R , Igra, A., & Leonard, A.R. (1988). Hypertension and related health issues among Asians and Pacific Islanders in California. *Public Health Reports, 103*(1), 28-37.

Stavig, G.R., Igra, A., Leonard, A.R., McCullough, J., & Oreglia, A. (1986). Hypertension-related mortality in California. *Public Health Reports, 101*(1), 39-49.

Urban Associates, Inc. (1974). *A study of selected socioeconomic characteristics of ethnic minorities based on the 1970 census* (Vol. 2). HEW Publication No. 5, Arlington, Va.

U.S. Department of Commerce, Bureau of the Census. (1988). *We, the Asian and Pacific Islander Americans*. Washington, D.C.: U.S. Government Printing Office.

Wager, N. (1973). Filipinos: A minority within a minority. In S. Stanley & N. Wagner (Eds.), *Asian-Americans: Psychological perspectives*. Palo ALto, Calif.: Science & Behavior Books.

Wallerstein, R. (1976). Blood. In M. Krupp & M. Chatton (Eds), *Current diagnosis and treatment*. Los Altos, Calif.: Lange Medical Publications.

Weisse, A., Abiuso, P, & Thind, I. (1977). Acute myocardial infarction in Newark, New Jersey: A study of racial incidence. *Archives of Internal Medicine, 137,* 1402-l405.

Woo, J.M., Rutherford, G.W., Payne, S.F., Barnhart, J.L., & Lemp, G.F. (1988). The epidemiology of AIDS in Asian and Pacific Islander populations in San Francisco. *AIDS, 2*(6), 473-475.

Wooley, P. (1972). *Syncrisis: The dynamics of health—An analytic series on the interactions of health and socioeconomic development: Vol. 4. The Philippines*. Washington, D.C.: U.S. Department of Health, Education, and Welfare.

Yamase, H., & McNamara, J. (1977). Geographic differences in the incidence of gallbladder disease: Influence of environment and ethnic background. *American Journal of Surgery, 123,* 667-670.

Young, F., Lichton, I.J., Hamilton, R.M., Dorrough, S.A., & Alford, E.J. (1987). Body weight, blood pressure, and electrolyte excretion of young adults from six ethnic groups in Hawaii. *American Journal of Clinical Nutrition, 45*(1), 126-130.

Young, J.L., Ries, L.G., & Pollach, E.S. (1984). Cancer patient survival among ethnic groups in the United States. *Journal of National Cancer Institute, 73*(2), 311-352.

Zahilka, G. (1967). *Customs and culture of the Philippines*. Rutland, Vt.: Charles E. Tuttle.

Zaide, G. (1961). *Philippine history: Developing of our nation,* Manila, Philippines: Bookman.

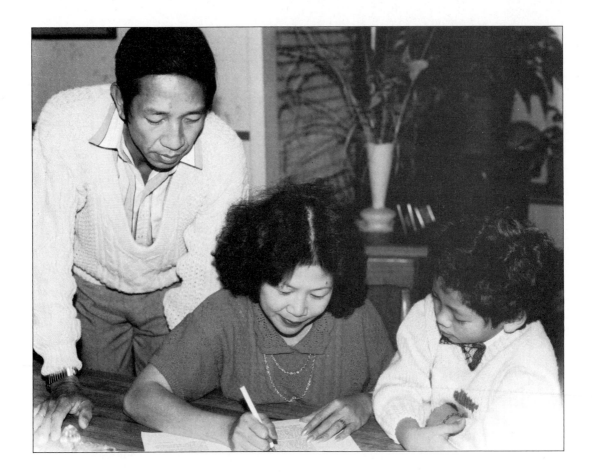

CHAPTER 18

▪▪▪

Vietnamese Americans

Ruth Yoder Stauffer*

BEHAVIORAL OBJECTIVES
After reading this chapter, the nurse will be able to:

1 Identify two important Vietnamese cultural values that influence all Vietnamese behavior.

2 Describe the organization of the Vietnamese family.

3 Articulate at least three explanations for the cause of illness that influence traditional Vietnamese thinking.

4 Discuss briefly the basic yin and yang theory of Chinese medicine and how it is expressed in the cause and treatment of disease.

5 Identify four barriers for Vietnamese people using the U.S. health care system.

6 Describe possible sources of conflict that may be experienced by a Vietnamese American working as a translator/interpreter in a clinic serving recently arrived refugees.

7 Articulate ways the nurse might modify "routine" procedures in a clinic or hospital to accommodate a Vietnamese American patient.

OVERVIEW OF VIETNAM

Vietnam is situated on the eastern coast of the Indochinese Peninsula, bordered on the north by China, with the Gulf of Thailand surrounding the Mekong Delta on the south. On the west, Vietnam is bordered by Kampuchea (Cambodia) and Laos, and on the east, Vietnam is bordered by the South China Sea. The country is slightly smaller than Japan, with 127,000 square miles. The country of Vietnam,

*Former Mennonite Central Committee relief worker in Vietnam; more recently worked with the Mennonite church in the Vietnamese community in the Washington, D.C., area; and presently working with the Mennonite church in Hawaii in resettlement.

along with Laos and Kampuchea, is often referred to as Indochina or Southeast Asia.

The northern part of Vietnam is mountainous with deep valleys and the industrial Red River Delta. The central ribbon is a long, narrow corridor with a mountain range, coastal plain, and miles of beautiful white sand beaches. The southern part of Vietnam is mostly the flat Mekong Delta, the agricultural area where most of the rice for the country and for export is grown. Vietnam is considered a tropical country, although the north has four distinct seasons and the south has two seasons: rainy and dry.

The population of Vietnam is approximately 56 million people, which includes "lowland people" (often urban and more educated), rural village people (with varying degrees of sophistication and education), and mountain people (made up of at least 30 different groups or tribes with a culture all their own). The Chinese are the largest minority, with 1½ million people (based on pre-1975 figures). The mountain people number approximately 1 million.

Vietnam has a recorded history of over 2000 years, with legends that cover an additional 2000 years. Earliest records are of dynasty rule and domination by the Chinese (111 BC to 938 AD). There were 900 years of independence until the French came in 1858. Throughout the French domination (until 1954), the Vietnamese continued to work toward independence.

The country was divided into the Communist north and the non-Communist south by the Geneva Accords in 1954 when it became clear that the "Nationalist" movement in the north had been monopolized by leaders leaning toward Communist ideology. The struggle between the Soviet-assisted North Vietnam and the U.S.-assisted South Vietnam ended in 1975 when Vietnam was reunited under the victorious Republic of North Vietnam. More than 30 years of war had physically, economically, and socially devastated the country. Thousands of people left Vietnam during the next 10 years for various countries in the free world, particularly the United States, France, Canada, and Australia.

IMMIGRATION TO THE UNITED STATES

There are 245,025 Vietnamese persons in the United States today (*Statistical Abstracts,* 1988). The highest concentrations of Vietnamese Americans are found in California, Virginia, Texas, and Florida (Lan, 1988). Approximately 90.5% of Vietnamese persons in the United States today were born in a foreign country (*Statistical Abstracts,* 1988). The median age for Vietnamese Americans is 21.5 years as compared with 30.9 years for the rest of the U.S. population. Approximately 48% of Vietnamese Americans are females as compared with 51% for the total nation.

Waves of Refugee Arrival

First wave

The first group of refugees, who began arriving in 1975, included many lowlanders, professionals, ranking South Vietnamese military, and those with close U.S. connections. This group also included those who had the means to get out of the country and those who would stand to lose the most under the new regime. A high percentage of these immigrants were educated in Vietnam or abroad, and some spoke

English. Many were young and single, or married with small children. The children moved into the school systems and could soon speak English more fluently than their parents, indeed more fluently than they could speak Vietnamese. (Today, some Vietnamese communities are sponsoring classes in Vietnamese for their children to study Vietnamese.)

Some of these persons had been exposed to European cultures or to the American culture for years and had economic or vocational assets. They generally did not go through a long stressful period of economic and psychological deprivation that affected their health and psyche. Of the 145,000 Vietnamese persons who came to the United States in 1975, 14% lived in single-family households, 42% were under 18 years of age, and 11.6% were over 44 years of age. One year after arrival, approximately 90% were employed (Coelho & Stein, 1980).

Second wave

A higher percentage of the second-wave refugees (1979 to 1980) were Chinese-Vietnamese extended family groups who left Vietnam under duress and pressure from the government. Again, these people often were educated and part of the business community in or near Saigon, with as much social status as was permitted under the new regime. For many persons in the second wave of refugees, however, Vietnamese was a second language, and fewer spoke English than in the 1975 group. These immigrants also included elderly persons and other extended family members who had varying health needs and problems.

Third wave

Most of the Vietnamese refugees during the 1980s were "boat people," who in many cases had lived through not only economic struggles, but also political and social change while at home. In addition, the boat people had survived life-threatening situations for days at sea. Persons in the third wave often spent months or even years in refugee camps along the way, and these earlier experiences caused turmoil that needed to be dealt with once they arrived and got settled in the United States. Third-wave immigrants were even more diversified than those in the two former groups. Many were in poorer physical condition than those arriving earlier, and generally the adjustment was more difficult and more complex. While many refugee education programs and school systems had organized effective programs to absorb the newly arrived children and adults in the first and second waves (and these persons tended to be motivated, highly literate, and able to do well quickly in the school system), the programs were not as effective with persons in the third wave. Life in camps did not encourage rigorous study habits or academic excellence, and many children in the third wave were not able to read or write well in either Vietnamese or English. For the boat people education needed to be much more comprehensive in order to assist adjustment to the new environment.

In the years following 1975, approximately 100,000 persons from Vietnam settled in the United States. After 1986 the countries surrounding Vietnam tightened laws regarding illegal immigrants on their shores, and the traffic from the boat people slowed markedly. Changes in government policy within Vietnam also eased the pressure to leave the country.

COMMUNICATION
Dialect

Vietnamese is the national language of most of the 56 million people who call or have called Vietnam their home. Vietnamese is not mutually intelligible with any other Asian language. It is monosyllabic and polytonal (five to six tones), and the words may be spoken in different intonations, each meaning something entirely different. The language is flowing and musical, and, for the most part, pronunciation is consistent and grammar is simple.

Until the 1960s French was the language of educated Vietnamese people, along with Vietnamese; therefore much of the scientific and technical vocabulary was borrowed from French or, more recently, English. Until 1975 in Vietnam, English was more common as the choice for a second language in high schools and colleges. Three distinct dialects of Vietnamese separate the northern, central, and southern regions of Vietnam. Dialects identify the speaker's origins and are understood by others regardless of region.

For many years before the Vietnam war, Vietnam had a large Chinese minority with their own schools conducted in the Chinese language. In the Chinese suburb of Saigon, called Cholon, many older Chinese persons spoke only Chinese, and the children learned Vietnamese as a second language. This explains why many persons in the large Chinese-Vietnamese refugee group can speak both Chinese and Vietnamese or only Chinese. In contrast to this, the ethnic mountain people, or *montgnards,* usually have their own tribal languages and often do not understand Vietnamese.

Style

As a cornerstone of Vietnamese society, respect is very evident in communication (Huynh, 1987). The Vietnamese language demonstrates the cultural focus on respect by a proliferation of titles. For example, when describing family relationships, English users have titles reserved for family members that include "mother," "father," "sister," "brother," "uncle," "aunt," "cousin," "grandmother," and "grandfather." However, the language and style of the Vietnamese not only encompass family descriptors such as "uncle," but also designate which side of the family a family member represents (mother's or father's) and further indicate whether a relative is the eldest brother or sister. Grandparent titles also reflect paternal or maternal side. When a sister or brother is being described, the term used indicates if the sister or brother is younger (*"em"*) or older (*"chi"* or *"anh"*).

Context

The word *yes* is used in English to express agreement and does not reflect an attitude of respect or disrespect. For Vietnamese people *ya* indicates respect and not necessarily agreement. Therefore a troubling verbal communication between health workers and Vietnamese American patients is the polite *"Ya, ya, Thua Ba, ya, ya,"* response, which Americans interpret as "Yes, yes, I understand, and I'll do it." For the Vietnamese the "yes" of *"ya"* is simply being respectful, indicating "I'm listening, and I respect what you're saying" (even though the request may not be within the realm of possibility). Nurses often reflect later, "But he said, 'Yes, yes,' and agreed to . . ."

Noncompliance by Vietnamese Americans can often be traced to this misinterpretation of *"ya."*

The Vietnamese person will often use personal pronouns to describe various roles held. For example, the speaker may refer to self as *"Em"* (referring to a child) when addressing parents, the nurse, or any superior. However, this same individual may refer to self as *"Thay"* (teacher) when addressing students. Except with family and close friends, it is very common for Vietnamese persons to use only the title of a person: "Uncle," "Teacher," etc. Especially when there is considerable distance between the speaker and the listener, the title alone is most correct. This custom is even practiced in the United States. For example, people often say "Madam Chair" or "Mr. President," indicating that the title is more important than the name.

A distinct feature of the Vietnamese culture, and consequently the language, is moderation and caution (Huynh, 1987). Vietnamese people are taught from childhood to think before speaking. High value is placed on modesty of action and speech. A Vietnamese proverb suggests that "bragging reflects an empty soul." There is also concern that a slip of the tongue may bring discord and be disruptive to harmony and respect.

Touch

Traditionally, the high value of emotional self-control and the general esteem for correct behavior has limited the use of touch in communicating. Physical behavior, including backslapping, is not considered proper for the well-bred. The young people have been less formal, and in the 1970s in Vietnam it was not uncommon to see groups of Vietnamese boys jostling each other in the street or girls walking arm-in-arm on the sidewalk. Today in the United States, many Vietnamese youths are taking some cues from their American counterparts.

Kinesics

In the Vietnamese culture respect is also conveyed by nonverbal communication. By the time they can stand alone, children are taught to cross their arms over their chest, lower their head, and bend their upper torso slightly forward when greeting an elder or a guest coming into the house. Forms of this behavior continue throughout life in situations requiring respect. Deference to others shows a Confucian and Buddhist influence in that how something is done is often more important than what is done (Hoang & Erickson, 1982).

Respect is also shown by avoiding eye contact when talking with someone to whom one is not equal in education, social standing, age, or sex. A student avoids eye contact with a teacher, an employee with the boss, a younger member of the family with the elders, and so on. Direct eye contact in these settings generally means a challenge or an expression of deep passion.

The head is considered sacred, and it is not polite to pat the head in communication. Feet are the most lowly of the body members, and it is best if toes are pointed slightly inward when a person is seated, or downward if the legs are crossed. The toes should not be pointed toward others, and it is never proper to put one's feet on a coffee table or desk.

In contrast to the usual palm-up position used by persons in the dominant culture in the United States, Vietnamese persons beckon for someone to come by turning the palm downward and waving the fingers. The upturned palm is used to call a dog or other animal, or as an insult. It is never proper to snap one's fingers or wave violently to gain the attention of another

Open expression of emotions is considered in bad taste, except in very private circumstances. Emotions interfere with self-control and can be considered weaknesses. Romantic overtures are reserved for home or private settings, and wildly joyous scenes in public are not considered appropriate. One exception to the usual restraint is the expected behavior of a widow at the grave on the burial of her husband, when she may wail or attempt to throw herself into the grave.

Implications for Nursing Care

Since respect and harmony are highly valued in relationships, there is a great desire in the Vietnamese culture not to disappoint, upset, embarrass, or cause another person to lose face. The desire to maintain harmony takes precedence over what the actual truth of a situation may be. Particularly if the answer is negative, when a Vietnamese American patient is confronted with a difficult or delicate question, such as "Did you take your medication?" the patient may choose not to give a direct answer in favor of the higher good of keeping the peace with the nurse. In the Western culture this avoidance might be labeled as an attempt to avoid the truth; however, in the Vietnamese culture the answer would be considered the correct way to handle a delicate situation.

The nurse should recognize that negative emotions or expressions of disagreement are usually conveyed by silence or a reluctant smile. For the Vietnamese a smile may express joy, but more often it is used to convey a number of other messages, such as stoicism in the face of difficulty or an apology for a minor social offense. A smile may be a proper response to a scolding to show sincere acknowledgment for the wrongdoing and to convey that there are no ill feelings.

A smile is also a way to respond when it is not proper to verbally say "thank you" or "I'm sorry" because of age or status. The smile is often present in Vietnamese American clinic or hospital patients, regardless of their situation. Even if angry, neglected, or in need, the Vietnamese American patient will rarely express this to the nurse or physician but will speak quietly and smile. Instead of asking questions that allow an answer, "Are you having pain?" or "Do you want something for pain?" the nurse should acknowledge the likelihood of pain and state, "Please let me get you something for pain."

Since most Vietnamese American patients entering the health care system in the United States do not speak "medical" English, an interpreter or bicultural medical translator may be essential to assist in accurate communication. It is important that the translator be culturally aware and conscientious in order to bridge the gap between the culture of the patient and members of the health care team. Accurate translation can be assisted if the interpreter is Vietnamese because of the built-in cultural awareness. However, the Vietnamese interpreter may be hesitant to translate certain complaints that are not acceptable to Western practitioners, for example, symptoms the patient states are "caused by the wind," a common problem. Other important factors to consider are the effect of differences in social class between interpreter and patient, the possible effect of a male interpreter if the patient is female, and the need for a female interpreter/companion when a physical examination is done on a female patient. When an interpreter is not available, it is important for the nurse to choose vocabulary carefully and to keep instructions simple and brief. Medical jargon should be avoided (Tran, 1980).

The nurse should be aware that English phonics applied to Vietnamese names often result in pronunciations that are unintelligible to the Vietnamese. "Naugen Thigh Hung" (pronounced "Wee-un T Hum") in no way looks like it sounds. In a clinic where patients must be called, it may be useful to have the patients take numbers, since numbers are more readily understood.

It is important for the nurse to appreciate that pronunciation may cause difficulties with questions regarding addresses and phone numbers. It may be easier for the patient to write answers to such questions. Such a patient should be encouraged to carry this information in written form.

A question about age may also be difficult for the Vietnamese American patient. A Vietnamese mother may be able to indicate the year a child was born but may not be able to state the child's exact age. In Vietnam and in the Orient, age has traditionally been calculated from the time of conception, so that a baby is already 9 months old at birth. Individual birthdays are not usually celebrated; rather, everyone becomes a year older at the beginning of each new year (Tet). Thus a newborn who arrives during the last half of the calendar year could be considered 2 years old following the first Tet celebration. Another reason for confusion about age, especially for persons who immigrated as teenagers, is that new birth certificates may show an earlier age adjustment of 2 or 3 years. This may have been done in Vietnam to avoid the draft or in the United States to facilitate entrance into high school, since after age 18 the student was much less likely to attend high school regardless of educational level in Vietnam. The slight build of many Vietnamese persons facilitates this age adjustment. Elderly Vietnamese persons without birth certificates usually know the year of their birth and are officially assigned, on arrival in the United States, a birthday on January 1.

Finally, the nurse should be cognizant of the fact that for many Vietnamese Americans the numerous questions asked by health professionals in the United States raise doubt about the competency of the health professionals. The nurse should attempt to communicate both acceptance of varying cultural practices and genuine concern in order to bridge the gap between the cultures and to increase the trust of the patient in the caregivers.

SPACE
Intimate Zone

Beliefs about space are rooted deep in the Vietnamese culture. For the traditional Vietnamese person, intimate-zone activities are carefully confined to private settings. Holding hands in public, especially with members of the opposite sex, is considered in poor taste, and hugging or emotionally touching in public, even by close friends or family members, is embarrassing to the traditional Vietnamese onlooker. For some Vietnamese people the head is considered the "seat," and touching it, even in the process of giving care, may cause some vital force to escape (Hoang & Erickson, 1982).

Beliefs about space also influence how Vietnamese people feel about care given to females. Until the early 1900s, traditional practitioners were not to touch the bodies of their female patients except to take their pulse. Figurines were used for the female patient to indicate where she was having problems. Today, many Vietnamese persons still place an emphasis on virginity at the time of marriage, especially for the woman, and continue to have strong feelings about unmarried young women having pelvic examinations.

Personal, Social, and Public Zones

Vietnamese individuals are likely to feel more comfortable with more distance during personal and social relationships than that required by persons in the dominant culture. Social exchanges generally do not involve physical contact other than handshaking, which may be practiced between men.

Living Space

In Vietnam extended families live comfortably in relatively small areas. The moderate or warm climate allows many of the family activities to be carried on outside. Often the kitchen is separate from the rest of the house, and the two or three main rooms double as living rooms and bedrooms, with the mosquito nets neatly tied back during the day. Even in spacious homes family members often prefer to spend much of their time in close proximity to each other. In Vietnam homes are typically arranged in communities and villages with several homes near each other.

While many Vietnamese persons were used to living in close proximity, refugee camps brought a new kind of cramped and confined closeness. As refugees, many Vietnamese persons lived for a period of several months to years with 8 to 10 persons occupying a one-room space, sometimes enclosed only by a blanket curtain. Special adjustment was required by most refugees when they received housing in the United States, because many well-intentioned sponsors made special efforts to provide single-home dwellings for the refugees, since "they've been so crowded so long." Unfortunately this space lacked the familiar sounds, smells, and people, and soon brought feelings of lonliness. Today, many Vietnamese Americans have homes with room for parents and additional family members and usually feel comfortable having relatives and friends in close proximity.

Implications for Nursing Care

When caring for Vietnamese American patients, the nurse should be cognizant of the effect that issues related to space may have on patient care. For example, the nurse should be aware that if a pelvic examination is to be conducted, it is important for a female translator to explain carefully why it is necessary and what will be done, and to remain with the patient during the examination. The nurse should also be aware that if the head of a Vietnamese American patient is accidentally touched or needs to be touched in the process of care and the patient feels that the head is sacred, touching the opposite side of the head or the shoulder (and thus preventing any vital forces from escaping) may take care of the problem (Hoang & Erickson, 1982).

The nurse should also be aware that a backrub could be an "uneasy" experience when given by a stranger. The nurse should use discretion in including the backrub as a routine part of nursing care if it is not a critical component of the care.

SOCIAL ORGANIZATION
Family

In the past in Vietnam, the family was the basic institution of society and provided life long protection and guidance to the individual. The roles and structure of the family were well defined, with extensive terminology designating kinship relationships. The father was the head of the household but usually shared the rights and authority with his spouse.

The immediate family included the parents, unmarried children, sometimes the husband's parents, and sons with their wives and children. In addition, the extended family included other close relatives (with the same family name and ancestors) who lived in the same community (see box on p. 412). The oldest son had the heavy responsibility of carrying on the family name, of taking over for the parents when they became elderly, and of following through with religious and ancestral observances.

The Vietnamese concept of family and extended family that has existed across generations past and future as a "superorganic unit" is profoundly different from the individualism of the nuclear family in the United States (Indochinese Refugee Action Center, 1980). For Vietnamese people the family has been the chief source of cohesion and continuity for hundreds of years. In the United States the family continues to be the basic unit of the Vietnamese society. Interestingly, today in their new locations, when Vietnamese individuals are asked for choices about associates, the highest percentage first choose family members or persons from their own village in Vietnam; second, they choose other Americans; and third, they choose other Vietnamese persons (Huynh, 1987).

Married-couple families account for approximately 73% of all family structures within the Vietnamese American population as compared with 83% for the rest of the general population in the United States. There are approximately 5.2 persons per family in Vietnamese American families as compared with 3.3 for the rest of the U.S. population. Today in the United States, 15.2% of all Vietnamese families have three or more members in the work force. The median family income for Vietnamese American families is $12,800 as compared with $19,900 for the rest of the general U.S. population. Therefore it is not surprising that 35% of all Vietnamese persons residing in the United States live in poverty as compared with 12% for the rest of the U.S. population. Nevertheless, 27% of all Vietnamese Americans own their own homes. This is not an impressive statistic if compared with the rest of the U.S. population, where 64% own their own homes. Despite this fact, the median value of homes for Vietnamese Americans is $56,800 as compared with $47,200 for the rest of the U.S. population (*Statistical Abstracts*, 1988).

Family rules and structure

The crux of family loyalty is "filial piety," which commands children to obey and honor their parents, an obligation that extends even beyond death in the form of properly remembering their parents and caring for their tombs. According to Huynh (1987), the worst insult a Vietnamese person can receive is to be accused of failure in fulfilling the obligation of filial piety. Filial piety is also encouraged and reinforced by Christian teaching, that is, "honor your father and mother."

NAMES

Many Vietnamese family names originated during the various dynasties that ruled in Indochina for periods during the past 4000 years. There were about 100 family names for over 56 million people, and of those 100 names, "only a score" are in common usage today (Huynh, 1987). "Nguyen" (near pronunciation is "Wee-un") is the family name for more than 25% of the Vietnamese family units in the United States and Canada. With so many persons having the same family name, it has limited usefulness in identification; therefore given names are used.

Names in Vietnam are always written family name first, middle name (or names) second, and given name last, for example, "Nguyen Thi Hong" or "Tran Van Hai." The same names may be used for males and females, and the middle name can be a clue as to gender. "Van" used as a middle name usually indicates male gender (Tran Van Hai) as compared with "Thi" (pronounced "Tee"), which is used for females ("Nguyen Thi Hong"). Sometimes several middle names are used, and therefore there is no gender indicator.

After marriage a woman keeps her maiden name and does not combine it with her husband's name. Informally she may be called by her given name or her husband's given name ("Mrs. Hai"), but formally she uses her full maiden name preceded by "Ba," which can be used as a respectful "Mrs." Children take their father's family name. Customs are changing in the United States, but to avoid confusion, many Vietnamese American wives are adopting their husband's family name. Either name may be used depending on the setting, and children have interesting choices when asked for "mother's name."

Given names usually have special meanings, often describing the baby or expressing the hopes of the parents for the baby. Names can be chosen from virtues or from nature or music; for example, "Hong" means "rose" and "Xuan" means "spring." At home or in the village, people may be called by their number in the sibling constellation, rather than by their given names, which explains the "nicknames" of "Nam" ("fifth") or "Bay" ("seventh").

Today, many babies born in the United States are given both an American name and a Vietnamese name. This is not a new practice for the Vietnamese. During the past half-century, for example, the Chinese-Vietnamese were commanded by law to change their Chinese given names to Vietnamese names. These persons may also have taken a Christian name when they converted to Christianity. In this resettlement period almost every Vietnamese child who has an English first name can also give a Vietnamese name if asked.

Except for close friends and co-workers, Vietnamese custom dictates that a person's name is used with a title, never alone. An example of this in English would be "Mr. Bill," "Mrs. Mary," "Director James," or "Uncle John." Titles are important and therefore should be selected carefully by the speaker to convey appropriate respect as well as sometimes to place emotional distance between the conversationalist and the listener.

Obedience and honor are shown in several ways: by obedient behavior and attitudes, by contributing to a good family name through outstanding achievement in some aspect of life, and by the use of the detailed kinship terminology that carefully designates the place of each person in relationship to the others. Parents consider it very important to train their children, and this responsibility is usually shared by members of the extended family living in the household, especially the grandparents. Personal interests and destiny are hardly considered outside the framework of the immediate and extended family. Behavior or misbehavior (juvenile delinquency, academic failure, mental disorders, etc.) reflects on the entire family and has great significance beyond the person involved. If personal feelings or ambitions might disrupt family harmony, the individual is expected to restrain from taking action and to sacrifice personal wishes.

Education

In Vietnam the Vietnamese experienced tremendous competition for the limited places in the high schools and universities. Before 1954 Hanoi was the educational center for Vietnam, and most of the institutions of higher learning, including the medical and dental schools, were there. Some 10 years after the Geneva Accords, South Vietnam had its own educational centers in Saigon, Hue, and Can Tho, but the demand far exceeded the supply, and many students had to either delay their education, go abroad, or, for the men, be drafted. Today in the United States, education continues to be highly valued in the Vietnamese community, and approximately 62.2% of all Vietnamese Americans 25 years of age or older have a high school education: 54% of Vietnamese women age 25 or older and at least 71% of Vietnamese men have at least a high school education. This compares with 66% of women in the same category and 67% of men in the same category for the rest of the general U.S. population. Vietnamese Americans are also gaining ground in regard to a college education. Today, at least 8% of all Vietnamese women, 25 years or older, and at least 18% of all Vietnamese men, 25 years or older, have a college education. This compares with 13% of women in the same category and 20% of men in the same category for the rest of the general U.S. population (*Statistical Abstracts,* 1988). This is remarkable, considering that either these students or their families have come to this country within the past 15 years.

Religion

Vietnam has a history of religious tolerance except for the period immediately before the French takeover, when Christians were suspected of being spies. Religious beliefs in Vietnam have been strongly influenced by several different religions, including Buddhism, Confucianism, and Taoism. Buddhism was introduced from China and India by the second century AD. It is considered less an organized orthodoxy than a state of mind using the Four Noble Truths taught by Buddha, which, simply stated, are (1) life is suffering; (2) suffering is caused by desire; (3) suffering can be eliminated by eliminating desire; and (4) to eliminate desire, one must follow the eightfold path of right understanding, purpose, speech, conduct, vocation, effort, thinking, and meditation.

The Buddhist Truths have played a large part in molding the Vietnamese characteristics of stoicism, strong self-control, and apparent passivity. Some patients, by implication, may attribute physical pain and suffering to failure to be righteous. There is much variation in specific application of Buddhist thought in Vietnam because of the many forms of Buddhism and a wide range of commitment.

Confucianism also came to Vietnam from China and is a code of ethics rather than a true religion. Confucianism emphasizes hierarchy of society, worship of ancestors, and respect for age, customs, teacher, and family.

Taoism originated from a Chinese philosopher in the sixth century BC and has been very influential in the Vietnamese culture. Tao, or "The Way," is a creative principle that orders the physical universe. Taoism emphasizes that when things are allowed to take their natural course, they move toward harmony and perfection. Therefore individuals should attempt to blend into the natural world rather than trying to conquer it.

Two minor religious sects, Cao Dai and Hoa Hao, began in Vietnam in 1919 and 1939. The former is a combination of the three chief religions (Buddhism, confucianism, and Taoism) along with teachings of Jesus, Victor Hugo, and others. Hoa Hao is a reformed Buddhist sect. In Vietnam these religions combine to claim about three million followers. Still another belief system, animism, continues to have a strong influence in Vietnam, especially among the tribal people. Animism includes many practices to deal with demons, evil spirits, angry Gods, and elements of the natural world that are not understood.

The first Catholic missionary arrived in Vietnam in 1513, and the Jesuits came in the early 1600s. Protestantism came to Vietnam in the early 1900s. Today in Vietnam, there are about 2 million Christians, and the majority of these are Catholics. Both Catholic and Protestant churches have grown since the Communist takeover in 1975.

The religious beliefs of many Vietnamese persons are often a rather vague synthesis of the three traditional "religions," along with one or more forms of ancestral worship or veneration of the dead. Through such rites as cleaning the ancestral graves and celebrations on the anniversary of a death, the family ties are reinforced and strengthened. Many of these practices are so woven into the fabric of Vietnamese life that it is difficult to separate them into either religious or cultural practices. In any case, since most of the ancestors are buried in Vietnam, the custom of gathering the family in the family home around the family altar or at the tombs in celebration is impossible to duplicate in another country, and this leaves a painful void for many refugee-generation Vietnamese persons who are serious about "filial piety" and properly honoring their ancestors.

Values

Respect and harmony are the two most important values in the Vietnamese culture and have their basis in the three major religious belief systems that have dominated the country. When the beliefs common to the Oriental or Eastern system found in Vietnam and those of the Occidental or Western system found in the United States are compared, the nature and extent of the conflict and frustration experienced by Vietnamese individuals who are undergoing acculturation in the United States become readily apparent (Cao, 1986; Nguyen, 1988):

Oriental or Eastern system	Occidental or Western system
Harmony with nature	Mastery of nature (skyscraper)
Tradition	Change, innovation
Hierarchy	Mobility, upward/downward movement
Age	Youth
Extended family (few family names)	Nuclear family, small, individualistic
Convergent thinking	Divergent thinking
Cyclic concept of time	Specific point, schedules, clocks
Group orientation and reward	Self-concept and self-actualization
Rote learning	Discovery learning
Conformity	Competition

Implications for Nursing Care

With the high priority on respect, harmony, "filial piety," and material sharing built into the Vietnamese family and extended family system, it should be readily apparent to the nurse that both the immediate and the extended family serve a significant role in providing emotional, physical, and economic support for Vietnamese individuals. It is essential that the nurse include family members in planning care and utilize the family to assist the patient in regaining physical and mental health. For the Vietnamese American patient, family members provide a network that provides a feeling of interdependence, belonging, and support (Cook & Timberlake, 1984).

TIME

The Vietnamese culture dates back thousands of years, and this antiquity is reflected in an orientation to time with an emphasis on the past. Emphasis is placed on ancestors and their wishes, memories, and graves. Most Vietnamese people have been oriented to think of time in terms of cycles, events, or occurrences (Hoang & Erickson, 1982). Many Vietnamese individuals, even those who are not Buddhist, have some belief in reincarnation. This cultural heritage makes time less of a fixed point (here and gone) and more of a recurring reality. In other words, there was yesterday, there is today, and there will be tomorrow . . . which will in fact be today, followed by tomorrow . . . and so on. This results in a less stressful and less time-conscious pace than that commonly experienced in the West. Being late or early is not considered a problem.

As refugees, Vietnamese people practiced a present and future orientation as they struggled to survive and focused on food, housing, a job, a car, child care, and education. Today, Vietnamese Americans have goals for the future and save for the future, and for many the motivation to live wisely may not only be to please the ancestors (past), but also may be connected with "the good life" (present) or the anticipation of heaven or reincarnation (future).

Implications for Nursing Care

The nurse should be aware that the concept of illness prevention requires both a future and a present time orientation, which is difficult for some traditional Vietnamese people to understand. Illness prevention is a difficult concept if a person lacks a scientific understanding of disease processes. The nurse should also be aware that Vietnamese American patients may feel that luck and fate play a significant role in suffering and that illness may be considered a result of spiritual failure or punishment. For Vietnamese Americans the act of seeking medical care is influenced by a number of factors, including time orientation.

Time orientation also affects a patient's tendency to return for clinic or medical appointments. Since for Vietnamese Americans time is thought of more in terms of cycles than as a specific point of reference, arriving at an exact time for an appointment may be considered less important than some other things. However, through assimilation and acculturation in the United States, many Vietnamese Americans have developed an understanding that punctuality is very important to persons in the United States and often arrive for appointments ahead of the designated time.

Noncompliance with keeping appointments is often a result of other factors in addition to time orientation. Some noncompliance can be traced to not understanding verbal or appointment card communications or not being able to read the instructions. It is important for the nurse to review carefully the appointment card and any instructions given to the patient to clarify what is written and to assure that the patient can read the information given. When a patient is given a phone number to call for an appointment or for assistance, it is important that the nurse ascertain whether the patient knows how to use the available telephone and has the clinic telephone number. Understanding and arriving at a clinic appointment on time can be a complex transcultural assignment for the Vietnamese American patient.

ENVIRONMENTAL CONTROL
Concepts of Illness

The medical system in Vietnam is a complex one, and there are various options for health care from which the Vietnamese person may select. Many traditional Vietnamese individuals tend to combine Chinese medicine with scientific techniques brought in from the West (Tran, 1972, 1980, 1989). For most the choice is usually deliberate and purposeful but rarely rigid or restricted in any single direction. "The baseline is often a set of time-honored beliefs, customs, and usages which are faithfully followed by some, fiercely contested by others, but more or less consciously incorporated by the majority. . . ." (Tran, 1989).

Tran (1980, 1989) has divided the explanations of cause of illness into three types: naturalistic (folk medicine), supernaturalistic (animistic beliefs), and metaphysical (the theory of hot and cold). None of these theories excludes the others, and a patient may explain illness by aspects of all three. A fourth explanation of illness (that is, germs) is offered by some.

Natural causes

The naturalistic explanation for illness encourages a search for a natural or obvious cause of the symptoms, such as rotten food, "poisonous water," or an obvious cause-and-effect relationship. To counteract the effects of these natural elements, an informal body of knowledge has been collected about indigenous medicinal herbs, therapeutic diets, and simple medical and hygienic measures. The information is usually transmitted orally and often treated with secrecy, remaining inside the clan or extended family. Vietnamese folk medicine may fall into the category of either *thuoc nam* (southern medicine) or *thuoc bac* (northern medicine), which more closely resembles Chinese medicine (see box on p. 417).

Supernatural causes

The supernaturalistic explanation for disease lays the blame on supernatural powers, such as gods, demons, or spirits. The illness is considered a punishment for a fault, for a violation of religious or ethical codes, or for an act of omission causing displeasure to a deity. In the supernaturalistic theory disease may be caused by black magic or an evil incantation of an enemy who has bought the services of a sorcerer (Westermeyer & Winthrop, 1979).

The supernatural explanation for illness is the most likely choice of Vietnamese persons who have limited education. Mountain tribes, as well as many of the peasants from the rural areas, tend to be more in touch with these beliefs.

COMMON FOLK PRACTICES

1. *Cao gio* (skin rubbing with a coin) is a folk practice used for diseases caused by wind entering the body, a common cold, flulike symptoms, etc. A layer of balm or ointment is spread on the skin over the affected area—often the chest, upper back, or shoulders. A coin (preferably the size of a nickel or quarter) is pressed on the skin and drawn in one direction, moving the coin a short distance on the skin without breaking the skin. This is repeated several times, and if dark blood appears under the skin, the treatment is considered to be working. Often these ecchymotic stripes are continued in symmetrical rows down the back or chest. The purpose is to create areas where the offending wind or air may escape from the body. It is usually not a painful procedure for children or adults, and most report feeling improved by the procedure (Lan, 1988; Rosenblat & Hong, 1989).

2. *Bat gio* (skin pinching) is a folk practice used for headache. Fingers and thumbs are pressed on both temples, attempting to move the blood across the forehead toward a spot between the eyes. After this has been repeated several times, the area on the forehead between the eyes is pinched between the thumb and forefinger and twisted slightly. If petechiae or ecchymoses appear, the treatment is considered successful. Skin pinching is also used on the neck for sore throat.

3. *Xong* is a folk practice in which Vicks Vaporub or a similar agent or herb is stirred into scalding water. Depending on the reason for the treatment, the patient may simply inhale the vapor or may be treated under a blanket as in a steam tent.

4. *Inhalation of aromatic oils or liniments,* such as menthol, eucalyptus, or mint-based aromatic oils, is used as a folk practice for symptoms such as motion sickness, indigestion, or cold or wind illness. The oils and liniments may be carried in vials in a pocket or purse for ready access and may be smelled when necessary; rubbed on the temple, under the nose, or on the abdomen; or taken internally in small amounts.

5. *Balm and medicated plasters* are a folk practice involving direct application to the skin. Many common balms, such as Red Tiger balm, Mac Phsu, Cula, or Nhi Thiem Duong oil, are available in Oriental shops, with certain balms obtainable only from an Oriental pharmacy. Salonpas is a Japanese preparation with widespread availability and use. Many of the ointments have a mild "deep heat" quality on application and are used for bone and muscle problems, as well as a variety of other ills.

6. *Herbal teas, soups, and condiments* are used as a folk practice for a variety of symptoms. The more complex, involving a variety of ingredients and combinations, are prepared by a pharmacist, whereas the simpler ones are prepared at home. The recipes may be generations old and have a mystical or secret quality about them. Many medicines are prepared to be given as soups. A treatment that may have a familiar ring is the use of garlic for hypertension. There is increasing interest and experimental evaluation of Eastern herbs in Western pharmaceutical firms.

7. *Giac cup suction* is a folk practice in which small, heated, cuplike forms applied to the skin cause a suction on the skin as the cups cool. The suction is used to remove unwanted wind or other elements from the body and is a favorite remedy for joint and muscle pains.

8. *String tying* is a folk practice to control spirits. This practice is more common among the mountain people. While the string, which stays on the arm, leg, or around the neck for long periods of time, may become dirty, it is relatively harmless and is a source of security for the wearer and significant others. Usually it can be left on without difficulty for anyone except health care workers, who may not understand the possible significance of this practice.

Metaphysical causes

A metaphysical explanation for illness may be found in areas of Vietnam heavily influenced by the Chinese (see box). The metaphysical explanation is built on the theory that nature and the body operate within a delicate balance between two opposite elements: the yin and the yang—for example, female and male, dark and light, or hard and soft. In medicine the opposites are expressed as "hot" and "cold," and health is the result of a balance between hot and cold elements. This results in harmonious functioning of the viscera, as well as harmony with the environment. An excess or shortage in either direction causes discomfort and illness.

All illnesses, foods, medications, and herbs are carefully classified along a continuum according to their hot or cold effects. Diarrhea and some febrile diseases are said to be due to an excess of the cold element, whereas pimples, boils, and various skin

---

CHINESE MEDICINE

"Any attempt at probing into the nature of Asian health practices must begin with a search into the age-old philosophy from which they, and indeed all Eastern concepts of health and illness, cure, and death evolved" (Branch & Paxton, 1976, p. 99).

Chinese medicine is a 5000-year-old system of medicine in which an 81-volume classic on the philosophy of life became the primary medical textbook. Body, mind, and soul are integrated, never separated, and man is seen in relationship to the environment. The system encompasses all of the following (in order of their importance as preventive concepts): philosophy, meditation, nutrition, martial arts, herbology, acumassage, acupressure, moxibustion, acupuncture, and spiritual healing (Branch & Paxton, 1976; Huard & Wong, 1968).

Part of the theoretical and philosophical basis for Chinese medicine comes from the Taoist concept that nature maintains a balance in all things and that as part of the universe, man interacts with this balance. The balance is measured in terms of energy and is articulated by the principle of yin and yang (negative/positive, dark/light, cold/hot, feminine/masculine, etc.).

A resultant important difference between Chinese and Western medicine has been the emphasis on prevention rather than disease and crisis intervention. This can be illustrated by the Chinese story of the "old days," when people would go to their physician to have their energy balanced. The physician, knowing the patient well, would prescribe the specific approach to life, type of meditation, exercise, diet, and occasional herbs to keep the patient healthy. For this service the doctor would be paid regularly. If the patient became ill, however, the patient stopped paying, and the treatment was free of charge. This may not be as true for Chinese medicine today, but it does underline a major difference in approach from Western medicine.

Disease theory and "germs" is another area where the basic approach separates the two systems. Western medicine has spent the past 200 years identifying disease-causing organisms under the microscope and finding ways of destroying them, in many cases with dramatic success. The goal of the treatment is to destroy the microorganisms causing the illness.

In Chinese medicine when illness results in an imbalance due to faulty diet or strong emotional feelings, body harmony can be restored through self-restraint and the use of a corrective diet, often aided by herbs. Action is taken not to kill organisms, but to restore a balanced state, countering the effects of unwise life-styles or food. When the yin/yang balance is disturbed, the body is more likely to become ill.

problems are thought to result from too many hot influences erupting through the skin. According to this belief system, vegetables and most fruits are cold; most spices are hot; sweets and candies are hot; water is cold. As a rule, all Oriental herbs are cold, and all Western medicines are hot. The medicinal value of medicines and herbs is strongly influenced by their hot or cold properties. Treatment consists of juggling the hot and cold qualities of medicines and foods to balance the hot or cold status of the body. This may cause no difficulty when used along with a more or less complementary or unrelated system of care (dealing with the supernatural, for example), but superimposing Western concepts of disease or treatment onto the theory of hot and cold can create major stress and conflict for the Vietnamese American patient and family.

Germs

Yet another option has been added by some Vietnamese individuals as a possible cause for illness: germs. Western medicine, with a germ disease causation philosophy, was introduced in Vietnam by the French in the nineteenth century. Western medicine was practiced and thus available in most cities and in the military but was expensive. By 1975 there were about 2000 Western-trained physicians in Vietnam, and 70% of these were in the military. The Indochinese modern medical model that evolved, which was often described as "shotgun therapy," was based more on clinical findings than on laboratory tests and was more pragmatic than strictly scientific. Often many medicines were prescribed in the hope of conquering the offending organism by one method or another. Generally, treatment plans included at least one or two injections. After the initial office visit, the patient would go to a pharmacy to purchase the medications. After purchasing the medications, the next step was to visit an "injection nurse," who gave the subcutaneous intramuscular or intravenous medication the patient had purchased. Tiredness or recuperation from surgery was reason enough to purchase a bolus of dextrose solution and have it injected intravenously.

Until 1975 many Vietnamese pharmacies sold any Western medicines they had, including antibiotics, over the counter without a prescription. Because Vietnamese people commonly treated themselves or were commonly treated by physicians with over-the-counter antibiotics, a high incidence of bacterial resistance to common antibiotics, as well as cases of agranulocytosis, developed. In the late 1960s chloramphenicol (Chloromycetin) was commonly bought to treat common colds and upper respiratory tract infections.

Implications for Nursing Care

It is important for the nurse to understand that Vietnamese American patients sometimes do not understand illness or diagnostic and treatment procedures encountered in the Western medical system (see box on p. 420). In addition, Vietnamese American patients who adhere to Eastern practices may explain illness by disease entities that may be totally unfamiliar to Western practitioners, such as problems caused by the wind, an encounter with an "evil eye," *phong* or toxic substance problems, bad karma, problems caused by spirits, or an imbalance of hot and cold. A patient who has such beliefs may utilize approaches that are contradictory to the recommendations of Western practitioners. For example, a patient who has a febrile disease or diarrhea will be encouraged by the Western practitioner to increase fluids, whereas the theory

COMMON MISUNDERSTANDINGS ABOUT ILLNESS AND DIAGNOSTIC OR TREATMENT PROCEDURES

1. *Drawing blood* for diagnostic purposes may cause a crisis for a Vietnamese American patient. The patient may complain, although often not to the health care worker, of feeling weak and tired for varying periods following the procedure. Such symptoms may last for months. A Vietnamese American patient may feel that any body tissue or fluid removed cannot be replaced and that once it is removed, the body will continue to suffer the loss, not only in this life but in the next life as well.

2. *Donating blood* may be a major decision for the Vietnamese individual. In one rural hospital in Vietnam, Western staff members made an effort not only to teach the Vietnamese staff the "facts" about donating blood, but also to have the Vietnamese staff assist as the Western staff donated blood and, after a short recovery time, again joined the medical team. Vietnamese staff members were invited to have their blood typed and to place their names on a possible donor list for emergency situations. Some did donate blood when the need arose (although since Vietnamese persons often weigh less than 100 pounds, only one half or three fourths of a unit was drawn).

3. *Donation of body parts,* such as the donation of an eye after death, is an act that is often viewed with much skepticism by many Vietnamese individuals, who have been heavily influenced by Buddhist beliefs that a body part cannot be replaced once it is removed and that the body may suffer in the next life. Even those who have been Christians for several generations may be very serious about care given to the body after death and are unlikely to feel comfortable with such practices.

4. *Hospitalization and surgery* were often considered a last resort in Vietnam. Unless insurance considerations are important, outpatient care for the refugee is likely to cause much less anxiety and should be offered as an option when at all possible.

5. *Clergy visitation* is usually associated with "last rites" by the Vietnamese, especially those who have been influenced by the Catholic religion. A visit by the clergy may be considered an indication that the situation is grave, and the common practice of chaplains visiting patients in hospitals in the United States can be quite upsetting for the Vietnamese American patient. It is important to provide the patient with a careful explanation of a visit by the hospital clergy person or chaplain.

6. *Giving flowers to the sick* is a practice that may surprise and upset a Vietnamese American patient who has not been given an explanation of this practice. In Vietnam flowers are usually reserved for the rites of the dead.

7. *American medicines* are considered by the Vietnamese to be much more concentrated than Eastern medicines. American medicine is likely to be given in tablet form, rather than in tea or soups. Also, Americans are often much larger than the average Vietnamese person; therefore medication needs to be carefully titrated so that it will not harm the Vietnamese American patient. It is important for the professional to let the patient know that small stature has been considered when the dosage was calculated. This can be done by either weighing the patient or by verbally discussing this when the prescription is written. It is not an uncommon practice for Vietnamese American patients to take only half of their prescribed dosage.

8. *The germ theory* is very confusing to Vietnamese individuals who have not been exposed to this concept. Many patients with animistic beliefs have a supernatural or spirit world disease-cause orientation. In an effort to move the patient's understanding into the scientific or natural world, germs are presented as the cause of disease because they are a component of the real Western world. For all practical purposes, however, germs also cannot be seen and are far less real to the refugee with animistic beliefs than the spirits and demons that the patient *knows* can cause trouble.

of hot and cold mandates that since these illnesses are cold diseases, fluids should be restricted. External use of either hot or cold water is also restricted according to this theory, and therefore a treatment such as a cold sponge bath may invoke dire consequences.

Another example of conflict between the theory of hot and cold and Western medicine is the requirement during illness of carefully restricting food in order to correct imbalance. Fresh fruits and vegetables, which are considered cold, are often banned. Meats such as pork or chicken, but not beef, are added to the diet slowly. Milk is usually not used. Maternity patients are told to eat a very salty diet with almost no fruits or vegetables. Especially during long illnesses, nutritional deficiency or starvation can inadvertently result.

Since the theory of hot and cold has been used by Vietnamese people for generations with some success, it is important for the nurse to understand that belief in this theory is not likely to be discarded simply because Western health care practitioners do not approve of it. Rather, the nurse should assist the patient and family in combining approaches from tradition with those from Western medicine in order to facilitate a high level of wellness.

The nurse who conducts physical assessments on Vietnamese American patients should be able to recognize ecchymotic areas that may result from *cao gio* ("coin rubbing") and should understand that this folk practice is not harmful. Yeatman and Dang (1980) reported a study that was done with 50 Vietnamese persons 4 years after their arrival in the United States to determine the prevalence of *cao gio* and problems created by it. The sample included students, professionals, housewives, etc. The data from the study suggested that 94% of the respondents had practiced *cao gio* before arriving in the United States and that all of the respondents claimed to have felt better after the treatment. None of the respondents reported any harm as a result of *cao gio*. All but one of the respondents reported having practiced *cao gio* in this country, and 26% of the respondents reported being criticized by physicians, teachers, spouse, or foster parents. One respondent had been reported by a teacher for child abuse. Today, the nurse should be aware that many Vietnamese Americans are refraining from practicing *cao gio* because of fear of societal condemnation, although many Vietnamese Americans continue to believe in its validity. Yeatman and Dang (1980) advocate that Western practitioners should accept *cao gio* as a "nurturant folk practice."

Although the benefits of folk beliefs are likely to outweigh the risks, the nurse who provides care to Vietnamese American patients must be aware of possible risks for patients, including the following:

1. Toxicity may result from the use of remedies containing heavy metals (lead, mercury, arsenic). (In 1983 24 H'mong children were found in the St. Paul, Minneapolis, area with excessively high lead blood levels.)
2. Inadequate labeling of Chinese medicines may result in excessive use of potentially harmful chemicals. (In 1984 four cases of agranulocytosis were diagnosed in one facility in patients who had been taking one or more Chinese medicines containing phenylbutazone or aminopyrine, neither of which was listed as an ingredient.)
3. Toxicity may result from human error. (For example, many herbs and plants such as mushrooms and seeds found in the United States are new to Southeast

Asians, and some have been mistaken for familiar ones "back home," resulting in poisonings.)

4. Problems may result from misidentification of folk medicine treatments when seen by Western health professionals. (For example, a child with ecchymotic areas on the back or abdomen caused by *cao gio* may be examined and diagnosed as having been abused [Lan, 1988; Yeatman & Dang, 1980].)

The nurse must be cognizant that the patient's use of folk medicine practices may cause delay in seeking Western medical treatment, with dire results. For example, if a Vietnamese American parent uses folk medicine practices for an extended period of time in the treatment of a baby, the baby may be brought for treatment too late for Western medical practices to be effective. If a Vietnamese American patient waits until gangrene has spread too far to save the limb or if oxygen deprivation has been severe for a lengthy period, it is unlikely that Western medicine will be beneficial. As Vietnamese American patients experience success with Western medicine and develop positive relationships with health care providers, these patients will be less likely to retain the "old ways" and more likely to seek help without waiting for symptoms to become severe.

BIOLOGICAL VARIATIONS
Body Size and Structure

Vietnamese people are generally small of frame and build, with average body weights between 80 and 130 pounds. An overweight Vietnamese person is uncommon except among the Vietnamese-Chinese population (Williams & Westermeyer, 1986).

Skin Color

The skin coloring is usually light to medium with yellow tones. Newborns are usually fair skinned. In the United States there appears to be a higher than average incidence of newborn icterus among Vietnamese Americans as compared with the rest of the general U.S. population.

Other Visible Physical Characteristics

Noses may be small and "classically oriental" or larger with a less-defined bridge. The eyelids usually have an epicanthic fold and a slight droop over the cartilage plate. Both variations are common to Orientals.

Teeth are usually proportionately large, with a high incidence of mandibular torus (lump on the inner side of the mandible near the second molar). Some dentists who have treated Vietnamese patients estimate that at least 40% of Vietnamese Americans have these tori as compared with 7% of the White U.S. population (N.B. Nguyen, 1988).

Enzymatic and Genetic Variations

The incidence of dizygotic twin births among the Vietnamese is only one half of 1% as compared with 2% for Whites and 4% for Blacks in this country (Overfield, 1985).

Although some Vietnamese people enjoy milk, cheese, and ice cream, an unknown percentage, possibly as high as 50%, have a congenital lactose deficiency. For most Vietnamese people, the intolerance is not a total one, and many Vietnamese persons can digest milk in small amounts without incidence. For some Vietnamese individuals with some degree of lactose intolerance, a glass of milk can be an inexpensive solution for constipation (Tran, 1989). Vietnamese babies indicate a lesser degree of the deficiency by their ability to accept the usual formula preparations without difficulty (Bayless, 1975).

Medical Problems among Vietnamese Refugees

Medical problems identified in 594 persons in two groups of refugees (400 in one; 194 in the other) studied by Hoang and Erickson (1982) included the following:

1. Skin: superficial fungal infections and scabies, 10% to 15%.
2. Teeth: moderate to severe dental problems, 90%.
3. Endocrine system: thyroid diseases, especially goiters, 10% in the group of 400 and 6% in the group of 194.
4. Cardiovascular system: mitral valve prolapse, 1.7%; hypertension, 7% of adults over age 30; rheumatic heart disease, 1%.
5. Renal system: microscopic hematuria may be present with no specific cause.
6. Blood: anemia, 16%.
7. Parasites: ascaris, hookworm infestation, giardiasis, trichuriasis (most common), and amebiasis.
8. Hepatitis B_s antigen (HB$_s$Ag), 13%.
9. Malaria: 2½% of the sample of 194 had a history of malaria, and 1% of this number developed an acute episode.
10. Psyche: 5% in the sample of 194 had "significant" psychiatric problems.

Tuberculosis Risk

Although bacillus Calmette Guérin (BCG) was widely used in Vietnam during the 1960s and was given to babies shortly after birth in birthing centers and maternity units in hospitals across the country, the living conditions and general upheaval during the past 25 years have reduced the long-term effectiveness of any type of preventive effort such as the administration of BCG. In the early 1970s there were an alarming number of active cases of tuberculosis in the South Vietnamese army, where "early TB" (stage 1) was rarely sufficient reason for discharge and almost all cases seen at private hospitals or tuberculosis clinics were either moderate or advanced (Stauffer, 1989).

Between 1968 and 1974, the movement of people from the less-secure countryside to the cities, with their accompanying overcrowding and poor nutritional status, simply exacerbated an already precarious situation. The caseload of children with active tuberculosis being diagnosed and treated in a private tuberculosis clinic in an area of Saigon (1969 to 1970) doubled in less than a year, partly from newly detected cases and partly from new cases developing in crowded rooms shared with adults with active disease. Hoang and Erickson (1982) recommended the use of isoniazid prophylactically for 1 year for all refugees under 35 years of age with positive skin tests, and that children with negative skin readings on arrival in the United States be checked in 3 to 6 months to single out false negative readings.

Nutritional Preferences

A common staple in Vietnam is rice, which is eaten from large bowls with chopsticks several times a day, often with dark green leafy vegetables. Fish sauce is added for saltiness and flavor. One way a patient may describe a medical problem to a doctor is to hold a hand up in the form of a bowl and say, "Now I eat only one bowl of rice at a meal instead of three as I used to do."

Rice, as well as many other cooked dishes, is seasoned with the unique Vietnamese condiment, nuoc mam, which is made by marinating small fish in salt in kegs for a month or more. When this condiment is used on rice, water, sugar, fresh lime juice, garlic, and chili peppers are added. In Vietnam dark green leafy vines or plants are gathered from the countryside or from gardens and brought in to the local village or small-town markets in truckloads each morning. Although not served in large quantities, the regular presence of these greens with rice contributes to a diet with adequate nutrients despite the lack of meat or meat substitutes. Meat, when served, is cut into slivers and eaten with rice and vegetables. Chicken and duck eggs are used as available. Bean curd is used, but (dry) bean dishes are not common. For the most part, milk and milk products are imported, expensive, and generally discouraged, since a large percentage of the population have lactose intolerance.

During the long French occupation, bread was introduced in Vietnam and was widely consumed in the form of small tasty French rolls, available fresh daily on the street corners in cities and towns. French pastries were also available. Today, many of the Vietnamese people replace some of their rice with fresh white bread.

According to the U.S. Department of Agriculture, Food and Nutrition Service, the traditional Vietnamese diet is low in fat and sugar, high in complex carbohydrates, and moderate in fiber. This compares very favorably with the dietary guidelines of the U.S. Department of Agriculture and the U.S. Department of Health and Human Services (Burtis, Davis, & Martin, 1988).

Depending on where the Vietnamese refugees are living in the United States or Canada, the traditional diet has changed considerably. With more meat and fat available, many Vietnamese persons are increasing their fat intake. In cities with large concentrations of Vietnamese Americans, the ingredients to prepare almost all of the ethnic foods, including nuoc mam, are likely to be available. Many Vietnamese Americans enjoy preparing native Vietnamese dishes, as well as dining in Vietnamese restaurants. In Vietnam brown, unpolished grains were considered the food of the mountain people and were almost never eaten by the more sophisticated lowlanders; in the United States, because of the stigma attached to brown bread and brown rice, with the exception of those Vietnamese Americans who take nutrition facts seriously, polished rice and white bread continue to be a favorite among Vietnamese people (Tien-Hyatt, 1989).

A favorite Vietnamese dish is a variation of Chinese noodle soup called *pho* (pronounced "phuh"), which is made by placing cooked rice noodles in a delicately flavored, clear, boiling broth, adding rare and/or cooked thinly sliced beef or chicken, and finally topping the mixture with scallions and black pepper. At the table a lime slice, bean sprouts, and que leaves may be added to taste. Although pho was a forenoon meal in Vietnam, in the United States it may be served in pho shops at any hour of the day.

While tea was associated in Vietnam with social etiquette (all guests were served tea) and potable cold water was a luxury many did not enjoy, since immigration many Vietnamese Americans have begun to drink water, as well as cola, other soft drinks, coffee, and some milk, and have begun to drink less tea. Among Vietnamese people in Vietnam and Vietnamese immigrants, poor liquid intake has been related to bladder stones in small boys as well as in men (Hoang & Erickson, 1982).

Unexplained Death

Sudden, unexplained nocturnal deaths have also been reported among adult Southeast Asian refugees, mostly H'mong tribespeople. Hoang and Erickson noted in 1982 that 38 cases of unexplained death had been reported, all but one of which involved men. The median age for these unexplained deaths was 32.5 years. These deaths usually occurred at night and were preceded by groans, unusual respiratory sounds, and sometimes seizurelike activity. All victims had apparently been in good health, and autopsy in 30 of the cases revealed no apparent cause (Hoang & Erickson, 1982).

Psychological Characteristics
Mental health

The term *psychiatrist* or "mental doctor" has no direct Vietnamese translation. There is slightly better understanding with the term that translates as "nerve doctor," but by far the best comprehension comes with an explanation of "a specialist who treats crazy people" (Tran, 1989).

In the Vietnamese culture there is recognition of two possible sources of mental disease: the organic model, which considers damaged nerves or brain, and the inorganic model, in which the less comprehensible phenomena of bizarre behavior may be attributed to various causes such as disobedience, sin, or demon possession.

Often the Vietnamese understand the nervous system to be the source of all mental and physical activities. Therefore when there is a disturbance in mental or physical activity, the nervous system is considered central to the malfunction. Neuroses are called "weaknesses of the nerves," which is used to describe many kinds of anxiety, depression, weariness, mental deterioration, and retardation. Psychoses, on the other hand, are known as "turmoil of the nerves," more accurately reflecting the patient's behavior or feelings (Tran, 1989).

For some Vietnamese people, most illnesses associated with the nerves precipitate optimistic feelings about the possibility of treatment with folk remedies: a nerve tonic to restore strength to weak nerves or a calming medicine to quiet inner turmoil. For some Vietnamese people, medication is the logical answer, though there is concern about dependency, oversedation, or mind-changing medicines. Most Vietnamese refugees bring mental problems to a Western psychiatrist or health professional only after these problems have become too obvious to be ignored (Westermeyer & Winthrop, 1979).

Treatment of a psychiatric problem of a Vietnamese refugee by Western psychiatric professionals is extremely difficult because of the language barrier. Although this difficulty persists even with the use of an interpreter who can identify, with the patient, "normal behavior" specific to the Vietnamese culture, assessment of the severity of a psychiatric problem is an especially difficult task for a psychiatric professional when a language problem exists. In response to problems created by the language barrier in assessing Vietnamese American patients, Kinzie et al. (1982) developed a Vietnamese Language Depression Rating Scale that can assist the practitioner in evaluation of the severity of the depression. Because many Vietnamese refugees are not used to verbal expression of emotion and thought, "amobarbital interviews" are used by some psychiatric practitioners to both assess and treat symptoms of depression (Lee, 1985; Owen, 1985). The variables affecting the mental health of Vietnamese refugees arriving in this country are profound and complex, and establishing a healthy equilibrium takes time and effort.

Emotional and behavioral manifestations of distress in refugees

Immigration is a complex circumstance that exacts a serious toll in terms of mental turmoil and distress, which may be referred to as cultural shock (Pickwell, 1989; Williams & Westermeyer, 1986). Hoang and Erickson (1982) reported that psychiatric problems may become more obvious 6 to 12 months after immigration. Psychologically, the distress is often experienced as a combination of depression and anxiety (Lin, Masuda, & Tazuma, 1982; Rumbaut, 1977; Tyhurst, 1977). As is often noted, individuals going through a life crisis, such as immigrating to a new land as a refugee, tend to exhibit behavioral disturbances (Lin, Masuda, & Tazuma, 1982; Nguyen, 1981). Somatic preoccupations, marital conflicts, intergenerational conflicts, substance abuse, and sociopathic behavior may all be manifestations of the stress of adjustment to a new culture.

The emotional and behavioral problems of refugees are often related to (1) loss of immediate and extended family, (2) overemployment or underemployment, and (3) the stresses of adaptation. Because of the marked differences between the Eastern and Western cultures and the traumatic conditions under which the immigration occurred, the "culture shock" experienced by many Vietnamese refugees is profound. Since Vietnamese people place a high value on self-control in speech and behavior and are used to dealing with family problems within the family structure, the refugee situation, in which family structure is incomplete or missing, has contributed to feelings of isolation, helplessness, and disorganization. Additional problems are found when families go through the acculturation process together, yet members react individually. D. Nguyen (1988) stated:

Prolonged closeness often creates friction; compulsory intimacy may generate irritation; exposure of the younger generation to the American culture often is the origin of conflict, and constant expectations of mutual dependency may turn into hateful obligations and be a source of mental illness.

Often compounding this problem is the language barrier between Vietnamese refugees and those who try to help them. With so much change and with often the very foundations of the Vietnamese society under attack (that is, deterioration of the ties with the family unit: the ancestors, grandparents, or parents), the conflicts may become overt crises that move "toward outcomes which are more likely to be radical and disruptive" (D. Nguyen, 1988).

General patterns of coping/adaption

A general pattern of coping/adaptation is experienced by many persons in their cultural adjustment to immigration (Cook & Timberlake, 1984):

Stage I. For the first few months there is a positive attitude and high expectations; energy is focused toward language, employment, and meeting basic needs. The excitement of a new physical environment and "things" helps suppress the pain of the multiple losses.

Stage II. The period of "psychological arrival" occurs 6 to 18 months after immigration, when the person becomes more aware of losses and "the past" becomes idealized. Survivor's guilt must be faced. (Why did I survive and my child did not?) Posttraumatic stress disorder (PTSD) is common, and all the normal tensions of close family life are magnified. Interpersonal conflict is common. Other symptoms may be feelings of hopelessness, acute distress and grief, fatigue, and mood instability. The period may be transitory or long-lasting, mild or severe, and seems to occur regardless of how much help or support has been given. It is usually a very frustrating time for sponsors and "helping persons," who feel inadequate to help. During this period somatization is common.

Stage III. After 18 to 24 months the person is able to reformulate the grief and get involved again with the tasks at hand. There is less idealizing of the past, and helping those left behind becomes important. Adaptation moves ahead at a more rapid rate as former ways of coping are given up for more effective ones. A new self-identity emerges.

Cook and Timberlake (1984) list denial as the defense mechanism most often used by Vietnamese refugees. These authors believe that denial is congruent with the values of the culture: submission to the common good (and to fate), and harmony and self-sacrifice. Denial is needed to lessen the impact of losses and allow the refugees to go on with the task of survival. When denial fails, facing the hard realities without the needed support systems sometimes causes "uprooting psychosis," withdrawal, and inappropriate behavior (Cook & Timberlake, 1984).

Somatic preoccupation

Somatization is viewed as being common among Southeast Asian refugees. In a Chinese-influenced culture where overt expression of anxiety, disappointment, or anger is considered failure, a high value is placed on suppressing negative feelings; therefore expressing mental distress through various physical ailments may be an acceptable option. One study reported that among Chinese patients with mental disorders, as many as 88% of the respondents complained of somatic ailments without admitting to feelings of anxiety or mental discomfort as compared with 4% in a group of patients without the influence of the Chinese culture (Eyton & Neuwirth, 1984). This data suggest that among Vietnamese immigrants it may be more acceptable to see a physician for physical problems (Eyton & Neuwirth, 1984).

Alcohol use

Alcohol consumption has rarely been a problem among the Vietnamese people. A major sociological and cultural reason for this is the high value placed on self-control, moderation, and correct behavior. A physiological reason is the "Oriental syndrome," or the accentuated facial flushing and pronounced neurovegetative symptoms, including trembling, palpitation, and rapid breathing, that result from an apparent genetic aberration in alcohol metabolism by Vietnamese people (Tran, 1980).

Implications for Nursing Care

The small body size of many Vietnamese American patients has an important implication in terms of nursing treatment. Some nurses have delayed giving pain medication to a Vietnamese American patient in pain "since the patient is so tiny" (Tien-Hyatt, 1989). Since Vietnamese American patients may be stoic, it is important for the nurse to evaluate carefully the need for pain medication and to provide sufficient medication without undue delay (Lin & Finder, 1983; Tien, 1984; Tien-Hyatt, 1989). Some studies have suggested that Vietnamese individuals have a pharmacodynamic difference in therapeutic response to psychotropics. In a study by Lin et al. (1989), the Asian patient's mean required dose was significantly lower than the average for optimal clinical therapeutic response, as well as the emergency of extrapyramidal symptoms, when haloperidol was administered. This study and others have suggested that Asian patients generally respond to substantially lower doses of neuroleptics (Murphy, 1969; Rosenblat & Tang, 1987).

Smither and Rodriguez-Giegling (1979) have noted that within the first 5 years after leaving Vietnam, personality and coping are the more important determinants of which acculturation patterns develop. Other significant factors are level of income and social class (Smither & Rodriguex-Giegling, 1979). Crystal (1989) has suggested that an additional complicating factor is the "myth of the model minority." According to the "model minority" myth, Asian Americans' cultural traits, which include diligence, frugality, and willingness to sacrifice, propel their upward mobility and win them public accolades. In reality, the "model minority" myth has obscured many serious problems in the Asian community and has been used to justify omitting Asian Americans from federal funding and some special minority programs. The Asian American success story for some has been an obstacle rather than the norm.

The nurse should also be cognizant of the fact that for many Vietnamese American patients, food is medicine. Although many Vietnamese Americans are able to practice their food beliefs without difficulty, if a patient develops a health problem and encounters Western medical practitioners, the need to adopt Western food practices may be considered necessary for survival, for example, the need for fluids, the restriction of salt, the need for specific medications (for example, cardiac medications), and the need for specific nutrients in the diet. Helping the patient to understand why dietary restrictions have been recommended is essential. A patient may be willing to limit the amount of nuoc mam in the diet when health care professionals carefully explain the reason for this request. For many Vietnamese Americans, eating habits are changing. Children are learning to eat hamburgers, french fries, pizza, spaghetti, and tacos in school lunch programs. Vietnamese Americans are pragmatists, and teaching about dietary practices in relation to Western medicine can result in changed behavior.

Another important health care issue for the nurse who provides care for Vietnamese American patients is utilization of health care resources. Tran (1980) suggested that utilization of health care services is related to the identification of a problem and the availability of an appropriate service. A study by Strand and Jones (1983) found that health services utilization is not directly correlated with education and English language skills but is related to a variety of factors. For example, working two jobs makes it difficult to take time for a clinic appointment. The person who speaks English best, as well as those persons who should accompany the patient to the health facility, is usually at work or school. A car or a baby sitter may not be available.

Choosing health care may be difficult. The options for health care are fewer than they were in Vietnam, and even wealthy Vietnamese persons may have problems finding health care providers who understand the Vietnamese language.

Another deterrent for some Vietnamese Americans in the utilization of health services is integration into ethnic subcommunities. For a minority group who have found learning English, and the process of acculturation, difficult, surrounding themselves with familiar life-styles, language, friends, or family has made loneliness less of a problem. For such individuals, traditional beliefs and/or superstitions survive far more readily in these subcommunities than in the "outside world." In such situations decisions are more likely to be made by the patient's extended family and community.

The majority of health care problems do not occur, or at least are not reported by Vietnamese refugees, during the initial settlement period. This may result from the fact that immediately before or after arrival the refugees are routinely screened and treated for existing problems. After the excitement of arriving and getting settled, however, previously untreated health problems often become evident. Silverman (1977) reported that in Denver 80% of Vietnamese American patients waited 5 days after the initial onset of illness before seeing a physician and at least 75% failed to return for follow-up care.

SUMMARY

It is important for the nurse to recognize that although many similarities exist among Vietnamese Americans, many variations also exist among subgroups and generations. Geographic origin, sex, age, and individual idiosyncrasies may all contribute to variations in response to the American health care system. The customs, values, and health beliefs and practices of Vietnamese American patients are an important consideration for the Western health care professional (Tripp-Reimer & Thieman, 1981). Most Vietnamese Americans have retained some folk medicine beliefs that affect not only explanations for causes of symptoms, but also the type of treatment that will be selected. The nurse who develops a knowledge and understanding of these beliefs, as well as sensitivity to the refugee's lack of familiarity with the American health care system, will promote more effective health Care delivery and will ease the Vietnamese American patient's adjustment to the new homeland.

CASE STUDY*   Mr. Yen Van Nguyen is a 26-year-old man who has recently arrived in the United States from Vietnam with his wife and 2-year-old son, Tran. Yen arrives at a local emergency room one evening carrying his son, Tran, and gesturing that his son needs medical attention because he has been running a low-grade fever, sneezing, and coughing for the past 2 days. Yen speaks very poor English and appears to be somewhat excited.

The emergency room nurse takes Tran back to an examination room where she can get him undressed and into a gown for examination by the physician. While undressing Tran, the nurse notices bruising over the sternum and along the spine, and immediately summons the physician. On examination the physician notices that the bruised areas do not appear tender but nevertheless suspects child abuse. The child's father, Yen, is escorted back to the child's room by a hospital security officer, where he is questioned by the physician. Yen speaks very

---

*Case study by Dale Moore, B.S.N., R.N.

poor English, and communication is difficult. The harder the physician tries to communicate with Yen, the more frustrated both the physician and Yen become.

A young Vietnamese woman who works in housekeeping is requested to report to the emergency department to help with the communication problem between the emergency room staff and Yen. After a short discussion with Yen, the young Vietnamese woman explains the custom of *cao gio,* or "coin rubbing," to the emergency room staff. On further examination the physician can find no other evidence of child abuse. The emergency staff realize that the bruising is from the coin rubbing and not from child abuse as initially suspected. The child is given an injection of an antibiotic and discharged.

CARE PLAN

Nursing Diagnosis   Communication, impaired verbal, related to foreign language barrier.

Patient Outcome

Parent will be able to communicate more effectively customs and beliefs used in treating illnesses, and nurse will better understand these customs.

Nursing Interventions

1 Determine parent's understanding and ability to communicate in the English language.
2 Talk slowly, enunciating words.
3 Face parent and speak in a slow, clear voice.
4 Use gestures to convey meanings, while not using excessive "touching."
5 Attempt to locate a translator for assistance.
6 Provide parent adequate space to communicate without "crowding him."
7 Keep language simple.

Nursing Diagnosis   Fear related to Americans' misunderstanding of Vietnamese culture with a potential for prosecution for child abuse.

Patient Outcome

Parent will experience reduced fear with awareness of nurse's understanding of Vietnamese cultural folk medicine.

Nursing Interventions

1 Allow parent to explain Vietnamese traditional folk medicine.
2 Provide parent with a quiet area to help reduce fears.
3 Attempt to communicate in a nonthreatening manner.
4 Recruit others familiar with Vietnamese culture to help parent explain.
5 Remove persons perceived as threatening to parent.

Nursing Diagnosis   Knowledge deficit related to modern medical practices secondary to cultural differences.

Patient Outcome

Parent will demonstrate an understanding of importance of modern medical treatment in conjunction with traditional folk medicine.

Nursing Interventions

1 Explain to parent importance of modern medical care in conjunction with cultural folk medicine.

2 Determine parent's perception of medical model of treatment.
3 Keep language simple; avoid long medical terms.
4 Explain importance of compliance with medical treatment ordered.
5 Keep instructions simple and brief.
6 Arrange for an interpreter to help explain importance of seeking medical attention for illness or injury.

Nursing Diagnosis   Parental role conflict related to child's present illness and need to seek "foreign" medical attention.

Patient Outcome	*Nursing Interventions*
Parent will demonstrate an understanding of importance of seeking qualified medical attention for betterment of his child's well-being.	1 Educate parent on importance of seeking medical attention to treat illnesses. 2 Provide parent the opportunity to describe how similar situations were handled. 3 Assess past medical practices and folklore the parent normally uses in similar situations. 4 Allow parent time to ask questions related to child's health care. 5 Provide information in a clear, concise, easy-to-understand manner.

Nursing Diagnosis   Noncompliance (potential for) related to misunderstanding of the prescribed treatment secondary to the belief that medications in the Western World are much stronger than those found in the Far East.

Patient Outcome	*Nursing Interventions*
Parent will demonstrate an understanding of prescribed treatment and importance of following prescribed medical regimen.	1 Assess parent's fear of prescribed treatment. 2 Promote health teaching to educate parent on the effects, desired outcome, and side effects of prescribed medicine. 3 Warn parent that some medications may make the patient sleepy and that this is an expected occurrence. 4 Teach parent about importance of adhering to prescribed medical treatment. 5 Reassure parent that prescribed medication is appropriate and safe for patient. 6 Review medication, dosage, and proper administration technique with parent to help him feel more comfortable with the treatment.

Nursing Diagnosis   Coping, ineffective family: compromised, related to illness of a family member and the necessity to seek culturally unfamiliar medical treatment.

Patient Outcome	*Nursing Interventions*
Family members will be better able to cope with illness-related problems after obtaining information on prescribed medical treatment.	1 Reassure parent of appropriateness of prescribed medical treatment. 2 Provide parent the opportunity to express fears and concerns. 3 Encourage parent to verbalize familiar treatments that family sought in Vietnam, including customs and folk medicine. 4 Direct parent to areas of potential help (e.g., churches, Vietnamese communities, social workers). 5 Instruct parent on how to perform prescribed treatment to increase his feelings of being needed.

Nursing Diagnosis   Role performance, altered (potential for), related to undue stress of an ill family member in an unfamiliar culture.

Patient Outcome	*Nursing Interventions*
Parent will discuss feelings of altered role performance and identify areas of undue stress.	1 Encourage parent to talk openly about actual or potential areas of stress. 2 Provide quiet area for parent to gather thoughts. 3 Help parent to understand what resources are available to him within the community (e.g., self-help groups). 4 Reassure patient. 5 Avoid negative criticism. 6 Encourage parent to discuss openly his concerns about the health of his child and about the care that his child will receive.

STUDY QUESTIONS

1. List several ways that the nurse and the emergency room staff might better communicate with the patient from Vietnam.
2. Should the client be told that his folk medicine treatment is foolish and that he should abandon it? Why or why not?
3. How could the nurse effectively teach the patient about the benefits of seeking conventional medical treatment in the United States?
4. When asked questions, Yen answers, "Yes." Does this always indicate that Yen necessarily means "yes"?
5. List some strategies and techniques to help the nurse communicate more effectively with the Vietnamese family.
6. Describe the misconceptions that Vietnamese Americans have concerning Western medical practices and medications.

7. In American society hospitalization and visitation by clergy is a common, almost expected act by some. How do the Vietnamese view hospitalization and clergy visitation?
8. Describe the importance of folk medicine and folk healers to Vietnamese Americans.

REFERENCES

Bayless, T. (1975). Lactose-milk intolerance: Clinical implications. *New England Journal of Medicine, 292*(5), 1156-1159.

Branch, M., & Paxton, P. (1976). *Providing safe nursing care for ethnic people of color.* East Norwalk, Conn.: Appleton-Century-Crofts.

Burtis, G., Davis, J., & Martin, S. (1988). *Applied nutrition and diet therapy.* Philadelphia: W.B. Saunders Co.

Cao, A.Q. (1986). Linguistic and cultural issues in refugees. In *The next decade: The 1986 conference on refugee health care issues and management. 1986 Refugee Health Care Conference Proceedings,* pp. 70-75.

Coelho, G., & Stein, J. (1980). Change, vulnerability and coping: Stresses of uprooting and overcrowding. In G. Coelho & P. Ahmed (Eds.), *Uprooting and development.* New York: Plenum Press.

Cook, K., & Timberlake, E. (1984). Working with Vietnamese refugees. *Social Work, 29*(2), 108-113.

Crystal, D. (1989). Asian Americans and the myth of the model minority. *Social Casework, 70*(7), 405-413.

Eyton, J., & Neuwirth, G. (1984). Cross-cultural validity: Ethnocentrism in health studies with special reference to the Vietnamese. *Social Science and Medicine, 18*(5), 447-453.

Hoang, G., & Erickson, R. (1982). Guidelines for providing medical care for Southeast Asian refugees. *Journal of the American Medical Association, 248*(6), 710-714.

Huard, P., & Wong, M. (1968). *Chinese medicine.* New York: McGraw-Hill.

Huynh, T.D. (1987). *Introduction to Vietnamese culture.* San Diego, Calif.: Multifunctional Resource Center, San Diego State University.

Indochinese Refugee Action Center. (1980, March 20). *Special report: Physical and emotional health care of Indochinese refugees.*

Kinzie, J.D., Manson, S.M., Do, T.V., Nguyen, T.T., Beui, A., & Pho, N.P. (1982). Development and validation of the Vietnamese language depression rating scale. *American Journal of Psychiatry, 139,* 1276-1281.

Lan, L.V. (1988, Sept.). Folk medicine among the Southeast Asian refugees in the U.S.A.: Risks, benefits, and uncertainties. *Journal of the Association of Vietnamese Medical Professionals in Canada, 98,* 31-36.

Lee, E. (1985). Inpatient psychiatric services for Asian refugees. In T. Owen (Ed.), *Southeast Asian mental health.* Washington, D.C., U.S. Department of Health and Human Services.

Lin, K.M., & Finder, E. (1983). Neuroleptic dosage for Asians. *American Journal of Psychiatry, 140,* 490-491.

Lin, K.M., Masuda, M., & Tazuma, L. (1982). Adaptational problems of Vietnamese refugees: Part 3. Case studies in clinic and field: adaptive and maladaptive. *The Psychiatric Journal of the University of Ottawa, 7,* 173-183.

Lin, K.M., Poland, R., Nuccio, I., Matsuda, K., Hathus, N., Su, T., & Fu, P. (1989). Longitudinal assessment of haloperidol doses and serous concentrations in Asian and Caucasian schizophrenic patients. *American Journal of Psychiatry, 146*(10), 1307-1311.

Murphy, H.B. (1969). Ethnic variations in drug responses. *Transcultural Psychiatric Research Review, 6,* 6-23.

Nguyen, D. (1981, Sept.). *Psychiatric and psychosomatic problems among Southeast Asian refugees.* Paper presented at the Sixth World Congress of the International College of Psychosomatic Medicine, Montreal, Canada.

Nguyen, D. (1988, Sept.). Culture shock: A study of Vietnamese culture and the concept of health and disease. *Journal of the Associates of Vietnamese Medical Professionals in Canada, 98,* 26-30.

Nguyen, N.B. (1988). Personal communication.

Overfield, T. (1985). *Biological variations in health and illness.* Reading, Mass. Addison-Wesley.

Owen, T. (Ed.). (1985). *Southeast Asian mental health.* Washington, D.C.: U.S. Department of Health and Human Services.

Pickwell, S. (1989). The incorporation of family primary care for Southeast Asian refugees in a community-based mental health facility. *Archives of Psychiatric Nursing, 3*(3), 173-177.

Rosenblat, H., & Hong, P. (1989). Coin rubbing misdiagnosed as child abuse. *Canadian Medical Association Journal, 140*(4), 417.

Rosenblat, H., & Tang, S.W. (1987). Do Asian patients receive different dosages of psychotropic medication when compared to Occidentals? *Canadian Journal of Psychiatry, 32*, 270-274.

Rumbaut, R.D. (1977). Life events, change, migration and depression. In W.F. Fann, I.J. Faracan, A.D. Pokorny, & R.L Williams (Eds.), *Phenomenology and treatment of depression.* New York: Spectrum.

Silverman, M.L. (1977). *United States health care in cross-cultural perspective: The Vietnamese in Denver.* Master's thesis, University of Denver, Denver, Colorado.

Smither, R., & Rodriguez-Giegling. (1979, Dec.). Marginality, modernity, and anxiety in Indochinese refugees. *Journal of Cross-Cultural Psychiatry, 10*, 469-478.

Statistical abstracts of the United States. (1988). Washington, D.C.: U.S. Department of Commerce, Bureau of the Census.

Stauffer, R. (1989). Personal experience.

Strand, P., & Jones, W. (1983, Nov.). Health service utilization by Indochinese refugees. *Medical Care, 21*(11), 1089-1098.

Tien, J.L. (1984, Dec.). Do Asians need less medication? Issues in clinical assessment and psychopharmacology. *Journal of Psychosocial Nursing and Mental Health Services, 22*, 19-22.

Tien-Hyatt, J. (1989, May). Keying in on the unique care needs of Asian clients. *Nursing and Health Care, 11*, pp. 269-271.

Tran, T.M. (1972). The family and the management of mental health problems in Vietnam. In W.P. Lebra (Ed.), *Transcultural research in mental health.* Honolulu: University of Hawaii Press.

Tran, T.M. (1980). *Indochinese patients.* Falls Church, Va.: Action for Southeast Asians.

Tran, T.M. (1989, Oct.). Personal communication.

Tripp-Reimer, T., & Thieman, K. (1981). Traditional health beliefs/practices of Vietnamese refugees. *Journal of Iowa Medical Society, 71*(12), 533-535.

Tyhurst, L.J. (1977). Psychosocial first aid for refugees. *Mental Health and Society, 4*, 319-334

Yeatman, G., & Dang, V. (1980). Cao gio (coin rubbing). *JAMA, 244* (24), 2748-2749.

Westermeyer, J., Lyfoung, T., Wahmenholm, K., & Westermeyer, M. (1989). Delusions of fatal contagion among refugee patients. *Psychosomatics, 30*(4), 374-381.

Westermeyer, J., & Winthrop, R. (1979). Folk criteria for the diagnosis of mental illness in rural Laos. *American Journal of Psychiatry, 136*, 136-161.

Williams, C., & Westermeyer, J. (1986). *Refugee mental health in resettlement countries.* New York: Hemisphere.

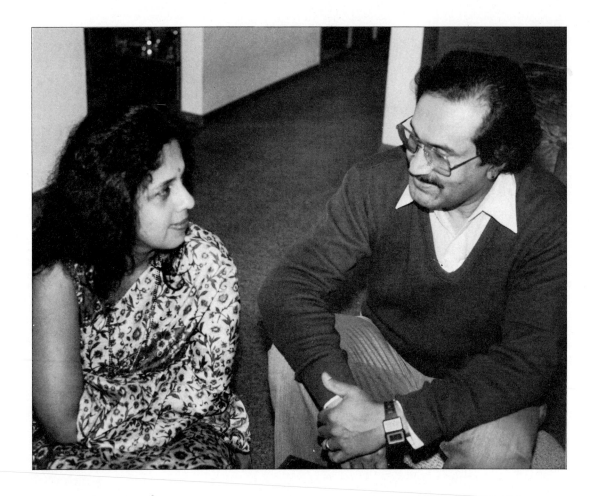

CHAPTER 19

■■■

East Indian Hindu Americans

Scott Wilson Miller and Jill Nerala Supersad

BEHAVIORAL OBJECTIVES
After reading this chapter, the nurse will be able to:

1 Identify two important East Indian Hindu cultural values that influence the behavior of East Indian Hindus living in the United States or Canada.

2 Describe concepts of health and illness influencing East Indian Hindus in relation to illness and health-seeking behaviors.

3 Outline the characteristics of the three waves of immigrants who have come to the United States and Canada from India.

4 Describe the effect culture has had on symptoms of mental illness experienced by the East Indian Hindu in India and after immigration.

5 Understand the unique beliefs about touch held by East Indian Hindus and explain how this may influence attitudes and reactions of East Indian Hindu Americans to care-givers.

6 Describe the beliefs and values held by East Indian Hindus concerning the family.

7 Explain the past, present, and future time orientation that may be held by East Indian Hindus.

8 Describe the Ayurvedic system and the way this system explains illness.

OVERVIEW OF INDIA AND HINDUISM

India is a subcontinent that is a vast, wedge-shaped triangular peninsula jutting south from the mainland of Asia into the Indian Ocean. India includes an area of about 1,262,000 square miles and stretches about 2000 miles from north to south. It has three major land regions: the Himalayas and associated mountain ranges to the north, the Indus-Ganges-Brahmaputra Plain in the north-central part of India, and the Deccan Plateau in the south.

The climate of India varies according to region. The Himalayas shield the Indian subcontinent from the main body of the Eurasian land mass, resulting in a unique climate. In winter high-pressure winds moving down the Gangetic Plain into the Bay of Bengal result in winters that are generally dry in most of the continent. The Ganges River Valley is noted for summer monsoons and rain, although rainfall may vary considerably. In the Ganges-Brahmaputra Delta and surrounding areas, rainfall may exceed 80 inches a year, whereas in the northeast portions of the Deccan region and along the southeastern coast, the total ranges from 40 to 80 inches. In the areas around the western half of the Deccan region, the annual rainfall is 20 to 40 inches. In the southern half of the country, temperatures are tropical and vary little from month to month. In northern India, however, the annual range is considerable, and in January the average temperature in the north may be 30° F lower than in the south (Simons, 1976).

About 70% of India's working population are engaged in agriculture. Living in small villages, working farms that average 2 acres per family, and using age-old cultivation techniques based on human or animal power, the average Indian farmer lacks efficiency and is seldom able to provide more than bare subsistence for the family. Cultivation potential is further handicapped by lack of water allowing only 50% of the land to be cultivated (McKay, Hill, & Buckler, 1988; Simons, 1976). The Indian constitution prohibits the slaughter of cattle. India has one of the largest livestock populations in the world, yet most of the animals are undernourished and diseased.

India is a democratic republic with a parliamentary system of government. The head of the state is a president who is elected for a 5-year term by the members of the national and state legislatures. Effective executive power is exercised by a prime minister who is normally the leader of the majority political party. Prime ministers have included Jawaharlal Nehru (1889-1964), Nehru's daughter, Indira Gandhi (1966-1984), and Indira's son, Rajiv Gandhi (1984-). Today, some unity seems to exist in India as a result of Rajiv Gandhi's skill in reconciliation of a large majority of the Sikh population, which for years has been fighting for a Sikh national state (McKay, Hill, & Buckler, 1988).

In spite of a large land mass, India is overpopulated. Most of the population, crowded into the Ganges River Valley and the eastern and western coastal regions, are of diverse racial genotypes. The people of India speak approximately 200 different languages, including 630 dialects. In 1981 the population of the Indian subcontinent numbered more than 685 million (United Nations, 1989). The Hindu population is increasing at the rate of 1.8%, or almost 13 million people, each year. In the slums of Calcutta, Bombay, and other large cities, thousands die yearly from malnutrition and disease. Under the pressure of population increases, the economic, political, and social aspects of life are strained (Warshaw, 1988).

Today, the situation in the region is further complicated by the forces of religion and nationalism. The people of the subcontinent are deeply divided by the Hindu and Muslim faiths. Their loyalties are divided between the nation-states of India, Pakistan, and Bangladesh, which share the subcontinent. Indian society is composed of many separate fragments coexisting through mutual tolerance and general agreement on the status and functions of various groups. The regions vary considerably in their historic traditions, cultural patterns, and complement of castes. Within each region contrasts in customs and traditions parallel class and caste differences. Cutting across linguistic and class divisions are the "communities," which are large aggregates of people defined by some common denominator, such as religion, ethnic affiliation or area of origin (Melendy, 1977). Some Indian people believe that there is no need for people in these diverse groups to conform to a single set of practices and beliefs. The underlying unity of the country is derived from the larger arena of cultural traditions shared by most groups and from the dominance of certain national elites.

Hinduism is the title given for convenience to the religion of the vast majority of the population of the Indian subcontinent (Warshaw, 1988). Consequently, approximately 85% of the population are classified as Hindu. Hinduism is a culture as much as it is a religion, and the balance of culture and religion forms the social structure of the Hindu society. Social and religious mores are so predominant that if the Orthodox Hindu were to abandon Hindu belief for another religion, this individual, like the Orthodox Jew, would become an outcast from the people.

Hindus agree on a philosophy rather than a doctrine. Although Hindus built magnificent temples, they developed no church. The priesthood is hereditary and can be achieved only through reincarnation. Of the few beliefs shared by all Hindus, respect for a priest is among the foremost. Hinduism evolved over the last 4000 years and has no single founder or creed; rather, it consists of a vast variety of beliefs and spiritually based health practices and customs. Formal organization is minimal, and a religious hierarchy is nonexistent.

A common belief shared by most Hindus is veneration of life, especially regarding the cow, which is thought to embody fertility. Although rivers, trees, and other forms of life are also regarded as sacred, the cow is considered the holiest life form.

Early Hindus were united in other philosophical respects. The transmigration of the soul represented one essential element of faith. In the backward or forward movement of the soul, there existed an underlying moral responsibility (*dharma,* which may also be translated as law, religion, virtue, morality, or custom). It was dharma that obliged each member of society to maintain the role that was assigned at birth. On the individual level, dharma required the pursuit of Nirvana in ways that were defined by the priests (Warshaw, 1988).

The doctrine of reincarnation, of which transmigration is an integral part, provided a vital link between the religion of Brahmanism and the social order in which it was practiced. The religion claimed a divine mandate to separate people by castes, otherwise known as the *varna* (color) system. At the same time, it suggested to members of the toiling lower castes that they might become reincarnated at a higher level in another life. To attain advancement in the other life, it was believed that the individual must fulfill moral obligations in the present one. Thus the doctrine of reincarnation was an incentive for members of the lower caste to be dutiful. The ultimate bliss of final union with Brahma, although dim and distant, was a realizable goal. While this union might be achieved through correct actions, the nature of action was limited by each caste (Warshaw, 1988).

The relationship between the people's belief concerning etiology of illness and attempts to seek relief from its effects is learned from local folk practitioners. Illness and its treatment are perceived as a biological, as well as a social, phenomenon (Kakar, 1977). Today, enormous amounts of money are allocated to government-operated medical and health programs, yet these programs often fail to attain the desired goals and expectations because of lack of understanding of the integrative nature of the rural culture.

Many health care professionals show little or no recognition of the fact that the health beliefs and practices of Hindus evolved over the centuries and that every cultural trait has direct relevance to the environment. However illogical beliefs concerning the etiology of prevalent diseases appear, they are difficult to dismiss or substitute with Western medical practices. Adequate knowledge about these beliefs can assist nurses in the formulation of nursing diagnoses and nursing interventions, and guard against undue conflicts with the practice of folk medicine.

IMMIGRATION TO THE UNITED STATES AND CANADA
First-Wave Immigrants

The arrival of East Indians from the Indian subcontinent during the first two decades of the twentieth century caused considerable uproar along the Pacific coast of Canada and the United States (Melendy, 1977). Although East Indians immigrated to these countries in very small numbers, their immigration coincided with increasing American and Canadian hostility against the Japanese. Before the nineteenth century, very few Hindu Indians migrated overseas from the Indian subcontinent because most Hindu Indians believed that crossing the "black waters" was dangerous to a Hindu soul. By 1900 the U.S. Census Bureau reported that 2050 East Indian residents had immigrated to the United States. Many of the immigrants in this group were non-Indians who were born in India, some were Indian students, and some were Indian businessmen (Melendy, 1977).

In 1901 East Indian students began arriving in the United States to enroll in various colleges and universities throughout the East Coast area. Many of these students enrolled in such prestigious institutions as Cornell University. It was not until about 1904 or 1905 that East Indian students began to immigrate to the western portion of the United States to enroll in such universities as the University of California and California Polytechical Institute.

Students were not the only immigrants who were included in this first major wave of Hindu Indians. During this period the U.S. ports of entry began to register major increases of East Indian immigrants; from 1904 to 1906, 674 East Indians immigrated as compared with only 9 in 1900. The bulk of East Indian immigrants were unskilled agriculturalists and small entrepreneurs from the arid lands of the Punjab, the United Provinces, Bengal, and Gujarat (Melendy, 1977).

From the onset of the first wave of East Indian immigrants, these people were classified as Hindus (or Hindoos) regardless of their home, culture, or religion. The U.S. Immigration Commission in 1911 mandated that any native of India was to be considered a Hindu for immigration purposes (Divine, 1957; U.S. Immigration Commission, 1911). In 1917 Congress passed, over President Wilson's veto, an immigration restriction act for East Indians. This new law required a literacy test and also encompassed a barred zone for immigration. All Asians who resided in India, Southeast Asia, the Indonesian Islands, New Guinea, or regions of Arabia, Afghanistan, or Siberia were excluded by the new immigration law (Melendy, 1977).

Second-Wave Immigrants

In 1909 Canada closed its doors to East Indian immigrants; however, immigration of East Indians to the United States continued for another 5 years. The Immigration Exclusion Act of 1917, which excluded most persons of East Indian descent, including Hindu Indians, severely curtailed the number of Hindus in the United States. The number of East Indian immigrants residing in the United States began to sharply decline in 1910. In 1910 the U.S. Commission reported that there were some 5000 East Indians residing in the United States, but in 1930 this number was disputed by the U.S. Census Bureau, who reported that there were only 2544 East Indians residing in the United States, with the vast majority of these people residing in California. In 1946 President Harry Truman signed into law a bill that allowed East Indian immigration by virtue of a quota and at the same time allowed naturalization of East Indians. It was this law that is credited with beginning the second wave of migration of East Indian Hindus to the United States.

These new immigrants, who arrived after World War II and before 1965, were mostly made up of professional Hindu people and their families. These immigrants came mostly from the large cities of Bombay and Calcutta.

Third-Wave Immigrants

In 1965 an immigration law was enacted marking the beginning of a third wave of immigrants to the United States. While the first-wave immigrants were primarily agriculturalists, with some students, and the second-wave immigrants were primarily businessmen with their families, this third wave of immigrants from India were entirely different. This new generation of immigrants were very young, with three out of five under 30 years of age and one out of seven less than 10 years old. In 1974 the United States reported that there were approximately 12,777 East Indians residing in the United States (U.S. Immigration and Naturalization Service, 1974).

According to the U.S. Department of Commerce, Bureau of the Census (1988), 387,223 persons of Hindu descent resided in the United States in 1980, approximately 74% of whom were born in a foreign country. Of the number of Hindu Indians residing in the United States in 1980, approximately 15.4% resided in California, 17.5% in New York, 9.7% in Illinois, and 6% in Texas. The median age of East Indian Hindus in 1980 was 30.1 years, and the number of married-couple East Indian Hindu American families represented 91% of that population as compared with 83% for the rest of the U.S. population.

COMMUNICATION
Origins of Hindustani Dialect

Language is a means of communication and disseminates new ideas. It is the storehouse of tradition and literature that provides a people with a sense of pride, self-confidence, and emotional unity. The national elite groups of a culture emphasize the value of a common language as a unifying force and the necessity for the development of language and literature. The study of linguistic heritage is not only an end in itself, but also serves to establish the conditions for nationhood (Pye, 1962).

Hindustani (the name given by Europeans to an Indo-Aryan dialect) owing to political causes, has become the great "lingua franca" of modern India. The name is not employed by natives of India, except as an imitation of the English nomenclature. Hindustani is by origin a Hindi dialect of western India.

It is often said that Hindustani is a mongrel pidgin form of speech comprising contributions from the various languages spoken in a Delhi bazaar. This theory has not been disproved because of the discovery of the fact that the language is the actual living dialect of western India, which has existed for centuries in its present form (Singh, 1966).

Hindustani is the natural language of the people of Delhi. Since the origin of Hindustani began with the people in the Delhi bazaar, it became known as the "bazaar language." From the inception of Hindustani, this language became the lingua franca of the mongrel camp and was transported everywhere in India by the lieutenants of the empire. Several recognized forms of the dialect exist, among which are Dakini, Urdu, Rekhta, and Hindi. Dakini, or "southern," is the form in current use in the south of India and was the first to be employed for literature. It contains many archaic expressions now extinct in the standard dialect. Urdu, "the language of the camp," is the name usually employed for Hindustani by natives and is now the standard form of speech used by Muslims. All the early Hindustani literature was written as poetry, and this literary form of speech was named Rekhta, or "scattered," from the way in which words borrowed from Persia were scattered through it. Hindustani is a name that is now reserved for the dialect used in poetry, with Urdu being the dialect of prose and conversation (Singh, 1966).

Style

The term *Hindi* is ambiguous and the source of much controversy because it is not easily defined. It is considered a regional dialect with a variety of common structural and interchangeable content elements. Its usage is dependent on both the regional affiliation and the social background of the speaker. Hindi is a highly open language closely related to other Indo-Aryan languages; therefore the degree of stylization is determined by the degree of language orientation consciousness in the speaker's mind (Corlett & Moore, 1980).

Hindi encompasses three areas of stylization: high, medium, and low. An individual may shift between high and low stylization according to situational requirements, such as in formal discourse, during conversation with equals, and in giving instructions to subordinates.

Volume and Kinesics

East Indians are generally noted for their soft-spoken manner, almost considered mumbling by some. Frequently, head movements and hand gestures accentuate conversations, adding vitality to the speaker's content. Men maintain direct eye contact with each other when conversing, but women usually draw their eyes downward when addressing their husband, father, or grandfather. This gesture demonstrates a sign of respect.

Touch

Any display of public affection is prohibited and viewed as disrespectful in the eyes of the gods. Married East Indian couples may show signs of affection in the privacy of their own home, but not in view of children or elders. Affectionate touching among friends, relatives, and acquaintances is not a socially acceptable Hindu practice.

Implications for Nursing Care

The use of Hindi among East Indian Hindus is the one culturally unifying trait these people possessed after immigration to the United States or Canada. Reluctantly, East Indian Hindus have recognized the need for adoption of English as a communicative norm in the Western culture. Still, most elderly family members are unwilling to abandon the native language, which is regarded as meaningful to their cultural identity, and find it difficult to learn and communicate in English. On the other hand, younger family members, especially children, easily adapt to the Western culture and are more inclined to incorporate English into their language skills. Whenever possible, translators, as well as younger family members who have a better conceptualization of English, should be utilized by the nurse and other health care personnel when administering care to persons in the East Indian Hindu American population.

When obtaining a health history from an East Indian Hindu American patient or family, both Hindi- and English-speaking family members should be utilized. Because of uncertainty with the English language, the patient may feel frustrated and not communicate conditions thoroughly. When a Hindi-speaking patient becomes frustrated, the patient may first attempt to translate needs by using Hindi; therefore it may be necessary to translate Hindi responses into English. This process preserves the patient's own cultural identity while promoting patient confidence.

It is important for the nurse to remember that it is considered taboo for a man other than the woman's husband to extend his hand toward a woman in greeting. In introducing oneself to the female Hindu patient, the greeting is first addressed to the husband or eldest female companion.

It is also considered taboo for a man other than the woman's husband to initiate or maintain direct eye contact with a woman. This may be perceived by the husband as a seductive gesture. The wife, as a show of respect and out of fear of reprisal, will divert her eyes downward during conversation.

SPACE

In countries that are vastly overpopulated, such as India, the time lag between a decline in the death rate and the acceptance and practice of rational control of fertility presents a serious strain on the economy of the country. India is making positive efforts to reduce the birth rate and thus reduce the phenomenon of overcrowding that currently exists (Moore, 1963). The automobile has been poorly adapted in India because the cities are so physically crowded, and the society has elaborately architecturally designed buildings (Hall, 1966). Most Hindu Americans who come to the United States are surprised to find that internal ornaments such as ceiling fixtures do not fit American houses because the ceilings are too low, the rooms are too small, and privacy from the outside is viewed as inadequate (Hall, 1966).

Most East Indian Hindus have become accustomed to extremely crowded spaces, and therefore the assimilation of these people into the Western culture, where crowding is not the norm, may be difficult. Some East Indian Hindu Americans may perceive that their personal space is greatly overextended and may sense a need to have their personal space collapse inward in order to feel more in control of their environment.

Implications for Nursing Care

East Indian Hindus are a family-oriented people who do not view family as intrusive in personal space parameters. When an East Indian Hindu American patient becomes ill and is hospitalized, the entire family may gather at the bedside. It is important for the nurse to remember that the patient may feel that the space in the hospital is overextended and that the family's presence is essential to collapse the space inward. In this case it is important for the nurse to involve family members in the plan of care and to ascertain which family member will provide personal care. This may possibly eliminate feelings of overcrowding on the part of the nurse and other health care professionals.

SOCIAL ORGANIZATION
Family

In a traditional East Indian Hindu household, married sons live with the family under the parental roof and are subject to parental authority. Frequently the joint family includes approximately 25 individuals, and it is not uncommon for the members to number up to 200. The average joint family is composed of six or seven family members, and the family may comprise several generations. The patriarch controls the finances of the group, giving the sons allowances from their earnings. The matriarch is the autocrat of the home, and her daughters-in-law are subject to her rule. Although this system provides the members of the family with security and sustenance, it has been suggested that it encourages dependence and lack of initiative among many family members (Reddy, 1986). In the past East Indian Hindu girls have wept at the prospect of marriage, not because of objections to little-known bridegrooms, but in fear of their future mothers-in-law (Reddy 1986). The joint family is a powerful social unit, whose pressures on the individual are greater than most Westerners can imagine. It has also been suggested that the East Indian Hindu family demands much sacrifice and devotion and consequently fosters timidity and lassitude on the part of its members (Reddy, 1986).

The hierarchy of the joint family places the father or eldest brother at the highest level. However, the family relies heavily on a democratic system of governance, and decisions of prime importance are determined by a vote in which the heads of the family may be overruled. While the head of the family (the patriarch) is the undisputed overseer of other male members of the household, the matriarch is responsible for the family's female members and is instrumental in determining other domestic concerns. Recent efforts to promote family planning to reduce the burden of the mushrooming population for the most part has resulted in action by women. Indian men appear to reject sterilization for both psychological and religious reasons, fearing it will destroy their male power or will interfere with God's will (McKay, Hill, & Buckler, 1988; Nossiter, 1970).

The East Indian Hindu father is perceived as being distant from his children, who prefer to bond closely with the mother (Kurian & Ghosh, 1983). The eldest son is destined to continue the family name and perform the holy death rites that will ensure peace for his father's soul. It is this expectation that places the eldest son in the position of being one of the closest family members to the patriarch. Throughout his life the eldest son, even when fully mature, rises when his father enters a room or is near him, and greets his father with the *pranam,* the sign of deference in which one touches the feet of a highly respected figure. East Indian Hindus tend to be respectful of authority figures but are more distant with male superiors than with their female counterparts. These people cherish courtesy, which is reflected in the traditional greeting, wherein the head is bowed, the hands are clasped, as if in prayer, and the Hindi word *"namaste"* ("I bow to thee") is uttered softly.

It is the family, above all other institutions, that is responsible for the implantation of social mores and values in the Hindu culture. Ancient traditions that suggest the existence of external rituals are still strictly practiced, and it is the adherence to these ancient traditions that determines whether young East Indians become conservative or rebellious (Warshaw, 1988).

Marriage

In India marriages of Hindu Indians have always been arranged by the parents or other intermediaries. Because marriage was regarded as a union of families rather than of individuals, the marriage traditionally took place when the husband and wife were only children. In 1955 in India, it became illegal to arrange for the marriage of girls under 15 and of boys under 18. Even today, however, this law is not easily enforced, and almost 20% of girls are married before they reach the age of 18.

The long-standing practice of courtship rituals, which is primarily a Western phenomenon, is beginning to gain wide acceptance as traditional arranged marriages are being displaced. Now, only the educated elite in India are able to personally arrange marriages, and these marriages account for less than 10% of the total marriages in India (Warshaw, 1988). Indians have long considered marriage a financial and social arrangement designed to strengthen the position of the whole family, and, traditionally, one of the most important factors determining the choice of a bride has been the size of the dowry, that is, the property a woman brings to her husband at marriage (Warshaw, 1988). In India marriage proposals traditionally have been elicited through a third party who may or may not be a member of the immediate or extended family. In contrast to this, today in the United States, East Indian Hindus frequently place a classified advertisement in their search for a suitable candidate for a prospective bride and groom (Warshaw, 1988).

Position of Women in the Family and in Society

In the past East Indian Hindu women ranked far below men in social status. Marriage became obligatory, since the unmarried woman was thought to have no place in heaven. Traditionally, the belief has been held by East Indian Hindus that the role of a woman is faithfulness and servility to her husband. Since women were deprived of inheritance, a male descendant (and thus the birth of a son) was essential (Reddy, 1986).

Traditionally, the wife had few legal rights and could not publicly contradict or challenge her husband. Mentioning her husband's name in public was also not permitted. This taboo proved particularly confusing when she was required to identify herself for legal purposes (Warshaw, 1988). Among the upper class in the Hindu communities of the northern regions of India and in some areas of southern India, many wives practice *purdah,* meaning "veil." This tradition decrees that in public a wife hides her face behind a veil to ensure that she will be seen only by her husband. This custom is intended to protect her husband's rights over her (Warshaw, 1988).

Mahatma Gandhi was one of the first champions for women's political and social rights in India. In addition, the Women's Indian Association (1917) and the All-India Women's Conference (1927) were organized to unite women in their quest for status attainment through education, social reform, and politics. The association and conference included political picketing and voluntary social work. Although the Indian women's organizations provided tremendous support for the independence movement, it has been reported that they were unable to promote the essential issues related to women's emancipation. It has even been alleged that these organizations were a means of maintaining and gaining status to move into higher echelons of power, and that only upper- and middle-class women benefited from them (Reddy, 1986). Cumulatively, change in the status of women in postindependence Indian society has been moderate and not far-reaching in its influence. For example, the issues of marriage (particularly regarding the remarriage of widows), divorce, and property inheritance all serve to illustrate the inequities still occurring today in India where women are concerned (Mukherjee, 1983; Sinha, 1977).

Caste System in India

For centuries East Indians had divided themselves by caste, by language, and by religion (Spear, 1972). The Hindu population was divided into four *varnas* (colors), which became castes. These segregated castes were the Brahmin, or priestly caste; the Kshatriya, or warrior caste; the Vaisya, or trading and farming caste; and the Sudra, or artisan caste. Approximately 60% of the population held membership in one of these four castes. Outside the caste system, another group of people were referred to as "untouchables." Gandhi renamed the "untouchables" the Harijans, or "children of God." These people were the handlers of slaughtered animals, garbage, and the dead. While the members of the highest caste, the Brahmins, were regarded as pure, Harijans were thought of as polluted and defiled (Spear, 1972). See box on p. 447 for a description of each caste's or noncaste's role in Hindu society.

An individual became a member of a caste at birth, and it was believed that only death could release an individual. It was expected that individuals would not marry outside of the caste. The exception to this rule was when a man took a bride from a lower caste. Work, acquisition of property, and education could not enable an individual from a lower caste to move to a higher caste.

Historically in India, an intricate system of subcastes, known as *jatis,* interlaced with the four main varnas. The members of a jati were closely united by family, village, and region. A jati had more prestige and gained greater rewards for services than did other people. Often the members of a jati would claim to have descended from a common ancestor, whether they had or not, to proclaim kinship with one another. These people shared customs, traditions, and usually a dialect. Based on an occupation or a set of related occupations, the jati did not encourage members to seek social relationships outside of the group. Tailors, sweepers, or moneylenders (some of the

---

CASTE SYSTEM IN INDIA

1. *Brahmins.* The Brahmins were the priests and occupied a position of prestige and influence. These priests performed scholarly pursuits. The distinguishing color of the Brahmins was white.
2. *Kshatriyas.* The Kshatriyas were the warriors, who in ancient times had been the head of society and later were ranked second to the priests. The color of their dress was red to symbolize their work of providing military and political leadership. Warfare was considered a duty of the Kshatriyas, and any hesitancy to fight, even against one's own kin, was considered a violation of the *dharma,* or law, of the caste.
3. *Vaisyas.* The Vaisyas, who made up the largest caste, were involved in commerce. The ritual color of this caste was yellow. The members of this caste had the more mundane tasks of raising cattle, tilling the soil, shopkeeping, and lending money. Although the Vaisyas lacked the social, ritualistic, and political privileges associated with the Brahmins and the Kshatriyas, they ultimately gained great power and wealth as a mercantile order.
4. *Sudras.* The function of the Sudras was to perform menial tasks for the higher groups. Most members of this caste were poor tenant farmers and artisans. The most the Sudras could hope for was that they would be reborn in a higher caste. The ritual color of this lower caste was black.
5. *Untouchables.* Untouchables were not allowed to live within the boundaries of a community or to have access to the village well. They had to perform those duties that were considered unclean, such as tanning leather, cremating the dead, and executing criminals (Spear, 1972).

---

occupations that compromised jatis) did business with one another but maintained a social distance from one another (Spear, 1972).

The caste system was officially abolished by the Indian constitution in 1950 (Warshaw, 1988). Today in most large cities, educated workers and professionals of many castes intermingle. Caste taboos on eating and drinking with others tend to be ignored. Schools, public transportation facilities, restaurants, and apartment houses have been almost entirely desegregated. Caste lines in major cities are so blurred that a person of the merchant caste may be an officer in the army, whereas a person of the military caste may be a prosperous business executive. However, while commercial practices are forcing East Indians to abandon the old castes, family life continues to employ them.

Religion

The Hindu religion may be the oldest religion in the world. There are over 300 million practicing Hindus in India and 254,600 practicing Hindus in the United States and Canada (Boyle & Andrews, 1989). The Hindu religion is polytheistic in the sense that there are numerous gods and goddesses, but there is an overriding sense of a supreme spirit. The origin of Hinduism is based on the Vedas, the sacred written scriptures. In Hinduism the belief is that Brahma is the principle and source of the universe, and the center from which all things proceed and to which all things return. Reincarnation is a central belief in Hinduism. Life is determined by the law of Karma. According to the law of Karma, rebirth is dependent on moral behavior in a previous stage of existence. In Hinduism life on earth is transient and a burden. The goal of existence is liberation from the cycle of rebirth and redeath, and entrance into Nirvana, a state of extinction of passion.

Hinduism is a common part of life for most Hindu Indians. Religious shrines are prevalent within many Hindu households and are located in various parts of the home, based on family preference. Each family has a set of specific gods and goddesses to whom they pray, and by popular account the Hindu pantheon numbers some 33 million gods. The shrines contain statues and pictures of the chosen gods, candles, incense, and offerings of milk, flowers, and fruits. Times for prayer and meditation are reserved for the early morning (after bathing) and early evening, as time permits.

The common Hindu custom of fasting is observed on specific days of the week, depending on which god the individual worships. This practice is predominant among the women of the family, and children are not allowed to participate. Based on the family's degree of compliance to Orthodox Hindu law, fasting rituals may vary from absolute abstinence to consuming only one meal a day. This practice may span over a 1-month period of time or merely be an observance of a holy day.

Impact of Immigration to the United States on Social Organization

The restricted immigration policies that were in place prior to 1965 in the United States created fear for many East Indian Hindu Americans because it appeared that the culture was losing its significance. Prior to 1965 there were so few East Indian Hindus residing in the United States that the few who did chose to remain culturally isolated. Those Hindu Indians who did choose to assimilate believed that there was no free access to the White community and therefore chose to assimilate the Mexican American culture, particularly in light of the fact that there were so few East Indian Hindu women residing in the United States prior to 1965. Some sociologists concluded that the assimilation between East Indians and Mexicans occurred as a result of their similarities in physical characteristics. In addition, some sociologists believe that the East Indian Hindus may have lost their ethnicity entirely in the Mexican subculture, but others regard the fact of intermarriage between East Indian Hindu Americans and Mexican Americans as evidence of mutual acceptance (Melendy, 1977). A classic study concluded that of 50 East Indian Hindu American men interviewed, 26 had wives in the United States, of which 22 were Mexicans. Consequently, the children from these Mexican–East Indian marriages were raised predominantly in the Mexican culture (Dadabhay, 1954).

As a new wave of East Indian Hindu immigrants began to assert themselves in the 1960s, the sagging Hindu culture and traditions were revived and prospered. This was due in part to the fact that after 1965 more East Indian Hindu wives and families began to arrive in the United States, which facilitated a revival of the traditional culture. On arrival this new breed of wives continued to wear saris, the traditional dress, whereas only about 10% of the men continued to wear traditional garb, since many of the men felt the need to conform to the business community in the United States (Wenzel, 1965). Most of the newer immigrants were more adaptable and moved more easily into the American way of life, whereas the older generation remained apart from the mainstream of American society. Although the older group of East Indian Hindus, who continued to live in rural areas, managed to adjust to economic demands, the social acculturation of this group remained significantly behind that of the newer generation of immigrants (Melendy, 1977). Today, some East Indian Hindu wives in the United States continue to practice the application of a colored dot on the forehead as a sign of the husband's well-being and prosperity (Reddy, 1986).

Urbanization, industrialization, and education are major interacting forces disrupting the framework of the joint family system traditionally found in the East Indian Hindu culture and consequently are affecting the East Indian Hindus' family value system in the United States. Education is so highly valued among East Indian Hindus that approximately 80.1% of East Indian Hindu Americans 25 years or older have a high school education as compared with 66% for the rest of the general U.S. population. Of the U.S. population 25 years of age or older, East Indian Hindus have the highest percentage of college graduates, with approximately 68% of Hindu men and 36% of Hindu women age 25 or older obtaining a college education as compared with approximately 20% of men and 13% of women in the rest of the U.S. population (U.S. Department of Commerce, Bureau of the Census, 1988).

Since the third-wave immigration period, East Indian Hindus have integrated into the U.S. labor force, with approximately 65.4% of all East Indian Hindus in the United States working. The median family income for East Indian Hindu Americans is $25,000 as compared with $19,900 for the rest of the general U.S. population. Consequently, the poverty rate of East Indian Hindu Americans is considerably lower than that of the rest of the general U.S. population, with only about 9.9% of East Indian Hindu Americans residing in poverty. In addition, 51% of East Indian Hindu Americans own their own homes, which have an average value of $74,300, as compared with 64% of the general U.S. population owning their own homes, which have an average value of $47,200 (U.S. Department of Commerce, Bureau of the Census, 1988).

An increasing number of young East Indian Hindu Americans are relocating to crowded cities and are living in apartments, and as a result, the joint family system has been rendered impractical. In school and at work, more East Indian Hindu Americans have learned to depend on ability rather than the caste system formerly found in India. The development of individualism among family members has resulted in uncertainty about the need for the elaborate rituals of the past. Some of the values learned from the family are therefore becoming extinct, especially as more young people detach themselves from the traditions that previously controlled them.

Implications for Nursing Care

It is important for the nurse to appreciate that the traditional East Indian Hindu family is the basic unit wherein values, manners, and morals are learned as part of its social structure. The pursuit of individualism, which is so predominant in Western culture, is not the accepted norm. The nurse should appreciate that the father is highly regarded as the head of the family and is the primary spokesman concerning important family matters, including the health care of the individual members. It is unusual for East Indian Hindu Americans to seek medical care outside the confines of the family because of fear that the family will be subjected to public scrutiny by strangers.

The nurse who cares for East Indian Hindu American patients should expect that the wife will usually sit passively by her husband, expecting all questions and inquiries to be directed toward him. He in turn may consult with his wife regarding the health status of other family members. The nurse who ignores the husband and seeks information directly from the wife may precipitate, on the part of the husband, feelings of personal humiliation and disrespect in the eyes of his family. The major objective in developing an effective nurse-patient relationship is to develop trust by gaining the husband's confidence so that the husband no longer views the nurse as an intruder but, instead, as a health care advocate.

TIME

The sense of time is an important concept for East Indian Hindus, who are past, present, and future oriented. East Indian Hindus are perceived as past oriented because of the traditions and rituals that are inherent to the culture. On the other hand, they are perceived as present oriented because of the view that they are "beings-in-becoming" (Klockhohn & Strodtbeck, 1961). Finally, they are perceived as future oriented because life in the present is lived with an emphasis on the hereafter.

At the highest intellectual level, Hindus seek the one reality, whether this is conceived impersonally or theistically. Once they succeed in reaching this reality, they may continue to live in the world, but without emotional attachment to it. They will have passed beyond sorrow and joy, pain and pleasure, and good and evil (Warshaw, 1988). In other words, the present is transcended by concern for the future and future reward.

Hindus, through the cremation of their dead, hope to release the individual's spirit for union with an all-pervading one. The act suggests the existence of a timeless presence in which all Hindus may share. The doctrine of rebirth—that every living being, animal or heavenly, will again be reborn and for all eternity—is a popular Hindu belief. The precise form of each rebirth is determined by the balancing of the being's deeds, good and evil, in previous existences. Escape from the cycle of rebirth constitutes salvation, a state of perfect, blissful, consciousness, which may be gained by acquiring perfect knowledge and performing one's duty flawlessly. Most Hindus aim only to improve their condition in the next existence.

Implications for Nursing Care

Since East Indian Hindu Americans are perceived as being past, present, and future oriented, it is important for the nurse to remember that the patient may place little or no value on some present things, such as being on time for appointments, but may place considerable importance on other present-oriented concepts, such as the spiritual atonement of the self. At the same time, the same patient may place equal importance on past-oriented things, such as traditions and rituals, and on future-oriented concepts, such as the preparation of the soul for the life hereafter.

ENVIRONMENTAL CONTROL

According to Klockhohn and Strodtbeck (1961), it is essential for a people to answer the question of whether or not humans are innately good or bad. In regard to this question, there exists a range of variabilities, including evil, good and evil, and good. Hindus believe that the goodness in the soul of man is recaptured by virtue of the process of reincarnation. In addition, they believe in the man-to-nature orientation, as proposed by Kluckhohn and Strodtbeck, that man is not only subjected to nature but also has a need to live in harmony with nature. Being a past-, present-, and future-oriented cultural group that subscribes to a multiple man-to-nature orientation, some Hindus believe that since man is a mixture of good and evil, there is a need for constant control and discipline of the self if any real goodness is to be achieved.

Hindus are viewed as having both an internal and an external locus of control, meaning that some Hindu people believe that while external forces control destiny, internal forces, such as feeling states or misuse of the body, can also control destiny. For example, Hindu Americans who subscribe to both an internal and external locus of control believe that internal conditions are influenced by psychological factors, such as anger, jealousy, envy, fright, and shame. This belief is supported by the premise that when an individual is unable to control internal conditions that are self-perpetuated, there exists a possibility for susceptibily to disease (Henderson & Primeaux, 1981). The external locus of control is evident in the view that illness is an external event or misfortune, the cause of which may be related to the fault of a family member or the wrath of a disease goddess against the entire family. It is not uncommon for Hindus to believe that malevolent spirits of dead ancestors, sins committed in a previous life, or jealous living relatives are responsible for one's ill health. Such phenomena as "soul loss," "breach of taboo," and "wrath of a goddess" are viewed as symbolic expressions of internal conflict. Hindus believe that people make themselves vulnerable to such calamities through conscious or unconscious transgressions against the ghosts and spirits. Agents empowered by evildoers to precipitate illness are numerous and varied; thus to avert the evil intentions of these demons, Hindus wear charms, make offerings to the saints and their ancestors, and avoid visiting areas in the village where spirits are believed to reside.

Perception of Illness

According to classical East Indian theory, the human body is made up of five natural elements: earth (bones and muscles), water (phlegm or *kapha*), fire (gall or *pitta*), wind (breath or *prana*), and space (in hollow organs) (Boyle & Andrews, 1989). Water, fire, and wind are the three elements that interact in harmony to produce wellness. Illness results from an excess or deficiency of one of these elements, which are also referred to as the *tridosha*, or the "three troubles." *Prana* deals not only with respiration, but also with a pneumatic element circulating in channels, distributing the "humours" and body fluids (bile, blood, and phlegm) throughout the body. In contrast to this view is that held by some other cultural groups, such as Puerto Ricans, that there are four bodily humors (blood, phlegm, black bile, and yellow bile) that must be in a state of balance for the individual to stay at an optimal level of wellness (Harwood, 1971). In addition to giving attention to the five natural elements, East Indian theory also identifies bone, flesh, marrow, fat, chyle, blood, and sperm as seven essential constituents of the body. Although the nomenclature of bones is extensive, the viscera is given less attention in East Indian theory.

A great deal of attention traditionally was devoted to the source of diseases and to hygienic prescription. The intention of medical treatment addressed not only the disease symptomology, but also the diagnosis of causes. For example, the treatment of fever consisted of giving antithermic drugs in addition to prescribing medication against *pitta* or the causative element involved (Dash, 1974).

Hindus believe that praying for health is the lowest form of prayer; it is preferable to be stoic rather than pray for recovery (Peck, 1981).

Folk Medicine

Significance of folk beliefs in the Hindu culture

Today there is growing sense among psychologists, sociologists, and biologists that illness and its treatment are both a biological and a sociological phenomenon (Kakar, 1977). It is thought that there are at least three different types of medical systems practiced at three different cultural levels. On the first level are primitive or preliterate people, who practice a form of primitive medicine based predominantly on a supernatural theory of disease causation. These people are thought to seek treatment through magico-religious means. On the second level are people who belong to the folk culture level and practice folk medicine, which encompasses a theory of illness that involves both supernatural and physical treatments, as well as causations. Finally, on the third level are people who subscribe to a modern theory of treatment and disease causation. At this level people recognize natural rather than supernatural causes of disease. When East Indian medicine is traced back historically, there is a magico-religious mixture of theology. In early East Indian history, disease causation was attributed to gods and goddesses and was explained on the basis of a cause-and-effect relationship with these gods and goddesses or with ghosts and evil spirits. However, Indian folk beliefs have undergone centuries of transition and now include herbal medicines and the Ayurvedic system (Kakar, 1977).

The belief that certain diseases have natural or physical origins does not preclude the simultaneous role of a supernatural antecedent. For example, diarrhea in a child is generally attributed to consumption of a combination of incompatible foods. However, the possibility of someone casting an "evil eye" or "evil mouth" on the child is also recognized (Kakar, 1977).

Another system of beliefs is the Ayurvedic doctrine, which dictates that disease not only has a germ causation, but also occurs because of an imbalance of the essential body elements. *Ayurveda* is a term that is composed of two words: *ayus* and *veda*. The literal translation for the word *ayurveda* is "science of life." A primary concern for East Indian Hindus is knowledge of favorable or unfavorable conditions that assist in the introduction or resistance of the growth of harmful or nonharmful germs. East Indian Hindus believe that there are three fundamental elements in the body—*dosa, dhatus,* and *malas*—which must be in balance if a state of optimal equilibrium is to exist. *Dosa* governs the physiochemical and physiological activities of the body; *dhatu* forms the basic structure of the body cell; and *mala* consists of substances partly utilized in the body and partly excreted in modified form after their physiological function has been completed (Kakar, 1977).

There are many medications that may be prescribed in the Ayurvedic system of medicine. For example, drugs for rejuvenation may be prescribed by an Ayurvedic physician (Dash, 1974). Another example of Ayurvedic medicine is found with the treatment of amebic dysentery, which is caused by the organism *Entamoeba histolytica*. In Ayurvedic medicine the belief is that the organism is not the major etiological cause of the condition; rather, the major cause is attributed to irregularity of diet; intake of heavy, indigestible foods; and emotional factors such as worry, anxiety, and anger (Dash, 1974). As a folk remedy for amebic dysentery, the drug *cyavana prasa* is used, but this drug is considered more a food than a medicine. Two tablespoons of this medication is taken in a glass of milk, and the patient is instructed to avoid salt in excess, as well as sour things. Another part of the treatment includes avoidance of anxiety, worry, and sexual indulgence (Dash, 1974).

Emphasis on the diet of a patient is a unique feature of Ayurvedic medicine. The popular belief is that the patient does not require any medication if he or she has a wholesome diet. According to this belief system, even if errors in diagnosis are made, most of the Ayurvedic herbal medicines will not produce any harmful effect; however if a diagnosis of a disease is correct, these herbal medications will act instantaneously.

Diseases in Ayurvedic medicine are considered to be psychosomatic in origin, involving both the body and the mind. This point is always kept in mind when medicines and regimens are prescribed for the patient (Dash, 1974).

Types of folk practitioners

A majority of East Indians obtain their beliefs in relation to the etiology, prevention, and elimination of illnesses from their families, their parents-in-law (particularly the mother-in-law), elderly women of the neighborhood, indigenous midwives, other folk practitioners, and government health care workers. Usually the decision to seek medical treatment is influenced by factors such as a patient's sex, the economic condition of the family, the family's perception about the etiology of illness, and the family's relationship with the local practitioner (Kakar, 1977).

Therapeutic advice is generally obtained at five different levels: family level, *Mohalla* level, caste level, village level, and beyond the village level (Kakar, 1977):

1. *At the family level,* the mother-in-law, regarded as the family practitioner and well versed in the use of home remedies, is the source of treatment for any illness. Her authority is highly regarded and usually unchallenged in the scope of maternal and child care. Acting as diagnostician and therapist, her healing techniques include such practices as the use of purgatives, massages, and various body-stretching devices.

2. *At the Mohalla level,* there exist two or three highly respected *sianas or sianis* (holy men), who are readily available and consulted only for certain illnesses. Intervention by the *sianas* is decided by the mother-in-law, and it is assumed that the importance of not relinquishing the family's secrets and affairs to the community is understood.

3. *At the caste level,* the intervention by one or two *sianas* is often sought. These practitioners cater to people's needs, especially members of their own caste. They are highly respected members of the caste and recipients of special treatment on socially important occasions.

4. *At the village level,* the faith healer, the most religious member, is a popular practitioner of choice and is employed for his free services regardless of caste or creed.

5. *At beyond the village level,* consultation is sought with a variety of folk and indigenous practitioners, ranging from exorcists to spirit mediums. There have been instances where a simple reassurance of the patient by the spirit medium, without any actual medication, has resulted in instant relief (Kakar, 1977).

Principles of Hygiene

Personal hygiene is extremely important to East Indian Hindus. As part of the religious duty, a bath is required at least once every day. Some Hindus believe that bathing after a meal is injurious and that a cold bath may prevent a blood disease, whereas a hot bath may cause an alterative effect on blood diseases. East Indian Hindus also believe that if the bath is too hot, injuries to the eyes may occur. Hot water may be added to cold water, but cold water is not to be added to hot water when one is preparing a bath. When the bath is completed, the body is to be carefully rubbed dry with a towel and properly dressed (Jee, 1981).

Perception of Death

Death, according to the Hindu belief, is perceived as a passage from one existence to another. From the scriptures and the inspiration of "seers," the Hindu learns that all creatures are in a process of spiritual evolution extending through limitless cycles of time. A person's lifetime is like a bead on a necklace whose other beads represent past and future lifetimes. Each *atman* (basic self) strives through successive rebirths to ascend the scale of merit until—after a life of rectitude, self-control, nonviolence, charity, reverence for all living creatures, and devotion to ritual—it wins liberation from worldly existence to achieve union with Brahma (Chakravarty, 1978).

In India the preparation of the body for cremation involves bathing the remains with a milk and yogurt solution, which symbolically cleanses the soul of the deceased. When a married woman dies, she is attired in a traditional white wedding sari, devoid of make-up or jewelry, the wearing of which is considered a bad omen. A man is attired in a plain off-white East Indian suit. Religious prayers and chanting are continually offered by friends, family members, and priests before and after death to promote safe passage of the soul. Outward displays of grief are accepted practices within the Hindu faith. Open grieving by family, friends, and acquaintances encompasses wailing, crying, and even fainting. Men are as expressive in their grief as women and do not project a stoic demeanor (Chakravarty, 1978). The eldest son of the deceased carries the body to the funeral pyre, and all other children are prohibited from approaching the funeral site. During the cremation ceremony a priest chants prayers while the body is cremated. The ashes are then placed in a container and transported by the eldest son to a designated holy ground and scattered .

Implications for Nursing Care

It is important for the nurse to remember when working with Hindu Americans that there may be a belief that self-control of strong feelings is one of the keys to balancing health or a wellness state. In addition, some Hindu Americans believe in a value orientation that encompasses the belief that man is subjected to nature and at the same time is expected to live in harmony with nature. Because of this belief, it is important for the astute nurse to keep in mind that the patient may believe that illness has a two-fold causation that may include ill favor or overindulgence of self.

Because Hindu Americans have very strict beliefs regarding such things as bathing, it is important for the nurse to remember that a Hindu American may refuse to take a bath after breakfast, which may be a common hospital policy in some institutions. In addition, since some Hindu Americans subscribe to a belief that holds that it is not permissible to add cold water to hot water, if the water is too hot, the nurse should pour the water out and begin the process again rather than risk offending the Hindu patient.

Since some Hindu Americans subscribe to a theory that encompasses the belief that there are three elements in the body that must be in harmony to produce wellness, it is important for the nurse to identify with the patient those beliefs that are beneficial, those that are harmful, and those that are neutral. If the patient has beliefs that are beneficial, it is important for the nurse to identify these beliefs and practices and incorporate them into the plan of care. It is equally important for the nurse to identify those beliefs and practices that are considered neutral, having no effect one way or the other on the outcome of treatment, and that therefore do not need to be eliminated from the daily rituals of the patient. Finally, it is extremely important for the nurse to identify those practices that could be considered harmful and that therefore need to be eliminated from the practices and daily rituals of the patient.

In a study reported by Kakar (1977), 98% of East Indian Hindus in a small village attributed specific diseases to the wrath of God. In this case many of these respondents believed that herbal preparations such as neem tree leaves and twigs were useful in the treatment of these diseases. It was difficult to convince these people that these practices did not alleviate or prevent the conditions. Although a successful vaccination program was launched, it was only successful because of education of the local leaders and folk practitioners. Therefore it is important for the nurse to remember that education of the patient and the family is extremely important in order to develop shared goals about health and wellness.

When a Hindu American patient dies, the nurse should not be surprised by the religious rites following death. For example, the priest may tie a thread around the neck or wrist to signify a blessing, and this thread should not be removed. The nurse should expect that after death a priest will pour water into the mouth of the body and that the family will request to wash the body. Since Hindus are particular about who touches the body after death, it is essential that the nurse communicate respect and provide privacy for the family so that these rites can be carried out (Murray & Huelskoetter, 1987; Potter & Perry, 1989).

BIOLOGICAL VARIATIONS
Variations According to Racial Strain

The modern population of India can be classified into six major racial strains. Two of the six racial groups can be related to a geographic region, whereas the other four groups may be found throughout India. Persons in the upper classes are different in physical type from those in the lower social strata. East Indians can be regarded as a separate racial group occupying an intermediate position between the peoples of Asia on the one hand and those of Europe on the other:

1. *Mediterranean strain.* These people are characterized by a long head, moderate stature, slight build, and dark skin. The face is narrow, the nose is small and moderately broad, and the hair is wavy or curly. These are the dominant features among the Dravidian-speaking people of southern India.

2. *Broad-headed strain.* This section of the population varies in stature from short to medium, and in skin color from light to dark brown. The head is broad and

sometimes high. The nose is prominent, and the hair is straight and usually abundant on the face and body.

3. *Nordic strain.* A distinguishing characteristic of these people is their long head. They are tall, long faced with a straight and narrow nose, and light skinned. This type of strain predominates in the upper castes in northern India.

4. *Mongoloid strain.* The head on these people varies from long to medium, and the skin color varies from light to dark brown. Their stature is medium, and the hair is sparse on the face and body. The face is short with predominant cheekbones, and the eye sockets are slanted, giving a slitlike appearance to the eye.

5. *Negrites.* These people represent earlier inhabitants of India. Their stature is less than 5 feet, and frizzy hair is among the chief distinguishing features.

6. *Prote-Australoids.* This strain is predominant with tribal people of central, western, and southern India. A long head, short stature, broad, short face with strongly marked brow edges and a small, flat nose, and wavy to curly hair are features of the lowest social strata of the population. The skin is dark to black. The strain is so named because of certain resemblances between people of this type and the Australian aborigines (Guha, 1945).

Enzymatic and Genetic Variations

Thalassemia, a genetic condition that can result in various degrees of anemia, is thought to have a high incidence in people from the Mediterranean region, the Middle East, and Southeast Asia. It is thought that thalassemia has a range of variability in occurrence in people of Indian descent (Overfield, 1985). In addition, glucose-6-phosphate dehydrogenase (G-6-PD) deficiency, which is also a condition causing anemia, is thought to have a high occurrence among people in high-risk malarial areas. What is believed to occur in high-risk malarial areas is that the malarial parasite attacks red blood cells that contain the G-6-PD enzyme. In this case cells with the deficiency are less likely to be parasitized, and therefore this lowers the parasite load and consequently lessens the severity of G-6-PD deficiency.

Lactose intolerance is another condition that affects persons of East Indian descent. Lactose intolerance is thought to have a causation that occurs among African and Asian populations because of genetic selection that may lead some groups of people to have adequate levels of intestinal lactase and others to have inadequate levels (Bayless & Rosensweig, 1975; Overfield, 1985). It is thought that while lactose intolerance varies by race, at least 80% to 90% of the world's population become lactose intolerant in adult life with the exception of some Whites (Overfield, 1985).

Susceptibility to Disease

Presently the U.S. data on life expectancies and susceptibility to disease by race do not allow an adequate perspective of all racial groups residing in the United States. The data available on life expectancy suggest that White women in the United States have a life expectancy of 74 years and White men have a life expectancy of 70.5 years, as compared with non-Whites such as Asian Americans and East Indian Americans, who have a lower life expectancy than White Americans but a higher life expectancy than Black Americans, Native American Indians, and American Eskimos (Overfield, 1985). However, statistical data giving empirical support to this contention are limited.

It is thought that susceptibility to heat stress is influenced by such factors as age, race, body build, body fat, climatic experience, and possibly sex (Wagner, 1972). According to Frisancho (1981), there is a possibility that certain races have the ability to withstand heat stress better than other races; however, the racial effect is compounded by climatic exposure. Frisancho (1981) concluded that persons brought up in hot climates, such as that found in India, are better able to tolerate heat than those persons raised in cooler regions, such as certain regions of the United States. In general, it is believed that Blacks, southwestern American Indians, Asian Indians, East Indians, and Australian aborigines have the ability to withstand heat better than their White counterparts (Frisancho, 1981; Riggs & Sargent, 1964). The belief is that these people have lower sweat rates than Whites with similar body temperatures and therefore may possibly have more efficient sweat production (Dill, Yousef, & Nelson, 1983). It is thought that part of the climatic influence on heat tolerance is directly related to the effect of heat on the development of the body during childhood. Eveleth (1966) concluded that children who grow up in hot climates such as the conditions found in India have a tendency to be more slender than their counterparts raised in more temperate areas. In addition, these children also have thinner arms and legs.

Nutritional Preferences and Deficiencies

Most caste Hindus are vegetarians. However, strictness in adherence to the vegetarian diet varies. In most cases the vegetarian diet consists primarily of grains (wheat, rice, millet, and barley), and legumes (grains, beans, and pulses, the edible seeds of plants having pods). In northern and western India baked or fried cakes made with wheat are common. Chapati, a popular form of bread, is a round, flat cake made of whole wheat flour and water and baked on a convex iron plate. Puri is similar to chapati, except for the addition of shortening and being fried in deep fat. Paratha, a third form of bread, is cooked on a convex metal pan.

In eastern and southern India, rice is the staple food. It is usually boiled, but it can be combined with ghee (clarified butter) and spices to become pilau. Corn, barley, and millet are served alone or as supplements to wheat and rice dishes. The primary sources of protein are the grains and pulses, which include channa (chick-pea) and arhar (pigeon pea), which when split and dried is referred to as *dal*. Vegetables include most of the green leafy vegetables, especially spinach, mustard and radish greens, as well as gourds, eggplant, okra, cucumbers, cabbage, turnips, and potatoes.

Most East Indians eat a very light breakfast on rising in the morning, a heavy meal at midday, and a lighter meal between 7 and 9 clock in the evening (Ashraf, 1970). Traditional Hindus, before partaking of the meal, chant the name of their god of preference, as if offering food to him or her before they eat. East Indian Hindu dietary law dictates that the right hand is used for eating, whereas the left hand is used for personal hygiene and toileting.

Psychological Characteristics

Community tolerance for mental illness is high in India, and in many cases personal idiosyncrasies are channeled into occupations or life-styles in which the behavior can be carried out. For example, a marginally schizophrenic Indian person may wander around the country doing odd jobs and living from handouts. Approximately 500 years ago *ambalams* were built throughout India to house travelers. Today, these ancient buildings are used by many persons who wander through India, including the mentally ill, as places to obtain food, beg, get water, and bathe.

For the East Indian Hindu, environment has a significant effect on mental illnesses that may develop (Ali, 1989). For example, because of the strong belief in supernatural forces, when a patient becomes psychotic, delusions and hallucinations are often related to possession by a god, demons, or a witch, rather than to the mind being influenced by equipment being placed or fears that the place is "bugged," which is more often the case in Western societies. An East Indian immigrant to the United States who has difficulty with English and with understanding what is occurring in the environment and who becomes psychotic will often manifest a paranoid reaction rather than one of the other psychotic illnesses. The delusions of the new immigrant frequently relate to the supernatural and reflect the culture of India. However, as East Indian Hindus have become assimilated into the Western culture, the nature of these delusions have changed to more "Western" symptoms.

As mental illness is consistent with the sociological beliefs of the people, the treatment is also sociologically based and must be appropriate for the belief about the cause of the illness, for example, exorcism of a spirit, demon, or god. The most effective exorcism is dramatically performed in a room with others in the family or in front of neighbors and friends (Ali, 1989).

Many drugs that are restricted in the United States are legal in India, such as cocaine, opium, and marijuana. While these drugs are cheap and available, abuse is much less common. Drugs found in the United States as drugs of abuse may be used in India for therapeutic purposes; for example, marijuana leaves in water may be used for a baby's cramps, and opium may be used for diarrhea. While Judeo-Christian beliefs pronouncing drug use as wrong have been present in India since the British entered the continent and to some extent have been adopted by the upper class of people, most East Indian Hindus still retain the value that while drug use may not be "good," it is not "wrong." Indians tend to frown on foreign "hippies" who come to India and support drug habits by stealing. Foreigners who are caught may be deported for such behavior (Ali, 1989).

Implications for Nursing Care

The most crucial aspect for practicing proper nutrition is to make Hindus aware of the advantage of diet in relation to the survival of children. As East Indian Hindu Americans become assimilated into the Western culture, it is important for them to understand the significance of using available foods in a nutritious manner. The nurse must keep in mind that a Hindu person may be reluctant to use Western foods because of sociocultural restrictions. Therefore since dietary considerations are of utmost importance to some Hindu Americans, the astute nurse will involve the nutritionist or dietitian in the development and implementation of a culturally appropriate plan of care. The nurse should also be aware that fasting is an important part of religious practice and that this practice can have consequences for persons on special diets or with diabetes or other diseases related to food (Murray & Huelskoetter, 1987).

Nurses and other health care workers need to know that the joint family continues to be an important characteristic of the East Indian Hindu community and that the authority of the paternal grandmother cannot be ignored because of her important role in decision-making matters related to health and nutrition. In planning culturally relevant nutritional programs for East Indian Hindu Americans, the nurse needs to understand the nutritional patterns in relation to other aspects of the culture and to identify those elements that can be changed without disorganization of the whole cultural scheme. The nurse also needs to explore the beliefs and attitudes of not only the people, but also the authorities from whom these beliefs are derived. It is also important for the nurse to remember that since some East Indian Hindu Americans have a genetic predisposition for G-6-PD deficiency, thalassemia, and lactose intolerance, alternative methods of supplying calcium in the adult diet may be necessary. In this case the nurse may need to teach the patient to supplement calcium by incorporating such food items as buttermilk, yogurt, and sharp cheeses in place of whole milk. Another consideration for the nurse is the theory that people from warmer climates have a more efficient heat production system and thus can tolerate heat better. It is important in this case to teach the patient that overexposure to heat does have profound effects on the body. East Indian Hindu Americans must be taught to recognize the signs and symptoms of heat exhaustion regardless of this biological or climatic adaptation.

Because of the concept that health results from the body's ability to help itself, the traditional East Indian Hindu American may discount Western medical practices while responding positively to traditional folk healing practices. It is important for the nurse to appreciate that these patients may believe that the treatment they receive for an illness is more likely to be effective if both a pill and a solution are prescribed. A physician who is aware of this belief may prescribe both types of medication, since this is what the patient expects will effect a cure (Ali, 1989).

SUMMARY

Nurses who work in a transcultural setting providing health care services to patients of East Indian descent and Hindu affiliation are challenged by the multiplicity of norms, mores, and values, all of which influence and shape the delivery of nursing care. It is essential that the professional nurse and other health care providers use a holistic approach toward the assessment, planning, intervention, and evaluation of nursing care activities.

CASE
STUDY

Vaidya Chuttani is admitted to the hospital with a diagnosis of Cooley's anemia (thalassemia major). Although Vaidya is only 14 years old, she is a student at the local university. Vaidya speaks English, but she is experiencing difficulty communicating her needs to the health care team. Her family, which consists of her mother and father and five brothers and sisters, all reside in Bombay, India. Vaidya has not seen her family or talked with them for the 3 months that she has been enrolled in the American school. She tells the nurse that it is not unusual for some Indian families to allow their children to come to America to study at such a young age. In addition, she relates to the nurse that after she receives her degree, she will return to her country to assist her family by working and contributing to the family's monetary resources.

On admission, Vaidya's presenting complaints include (1) cholelithiasis as revealed on radiographic examination, (2) a right leg ulcer about 1½ inches in diameter, (3) jaundice, and (4) an enlarged spleen as revealed on radiographic examination. The nurse notes the following on examination: blood pressure 140/70, pulse 88, respirations 20, and temperature 99.2° F.

CARE
PLAN

Nursing Diagnosis Communication, impaired verbal, related to recent migration from India and use of English as a second language.

Patient Outcomes	**Nursing Interventions**
1 Patient will be able to communicate basic needs to health care personnel.	1 Use gestures or actions instead of words to communicate information.
2 Patient will relate feelings of acceptance, reduced frustration, and decreased feelings of isolation.	2 Use visual aids that will communicate to patient necessary procedures to be done.
	3 Write down messages in the hope that patient can understand written English better than spoken English.
	4 Obtain a translator, if necessary, to communicate important information.

Nursing Diagnosis Tissue perfusion, altered peripheral, secondary to Cooley's anemia.

Patient Outcomes	**Nursing Interventions**
1 Patient will define peripheral vascular problems in own words.	1 Assess causative and contributing factors of right leg ulceration as related to Cooley's anemia.
2 Patient will identify factors necessary to improve peripheral circulation.	2 Promote factors that will improve arterial blood flow.
3 Patient will verbalize an understanding of medical regimen, diet, and medications.	3 Encourage patient to keep right leg in a dependent position.
4 Patient will verbalize an understanding of activities that promote vasodilation.	4 Encourage patient to change position every hour when in bed.
5 Patient will verbalize an understanding of factors that inhibit circulation.	
6 Patient will communicate existence of pain from right leg ulceration to health care professionals.	

Nursing Diagnosis Health maintenance, altered, related to lack of information about Cooley's anemia (thalassemia major).

Patient Outcomes	**Nursing Interventions**
1 Patient will verbalize desire to learn more about condition and preventive techniques to reduce symptomatology.	1 Identify sociocultural factors that impact health-seeking behaviors.
2 Patient will verbalize a willingness to comply with treatment regimen.	2 Determine present knowledge of illness severity and prognosis.
	3 Determine patient's level and stage of adaptation to present condition (e.g., disbelief, denial, depression).
	4 Using appropriate visual aides, describe necessity for blood transfusions to correct Cooley's anemia.

Nursing Diagnosis Family processes, altered, related to separation from family because of schooling in another country.

Patient Outcomes	*Nursing Interventions*
1 Patient will verbalize fears and anxiety related to separation from family.	1 Determine patient's understanding of present condition.
2 Patient will identify support systems available within school and community, and from external resources that will facilitate return to optimal health.	2 Determine support systems available in school and community and from external outside resources that will facilitate return to optimal functioning.
3 Patient will verbalize desire to be involved in health care and scheduling of patient-centered activities.	3 Involve patient in care and scheduling of patient-centered activities (e.g., wound care for right leg ulceration).

STUDY QUESTIONS

1. List other nursing interventions that can be implemented to facilitate communication between Vaidya and the health care team.
2. Describe the family structure of some East Indian Hindu families and the effect the family organization may have on health-seeking behavior, as well as how this may affect nursing interventions for Vaidya.
3. Describe why Cooley's anemia is perceived as a biological variation for persons of East Indian descent.
4. Identify at least two other biological variations that are common to persons of East Indian descent.
5. Identify how Vaidya's health-seeking behavior may be affected by time and space variables.

REFERENCES

Ali, S. (1989, Nov. 1). Personal communication. (Dr. Ali is former district medical officer in Silon, India.)

Ashraf, K.M. (1970). *Life and conditions of the people of Hindustan*. Delhi, India: Munshiram Manoharial.

Bayless, T.M., & Rosensweig, N.S. (1975). Lactose and milk tolerance: Clinical implications. *New England Journal of Medicine, 292,* 1156.

Boyle, J., & Andrews, M. (1989). *Transcultural concepts in nursing care*. Glenview, Ill.: Scott, Foresman/ Little, Brown College Division.

Chakravarty, A. (1978). Quest for the universal one. In *Great religions of the world*. Washington, D.C.: National Geographic Book Society.

Corlett, W., & Moore, J. (1980). *The Hindu sound*. New York: Bradbury Press.

Dadabhay, Y. (1954). Circuitous assimilation among rural Hindustani in California. *Social Forces, 33,* 141.

Dash, V.B. (1974). *Ayurvedic treatment for common diseases*. Delhi, India: Delhi Diary.

Dill, E., Yousef, M., & Nelson, J. (1983). Volume and composition of hand sweat of White and Black men and women in desert walks. *American Journal of Physical Anthropology, 61*(1), 67-73.

Divine, R. (1957). *American immigration policy, 1924-1952*. New Haven, Conn.: Yale University Press.

Eveleth, P. (1966). The effects of climate on growth. *Annals of the New York Academy of Sciences, 134*(2), 750-759.

Frisancho, A. (1981). *Human adaptation*. Ann Arbor: University of Michigan Press.

Gobal, R. (1966). *Linguistic affairs of India*. Delhi, India: India Publishing House.

Guha, B.S. (1945). *Racial elements in the population of India*. New York: Oxford University Press.

Hall, E. (1966). *The hidden dimension*. New York: Doubleday.

Harwood, A. (1971). The hot-cold theory of disease. *JAMA, 216*(7), 1153-1158.

Henderson, G., & Primeaux, M. (1981). *Transcultural health care*. Reading, Mass: Addison-Wesley.

Jee, H.H. (1981). *Aryan medical science: A short history*. Delhi, India: Maharaja of Gundal (Rare Reprints).

Kakar, D. (1977). *Folk and modern medicine*. New Delhi: New Asian Publishers.

Klockhohn, F., & Strodtbeck, F. (1961). *Variations in value orientations.* Evanston, Ill.: Row, Peterson.

Kurian, G., & Ghosh, R. (1983). Child-rearing in transition in Indian immigration families in Canada. In Overseas Indians: A study in adaptation. *Journal of Comparative Family Studies, 83,* 132-133.

McKay, J., Hill, B., & Buckler, J. (1988). *A history of world societies.* Boston: Houghton Mifflin.

Melendy, H. (1977). *Asians in America.* Boston: G.K. Hall.

Moore, W. (1963). *Man, time and society.* New York: John Wiley & Sons.

Mukherjee, P. (1983). The image of women in Hinduism. *Woman's Studies International Forum, 6,* 375-381.

Murray, R., & Huelskoetter, R. (1986). *Psychiatric nursing.* East Norwalk, Conn.: Appleton & Lange.

Nossiter, B. (1970). *Soft state: A newspaperman's chronicle of India.* New York: Harper & Row.

Overfield, T. (1985). *Biological variation in health and illness.* Reading, Mass.: Addison-Wesley

Peck, M.F. (1981). The therapeutic effect of faith. *Nursing Forum, 22*(2), 153.

Potter, P.A., & Perry, A.G. (1989). *Fundamentals of nursing: Concepts, process, and practice* (2nd ed.). St. Louis: C.V. Mosby.

Pye, L. (1962). *Politics, personality, and nation building: Burma's search for identity.* New Haven, Conn.: Yale University Press.

Reddy, G. (1986). Women's movement: The Indian scene. *The Indian Journal of Social Work, 46*(4), 507-514.

Riggs, S., & Sargent, F. (1964). Physiological regulation in moist heat by young American Negro and White males. *Human Biology, 36*(4), 339-353.

Simons, B. (1976). *The volume library.* Nashville, Tenn.: Southwestern Company.

Singh, B. (1966). *The dialect of Dehli.* South Asia Institute, University of Heidelberg. New Delhi: Lakherwal Press.

Sinha, D. (1977). Ambiguity of role-models and values among youth. *Indian Journal of Social Work, 38,* 241-247.

Spear, P. (1972). *India: A modern history.* Ann Arbor: University of Michigan Press.

United Nations. (1989). *Population and vital statistics report.* New York: Author.

U.S. Department of Commerce, Bureau of the Census. (1988). *We, the Asian and Pacific Islander Americans.* Washington, D.C.: U.S. Government Printing Office.

U.S. Immigration Commission. (1911). *Dictionary of races of people.* 63rd Congress, 3rd Session, pp. 52-54, 75-76.

U.S. Immigration and Naturalization Service. (1974). *Annual report,* pp. 3, 59.

Wagner, J. (1972). Heat intolerance and acclimatization to work in the heat in relation to age. *Journal of Applied Physiology, 33*(5), 616-622.

Warshaw, S. (1988). *India emerges.* Berkeley, Calif.: Diablo Press.

Wenzel, L. (1965). East Indians of Sutter County. *California Living, 17,* 3-15.

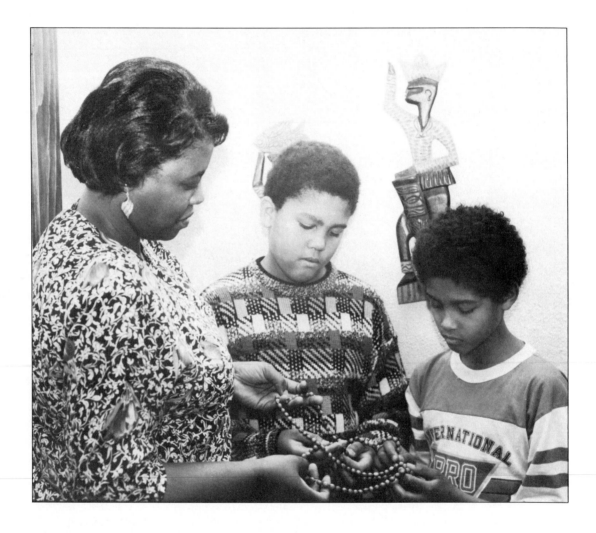

■ ■

CHAPTER 20

Haitian Americans

Robert E. Cosgray

BEHAVIORAL OBJECTIVES
After reading this chapter, the nurse will be able to:

1 Understand the dynamics of employing culturally appropriate nursing care to persons of Haitian descent.

2 Understand the Haitian family structure and the relevance to assimilation of Haitian Americans into the Western culture.

3 Identify diseases that are prominent in persons of Haitian descent.

4 Identify the religious beliefs of the Haitian culture and how they pertain to healing.

5 Understand beliefs related to the postpartum period.

6 Formulate a workable nursing care plan for a Haitian American patient with tuberculosis.

The small republic of Haiti in the West Indies has a colorful but tormented history. To provide appropriate care to Haitian American patients, the nurse needs to have knowledge about the social and political turmoil that Haiti has experienced. In addition, the nurse should be aware of the difficulties that have surrounded migration as Haitians have sought sanctuary from their troubled homeland. It is only through an understanding of Haitian culture and health beliefs that the nurse can adequately meet the needs of Haitian American patients. In addition to discussing the land of Haiti and the immigration process, as well as the impact of the six cultural phenomena on nursing care of Haitian American patients, this chapter explores the struggles Haitians have experienced in their attempts to assimilate cultural traits of the dominant culture in North America.

OVERVIEW OF HAITI
Social History

Columbus discovered the island of Hispaniola on Christmas Eve in 1492 when his flagship, the Santa Maria, ran aground and was wrecked at Cap Haitien, a historic town on Haiti's northern oceanfront. Today, both Haiti and the Dominican Republic are located on what was Hispaniola. As the French moved in to take over this island paradise, the native Indians were either exterminated or removed to Mexican gold mines. Black slaves were imported from Africa as the French became owners of flourishing sugar cane plantations. By 1681 there were 2000 slaves in St. Domingue, the French name for Haiti. A little more than a hundred years later, there were at least 500,000 African slaves and some estimate as many as 700,000, as compared with 40,000 Whites and 28,000 freemen of color—offspring of masters and slaves (Wilentz, 1989). Many slaves were newly imported, since many died of overwork, beatings, disease, and undernourishment. The masters were obviously outnumbered, necessitating harsh measures to keep the slaves in line.

Interestingly, the African religions were seen as a source of resisting the French, and while night ceremonies and dances were often forbidden, they continued and fomented the desire for power and freedom. Legend has it that one night the slaves on half a dozen plantations rose up and burned down their masters' homes, killing their masters. This revolt spread throughout the country, continuing for some 13 years. In 1802 Napoleon's troops landed at Cap Haitien, planning to recapture the island from the slaves and use it as a jumping-off place for an invasion of the United States. However, because of yellow fever epidemics, which assisted the Haitians in killing the French soldiers, the Haitians altered the course of world history, and the French admitted defeat. In 1804 Haiti was freed from France and became the second independent nation in the Western Hemisphere and the first independent Black republic in the world. According to Hobsbawm (1962), the failure of Napoleonic France to recapture Haiti was one of the main reasons why France liquidated its entire remaining American empire, which was sold by the Louisiana Purchase to the United States. Thus a consequence of the revolution in Haiti was to make the United States a continent world power.

Unfortunately, independence from France did not end the misery for the poor in Haiti. Although they were no longer slaves, the poor soon found that the oppressive French rulers had been almost immediately replaced by equally oppressive new Black rulers, the mulattos. With the advantage of money inherited from their French fathers, the mulattos became educated and wealthy and continued to monopolize Haiti's resources with little regard for the social conditions of the poor (Seligman, 1977).

The American occupation, from 1915 to 1934, resulted in reorganization and improvements of the country in regard to its road system, telecommunications, health care system, universities, banking system, etc., but did not effect permanent change. This assistance failed to solve the economic and social problems, and when the majority of Americans left in the 1930s, the country once again regressed.

In addition to the attempt at revitalization by the Americans, François Duvalier, who came to power in 1957 and was the self-proclaimed "president for life," can be credited with initiating comprehensive programs to alleviate economic and technological problems. Unfortunately, Duvalier, preoccupied with wealth and power and the programs that were initiated, failed to have long-lasting effects, and the country's money was squandered. In 1963 Duvalier murdered countless enemies and managed to incur the wrath of Haiti's neighbor, the Dominican Republic, by harboring enemies of its new president. When François Duvalier died in 1971, his son, Jean-Claude, came to power (Wilentz, 1989). In 1980 a sizable portion of the country's financial resources were spent on the wedding of Jean-Claude Duvalier and Michele Bennett, a mulatto whose large family suddenly started to do better socially and economically. Michele Duvalier's lavish spending contributed to her total alienation by the people, and resentment toward the new dictator increased. Eventually, Jean-Claude Duvalier and his wife were forced to flee the country because of massive rioting and murders occurring throughout the country. Today, Haiti continues to be desperately poor, torn by economic insecurity, and revolutions and political turmoil continue (Bordeleau & Kline, 1986).

Life in Haiti

Today, Haiti is an independent republic of more than 4,000,000 inhabitants. Some 92% of the population live in small, rural hamlets. Between 90% and 95% of the Haitian population are descendants of West African slaves. While the issues and problems confronting the people of Haiti are similar to those of many other countries, they seem to be more numerous and more intensified. The country is drastically overpopulated, with 157 inhabitants per kilometer, which is a population increase index of 16.1 per 1000. There also is a high mortality rate among children of less than 4 years of age (250/1000) and a shortened life expectancy of 40 years (*National Catholic Reporter,* 1983).

The average per capita income is less than $75 per year (Bordeleau & Kline, 1986), causing many persons in Haiti to live in straw shacks with no light, water, or windows. Because of the wider range of employment opportunities, women have tended to have more steady employment than men (Racine, 1984).

Haiti has numerous unresolved obstacles to public hygiene, including an inadequate water supply for 88% of the population. In addition, Haiti has an inadequate food supply, resulting in 80% of the population suffering from malnutrition (Wilk, 1986). Health care services are lacking throughout Haiti. A national health service is responsible for the medical care of the population. Most of the 450 physicians are on the government payroll and are disproportionately concentrated in the capital city, Port-au-Prince (1:1,500), as compared with the rural areas (1:75,000) (Bordeleau & Kline, 1986). The lack of available medical care or economic resources to pay for it has contributed to infrequent use of medical care by the general population.

Health care is also provided by private foundations such as the Mellon Foundation, which sponsors the Hospital Albert Schweitzer in central Haiti. To make health care more available to the people, small medical teams go out from this hospital into the rural areas to provide village-based health services. In this program rural farmers, both men and women, are trained in primary health skills and provide direct services to patients. Health service delivered to the natives has resulted in a significant decrease in tetanus, which formerly ranked with tuberculosis and malnutrition as the three major health problems (Grant, 1989; Reichman, 1989; Stauffer, 1989; Westphal, 1989).

Many Haitians, dissatisfied with the Duvalier regime and seeing little chance for improvement in the miserable economic situation, have fled their country in search of freedom and opportunity elsewhere. During recent times of unrest, poor Haitians have given all their money to private entrepreneurs and boarded barely seaworthy crafts for a chance to escape to a better life (Portes & Stepick, 1985).

IMMIGRATION TO THE UNITED STATES

Haitian immigration to the United States has been occurring for many years. In 1975 Haitians could be found in 45 of the 50 states (Seligman, 1977). Large settlements of Haitian people are located in the southern and eastern parts of the United States, with from 75% to 95% presiding in Florida (Boswell, 1982; Wilk, 1986). Cities such as New York (especially Brooklyn) and Montreal have large, established Haitian communities that have mushroomed during times of revolution and political unrest in Haiti. For example, in 1960 there were reported to be 2584 Haitians living in New York City (Rosenwarke, 1972). In 1968 it was estimated that 34,000 Haitians had arrived in the United States during that year, and in 1970 it was estimated that 50,000 Haitians were living in New York city alone (McMorrow, 1970). According to the U.S. Department of Commerce (1980), there were 90,000 registered Haitians in the United States in 1980, with approximately 72% residing in the northeastern area, 21% residing in the southern regions, 4% residing in the north central area, and 2% residing in the western regions of the United States. This census figure may be underrepresented because of the number of illegal aliens from Haiti.

Most of the immigrating Haitians in the early years were upper-class individuals who come to the United States as resident aliens. These upper-class Haitians were able to obtain permanent residence and citizenship with little difficulty and became assimilated into the dominant culture.

In 1980 an explosion of Haitian immigration took place as a result of a short-lived (April to October 1980) change in the U.S. immigration policy. More than 14,000 Haitian refugees landed on the shores of southern Florida during 1980 (Dempsey & Gesse, 1983). This was the period of the Mariel boatlift from Cuba, and the influx of Cuban refugees required that a special status be created by the State Department, called "Cuban-Haitian entrant, status pending." Haitian refugees were included in this status to prevent the policy from being discriminatory (Metropolitan Dade County, 1981; Walsh, 1980). The "entrant" status described a temporary status and was used rather than granting the new arrivals political asylum. However, this "entrant" status placed the Haitian immigrants in a bureaucratic limbo that cannot lead to citizenship (Wilk, 1986).

In October of 1980 the immigration policies changed. A maritime interdiction program was initiated to turn back Haitian refugees at sea. Haitians who arrived in the United States were not classified as entrants but as parolees and were subject to deportation. Haitians were kept in detention along with Cubans, where their cases were processed in the courts. Unlike other refugees arriving at the time (such as Indochinese refugees), resettlement was not guided by the federal government. The federal government's refusal to grant asylum deprived the refugees of benefits under the new 1980 Refugee Act. Emergency aid was limited, and most of it had lapsed by 1983. Lacking either jobs or government assistance, many refugees were compelled to rely on private charity and to invent jobs in a burgeoning "informal" economy in Miami.

These waves of immigrants have resulted in four classifications or categories of Haitians now present in the United States: (1) citizens, (2) residents or legal aliens, (3) entrants, and (4) illegal aliens. Illegal aliens have all the pressures and fears of discovery, which could result in sudden deportation. Entrants, on the other hand, suffer from the uncertainty of whether they will be able to remain and from being unable to make permanent plans or feel entirely settled (Wilk, 1986). Since possibly half of the Haitians in the United States are here illegally, this may account for the lack of programs available to provide assistance. Some Haitians are understandably reluctant to discuss their difficulty and attempt to maintain a low profile with government agencies that might return them to Haiti. Another effect of an uncertain status in North America is infrequent use of health care services after migration. The nurse should be aware that the Haitian immigrant probably will not seek medical treatment until the condition is severe or has become chronic (Bryan, 1988).

In spite of these difficulties and the possibility of deportation, many, primarily poor, Haitians continue to try to enter the United States. Those who do make it to North America are in one of the most at-risk populations now living in the United States. This high risk becomes actualized in a number of ways; for example, a study by Moskowitz et al. (1983) reports unusual cases of death among Haitians residing in Miami and a high prevalence of opportunistic infections. It is important for the nurse to expect, when caring for a Haitian patient, that the patient may never have had immunizations. If a patient is in need of a tetanus immunization, it is unlikely that a tetanus booster is appropriate, since the patient more than likely has not received the series.

Adaptation of post-1980 Haitians to the dominant culture in the United States and Canada has been especially problematic, since the proportion of refugees having a high school or college education and skills in English has declined. With limited education and money, many Haitians arriving in North America have been restricted to occupations such as migrant agricultural work and service industry jobs in restaurants and hotels. Only a few of the more educated Haitians have been able to find work as mechanics and construction workers. Gaining the requirements needed to adjust to the urban, industrialized culture encountered in the United States and Canada is for most Haitians a stressful, overwhelming, and slow process because the people continue to cling to their cultural values and beliefs.

COMMUNICATION

Issues related to communication present a variety of problems for Haitians living in the United States or Canada. In Haiti there are two official languages: Creole and French. French is the official national language and is understood and spoken only by the upper or wealthy class. Although Creole is the language of the rural or poor population, it is also the primary language and is understood and spoken throughout the country (Weil, 1973). Speaking only Creole, a hybrid of old French vocabulary and African grammar, is perceived as a sign of poverty and a lack of education. Both Creole and French are often spoken so fast that one word is slurred into another. Because many Haitian immigrants in the United States continue to combine Creole and French, a dialect termed *creolization* has been created, which creates language barriers for some Haitian immigrants, since most people in the dominant U.S. society are not familiar with it.

Haitians frequently use hand gesturing to complement their speech. Hand gesturing, as well as the tone of voice, becomes more pronounced during the course of communication. Primarily, hand gesturing is used as an addition to verbalizations. Touch and direct eye contact are also used in both casual and formal conversation. The Haitians' use of touch in conversation is perceived as friendship and does not violate personal space. Direct eye contact is used to gain the attention and respect of the other person during conversation. The Haitian cultural uses of touch and direct eye contact, and the perception of friendship through conversation, are much like those used throughout America.

Implications for Nursing Care

Language is often an area where problems arise between refugees and providers of health care. One reason Haitians have received limited health care in the United States is because of the failure of many Haitians to speak either of the dominant languages: English or Spanish. Many schools in the United States have extensive bilingual programs for native Spanish speakers but have paid little attention to other non-English speakers. The problem of providing bilingual education for Haitians is complex and begins with a lack of materials for teaching English to Creole speakers. There are also varying opinions on the best way to teach literacy skills. Some persons believe that Haitians who have immigrated to the United States must be taught literacy in their native language. The view is that if Creole is used as a teaching tool, it can facilitate acquisition of reading and writing skills in English (Dejean, 1983).

The nurse should promote the Haitian American patient's interest in gaining English language skills to facilitate the patient's adjustment to the dominant culture. While most Haitians are eager to learn English, learning to read and write as an adult is often difficult and time consuming, and support from health care professionals can encourage the Haitian individual to stick with this difficult task. Many Haitians who use French as their primary language have retained it, even though they have made a permanent move to the United States or Canada. Although many in the United States and Canada share the French-speaking Haitian's view that French is the language of the culturally elite, it should be noted that French-speaking Haitians have as much difficulty learning English as do any other non-English speakers.

If the patient does not speak English, the nurse should first determine what language the patient does speak. If the nurse does not know Creole or French, an interpreter may be necessary. When possible, a bilingual family member can help convey to the patient and nurse information essential to health care. The nurse may find that Haitian Americans with children are more likely to speak correct English, since speaking correct English is a status symbol and parents who know English will usually role model correct English in the home. The nurse caring for a Haitian American patient should be aware that Haitians value a touch or a smile by the nurse as a sign of friendship. Nonverbal communication can assist in bridging gaps between the differences in language because it can facilitate an understanding of patient needs.

SPACE

Personal space to the Haitian can be defined as a public zone. Haitians as a cultural group are a sharing population. If they possess something that another person could or might benefit from, it will be shared. Another factor that tends to make the culture a public zone is the closeness of the living arrangements or dwellings. As a result, the Haitians are a public-oriented society. Haitians in the United States, for the most part, usually socialize with other immigrants arriving from their own town in Haiti and maintain primary loyalty to family members, many of whom remain in Haiti. Legal immigrants look forward to spending holidays in Haiti and regard the allowed time each year as a focal point. Illegal aliens are more isolated because they cannot maintain family contact. This represents a great change from the life-style led in Haiti, where extended family and the closeness of the community are emphasized.

Implications for Nursing Care

It is important for the nurse caring for a Haitian American patient to know that studies have shown that Haitians find touch by caregivers to be supportive, comforting, and reassuring (Dempsey & Gesse, 1983). In a study of ten women, Dempsey and Geese noted that there were diverse views on whether or not these women preferred to be touched during delivery and if the preference was for a man or woman to touch them. In the study two women specified a preference for being touched by a woman, three preferred to be touched by a man, and three did not have a preference. Nine stated that the father should be present. What is implied by this is that Haitian women may be less likely than women from some cultural groups to insist on having female nurses in the delivery room.

Although Haitians and African Americans share a heritage that extends back to Africa, the two groups do very little social mixing and tend to mistrust each other (Dempsey & Geese, 1983). It is important for the nurse to understand that just because two patients may be Black does not mean they will share common interests or find each other suitable companions for sharing a hospital room. Some Haitians, like some other people from other social groups, are not free of social prejudice. Appreciation of these cultural socioeconomic issues by the nurse will facilitate assignment of staff to care for Haitian patients as well as room assignments of patients.

Because of the large gap in classes, it is important for the nurse to consider also the economic background of patients before placing them in an area together. For example, a poor patient and a wealthy patient with a Haitian background, while being from the same country, may find a room assignment together in a hospital very distasteful.

SOCIAL ORGANIZATION
Social Class

The Haitian masses are essentially divided into two class structures: the wealthy and the poor. Statistically, 85% of the Haitian population are classified as poor, 10% are classified as middle class, and 5% are classified as wealthy (Bell, 1981). Class is demonstrated in many interesting ways. Wearing shoes is a requirement by law in the capital city, but many others, especially in the small towns and villages, go barefooted. This is by no means a matter of choice but a mark of social standing. As an illustration of this, a Haitian physician who was enjoying a little recreation in one of the small towns was told that a patient was waiting for him nearby. The physician asked if the patient had shoes on. What was implied in this question was that if the patient had shoes on, the physician would be obliged to go immediately. On the other hand, if the patient did not, the patient would be in for a wait (Jeanty, 1989). Regardless of class, Haitians are a proud and independent people. Although Haitians reside in one of the most densely populated countries in the world, and suffer and tolerate the effects of intense poverty, they are proud that they are economically independent from the rest of the world.

Education

Education in Haitian schools differs greatly from that in American schools. Until 1979 the only officially recognized language, and the language that was required to be used in school, was French. The educational system and schools are strict and authoritarian. Children who are financially able to attend must wear starched uniforms. The Haitian teacher has the right to use corporal punishment on a misbehaving child. Thus the lack of structure and discipline of many American schools meets with disapproval from Haitians. Much of the information given to students in the Haitian schools is memorized; memorization through repetition is the primary source of learning. Haitian children can be heard reciting multiplication tables through rhyme and song throughout the community. Sheer repetition of the same formula, problem after problem written on the blackboard, manages to register the information in the student's mind. Haitian teachers enunciate clearly when communicating with their students (Verdet, 1985).

Haitian immigrants in the United States, rather than attend the public high schools, prefer to remain out of the mainstream of education and often strive to accelerate the educational process and obtain the credentials they value by seeking a high school equivalency diploma. Haitian immigrants in the United States view a college education as a form of prestige and status.

Family

The commonality among Haitians in Haiti and Haitian immigrants in the United States, whether wealthy or poor, is family. The family structure or system is very different from the American system. The practice of common-law marriage is predominant, particularly among the poor. Most legal marriages occur among the wealthy as a result of their economic status. Common-law marriage gives the father of the family much freedom and imposes much of the responsibility of caring for and meeting the needs of the family unit on the mother. The father, perhaps dividing his time between several family units, becomes a powerful but unreliable figure. The concept of a single-parent family, primarily the single mother, is similar to that in the United States but is more prevalent in Haiti. The Haitian mother is commonly left to raise the children without the support system of the father.

The term *placage* may be defined as the union of a man and woman who desire to live together and who fulfill certain obligations and perform certain ceremonies at the home of the woman's parents, after which a new household is established. These unions are said to endure as long as recognized church marriages and constitute two thirds of all unions in Haiti (Herskovits, 1971; Schaedel, 1962).

Haitian women involved in *placage* can be classified into four groups according to their relationship with Haitian men:

1. *Femme caille* (common-law): a woman who shares her home with a man in a common-law marriage situation.

2. *Mama petite* ("mother of my children"): a woman who is the mother of some of the man's children but who does not share his house. This is similar to some *placage* unions with children, but in this situation the husband continues to live with his first wife while maintaining the second relationship.

3. *Femme placage* (woman whom a man "goes with" or a friend): a woman who neither lives with nor has had children by a man but who shares his bed intermittently and often maintains a garden, usually furnished by him.

4. *Femme avec* (woman who is lived with): a woman with whom the man cohabits for pleasure and without firm economic ties (Williams, Murthy, & Berggren, 1975).

Affection from both parents is readily given to children, while at the same time physical punishment is given as a form of discipline. Haitian mothers rely less on parent-child dialogue and more on physical punishment to effect changes in the child's behavior and to instill proper attitudes and values (Charles, 1979). Although Haitian mothers are extremely affectionate with their children, the children are taught from infancy that there is an unquestioned obedience to adult wishes. Haitian children do not presume to question parents or seek information concerning matters such as sex education, since this would be seen as disrespectful of adult authority (Bestman, 1979). Child rearing is shared by siblings, as well as by the parents.

The Haitian family is traditionally extended, with each dwelling or residence paralleling a small community. Outside of the extended family, godparents play a very important role in the family organization and are generally considered part of the natural family. Rural or poor families tend to be matriarchal and child centered, with parents exercising a strong influence and authority over their offspring, even when the children are grown. Haitians view their children as direct reflections of themselves and the family. If children fail to fulfill obligations or meet expectations, they are seen as having failed the family and as having brought disgrace on the parents (DeSantis & Thomas, 1987). Because of the parent-child ties, many Haitian couples separate only temporarily when immigrating. The wife usually immigrates with the younger children, and the husband remains in Haiti with the older children until the entire family can obtain authorization to relocate. One-parent families, then, are quite common among this immigrant group in the United States.

Haitian parents have a strong voice in their children's selection of a mate, as well as in their choice of a career. Haitians tend to be an extremely status conscious group and desire marriages or careers that enhance the status of the family. For most Haitian immigrants in the United States, home ties to Haiti remain strong. Even though there may be little opportunity for travel back and forth because of cost, and the illegal status of many, ties to the mother—and home—remain. Letters, packages, and money are sent regularly. Since many Haitians are illiterate, sending cassettes to relatives in the United States or home to Haiti is a common form of communication (Jeanty, 1989).

Implications for Nursing Care

Cultural factors related to social organization have an important impact on health and health care behavior. Fundamental norms, such as the desirability of having many children, and the traditional roles of men and women affect reproductive behavior. Since the legal status of many is either questionable, as for entrants, or undesirable, as for illegal aliens, Haitians frequently use different names, giving one name at one clinic and another name at another clinic. In addition to causing confusion to health care providers, this practice leads to people "falling through the cracks" because of records not being available. Consequently, there is a loss in continuity of care for some Haitian patients. In addition, because of the repeated intake procedures on the same patient, health care services may be delayed (Wilk, 1986).

An astute nurse will keep in mind that since the Haitian family is traditionally extended, the opinions and ideas of the family must be incorporated into a culturally sensitive plan of care. It is also important to remember that since Haitian children are taught from infancy to be unquestionably obedient to adult wishes, it is especially important to provide parents with adequate health education if children are to benefit from improved and knowledgeable health care.

TIME

Some Haitians in Haiti and Haitian immigrants to the United States are present time oriented, since they find it necessary to live from day to day, looking for food and trying to sustain a meager living. Because of their economic and educational status, the future for some of these people remains bleak. Thus it is unlikely that they will develop a future time orientation, since there is little to no chance of getting ahead without money, status, or a job.

On the other hand, wealthy Haitians in Haiti or Haitian immigrants may perceive time from a totally different perspective. For these people time orientation may be a combination of both present and future orientations. It would appear that as a result of adequate financial resources, upper-class Haitians and Haitian immigrants do make plans for the future. Because wealth may ensure educational attainment, which may translate into status and prestige, it is likely that a well-educated upper-class Haitian may have a future time orientation.

Implications for Nursing Care

Since Haitians may have different orientations to time, depending on their social status and class, it is important for the nurse to adequately assess each individual patient. It is also important for the nurse to remember that personal ethnocentric attitudes toward time may negatively affect the planning of care for patients. Persons with a present time orientation may view future-oriented tasks as irrelevant or unimportant to present situations. Thus a present time orientation may restrain a Haitian from gaining upward mobility, since future orientation is required in gaining an education and planning to achieve future goals. It is also important to remember that when a Haitian immigrant does not keep an appointment or does not arrive for a clinic appointment on time, it may be a result of a present time orientation but may also be because of economic constraints. It is important for the nurse to assess not only the time variable, but also other socioeconomic variables, including the availability of transportation to and from clinic appointments.

ENVIRONMENTAL CONTROL

Although Haitians and African Americans share a lineage that extends back to Africans who were seized from their countries and enslaved, some individuals have surmised that these two cultural groups fraternize very little socially and tend to mistrust and be suspicious of each other (Wilentz, 1989). It is thought that Haitians place a high value on personal liberty and therefore are resentful and at times indignant of American prejudice and critical of American Blacks, whom they discern as being too submissive and accepting of discrimination (Wilentz, 1989). At the same time, Black militancy and violent protest seem to be contrary to the Haitian personality and are generally regarded by Haitians with disapproval (Wilentz, 1989).

Traditionally, the upper classes in Haiti have been the lighter-skinned Blacks, whose skin color is due to crossbreeding with other, lighter-skinned people. Light skin traditionally has been regarded as more prestigious than dark skin in Haiti (Leyburn 1955), with the upper-class, lighter-skinned Haitians dealing with the darker-skinned persons in the lower class in an authoritarian manner. Therefore because of indoctrination regarding the color of the skin and its perceived relationship to social status or class, some Haitians have developed social prejudice that causes difficulty in the assimilation process in the United States. As a result of social prejudice formed by such variables as color grading and social status, some Haitians living in the United States or Canada continue to have trouble adjusting to other groups and thereby choose to remain in isolated areas, socializing only with other Haitians and family members.

Voodoo Practices

The practice of voodoo, the primary religion in Haiti, is prevalent throughout the country. Voodoo is a religious cult practice that dates back to the preslavery days of Africa. Christianity, particularly Catholicism, is becoming more prevalent but is slow to emerge because of the deep-seated roots of the voodoo culture and conviction. From their West African homelands, Haitians brought the belief that man is surrounded or enveloped by a variety of powerful, dominant spirits. Some Haitians believe it is essential to invoke spirits. In the Haitian culture the invoked spirits are called *loas, mysteres,* or saints. Some Haitians believe that voodoo spirits manifest and reveal themselves by possessing or "riding" the devoted believer. It is thought that the personality of the *loa* "mount" may change; he or she may be calm and subdued one minute and then suddenly become violent. Such transformations may be due primarily to nervous instability under the influence of compelling drum rhythms and mass emotion (Logan, 1975). Haitians trust and depend on their voodoo beliefs and also rely on "readers" or "diviners," who predict the future by reading cards or hands, and cure by means of being possessed by the voodoo spirit. The readers or diviners, also considered voodoo priests, are organized into independent cults.

Voodoo priests may be either male *(hungan)* or female *(mambo),* and there are five classes of such healers or priests that can be identified: shaman (voodoo practitioner), herbalist (*docte fey,* literally "leaf doctor"), midwife (*matronn* or *fam saj*), bone-setter *(docte zo),* and injectionist *(pikirist).* Healers are often not well defined, and a Haitian may go to a neighbor who has "extra" medicine or a healing practice in hopes of relief. In terms of the number of practitioners and frequency of use, the herbalists constitute the most significant class of healers. Herbalists are the most generalized car-egivers, and thus their role characteristics overlap to a certain extent with all other healer types (Coreil, 1983). Haitians often use home remedies and herbs for treating illnesses that are suggested by healers or priests. Many Haitians think that tea made from leaves of the Bible will cure rheumatism. In this case, the Bible serves as protection against black magic, which is thought to cause rheumatism (Nida, 1954).

Magic powers may be employed for purposes other than destroying enemies or healing the sick. The voodoo sorcerers of Haiti claim to be able to change themselves into animals, to pass through locked doors, and to raise the dead and make them slaves (zombies). Almost everyone who is a native Haitian claims to know someone who has been a genuine zombi. One man requested his family to cut his corpse into two pieces to be buried in separate graves for fear that the local sorcerer, who was his enemy, would bring him to life as a wretched slave. While the Haitian government has no valid evidence of the existence of zombies, it sanctioned the belief by passing a law against the supposed practice (Nida, 1954).

In Haiti voodoo is sometimes actualized as fetishes, which are shared by groups of native Haitians. For example, a Haitian might have a small bottle containing some reddish liquid and a small mirror backed by cardboard facing the bottle, and all this wrapped in coarse red cloth with yards of black thread. This object is safeguarded in the most remote part of the house, with its location kept secret from visitors. If the Haitian could be induced to talk about this, he might explain that his father, who was a kind of voodoo priest, captured his soul when he was very young and put it in the bottle. As long as the bottle is preserved, the person will live, but once the bottle is broken, the soul will depart and the man must die. Not only would this fetish be held by this individual, but identical or similar fetishes might be shared by others in the community (Nida, 1954).

Many Haitian influences regarding voodoo practices are evident in the main-stream of American society. For example, in some cities and towns in Louisiana, the Haitian influence is extremely prevalent and is perceived or felt by persons from other cultural groups as well. Louisiana is renowned for its voodoo society, which is a car-ryover from Haitian slaves who were brought to areas such as New Orleans for various domestic duties. Even today, because of early Haitian influence, voodoo and mys-tical thought remain evident regardless of ethnic or cultural background in cities such as New Orleans (Snow, 1981).

Childbearing Beliefs

While health care is a significant problem in urban Haiti, it is even more of a problem in rural Haiti, with pregnant and postpartum women being particularly vul-nerable (Wiese, 1976). Many Haitians know nothing about prenatal care and do not routinely seek such care. Some may never have seen or been to a physician in their life. Healers are related to protection, and physicians are related to sickness. Use of a midwife is culturally permissible and is much more likely among Haitian people. When a nurse is interacting with a pregnant Haitian woman or is providing care for a baby, using the phrase "We will help you have a strong baby" will often elicit cooperation. Staff who are willing to help the mother have a "strong baby" (rather than a "healthy" baby") are more likely to be accepted (Jeanty, 1989).

Pregnant women are viewed as special and are likely to be treated with more kindness and respect than nonpregnant women. Chants or sounds of a woman in labor include praying, singing, crying, and moaning in various combinations. This is done to call on their voodoo protectors (Dempsey & Geese, 1983).

A study conducted by Scott in 1974 identified the postpartum period as the most crucial and decisive period of childbearing for the Haitian woman. During the postpartum period of 6 to 11 weeks, the Haitian woman follows a cultural regimen of baths, teas, vapor baths, and dressing warmly. This practice is supposed to make the patient healthy and clean again after the birth. For the first 3 days the mother bathes in hot water in which herb leaves have been boiled. She also drinks tea made from boiled herb leaves. (Also during the first few days after childbirth, the mother takes "vapor baths." She sits above a pot of steaming water with leaves in it, especially orange tree leaves, and drapes a cloth over her head and shoulders.) For the next 3 consecutive days the mother takes her second series of baths, which are prepared with leaves in water warmed by the sun. At this point the mother drinks only water warmed by the sun or tea made with leaves steeped in water warmed by the sun. The mother takes constant special care to keep her body warm. She stays inside her dwelling for at least 3 days after the birth and keeps the doors and windows closed to keep out the cool air. She wears long sleeves, keeps her head covered, and wears heavy socks and shoes.

After 2 weeks to a month, the mother takes another bath. She may take a cold bath or perhaps jump into an cold stream. After this ritual, she may self-induce vomiting to cleanse her inner body. After all of this is completed, she can again resume normal activities and is considered clean (Harris, 1987).

The Miami Health Ecology Project (Scott, 1978) reported beliefs about menstruation among Haitians, a majority of whom believed the function of menstruation to be that of ridding the body of "unclean," "waste," or "unnecessary" blood. Many Haitians also described menstruation as "it means you are a woman," "woman" meaning that the individual has sexual feelings or needs and is not sterile. The Haitian girl reportedly learns about menstruation at a median age of 10 years. For 85% of the sample, this information was obtained from their mothers or in classes at school.

Implications for Nursing Care

It is important for the nurse to understand that for many Haitians leaves have a special significance. When the patient comes into the hospital or the clinic for an examination, leaves may be found in the clothes and on various parts of the body. Leaves are thought to have mystical power, and therefore keeping them close to the body is related to regaining or keeping health (Jeanty, 1989). The nurse should be accepting of this practice and avoid being shocked if leaves are found in the luggage or on the body of a patient being treated. If Haitian Americans do use conventional means of health care, they tend to use emergency rooms or clinics (Orque, Bloch, & Monrroy, 1983). Haitian Americans may also seek relief from their symptoms through a physician and at the same time consult a cultural healer. The patient's having both a faith healer and a physician should not be perceived as incongruent

(Jeanty, 1989). A patient's fear and anxiety that he or she has been "hexed" may be alleviated or reduced by combining conventional treatment with the assistance of a cultural healer who is believed to be able to remove the hex or spell. Nurses, as primary health care providers, must formulate and use a treatment plan that displays respect and understanding of the patient's cultural healing system or systems and accept that a Haitian American patient may use a variety of sources to obtain relief when sick.

Haitians have grown accustomed to receiving some direction from authority figures in their lives—parents as well as religious and social leaders. The nurse, as an authority figure, will usually find that Haitian Americans respond well to counseling approaches that foster self-help and independence and should take into account the need for heightened self-esteem, which is manifested by the pride and willingness to work that is present in most Haitians.

Haitian Americans need to have occupational options expanded for them and need to understand the steps involved in achieving an occupational goal. Since Haitians have not traditionally had the freedom to set goals, the nurse may be of assistance in goal setting, as well as problem solving, to achieve the goals that are established.

BIOLOGICAL VARIATIONS
Body Size and Structure, Skin Color, and Other Visible Physical Characteristics

Haitians and African Americans are similar biologically. As with some other racial groups, the body size and structure of Haitians vary greatly. Haitians have no specific or distinctive size that can be linked genetically. This phenomenon may be due to crossbreeding with other races throughout history. For this reason, Haitians can be short or tall, and light skinned or dark skinned. Haitians are characterized as having shades of brown to black skin, as well as brown to black eye color. The hair on the head is often tightly curled, and the body hair is sparsely distributed. The "true" Haitian is tall and exhibits an erect stature. The skull is infantile in form, being long and relatively narrow. The eyebrow ridges are scant or absent, and the forehead is moderately wide. The form of the orbits is almost square, and their margins are strongly built. The cheeks are wide and, with their supports or zygomatic arches, are bowed laterally in keeping with the powerful jaw musculature. The eyes are set widely apart by the broad and flattened nasal bones. The nose is flat, and the nostrils are widely expanded. The face is large and prominent. The jaws are prognathic and are covered by full, fleshy lips, whose prominent mucosa is reddish black or purple in color (Godsby, 1971).

Some years ago, anthropologists and scientists discovered that two different types of ear wax are present among the human race, and that the composition of the ear wax determines racial origin. Haitian ear wax is described as moist and adhesive (Godsby, 1971).

Susceptibility to Disease and Other Health Concerns

Several major areas of health concerns have been identified in the Haitian culture, including intestinal problems and/or malNutrition, venereal disease, a high birth rate, tuberculosis, and sickle cell anemia (Wilk, 1986). Acquired immunodeficiency syndrome (AIDS) has also become a health issue since the 1970s.

Intestinal problems and/or malnutrition

Intestinal problems stemming from malnutrition and ranging from stomach ailments to peptic ulcers are common. The peasant Haitian suffers more from these types of ailments than does the wealthy or elite Haitian. Typically, the Haitian diet tends to be very spicy and greasy. Haitians cook almost everything in oil or grease. Even after immigration to the United States, some Haitians continue to prepare foods that are spicy and greasy.

In Haiti the poor Haitian will consume virtually any type of food in order to sustain human life. Since many Haitians who have immigrated to the United States have remained at or below the poverty level, it is likely that these people will continue to consume any type of food available. Chronic abdominal discomfort is primarily caused from parasites that are common to the Haitian population (Wilk, 1986).

Venereal disease

Another problem is venereal disease. Haitian men tend to be more susceptible to different kinds of venereal diseases as a result of promiscuity (Jeanty, 1989). Since most marriages are common law in nature, the man of the family generally lacks commitment to one woman and usually has more than one sexual partner. In addition, the venereal disease is difficult to treat because the medication is usually taken only as long as the symptoms persist. Premature discontinuation of medication results in an incomplete cure. The problem of venereal disease is also extremely difficult to treat because Haitians do not equate venereal disease with sexual intercourse.

Since there are a number of illegal Haitian immigrants, the prevalence of veneral disease among Haitians in the United States is likely but the extent is unknown.

High birth rate

The high birth rate has many health and cultural implications for Haitians. One factor contributing to the population explosion is the lack of contraception, which is virtually nonexistent in the conventional manner. This is attributed to a lack of education and technology. An unusually large number of very young Haitian women have pregnancies (Jeanty, 1989), and Haitian women also tend to become pregnant at older ages. Pregnancy in women 35 and older in Haiti is not uncommon (Wilk, 1986). Williams, Murthy, and Berggren (1975) reported that Haitian women between the ages of 35 to 49 have an average of eight pregnancies. Because of this pattern, the nurse must be aware of the high-risk potential among Haitian women in relation to their childbearing habits. Furthermore, family spacing is not optional, and a series of pregnancies within a short time leaves the women's body unable to fully recover or to replenish iron levels.

Tuberculosis

Tuberculosis is another concern to this population. As a result of the poor economic levels, which lead to poor living conditions and malnutrition, Haiti has one of world's highest rates of tuberculosis (Wilk, 1986). Another factor is overcrowding, which results in poor sanitation. The majority of the population has no waste facilities. Garbage and human excrement are thrown into the streets or placed in community pits, and the water for drinking is contaminated, resulting in a vast majority of the diseases, including tuberculosis. Malnutrition complicates the situation. The poor cannot afford the cost of examination or the medication to treat the illness if it is diagnosed. Because of the high incidence of tuberculosis in Haiti, Haitians coming into the United States often bring this disease with them. Assessment for symptoms of tuberculosis is an important part of health screening when caring for Haitian patients.

Sickle cell anemia

Sickle cell anemia, or Hb SS disease, is a chronic hereditary hemolytic disorder mainly affecting the Black populations of the world and characterized by the presence of erythrocytes that primarily contain Hb S instead of Hb A. The red blood cell assumes a sickle shape when exposed to lower oxygen levels. Persons who are homozygous for Hb S are estimated to have erythrocytes that contain 80% to 100% abnormal Hb S and only up to 20% normal Hb A. The erythrocytes of persons with sickle cell trait contain approximately 25% to 40% Hb S and 60% to 75% Hb A.

Sickle cell anemia develops as a result of a genetic mutation that is transmitted from parent to child. Laboratory testing is available to determine if the sickle cell trait is present (Luckmann & Sorensen, 1974). It is important for the nurse to have a working knowledge of sickle cell anemia when assessing Haitian American patients and to be able to refer the patient to any associations for sickle cell patients. It is important to provide the patient with information about this illness, since most of these patients know little about it (Jeanty, 1989).

AIDS

Cases of AIDS in Haiti are believed to date back to the late 1970s and now number at least several hundred, though there are no reliable estimates. Information from Haiti is sketchy and obscured by poor medical recording and services. However, there is considerable evidence that the majority of cases occur in neither drug users nor men with homosexual histories; the latest figures suggest that a third of known cases occur in women (Gilmore et al., 1983; Perlman, 1984). Because of the publicity of AIDS originating in Haiti (which has never been proved), Haitians who have immigrated to the United States face constant discrimination, although the fear and stigma about AIDS in the Haitian population are gradually decreasing (Laverdiere et al., 1983). The nurse must keep in mind that Haitians are no longer classified as a "high-risk group" by the Centers for Disease Control (Fain, 1984).

Nutritional Preferences and Deficiencies

There is a critical problem with malnutrition in the agricultural areas of Haiti among the poor (Rodman, 1961). Some estimate that 80% of Haitians suffer from malnutrition (*National Catholic Reporter,* 1983). For the Haitian peasant, environmental, technological, and economic factors alone account for a substantial amount of poor nutrition.

Haiti's rugged topography combines with a generally limited system of mass transport to accentuate the regional and seasonal nature of many of the crops. The economic status of most Haitians confines their food expenditures to a survival level of foods chosen from among locally produced foodstuffs. In addition, the humeral medical beliefs that classify food into "hot" and "cold" categories further restrict dietary selection (Wiese, 1976).

The nurse should be aware of food preferences customary to the Haitian culture. As a result of the lack of ready availability of food items, Haitians have learned many poor nutritional habits, which have persisted even after immigration to the United States, particularly if similar economic conditions prevail. The foods customary to the Haitian culture are listed in the box below.

Dietary habits for childbearing Haitian Women

Childbearing Haitian women are very particular about their dietary habits both before and after delivery. These dietary cultural habits include foods that a women should and should not eat (see box on p. 482). The nurse should assess these foods to ensure that the patient maintains adequate nutrition.

Breast-feeding is common among Haitians; bottle-feeding is not considered natural (Jeanty, 1989). Thus dietary intake of the mother must be carefully assessed by the nurse after delivery as well as before.

Psychological Characteristics

Psychiatric care is also limited in Haiti. In 1956 Kline (Bordeleau & Kline, 1986) reported the presence of one psychiatrist and one psychiatric hospital in Haiti.

COMMON CULTURAL FOOD PREFERENCES

Fruits and nuts	Meat, vegetables, and other foods
Rice	Beef
Avocados	Beets
Cashew nuts	Okra
Coconuts	Biscuits (from imported white flour)
Grenadilia flesh	Cabbage
Mangos	Carrots
Pineapples	Imported cheese
Soursop fruit	Chicken
Star apples	Milled corn
Cassava bread	Eggplant
Bananas	Fish
Limes	Goat meat
Grapefruits	Kidney beans
Oranges	Lima beans
Tomatoes	Peas
Watermelons	Pork
	Sweet potatoes
	Pumpkin
	Sugar cane

Foods childbearing women may eat	Foods avoided by childbearing women
Cornmeal porridge with bean sauce	Lima beans
Rice and beans	Tomatoes
Plantains	Black mushrooms
	White beans
	Okra
	Lobster
	Fish

The first modern psychiatric hospital was opened in 1959, amid prejudice and resistance, by two psychiatrists from Canada and the United States. Since perphenazine (Trilafon) was donated by the three founding pharmaceutical companies and was used abundantly, the psychiatrists were called "Trilafon doctors." While psychiatric treatment has improved, the frequency of mental illness in Haiti is unknown and the psychiatric services remain undeveloped. Bordeleau and Kline (1986) have reported that psychiatric symptoms do not appear to be much different from those found in other counties. Projection has been identified as a frequent defense mechanism, since paranoid delusions often appear in patients who are psychotic. Delusions are profoundly colored by voodoo religious beliefs. Aggressivity is seldom directed toward others, with psychomotor hyperactivity being more often noisy than destructive. Affective disorders are more often of the hypomanic or manic type than depressive, and suicide among Haitians is rare. More recently, psychiatric care has advanced with the development of outpatient clients (Bordeleau & Kline, 1986).

Laguerre (1981) has studied patterns of bereavement among Haitian American families. Death arrangements are usually taken care of by a male kinsman of the deceased who has had experience with American bureaucracies. Death appears to mobilize the entire extended family, including matrilateral and patrilateral members. Since Haitians frequently believe that illness and death can be of a supernatural, as well as natural, origin (Metraux, 1953), death is often accompanied by feelings of guilt and anger. The surviving relatives may believe that the death was a result of failure to relate appropriately to the voodoo spirit. Recurrent dreams of the deceased person, so much a part of grief work, take on a particular meaning to the Haitian. The Haitian commonly evaluates illness in terms of symptoms previously experienced by close kin (Laguerre, 1981), and grief work frequently includes taking on symptoms of the deceased person's last illness (Eisenbruch, 1984).

Possession crisis, which has been diagnosed in some Haitian patients, is not unique to Haitian voodoo, but has also been observed in many African countries and on rare occasions among the American Indians. It has much similarity with the early Greek Dionysian mysteries, the evil possession of the European Middle Ages, the witch possession in the New England colonies, and the contemporary Black religious services of certain extreme groups in the South. See box on p. 483 for the conditions that must be present to have a possession crisis (Bordeleau & Kline, 1986).

POSSESSION CRISIS

1. The general population of the local community must believe that a human being can communicate with the deities.
2. The person being "mounted" by the spirit *(loa)* is one of a group involved in a religious ceremony where the drums control the rhythm of the dance and the *hungan* behaves at first as a ritualistic priest.
3. Some spirits "participate" only at a certain time of the year and with a similar type of personality; that is, a gentle *loa* mounts a calm person and a fighting *loa* chooses an aggressive person.
4. The group considers being possessed to be a privilege, not a shameful event.
5. The possession crisis is stereotyped in the sense that someone mounted by a specific *loa* will talk like the *loa,* ask for the needed symbolic ornaments, and generally behave and dance in the way traditions in the region have dictated.

Implications for Nursing Care

Because stomach ailments are a major problem for Haitians, the astute nurse will carefully assess the Haitian American patient for various stomach ailments, including worms, which may be the result of spoiled food. In fact, a nurse may assume that if a Haitian American family has poor nutritional habits and at the same time cannot afford nutritious food, the likelihood that the family members will have worms is increased. Garlic is considered a folk remedy for worms and is boiled and eaten both to prevent and to treat worms. When a Haitian American patient brings in a specimen and hands it to the clinic nurse, it is important for the nurse to understand that this may be a communication about a problem with worms and that the specimen should be analyzed with this in mind. The nurse will be better able to assist the Haitian American patient by not trying to convince the patient that garlic is not appropriate. The folk remedies should be accepted and combined with Western medicine.

It is important for the nurse to know that many Haitian Americans have very little information about disease or medical problems. Therefore an illness is more commonly considered a "hex" or the result of an evil curse. The nurse should collect information from the patient about the possible cause for the medical problem and should remain nonjudgmental even when voodoo is provided as a possible explanation. Health teaching (for example, regarding diarrhea or pneumonia) is essential to help the Haitian patient understand that the illness is not an evil curse imposed by a neighbor but an illness with natural physical causes.

The nurse cannot assume that the next Haitian American individual encountered will have the same beliefs as the last one to whom care was given. It is useful to ask Haitian patients the length of time they have been in the United States. This will provide an indication of how Americanized the patient may be. The age of the patient is also a consideration when health beliefs are being assessed. Younger people are more likely to have made an effective adjustment to the Western culture, whereas older people often continue to find such things as American food strange and unacceptable.

Haitian American patients are more likely to feel they are receiving effective treatment when a nurse is seen. In Haiti a nurse is given more authority and status than a physician, and the patient will often be more cooperative with directions given by a nurse (Jeanty, 1989). When nursing procedures are being implemented (for example, taking the patient's blood pressure), the nurse should tell the patient verbally what is being done and that this is for the patient's benefit. Actions by the nurse are related to being helped.

Some Haitian Americans associate wheelchairs with being sick. Therefore on discharge the patient who is allowed to walk out of the hospital will be more likely to feel that care has been effective (Jeanty, 1989).

Great stress has been placed on the Haitian people as they have attempted to adjust to life in the United States and Canada. Coming from a disadvantaged background and often arriving in the United States with a history of poor health care, Haitians have been hesitant to reach out for health care. For some of these people, going to the hospital is perceived as a place to go to die. This belief may contribute to large numbers of visitors when a Haitian person is ill, since many Haitians believe that only very sick persons go to a hospital and that death may therefore be imminent (Jeanty, 1989). Health professionals at all levels need to communicate a nonjudgmental attitude while trying to encourage the Haitian American patient to take advantage of health services that are available. Not only do Haitian Americans need to be educated regarding health care agencies, but they may also need information on health insurance, on how to use health benefits, and on finding a job that has medical benefits.

SUMMARY

Haiti is an independent underdeveloped republic that continues to face many critical issues such as a poor economy, lack of technology, high mortality, inadequacy in food and water supplies, and a lack of adequate or quality health care. With the ever-growing Haitian population migrating to the United States, the nurse must constantly keep these issues in mind when formulating a treatment plan for a Haitian American patient. The holistic approach must be a priority approach when assessing, treating, and evaluating the Haitian American patient. The Haitian cultural method of health care delivery must be included with conventional methods of treatment, and transcultural issues in nursing must be recognized before quality care can be rendered. Cultural behavior is meaningful and should not be ridiculed, judged negatively, or ignored. The nurse must be aware of cultural and behavioral considerations that affect the care of the Haitian immigrant and use this understanding in implementation of the nursing process.

CASE
STUDY

A 33-year-old Haitian man is admitted via the emergency room with symptoms of persistent coughing and spitting up small amounts of blood. Through the nursing assessment and by talking with the patient and his family members, it is determined that the patient has been experiencing a progressive lack of appetite and is visibly underweight. Radiographic examination reveals that the patient has an active and communicable case of tuberculosis. When the patient and the family are informed that the diagnosis is tuberculosis, there is little reaction. The nurse is informed by the patient's family members that the patient was initially diagnosed as having a positive Mantoux test in Haiti approximately 2 years previously. At that time the patient was given a prescription for isoniazid (INH) by a clinic physician but was noncompliant with his medication regimen.

CARE PLAN

Nursing Diagnosis   Gas exchange, impaired, related to tuberculosis as evidenced by viscous secretions and coughing.

Patient Outcome	*Nursing Interventions*
Patient will have no further coughing or viscous secretions.	1 Maintain adequate hydration (increase fluid intake to 2 to 3 quarts per day). 2 Maintain adequate humidity of inspired air. 3 Minimize irritants in inspired air (e.g., dust, allergens). 4 Provide periods of uninterrupted rest. 5 Administer prescribed medication such as cough suppressant or expectorant as ordered by physician.

Nursing Diagnosis   Nurtition, altered: less than body requirements, related to tuberculosis as evidenced by anorexia and weight that is below normal for age, sex, and body stature.

Patient Outcome	*Nursing Interventions*
Patient will gain weight to be within normal range for body size.	1 Maintain good oral hygiene (make sure patient brushes teeth, rinses mouth) before and after ingestion of food. 2 Arrange to have highest protein/calorie foods served at times patient feels most like eating. 3 Use dietition for meal planning.

Nursing Diagnosis   Medication noncompliance related to communication barriers as evidenced by previous noncompliance, cultural beliefs, and religious beliefs.

Patient Outcome	*Nursing Interventions*
Patient will take prescribed medication as ordered.	1 Allow patient an opportunity to make decisions about his own health care; assume an advisory approach when counseling, rather than one that is dictatorial. 2 Consult with an interpreter who speaks both English and Creole to provide instructions on how to take medication. 3 Consult with an interpreter who speaks both English and Creole to help patient vent his feelings of anxiety and frustration.

Nursing Diagnosis   Medication noncompliance related to referral process.

Patient Outcome

Patient will keep scheduled follow-up appointments.

Nursing Interventions

1   Whenever possible, allow patient to make own appointments.
2   Shorten referral waiting time.
3   Personnel handling referral appointment should inquire about transportation, suggesting help if needed.

Nursing Diagnosis   Family processes, altered, related to an ill family member as evidenced by ambivalent feelings of family members to the disease process and lack of support from family members.

Patient Outcome

Family will achieve functional support for patient.

Nursing Interventions

1   Include family members in group education sessions about tuberculosis.
2   Refer family members to support and self-help groups.
3   Obtain Creole-speaking interpreter to facilitate communication.
4   Facilitate family involvement with social supports.

STUDY QUESTIONS

1. If a Mantoux test is given incorrectly and no wheal appears (because the injection was made too deep), should the nurse repeat the test at another site that is at least 2 inches away from the first injection?
2. What does erythema without induration mean?
3. In tuberculosis, treatment is continued until when?
4. The physician says the patient has induration. What does this mean?
5. List the possible side effects of isoniazid (INH).
6. What preventive steps can be taken to avoid the spread of a diagnosed case of tuberculosis?
7. Why is proper nutrition important with a patient diagnosed as having tuberculosis?
8. Why is the Haitian population at high risk for being infected by tuberculosis?
9. What is the nurse's role when caring for a patient with tuberculosis?
10. Compare the similarities and differences in family structure between the American and Haitian cultures.
11. What are the contributing factors that lead to the high birth rate in Haiti and among Haitian immigrants?
12. Why are Haitian women at risk during pregnancy?
13. Describe the practice of healers and their importance to the Haitian population.
14. Describe the role of the Haitian man as it pertains to family.

REFERENCES

Bell, I. (1981). *The Dominican Republic.* Boulder, Colo.: Westview Press.

Bestman, E. (1979). *Cultural, linguistic and racial barriers in providing health services to Haitian refugees.* Paper presented at a workshop on improving health services to Haitian refugees, sponsored by the U.S. Health Service Administration, H.R.S., Metro-Dade County, Fla.

Bordeleau, J.M., & Kline N.S. (1986). Experience in developing psychiatric services in Haiti. *World Mental Health,* pp. 170-183.

Boswell, T. (1982). The new Haitian diaspora. *Carribbean Review, 11*(1), 18-21.

Bryan, S. (1988, summer). *Ethnic diseases.* Paper presented at a workshop sponsored by the U.S. Health Service Administration, Metro-Dade County, Fla.

Charles, C. (1979). *Anthropological consideration of barriers affecting delivery of health services to Haitian refugees in Florida.* Paper presented at a workshop on improving health services to Haitian refugees, sponsored by the U.S. Health Service Administration, H.R.S., Metro-Dade County, Fla.

Coreil, J. (1983, July). Parallel structures in professional and folk health care: A model applied to rural Haiti. *Culture, Medicine and Psychiatry, 70,* pp. 131-151.

Dejean, Y. (1983). *Revisiting the issues of the native language as a natural medium of instruction.* Thesis, Bank Street College of Education, New York.

Dempsey, P.A., & Geese, T. (1983). The childbearing Haitian refugee: Cultural applications to clinical nursing. *Public Health Reports, 98*(3), 261-267.

Desantis, L., & Thomas, J. (1987, Aug.). Parental attitudes toward adolescent sexuality: Transcultural perspectives," *Nurse Practitioner, 12,* 43-48.

Eisenbruch, M. (1984). Cross-cultural aspects of bereavement: Part 2. Ethnic and cultural variations in the development of bereavement practices. *Culture, Medicine and Psychiatry, 8,* 315-347.

Fain, N. (1984, Sept. 18). Health. *The Advocate,* pp. 6-9.

Gilmore, N., Beaulieu, R., Steben, M., & Laverdiere, M. (1983). AIDS: Acquired immunodeficiency syndrome. *Canadian Medical Association Journal, 128*(11), 1281-1284.

Godsby, R. (1971). *A race and races.* New York: Macmillan.

Grant, W. (1989, Aug. 6). *The prevalence of antibodies to HTLV-I virus in the Aribonite Valley.* Paper presented at the annual reunion of the Hospital Albert Schweitzer Alumni Association, Burlington, Vt.

Harris, K. (1987). Beliefs and practices among Haitian American women in relation to childbearing. *Journal of Nurse-Midwifery, 32*(3), 149-155.

Herskovits, M.J. (1971). *Life in a Haitian valley.* New York: Doubleday.

Hobsbawn, E.J. (1962). *The age of revolution: 1789-1848.* London: Weidenfeld & Nicolson.

Jeanty, M. (1989). Personal communication at Logansport State Hospital, Logansport, Ind. (Dr. Jeanty is a Haitian psychiatrist.)

Laguerre, M. (1981). Haitian Americans. In A. Harwood (Ed.), *Ethnicity and medical care.* Cambridge, Mass.: Harvard University Press.

Laverdiere, M., Tremblay, J., Lavallee, R., Bonny, Y., Lacombe, M., & Boileau, J. (1983). Aids in Haitian immigrants and in a Caucasian woman closely associated with Haitians. *Canadian Medical Association Journal, 129*(11), 1209-1212.

Leyburn, J.G. (1955). *The Haitian people.* New Haven, Ct.: Yale University Press.

Logan, M. (1975). Selected references on the hot-cold theory of disease. *Medical Anthropology Newsletter, 6*(2), 8-11.

Luckmann, J., & Sorensen, K. (1974). *Medical-surgical nursing: A psychophysiologic approach.* Philadelphia: W.B. Saunders.

McMorrow, T. (1970, Nov. 15). Haitians try to adopt U.S. with three strikes on them. *Daily News,* p. B1.

Metraux, A. (1953). Medecine et vodou en Haiti. *Acta Tropica, 10,* 28-68.

Metropolitan Dade County. (1981). *Social and economic problems among Cuban and Haitian entrant groups in Dade County, Flordia: Trends and implications.* Miami: Author.

Moskowitz, L., Kory, P., Chan, J., Haverkos, H., Conley, F., & Hensley, G. (1983). Unusual causes of deaths in Haitians residing in Miami. *JAMA, 250*(9), 1187-1191.

National Catholic Reporter. (March 2, 1983), p. 1.

Nida, E. (1954). *Customs and cultures.* New York: Harper & Brothers.

Orque, M.S., Bloch, B., & Monrroy,, L.S.A. (1983). *Ethnics in nursing care: A multicultural approach.* St. Louis: C.V. Mosby.

Perlman, D. (1984, Dec. 15). The search for a cure. *San Francisco Chronicle,* p. 15.

Portes, A., & Stepick, A. (1985, Aug.). Unwelcome immigrants: The labor market experiences of 1980 (Mariel) Cuban and Haitian refugees in South Florida. *American Sociological Review,* 493-515.

Racine, M. (1984). Why literacy in the native language: The case of adult Haitian illiterates. *Papers in the Social Sciences, 4,* 61-77.

Reichman, L. (1989, Aug. 5). *Treating tuberculosis in developing countries.* Paper presented at the annual reunion of the Hospital Albert Schweitzer Alumni Association, Burlington, Vt..

Rey, K.H. (1970). *The Haitian family.* New York: Community Service Society.

Rodman, S. (1961). *Haiti: The Black republic.* New York: Devin-Adair.

Rosenwarke, I. (1972). *Population history of New York.* Syracuse, N.Y.: Syracuse University Press.

Schaedel, R. (1962). *The human resources of Haiti.* Unpublished manuscript.

Scott, C. (1978, Nov./Dec.). Health and healing practices among five ethnic groups in Miami, Florida. *Public Health Report, 55,* 524-532.

Seligman, L. (1977, March). Haitians: A neglected minority. *Personnel and Guidance Journal, 2,* 409-411.

Snow, L.F. (1981). Folk medical beliefs and their implications for the care of patients: A review based on studies among Black Americans. In G. Henderson & M. Primeaux (Eds.), *Transcultural health care.* Reading, Mass.: Addison-Wesley.

Stauffer, R. (1989). Personal communication with the former Assistant Director of Nursing at Hospital Albert Schweitzer, Deschapelles, Haiti.

U.S. Department of Commerce. *Ancestry of the population by state: 1980.* Washington, D.C.: U.S. Government Printing Office.

Verdet, P. (1985, winter). Trying times: Haitian youth in an inner city high school. *Social Work in Health Care,* pp. 228-233.

Walsh, B. (1980, May 17). The boat people of South Florida. *America,* pp. 420-421.

Weil, T.E. (1973). *Area handbook for Haiti.* Washington D.C.: U.S. Government Printing Office.

Westphal, R. (1989, Aug. 5). *Transfusion transmitted infectious diseases.* Paper presented at the annual reunion of the Hospital Albert Schweitzer Alumni Association.

Wiese, J. (1976). Maternal nutrition and traditional food behavior in Haiti. *Human Organization, 35*(2), 193-200.

Wilentz, A. (1989). *The rainy season.* New York: Simon & Schuster.

Wilk, R. (1986, winter). The Haitian refugee: Concern for health care providers. *Social Work in Health Care, 11,* 61-74.

Williams, S., Murthy, N., & Berggren, G. (1975, Nov.). Conjugal unions among rural Haitian women. *Journal of Marriage and the Family, 37,* 1022-1031.

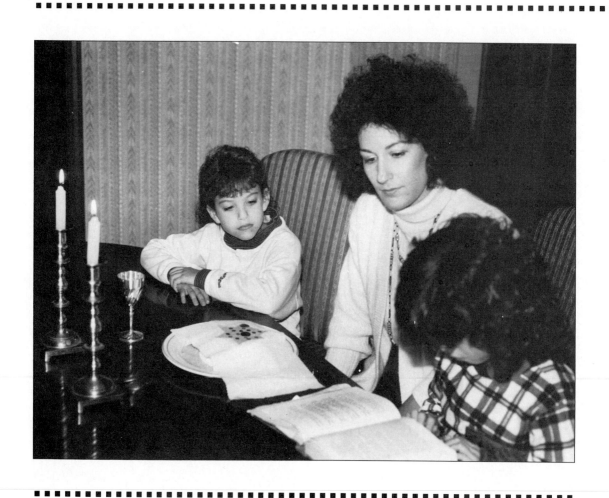

■ ■

CHAPTER 21

Jewish Americans

Enid A. Schwartz

BEHAVIORAL OBJECTIVES
After reading this chapter, the nurse will be able to:

1 Identify how the religion of Judaism affects the cultural behaviors of Jewish Americans.

2 Identify some of the differences between health-oriented behaviors demonstrated by various religious groups within Judaism.

3 Identify how the various ethnic backgrounds of Jewish Americans affect their cultural behaviors.

4 Describe attitudes and beliefs affecting health care within and across individuals in various Jewish groups.

5 Identify how the verbal and nonverbal communications of Jewish individuals may affect health care.

6 Identify implications and/or precautions for providing effective nursing care to Jewish Americans.

7 Recognize those health care practices that are mandated by Jewish law for people who are Jewish.

Explaining what it means to be Jewish is not easy. It is more than just belonging to a religious organization; it is also being a part of a specific people (Glazer, 1957; Popenoe, 1977; Trepp 1980). It is a shared feeling of "Jewishness." Jewish people are linked together by a common history, common ethical teachings, a common language of prayer (Hebrew), a vast quantity of literature, common folkways, and, above all, a sense of common destiny (Kertzer, 1978). Jewish people share centuries of history as a minority subjected to hostility wherever they go.

The Jewish American culture has many subcultures because of the different areas of the world in which Jews live, as well as a diversity of religious observances. Jews came to the United States predominantly from Spain, Portugal, Germany, and Eastern Europe. There are three main religious groups: Orthodox, Conservative, and Reform. Within the Orthodox group are the Chassidic and Lubovovitch subgroups. Although many other subgroups exist in the United States today, the Chassidic and Lubovovitch subgroups are the largest ones.

Despite differences, there are some cultural similarities that are indigenous to this group of people. To understand the culture, one must have knowledge of some of the religious dictates. Through a discussion of the six common variables found within and across cultural groups as they apply to Jewish Americans, this chapter attempts to clarify some behaviors that are commonly found among Jews in order to assist nurses in developing an effective plan of care for the Jewish American patient. Attention is also placed on Jewish rituals and the effects of assimilation on their cultural traits.

OVERVIEW OF THE JEWISH PEOPLE IN AMERICA

The history of American Judaism encompasses three distinct tides of immigration. The first tide of people, who began arriving in the middle 1600s, was relatively small in number. These were Sephardic Jews from Spain and Portugal, and they had little effect on the development of present-day American Judaism (Sachar, 1964). The beginning of the nineteenth century saw a steady German immigration, which swelled after 1836, when Jews sought to escape persecution in Bavaria and other German communities (Glazer, 1957). The last tide of immigration began slowly in 1845, when Polish Jews began arriving in the United States, but swelled to tens of thousands in 1881 as a result of a wave of pogroms and a series of new anti-Jewish decrees in Russia. This last tide, consisting of Eastern European Jews and German Jews, has had a profound effect on present-day Jewish American culture and religious practices.

To understand Jewish American culture today, it is necessary to consider Europe during the Middle Ages. At that time, most of the internal law in European Jewish communities was strongly controlled by the Talmud (the Rabbinic code). Talmudic law not only governed the religious behavior of Jews, it also governed almost every other aspect of life, such as birth, marriage, and death, as well as the proper foods to eat and the proper clothes to wear. The Jews were kept separate from the general population not only by persecution from others, but also by the rigidity of these laws.

In the nineteenth century not all German Jews were isolated in their communities; some were involved in non-Jewish communities. Many of these Jews were embarrassed by the ancient laws and found them distasteful, especially if they desired the status of full members of the German nation (Glazer, 1957). To maintain their beliefs and yet not appear different from the general culture, German Jews of high social status attempted to start the Reform movement.

The freedom experienced in America allowed the Reform movement to flourish. The German Jews who immigrated to the United States and wished to become part of the American community were willing to rid themselves of the old traditions and become increasingly "Americanized." They were insistent, however, that the Jews be maintained as a people.

The Eastern European immigrants came predominantly from Russia, Rumania,

Poland, and Austria. In contrast to many of the German Jewish immigrants who had lived predominantly in nonsegregated areas, most of the Eastern European Jews came from all-Jewish villages, known as *shtetls,* where a Jewish culture was created that was almost totally unaffected by the cultures of the people around them. Life was dictated by the religious traditions Eastern European Jews followed and was much the same as it had been during the Middle Ages.

Along with these pious Jews came the radical political and socialist Jews, who believed that the only way to survive was through abandonment of religion altogether. A third group who immigrated during this time represented the "middle of the road" Jews, who were both religious and radical (Glazer, 1957).

It is important to understand the differences in religious behavior when caring for Jewish patients. All Jewish beliefs derive from the Torah (the five books of Moses) and the Talmud (the Rabbinic code). From the Torah come 613 commandments. The combination of the Torah and Talmud results in codes of law. Rather than referring to a body of doctrine, Judaism refers to a body of practices (Glazer, 1957).

As mentioned earlier, there are three main religious Jewish groups today: Orthodox, Conservative, and Reform. The Orthodox Jew maintains a strict code of interpretation of the law; the Conservative Jew does not maintain as strict a code of interpretation, and the Reform Jew follows a more liberal interpretation of the law. An example of the differences deals with the head coverings worn by men: the Orthodox Jew is obligated to keep his head covered at all times in reverence to God; the Conservative Jew keeps his head covered during times of worship; and the Reform Jew is not obligated to keep his head covered.

The division between Jewish practices started in Germany in the nineteenth century, but it was not until Jews experienced the religious freedom of the United States that the Conservative and Reform movements thrived. The freedom experienced in America allowed the Jewish immigrant to question the narrow confines of Orthodoxy and led to a desire to express religious beliefs and traditional practices in a less confining environment. The German Jews had begun to practice Reform Judaism. However, to the Eastern European Jew, Reform Judaism seemed empty (Howe, 1976). A movement known as Conservatism, which had begun in nineteenth century Germany, had a small beginning but appealed to the children of many Eastern European immigrants. According to Glazer (1957), Conservatism offered a compromise between the blind religious teachings of the Orthodox and the scholarly endeavors of the Reform movement to break from tradition completely. Today, there are discussions among the Reform temples about returning to some of the traditional practices.

In regard to religion, Jewish identity has changed through the generations. In America today, the sense of Jewish identity does not lie in the Old World religious observances. Most Jewish Americans do not observe the traditional Jewish Sabbath, nor are they active in their temple or synagogue. According to Sowell (1981), their identity lies not with the historical religious aspects of Judiasm, but with their ethnic or racial identity.

Changes in immigration laws have decreased the number of Jews entering the United States. However, since the time of the large immigration of Eastern European Jews, other Jews from other countries have come to America under different circumstances. There are Jews who escaped or lived through the Holocaust, Jews who have immigrated from Communist Russia, and Jews who have arrived from many other countries of the world, including Ethiopia and Israel. Each group has added to the cultural diversity of the Jewish people.

All of these Jews have brought with them the culture of the land from which they immigrated. Because of the close ties that have developed between Jews of all nationalities, cultural traits have begun to blend. For instance, today, descendants of Eastern European Jews talk about their falafel, a food made from ground chick-peas, which originated in the Middle East.

A fear of many Jewish Americans is the effect of assimilation on their children. Jewish people do not want to appear different from other Americans, since being different has led to thousands of years of persecution. However, many Jewish Americans do not want to lose the common thread that binds them to one another.

Although Jews make up only about 3% of the American population, they are visible in many areas of the American culture. They are distinguished members of the arts, academia, sciences, medicine, law, and the political arena. Education is a large part of the Jewish culture, and this has helped Jews in America succeed as they never could in other countries.

The desire to succeed, plus intermarriage, has caused some loss of Jewish identity. There are Jews today in the United States who do not wish to be identified as Jewish for fear of discrimination in the workplace. Discrimination against Jews does exist in the United States, and many Jews are sensitive to anti-Semitism.

COMMUNICATION

Today the primary language of Jewish Americans is English. In the late 1800s the primary language of the Jews was Yiddish, which is a combination of German, Slavic languages, Old French, Old Italian, and Hebrew (Rosten, 1968).

The freedom experienced in the United States led to the desire for assimilation. Many Jewish Americans of German descent were embarrassed by the use of Yiddish. To them, Yiddish was vulgar, represented the lower socioeconomic class, and above all was un-American. The children of first-generation Jews, born to Eastern European parents, wanted to be accepted by the other children. Although Yiddish may have been spoken in the home, these children spoke English outside the home. Very few second-generation Jewish Americans understand Yiddish. However, almost all Jewish Americans know some Yiddish and many Jewish conversations are sprinkled with Yiddish words. Some of these words have become a part of American English, such as *shtick* and *tush*.

Hebrew, which is the language of Israel, is not spoken by most Jews. However, Hebrew is the language of the Torah, and many Jews can read it. An important part of Jewish religious education is the reading, speaking, and writing of Hebrew. *Shalom* is one Hebrew word that is commonly used by Jewish people to mean "peace," "hello," or "goodbye."

The Sephardic Jews have a language of their own, Ladino, which is similar to Old Spanish. It is not commonly spoken in the United States today.

Style

Jews tend to be expressive when communicating, and they tend to be very verbal about how and what they are feeling. Most Jewish people use their hands to express their thoughts; as they talk, their hands assist in emphasizing what is being said. They not only punctuate their conversations using hand and arm movements, but also use voice inflections. By changing the emphasis on certain words, the Jewish person changes the meaning of the message being conveyed (Rosten, 1968). This is done easily in Yiddish and has been carried over into English. As an example, changing the emphasis on the words, "Him you trust?" changes the meaning: "Him you *trust?*" versus "*Him* you trust?" The first questions a person's judgment; the second implies that anyone who would trust the character of such a scoundrel must be an idiot.

Humor is used frequently by Jews, and often the humor is directed at themselves. This self-directed humor has led to comments that Jewish humor comes out of self-hatred. Although Jewish humor may appear to be self-critical and sometimes self-deprecating, it does not stem from a form of Jewish masochism. One of the most popular beliefs is that Jewish humor arose as a way for Jews to cope with the hostility they found around them, sometimes using that hostility against themselves. It appears as if a Jewish person is telling enemies, "You don't have to attack us. We can do that ourselves—and even better" (Novak & Waldoks, 1981).

Jews today are sensitive to humor from "outside" sources. Jokes that are not appreciated when told by non-Jews include "JAP" (Jewish American Princess) jokes and those about "Jewing people down" (referring to Jews being cheap or unmerciful at bartering).

As Jews become more acculturated with each generation, the communication styles change. Jewish people who are third- or fourth- generation Americans will more likely demonstrate the same communication style as their neighbors rather than that of their parents, grandparents, or great-grandparents. This type of acculturation is part of the history of Jews all over the world (Patai & Wing, 1975).

Touch

The use of touch varies with Jewish people; however, the use or nonuse of touch can be a critical issue with Orthodox Jews and must be carefully considered by the nurse.

Because of the Jewish laws regarding personal space and touching others of the opposite sex, it is important to ascertain what religious group the patient belongs to. If the person is Orthodox, he or she will be very modest. Overexposure of or touching the parts of the body associated with sexual activities can cause a great deal of distress. When caring for very Orthodox Jewish patients of the opposite sex, the nurse should use touch only for hands-on care. To touch the person at any other time could be offensive because of the sexual connotations attached to casual touch by this group of people.

It is also important to note that according to Jewish law, religious observances are not to be followed if doing so will endanger the person's health.

Implications for Nursing Care

Because older Jewish patients may be very verbal about what and how they are feeling, they may appear to be chronic complainers. Although it is difficult to remain nonjudgmental with a patient who is considered a chronic complainer, it is important to remember that letting others know feelings is part of the Jewish culture. It may be difficult to assess pain levels of Jewish patients because they are very emotional when expressing their discomfort, and it may take persistence and patience to pinpoint the problem and its extent. Younger Jewish patients may be more articulate and may also complain less than their parents or grandparents as a result of acculturation.

SPACE

The Orthodox Jew is keenly aware of religious dictates regarding personal space that may or may not be invaded by members of the opposite sex. Many Orthodox Jewish men and women will not shake hands with a member of the opposite sex. This stems from the ruling in the *Code of Jewish Law* that forbids a man to smell the scent of a strange woman, to look upon her hair, or even to gaze upon her little finger (Kolatch, 1985). A very Orthodox Jewish man will not usually touch his wife in public.

Traditionally, Jewish people have also had practices about personal and social space. In times of sickness and during their elderly years, Jewish individuals have an acute desire to have members of their family and other Jews around them. This has been illustrated in studies of the elderly that indicate that elderly Jewish people in nursing homes adjust better if they have other Jews around them (Kaplan, 1970).

Implications for Nursing Care

Judaic laws can lead to some misinterpretation by nurses and other health care providers. For example, during childbirth, if a very Orthodox Jewish husband decides to participate in the delivery, his participation will only be verbal. He will not touch his wife during labor. This practice is associated with the laws of separation that dictate that avoidance is necessary during the time a woman has any vaginal bleeding. He will not view the birth, since he is not permitted to view his wife's genital area. After the birth, he may lean over his wife (being careful not to touch her), smile, and say, "*Mazal Tov*" (good luck, congratulations) (Bash, 1980; Lutwak, Ney, & White, 1988).

Some very Orthodox husbands elect to participate only spiritually. If this is the case, they will sit with their prayerbook and recite from the Book of Psalms. It is important to remember that this practice does not mean the man loves his wife any less than the man who actively participates. Orthodox men and women who fall into this subculture are often recognizable by their appearance. The men usually have long earlocks and beards, and wear yalmuchas (skull caps) or large black hats and long black frock coats. The women are modestly dressed in long-sleeved dresses and have wigs or scarves covering their heads.

With the increase of male nurses, the question arises regarding the assignment of a male nurse to a female Orthodox Jewish patient. The *Code of Jewish Law* (Ganzfried, 1927) states: "A male is not permitted to attend to a woman who is suffering with a belly ache . . . but a woman may attend to a male who is so suffering . . ." This passage may be interpreted to mean that a male nurse should not be assigned to care for a female patient. If, however, there are only male nurses available, this law would probably be waved because all laws are suspended in the case of severe illness.

There is also a law that addresses attendance of a male physician with a female patient. This law states that a physician is permitted to let blood and to feel the pulse or any other place of a woman, even if she is married, even the pudenda (external genital organs), as is customary with physicians, because he is merely following his profession (Ganzfried, 1927).

The nurse should be aware that since elderly Jewish patients, in non-Jewish hospitals or nursing homes, may adjust better with other Jews around them, it may be advantageous to have Jewish patients room together or at least be in close proximity. This will allow for increased comfort and offer the Jewish patient the chance to interact with someone who "understands" him or her.

SOCIAL ORGANIZATION

The foundation of the Jewish culture is the nuclear family and the greater Jewish community. Controversy exists as to whether the Jewish community or the Jewish family has had the bigger influence on maintaining the Jewish faith and the Jews as a people (Schneider, 1985).

Jewish families tend to be closely knit and child oriented (Schlesinger, 1971). Jewish parents tend to "want better" for their children than they had themselves. It is not unusual to hear a parent say they have given up something they really wanted for "the sake of the children."

Family life of the Jew in America has changed through the years. The earlier Jewish family was male dominated, and the father made the major decisions. The mother's job was to care for the home, the children, and her husband. Today the delineation of duties is more obscure. Usually both parents work, oftentimes at jobs of equal financial and/or professional status.

The Jewish family structure has been seen as protective. The Eastern European mother of the past got the reputation of being overbearing and overprotective. In the shtetls of Europe, the mother was the cohesive force in the home. This is still considered the case today, although the younger women are not viewed as being as overbearing or overprotective as their mothers and ancestors were.

In the Jewish family the child is seen as the means of maintaining Jewish existence. Therefore education of the child in the Jewish faith and traditions is often seen as the most important thing a community, as well as the family, can do. The fear of assimilation and annihilation increases the importance to the community of "sticking together" and educating the children.

Among the commandments Jews are expected to follow are those that dictate the social relationships expected toward family and community. These commandments dictate expected behavior toward parents and people within the community, such as the poor, teachers, rabbis, neighbors, ill people, the dying, and the dead.

It is social orientation that has helped maintain the Jewish people. When the Eastern European immigrants arrived in the United States, they were an embarrassment for the German Jews. However, commandments that control social behaviors dictated that the German Jews reach out to help the newcomers. This sense of kinship was so strong that Jews felt obliged to help one another, both in America and abroad.

Eastern European Jews brought with them a strong sense of community, which arose from their restricted lives within the shtetls. Furthermore, they were often held responsible for political events that occurred outside the Jewish quarters. Even though each Jew developed his or her own individuality, there was an intense feeling of groupness, an identification with a common cultural heritage (Kolatch, 1985).

When the immigration laws of the 1920s resulted in decreased numbers of Eastern European Jews entering the United States, increased assimilation began to occur. Several significant events have occurred in the world that have helped slow the rate of

Jewish American assimilation. The event that seems to have had the largest effect was the rise of Nazi anti-Semitism and its American counterparts. The Holocaust caused all Jews to realize they were indeed brothers (Janowsky, 1964), and the memory of the Holocaust continues to have this effect on the Jewish people.

Other events that have had an effect on Jewish identification were related to the development of the state of Israel and the struggle of Israel to continue to exist despite a hostile environment. I can remember the effect the famous "Six-Day War" had on the Jews around me. When Israel won the war, the feeling of pride in the Jewish State was almost tangible. There seemed to be a stronger sense of "Jewishness" and an increased willingness to admit to being Jewish.

The Jewish American community today is much more mobile than in the past. It is not unusual for the children to move away when they leave for college or marry. When a Jewish individual moves, often one of the first things looked for is Jewish affiliation. A Jew may not join a synagogue, at least not until the children are ready for Sunday school, but often desires the company of other Jews.

Implications for Nursing Care

When a Jewish person becomes ill, family and community resources are mobilized to assist the patient. In the Jewish faith it is a commandment to visit the sick. For this reason, friends, relatives and neighbors will visit the ill Jewish patient. If the patient is very ill, these individuals will act as patient advocates. It is important for the nurse to recognize the cultural implications of these visitors and to expect them to ask about the patient.

Because of the protective attitudes of Jewish parents, they will make arrangements to have someone with their child at all times if the child is hospitalized. Jewish parents may appear demanding and aggressive if they feel their child is not getting the care he or she "deserves." It may take patience on the part of the nurse to handle the concern of the parents. The nurse needs to remember that this is a culture of people who highly prize their children and who see the survival of the Jewish people as a responsibility of the next generation. This view places a large responsibility on the child to get well, and on the parents to see that the child gets well.

TIME

The best way to classify Jewish people in relation to time orientation is to say that they are past, present, and future oriented. Jews are aware of their past—all 5000 years of it. They are also concerned about the present and are very involved with present-day social concerns, both Jewish and non-Jewish. They also look toward the future by insisting that their children be educated, religiously and secularly, and by participating in philanthropic activities to help the future of Israel.

The Jewish concern with the past is very obvious in American society, especially in relation to the Holocaust. Almost every Jew believes that this kind of atrocity should never happen again. By continuing to remind the world of the horrors that happened, not only to Jews, but to people of all faiths and ethnic origins, the Jewish people hope the world will never again let that type of event occur to any other people.

During happy occasions, such as a wedding, there is always something to remind

Jews of their past. As an example, at the end of the wedding ceremony the groom breaks a glass. One reason for this custom is to symbolize the destruction of the Jewish temple during the Roman invasion.

Past orientation is also seen following the death of a loved one (such as a parent, sibling, or spouse). On the anniversary of the death each year, a candle is lit and a prayer—kaddish—is recited in honor of that person. In addition, the kaddish is recited at special times during the year for a loved one. In some congregations the kaddish is recited by the whole congregation in memory of those who have recently died or those who have died in years past and have no one to say the prayer for them.

In relation to present time orientation, Jews tend to be very social minded and are often involved in social movements. In a small southwestern community, Jews help run a soup kitchen. In a southwestern city a rabbi is involved with the sanctuary movement.

From the Talmud comes the requirement that Jews care for all who are in need whether they are Jewish or non-Jewish. Because the concepts of charity and righteousness are so intertwined, the Hebrew word for righteousness (justice)—*tzedaka*—has become the Hebrew word for charity (Kolatch, 1985). This concept has had an influence on the social system in New York City (Howe, 1976).

Another way that Jewish present time orientation is apparent is in relation to an afterlife. Although Jews may believe that the spirit continues to live or reside with God after death, they are not concerned about an afterlife. What is considered important is doing good deeds on earth. During an interview regarding the belief in a soul, one woman summed up what has been written by other authors when she stated that it is the memory of one's good deeds that causes one to be immortalized (Schwartz, 1984).

Future time orientation is apparent in issues concerning the education of children. Establishing schools, supporting schools, and furthering education are top priorities. Throughout the ages education of the children in the Torah has been regarded as a duty. Originally it was the duty of the parents. Eventually it became the duty of the community (Janowsky, 1964). Today, not only religious but also secular education is seen as important. In most Jewish households the children hear, from the time they are very young, that someday they will go to college. Education is highly prized as a way of securing the future for the child, as well as for the Jewish community as a whole.

Another way that future time orientation is apparent relates to concerns during illness. Jewish people not only want immediate relief, they also worry about what the future implications of their illness will be. They worry about the effect of their illness on the future of their family members, their jobs, and their lives. According to Zborowski (1969), the intensity of their concern is greater than that of other Americans.

Many Jews tend to be punctual when it comes to appointments and become very upset when they arrive on time and have to wait for their appointment to begin. However, some Jewish people also talk about "Jewish standard time," which is at least 10 to 15 minutes later than regular time. Although there are many Jews who are very punctual (especially when it comes to appointments), for general Jewish functions, such as weddings or Bar Mitzvahs, it is not unexpected for them to begin late.

Implications for Nursing Care

Because Jewish people are past, present, and future oriented, as well as emotionally expressive, they appear to feel joy, sorrow, illness, etc., with great intensity. They become very anxious when they do not feel well and may appear to be impatient regarding finding a cure. Jewish people have a tendency to worry about what the illness means in the present, as well as the implications it has for the future.

Patience and honesty are necessary qualities for a nurse to display when dealing with Jewish people. Demonstrating interest and concern will convey the message that the nurse cares about the ill person and may help decrease the amount of anxiety the person is feeling. Until a diagnosis is made, trying to help the anxious Jewish patient put events into proper perspective may not work, because the patient reasons that the nurse cannot know what the future will hold if the physician does not know what is wrong.

It is important to note that the high degree of outward anxiety the Jewish person may feel is probably more apparent with the older generation of Jews than with the younger generation, since assimilation has caused more "acceptable" behavior patterns to be exhibited in the younger generation.

ENVIRONMENTAL CONTROL

Many Jews tend to be fatalistic about life. Jewish people may believe that they do have some control over their health, but God has the final say. This is apparent every year during Rosh Hashanna and Yom Kippur (the New Year and the Day of Atonement), when Jews pray to be written in the Book of Life for another year.

Health Care Beliefs

It is a religious requirement to maintain the health of the body as well as the soul in Judaism. The origin of Jewish health care beliefs go back to the Torah. Many of the 613 biblical commandments appear to be hygienic in intent. There are several chapters in the Book of Leviticus (12 to 14) that are devoted to the control of disease, as well as others throughout the Bible (Kolatch, 1985). The Talmud continues to stress this concern for health. There are passages that deal with proper exercise, getting enough sleep, eating breakfast, and eating the proper diet.

Physicians are held in high esteem by people in the Jewish culture (Feldman, 1986). In biblical times the priests were physicians. When a Jewish person is ill, it is a duty to go to a physician, and it is the duty of the family to make sure the individual goes. The importance of health care is so great in this culture that Talmudic scholars stated that a person should not settle in a city without a physician (Feldman, 1986).

Jewish people realize that physicians cannot heal without the participation of the patient. It is permissible for the Jewish patient to question the physician if the patient feels the physician is wrong about a diagnosis or treatment (Feldman, 1986; Zborowski, 1969), and the Jewish patient may decide not to follow the physician's orders. However, if the patient chooses not to listen to the physician, or does not agree with the physician, this individual is expected to seek the knowledge of another physician (Feldman, 1986). Seeking the best medical care, even obtaining a second opinion, is a religious dictate.

Health is one of the most frequent topics of conversation among Jewish people.

With some Jewish people, especially older ones, health is seen as an exception rather than the rule. The older individual may become preoccupied with the issue of good health, since life may be viewed as a temporary lapse between one illness and another (Zborowski, 1969).

The Jewish person believes that prevention of illness is important. Each family member tries to protect and warn the other members of dangers that may cause illnesses, and this attitude can make patient teaching easier for the nurse. It is important to remember that patient teaching in the Jewish family requires the cooperation of all the immediate family members.

Illness Behaviors

When a member of a Jewish family is ill, the whole family suffers with the person. Each individual is expected to become a part of the process of helping the ill individual feel better.

Complaining about discomforts is expected and accepted, especially in the older generation. Complaining fulfills several important functions: it gives relief through its cathartic function; it is a means of communication; it mobilizes the assistance of the environment; and it reaffirms family solidarity (Zborowski, 1969).

When a Jewish patient is admitted to the hospital, this patient may continue to behave as though he or she were at home. The patient may attempt to mobilize the attention and sympathy of those in the new environment by using the same methods that worked in the home, so that what the nurse encounters may be a person who complains, cries, moans, and groans. When this behavior does not result in the reactions the person would receive from the family, the individual may attempt to temper reactions so that feelings of acceptance and being cared for are experienced.

If the ill member of the family does not verbalize pain, there is usually another member of the family who will verbalize it instead. The reasoning is that the person may be too ill to tell the physician or nurse and that it is the family member's responsibility to communicate in order to obtain the attention the family member thinks the loved one should have.

Zborowski's (1969) study of first-generation Jewish Americans in pain noted that these patients responded to questions in details that sometimes seemed to relate only marginally to the topic. In the study it was noted that a simple question released a flow of responses that led to information about pain, illness, anxieties, intrafamily relationships, etc. It was found that probing was necessary to pinpoint specific information rather than to elicit a fuller answer to a question.

Second-, third-, and fourth-generation Jewish Americans seem to be a little less expressive about their pain. However, they do consider it wrong not to express their feelings. The expressive behavior of the Jew indicates that there is a belief among Jewish people that one cannot get help unless a complaint is made.

If verbally complaining does not result in the type of behavior the patient wishes to elicit from those around him or her, crying may be used. Crying, with many first-generation Jewish Americans, is acceptable behavior. It is seen as an expression of frustration or pain and often results in the attention desired (Zborowski, 1969).

With increased American acculturation, each succeeding Jewish American generation appears to be less expressive when in pain. The women may cry easily, but the men have adopted the American view that crying is not proper behavior for men. Second-generation Jewish American male patients tend to be less verbal about their pain than their fathers (Zborowski, 1969). For some Jewish people, however, the meaning of pain does not change, just the outward signs. To the Jewish person, pain, discomfort, and change in the state of good health are seen as a warning that something is wrong and that the health care system needs to be utilized.

Utilization of the health care system may consist of getting the opinions of a number of physicians. The Jewish patient recognizes that the physician is only another human, with the possibility of being incorrect. By getting at least one other opinion, the patient can decide if the physician was correct or not. Not only is a Jewish patient likely to get a second or third opinion, the patient may also check the medical literature. Zborowski (1969) has noted that these activities seem to be based on a feeling that the patient is the final judge and authority in matters pertaining to his or her own health. In this case the physician is seen in the role of consultant and advisor.

Once the Jewish patient accepts the physician's opinion, the patient will also accept the prescribed treatment. The cultural belief is that to get well, one must cooperate with all therapeutic measures. Although the Jewish patient will follow the prescribed regimen, the patient expects the medication regimen to be individualized, because illness is viewed as being individualized.

In many cases, the patient will want to know all about the prescribed treatment: what is expected of the patient, what the side effects are, and, if a drug is being prescribed, the name of the drug. The patient is unlikely to be content with "It's good for you."

The Jewish patient tends to observe carefully the effects of the drug or treatment on the system. Since many Jews believe they are the ultimate judge of their condition, they may change the time they take a drug, increase or decrease the number of drugs taken, or reject the drug completely if they decide it is not helping or is harmful. Many times these decisions are made without consulting the physician. Careful, thorough explanations about the drug, its purpose, side effects, and why it was ordered are essential.

The future-oriented Jewish patient may become hesitant to take analgesics, since most drugs are viewed as "dope" and Jewish persons often fear addiction. This increases the problem for the patient in pain who wants to receive pain relief but is afraid of addiction (Zborowski, 1969).

Kosher Diet, Religious Holidays, and Illness

Maintaining a kosher diet may pose a problem for some Jewish patients. As mentioned in Chapter 7 on Biological Variations, kosher meat is usually salted to help drain all the blood. This presents a problem for a patient on a low-salt diet unless the meat is soaked in water to remove as much of the salt as possible.

It is important for the nurse to consider what can be done for the Jewish patient on a kosher diet if the hospital does not have a kosher supplier nearby. In this case it is possible to serve any fish that meets the dietary requirements of having fins and scales. It is also possible to serve dairy products as long as they are not contraindicated on the person's diet. These meals should be served on paper plates with plastic utensils, since meat and milk dishes should not be mixed.

If, because of medical dietary restrictions and unavailability of kosher food, maintaining a kosher diet is impossible, then the patient must decide to wave the dietary restrictions. All commandments are suspended whenever a life is in danger, no matter how remote the likelihood of death (Feldman, 1986). Food is essential to maintain life; therefore the person would be directed by the rabbi to eat whatever the hospital could provide that would help sustain life.

Yom Kippur (the Day of Atonement) and Passover are two holidays that require special consideration. On Yom Kippur a Jew is required to fast for 24 hours. If this fast is considered physically or medically dangerous, however, the Jew is required by law to put aside the law and eat.

Passover requires that special foods be served. Passover, which falls in or near the spring of the year, is an 8-day holiday that celebrates the freedom of the Jews from Egypt. During these 8 days there are certain foods that must be "kosher for Passover." In addition, there are other foods that are forbidden, including any foods with leavening (bread, cakes made with baking soda or powder) or foods made with even a small amount of a grain product or by-product that is not specifically prepared for Passover. This prohibition includes many drugs and medications, such as those containing starch or grain alcohol. These drugs may be refused by the patient unless they cannot be replaced and are urgently needed by the patient.

Procreation

The use, or nonuse, of contraceptives is dictated by Jewish law, which requires one to "be fruitful and multiply." This can cause special problems for the woman who is unable to conceive or the woman who may have physical problems making conception dangerous. There is a lengthy discussion of this issue in the Mishnah (a part of the Talmud containing the oral law). The final analysis is, the man is commanded to procreate, but the woman is not, because, it is believed, God would not impose on "the children of Israel" a burden "too difficult for a person to bear" (Gold, 1988). Since childbirth is painful and may be physically dangerous, it would be unfair for the Torah to impose the commandment for procreation on the woman.

When Jewish men were allowed two wives, this commandment was not a problem. Today, since monogamy is the rule in the Jewish community, procreation is seen as the couple's obligation. However, outside of the very Orthodox community, Jewish couples today decide on how many children they want, and most practice some form of birth control. Within the very Orthodox community, the use of birth control is discouraged unless pregnancy or delivery would be dangerous for the woman.

Couples who have a problem with fertility are encouraged to seek medical help. For the very Orthodox Jewish man, however, a problem arises in the collection of semen. Rabbis have declared that masturbation and the use of male contraceptives such as the condom are not permitted, because the Talmud outlaws the spilling of seed. For this reason, the woman is usually tested first and, if no problem can be detected, then the man may be tested. The very Orthodox Jewish husband will have to consult his rabbi before he consents to a sperm count. Since masturbation is considered taboo, it may be emotionally difficult for the man to collect his semen. This is not a problem for most non-Orthodox couples.

It is interesting to note that the role of companionship is given an equal place with procreation in the purpose of a Jewish marriage (Gold, 1988). To add to this idea of companionship, rabbis have also addressed the idea of sexual satisfaction being the right of both men and women within the bonds of marriage (Lutwak, Ney, & White, 1988).

Organ Transplants

According to Jewish law, all body parts should be buried with the body after death (Jakobovits, 1959). However, if an organ transplant would save the life of another human being, it is permissible to donate the organ (Feldman, 1986). Even removal of the heart for transplantation is allowed as long as the dying person has experienced total brainstem death (Feldman, 1986; Kolatch, 1985).

Life Support Measures

According to Jewish law, nothing may be done to hasten death; a patient must be given every chance for life. However, if the use of mechanical systems would help prolong death rather than life, they should not be used. If the systems have been connected and it is realized that they are not helping to prolong life but are prolonging death, they may be removed (Feldman, 1986).

The Dying Jewish Patient

As there are commandments that control living for the Jew, there are also commandments that control dying. These commandments are usually followed strictly only by Orthodox Jews, but some of the behaviors that the nurse may see in non-Orthodox Jews are due to the cultural knowledge that these commandments have created.

According to Jewish law, a person who is very ill and considered to be dying should not be left alone. One reason for this law is that the spirit is believed to depart from the body at the time of death, and if no one were present, the soul would feel alone and desolate (Sperling, 1968). To satisfy this commandment, family members will often take turns sitting with the critically or terminally ill patient. Asking family members to leave may cause family distress.

Jewish law also dictates that a patient should be informed that death is near. However, because of two controversial passages in the Torah, some rabbis have decided that it is important to inform a dying individual about serious illness, but not that death is near. Informing a person about a serious illness allows the individual time to put worldly affairs in order, as Isaac and Jacob did when they were told they would die (Heller, 1975). However, to tell a person that death is imminent removes all hope, and it is feared that this information may hasten death.

Judaism teaches that it is important to lead a good, decent, and helping life on earth. Since good deeds must be done on earth, the law requires a Jew to ask God to forgive those deeds that may have been against God or not in keeping with his commandments. To fulfill this commandment, the dying person is encouraged to recite the confessional. If the individual is too sick to say the whole confessional, the individual is encouraged to recite the affirmation of faith, the Shma. If the dying person cannot repeat any of the confessional, the law says it is up to the family or friends who are with the person to recite it for the patient.

Once death has been established, the eyes and mouth are closed by the son or nearest relative. In some Orthodox Jewish families it is customary to remove the body from the bed and place it on a straw mat on the floor with the person's feet toward the door through which the body will be taken. A candle is placed at the person's head to symbolize the "light," or joy and love the departed brought to others while alive (Trepp, 1980). A sheet is placed over the person's face, since it is disrespectful to the dead to permit others to see the ravages of death on the face (Sperling, 1968). The dead body is viewed as being contaminated by Orthodox Jews and is placed on the floor because the bed is viewed as being defiled by contact with the dead body; however, the ground is not considered defiled by contact (Sperling, 1968). It is important to note that this behavior is rarely seen in most hospitals or nursing homes today.

Autopsy is not allowed by Orthodox Jews unless (1) it is required by governmental regulations, (2) the person had a hereditary disease and autopsy may help safeguard the health of survivors, or (3) another known person is suffering from a similar deadly disease and an autopsy may yield information vital to that person's health (Jakobovits, 1959). If an autopsy is performed, all parts that are removed must be buried with the body. Autopsy does not pose a religious problem for the non-Orthodox Jew.

AIDS

It has been stated that "AIDS will cause psychological and social reactions that may change the character of human social life" (Edelheit, 1989). In the Jewish community AIDS poses a psychological, social, and religious problem. The problem lies in the traditional belief system of the Jewish people: according to the Torah, homosexuality is an abomination, and premarital sexual activity is not permitted by the traditional rabbinate. This belief system is a potential cause of distress for the Jewish homosexual, or for any Jew who tests HIV-positive. They not only have to live with their disease, but they also have to live with being an outcast of their culture.

Patient education in an Orthodox Jewish environment may be very difficult, and rabbis in all the religious groups are still trying to decide how to handle this situation. Some of them are addressing it and trying to teach about the disease and safe sex. It is not clear how Orthodox rabbis are handling the issue of "safe sex," since the use of the condom is prohibited by Jewish law, as is more than one sexual partner and homosexual behaviors.

AIDS and the Jewish patient is an area of great sensitivity for the nurse. The most important thing that the nurse can do for the Jewish AIDS victim is to be there for support. These victims not only need to deal with a terminal illness and rejection by the general society, they also need to deal with possible cultural and religious ostracization.

Wellness Behaviors

Jewish people tend to be more educated than most other American ethnic groups (Sowell, 1981), and the thirst for knowledge is apparent in their wellness behaviors. They tend to be well read on issues of health, and it is not unusual to hear Jews discussing the latest information on maintaining healthy diets, preventing disease, or following health-oriented regimens.

In years past, it was rare to see Jewish children involved in physical activities; Eastern European Jews tended to deemphasize physical activity in favor of more intellectual activities that kept the children closer to home. This may have stemmed from the fears of child abduction that they brought with them from "the old country" (Sowell, 1981). However, this trend seems to be changing. Jewish children are now involved with soccer teams, baseball teams, etc. Their parents are also more involved in physical exercise. Jogging, tennis, racquetball, and aerobics are some of the activities that are attracting more Jews since the importance of physical exercise has become talked about in the media.

Maintaining certain laws is included in the wellness behaviors seen in Orthodox Jewish people. Many of these laws have been incorporated into the everyday habits of most Americans because they are good hygiene and/or they have been proved to be medically prudent. The following are examples of these laws taken from the *Code of Jewish Law* (Ganzfried, 1927):

1. The hands must be washed on awakening from sleep, after elimination of bodily wastes, after hair cutting, after touching a vermin, and after being in proximity of a dead human body.
2. The proper way of washing oneself is to take a bath regularly every week.
3. It is advisable for one to accustom himself to having breakfast in the morning.
4. One is forbidden to eat or drink out of unclean vessels, and the individual should not eat with hands that are not clean.

Circumcision

According to Jewish teaching, God made a covenant with Abraham in which God promised to bless Abraham and make him prosper if Abraham would be loyal to God. This convenant was entered into and sealed by the act of circumcision. Jewish people honor this convenant by having a brit (which means "sign of the Covenant") on the eighth day of the baby's life. If the child is ill or was born prematurely, the brit is postponed until the infant is in good health.

The circumcision is usually done by a mohel, who is trained to do circumcisions. This is a time of celebration, and usually the entire family and some friends gather at the home of the baby's parents for this important occasion.

Since the circumcision is performed in the home, the nurse should review the principles of circumcision care with the mother before discharge. The postcircumcision care is usually managed by the mohel.

Implications for Nursing Care

The Jewish patient may be viewed as a difficult patient by the nurse. Jewish patients tend to be vocal about feelings, anxieties, and pain, but they may not be direct about what is bothering them. This type of verbalization can prove to be difficult for health care providers who expect the patient to be compliant, noncomplaining, and direct about needs. Nurses with judgmental attitudes may label the ill Jewish patient as childish, which leads to treating the patient as a child or ignoring the patient as much as possible. It is important for the nurse to remember that for the Jewish patient, this childlike behavior may be part of the culture. The nurse must be patient and let the patient know the nurse cares about needs, since this will lead to feelings of trust and may decrease what is seen as demanding behavior.

Demanding behavior is less likely to occur in second-, third-, or fourth-generation Jewish Americans, who are more aware of what is considered acceptable behavior by the general American culture. This does not mean that they feel pain or anxieties any less.

Illness is often viewed by Jews as a family affair. Because the whole family is involved with the ill person's suffering, the whole family wants to know what is happening with or to the patient. The family members often do not appear to trust the word of another family member and instead want to get the information directly from the physician or the nurse. To assist the family, and decrease the amount of time numerous explanations may take, it may help to have a family conference. However, not all the members may show up at the same time, and the nurse may still need to repeat the information. The most important message to convey to the family of a Jewish patient is that of caring, not only about the ill person, but also about each family member and the pain they are going through.

Assisting the patient who is dying, as well as the family, requires knowledge of Jewish cultural practices and beliefs. The nurse needs to remain sensitive to the need for a confessional if death is imminent and the patient is Orthodox. Studies have shown that following cultural practices helps decrease the amount of distress and disorganization felt by loved ones during the death and dying period (Dempsey, 1975; Ross, 1981). Therefore it is the duty of the nurse to assist families in following customs related to death and dying. When an Orthodox Jew dies, the body must not be touched by a person of the opposite sex. One nurse recounted the story of a young Chassidic boy who died and was washed by the nurses on the floor before the father arrived. The father became so upset that a female had touched his son's body that he told the nurses not to touch him, left the hospital, and returned a few minutes later with some dirt and a bag. He covered the boy's body with the dirt, put him in the bag, and carried him out of the hospital. He did this because the body was considered contaminated.

Jewish people are interested in health prevention and may ask in-depth questions to clarify what is being said. They may need to ask many questions in order to weigh information for personal impact, and these questions should not be misconstrued to indicate mistrust of the health care professional.

When caring for a Jewish patient, it is helpful for the nurse to know what form of religious practice is adhered to, since the Orthodox Jewish patient will follow religious practices more strictly than any other group. Unless the nurse works in an area that has a large number of Orthodox Jews, most Jewish patients cared for will be non-Orthodox and may not be affiliated with any group.

BIOLOGICAL VARIATIONS

Some people believe that a Jewish person can be recognized by physical appearance, and the "Semitic appearance" is occasionally related to cultural patterns (Goodman, 1979). However, Jews differ greatly in physical appearance depending on what part of the world they migrated to when forced out of Israel. Jews are not uniformly the same as far as height, hair and eye color, body structure, or shape of the nose is concerned. European Jews are White, Falashas (Ethiopian Jews) are Black, and Chinese Jews have Oriental features. The differences among Jews from different parts of the world are the results of biological adaptation to the area of the world resided in, intermarriage with non-Jews, and converts to Judaism (Goodman, 1979; Mourant, Kopec, & Domaniewsks-Sobczak, 1978).

To determine the extent of genetic similarity among Jews as opposed to non-Jews, studies of blood phenotypes have been done (Goodman, 1979; Mourant, Kopec, & Domaniewsks-Sobczak, 1978). As opposed to outward appearances, blood characteristics are unaffected by the environment.

Enzymatic and Genetic Variations

Although skin color, body size, and body structure vary depending on the part of the world resided in, fingerprint patterns indicate a relatedness among Jews from Germany, Turkey, Morocco, and Yemen. The patterns of fingerprint whorls, loops, and arches are similar to those of non-Jews living in the Mediterranean area. This seems to indicate that the Jewish people, although appearing to be diversified genetically, still maintain a remnant of the Mediterranean gene pool.

To classify genetic differences of peoples, polymorphic blood groups, serum and cell proteins, and enzyme variants that have altered catalytic activity, kinetic properties, stability, or electrophoretic mobility are used. Since anthropological structures and simple genetic traits of Jews are difficult to define, Jewish genetic studies have concentrated on the genetic polymorphisms (Rothchild, 1981) and have concluded that (1) Jewish groups from different parts of the world are very different genetically, (2) Jews of a certain area tend to resemble the surrounding non-Jews more than they resemble Jews from other parts of the world, and (3) European Jews have a residue of non-European genes that resemble Mediterranean genes (Patai & Wing, 1975).

A study by Stevenson, Schanfield, and Sandler (1985) on immunoglobulin allotypes had interesting results. The multivariate analyses indicated that the Jewish populations may be derived from a common gene pool. When the results were plotted, all the Jews, except the Yemenites group, were genetically similar to each other. The European Jewish cluster is the most closely knit in similarity and the Asian and North African Jewish clusters are closer to Middle Eastern groups than to European non Jews.

In relation to genetic disorders, the Jewish population is divided into Sephardic Jews, Oriental Jews, and Ashkenazi Jews. Since the largest number of Jews in the United States are Ashkenazi Jews (European), the rest of this discussion involves genetic disorders most prevalent in this group.

Of all the genetic disorders that occur most frequently in Eastern European Jews, the one receiving the most publicity is Tay-Sachs disease. This is a recessively inherited disease that is characterized by the absence of an enzyme involved in fat metabolism, resulting in the accumulation of fatty substances in the brain and leading to gradual neural and mental degeneration, with death occurring around the age of 3 or 4. Couples wherein both partners are Jews of Eastern European descent should be counseled to have genetic screening done to prevent the possibility of having a child with this deadly disease.

Susceptibility to Disease

Susceptibility to disease for Jewish people depends on geographic origin. Some beliefs about Jewish susceptibility have no real scientific basis, for example, the belief of some that Jews are more likely than others to have diabetes mellitus. Some studies have shown that Jews are no more susceptible to this disease than non-Jews from the same area of the world, as had been originally thought (Goodman, 1979).

Cancer

Certain cancers are more frequent in certain groups of Jews than in others. Stomach cancer is more prevalent among Jews from Europe and America. Breast cancer, the most frequent type of cancer for all Jewish female groups except those from Iran (Patai & Wing, 1975), has been found to be higher in Jewish women from Europe and America than in those from Asia. Cancer of the ovary is generally higher in Jews from Europe than in those from Asia or Africa.

Historically, cancer of the cervix has been lower in Jewish women than in non-Jews (Patai & Wing, 1975). However, as Jews become more acculturated and the incidence of multiple sexual partners, as well as partners who are not circumcised, increases, so does the incidence of cervical cancer. Cervical cancer is an area of concern for some Jewish individuals and is an area where patient teaching is helpful.

Heart disease

A 1952 study of serum cholesterol levels in New York found a higher frequency of elevated serum cholesterol levels among Jews than among non-Jews. It is believed that elevated serum cholesterol levels may be due to a single gene (Patai & Wing, 1975). If this is true, Ashkenazi Jews may have a higher frequency of the gene than do Oriental Jews, who seem to have a relatively low rate of elevated serum cholesterol levels.

It is commonly thought that Ashkenazi Jews are more prone to coronary heart disease than are other Jewish ethnic groups or non-Jews. In international comparisons of the rate of first-time myocardial infarctions among men, Israel ranks among the highest in the world if all types of infarcts (including clinically unrecognized infarcts) are included (Mourant, Kopec, & Domaniewsks-Sobczak, 1978) . Although there is a relatively high incidence of infarcts in Israel, there is a low fatality rate. After numerous studies, the conclusion regarding heart disease in the Jewish population is that further studies need to be done to determine the frequency of the disease among Jews, as well as the interplay between heredity and environment (Mourant Kopec, & Domaniewsks-Sobczak, 1978).

Polycythemia vera

There is evidence indicating that polycythemia vera is more common in Ashkenazi Jews than in other ethnic groups. In addition, there seems to be a higher prevalence of polycythemia vera in Jewish men than in Jewish women (Mourant, Kopec, & Domaniewsks-Sobczak, 1978).

Diabetes mellitus

Diabetes has been referred to as the "Jewish disease" in Germany. Through ethnic Jewish studies done in Israel, an interesting phenomenon has been noted. There is a slightly higher percentage of Ashkenazi Jews than Sephardic Jews who have diabetes. Also, in Yemenite and Kurdish newcomers to Israel, there are almost no cases of diabetes. However, in Yemenite and Kurdish settlers who have lived in Israel for more than 25 years, the same frequency of diabetes as with Ashkenazi Jews has been identified (Mourant, Kopec, & Domaniewsks-Sobczak, 1978; Patai & Wing, 1975). The results of this study indicate that dietary habits have an influence on the development of diabetes. The main dietary change in the older settlers as compared with the new arrivals has been an increased intake of sugar.

Although the incidence of diabetes in Jewish people has been indicated as being higher than in the general population, there have been no studies to confirm this belief. Most of the studies on diabetes among Jews have been done in Israel. For a truer assessment of the prevalence of diabetes in the Jewish community, further studies outside Israel need to be conducted (Mourant, Kopec, & Domaniewsks-Sobczak, 1978).

Crohn's disease

Studies indicate that Crohn's disease occurs in Jewish males more often than in Jewish females, and in Jews more often than in any other White ethnic group (Mourant, Kopec, & Domaniewsks-Sobczak, 1978). Although the number of young people diagnosed as having this disease has been increasing (Thompson et al., 1989), it is not known if the increase is due to a better awareness of the disease and improved diagnostic techniques or if there is an actual increase in the number of cases.

Ulcerative colitis

Uncerative colitis is seen more frequently in Ashkenazi Jews than in non-Jews or any other Jewish ethnic groups. It has many similarities to Crohn's disease and may even be seen in conjunction with Crohn's disease. The cause of ulcerative colitis is unknown, but familial tendencies have been noted; it occurs 10% to 15% more often in families of patients with ulcerative colitis than in families of control patients without the disease (Mourant, Kopec, & Domaniewsks-Sobczak, 1978).

Myopia

Jews seems to have a larger incidence of myopia than the general population, and it occurs more often in boys than in girls. It is important to note that myopia is not caused by close book work, as was thought many years ago, but by a prevalence of low hypermetropia and factors that allow for a greater or longer development of the length of the eye. Vision screening is an important part of a physical examination for Jewish people, particularly Jewish children.

Nutritional Preferences and Deficiencies

Jewish people tend to eat a lot of dairy products, which becomes a concern in patients with a history of lactose intolerance. Lactose intolerance has been identified among some Jewish ethnic groups, and a study done in Israel identified approximately two thirds of the Jewish population in Israel as being lactase deficient. However, the researchers also noted that most of these patients were not aware of their milk intolerance, leading to the conclusion that the condition was relatively benign and asymptomatic in the Jews studied (Mourant, Kopec, & Domaniewsks-Sobczak, 1978). Any Jewish patient with a history of diarrhea, nonspecific lower gastrointestinal symptoms, and abdominal pain should have a good dietary history taken to check for a history of milk intolerance. The nurse needs to determine any family tendency toward lactose intolerance, as well as the relationship between foods and the onset of abdominal symptoms.

It is important for the nurse to remember that not all Jews maintain a kosher diet and that some Jews are more strict about their diet than others. If the nurse is caring for an Orthodox Jewish patient who is not eating properly because of the conflict between maintaining a kosher diet and eating institutional food, the nurse should consult with the family about bringing food from home. If the family cannot help with this situation, the patient's rabbi may be consulted.

Psychological Characteristics

Jews have been labeled with certain personality traits for over 3000 years. According to the Bible, the Children of Israel, following their exodus from Egypt, were "stiff-necked," quarrelsome, disobedient, and rebellious. In Talmudic literature the Jews are described as "the merciful sons of a merciful father." Greek and Roman authors, who were usually anti-Semitic, made derogatory comments on the Jewish character.

It was not until the 1930s that studies began to explore Jewish personality characteristics (Patai & Wing, 1975). All of these studies involved Jewish Americans, and most involved college students. The conclusions derived from these studies are (Patai & Wing, 1975):

1. Studies indicate that Jews are superior in intelligence to comparable groups of non-Jews, especially in verbal intelligence. It is questionable whether Jews are genetically more intelligent than non-Jews; the apparent superiority in intelligence may be due to the pressures from the Gentile world for Jews to rely on their brains in order to survive.
2. In scholarly, intellectual, literary, and artistic pursuits, Jews seem to be proportionately overrepresented. Whether this phenomenon is proof of special Jewish talent or the result of extraneous circumstances that attracted Jews to concentrate on certain areas is open for debate.
3. As far as character traits are concerned, it is difficult to pinpoint differences between Jews and non-Jews. Character traits seem to be formed more by personal experiences in the immediate environment than by historical conditioning. As an example, Jewish Americans have been characterized as being aggressive, and this aggressiveness may be due to the pressure placed on Jewish children by their parents to "have a better life" than they did.

Anti-Semitism is a concern for Jewish people. Within the Jewish community mention is often made of Jewish paranoia in regard to anti-Semitism. Although the relative freedom experienced in the United States has led to a decrease in the practice of many Jewish rituals, and possibly to the increased numbers of nonpracticing Jews, there are constant reminders that Jews are different and not always accepted by the general public. Today, in addition to constant reminders of the Holocaust, some Jewish people are also concerned about events in Israel.

Mental health

The older medical literature indicates that the rate of occurrence of a variety of mental illnesses in Jews is high. In discussing this issue with numerous psychiatrists and leaders in the mental health field, Mourant, Kopec, and Domaniewsks-Sobczak (1978) have concluded that necessary data are lacking to confirm that the old medical literature is correct.

One concern among psychiatrists and mental health workers in Orthodox Jewish sections is the apparent need for, but lack of use of, mental health facilities. To determine what discourages Orthodox Jews from seeking psychiatric professional help, a study was conducted with 20 Orthodox Jewish mental health outpatients, which revealed that Orthodox Jews attach a stigma to mental health treatment and to Jews who avail themselves of it. This stigma is partly the result of an association of mental health treatment with insanity and partly because of the fear that this knowledge will have a negative effect on matrimonial prospects (Wikler, 1986).

It is important for the nurse to remember that Orthodox Jews do not enter mental health treatment easily. In the case of an Orthodox Jew who may need psychiatric counseling, there may be resistance to overcome before treatment can be started. The prospective patient may display a real concern about confidentiality that may be seen as paranoia. This paranoia needs to be understood within the context of the social risk involved.

Orthodox Jews who do seek mental health care usually choose the agency or therapist because of the reputation of the agency or therapist. One agency that opened its office in the Williamsburg section of Brooklyn, New York, in the heart of the Chassidic and Orthodox Jewish section, was picketed and threatened. Today, however, this center has earned the "grudging" respect of the community (Meer, 1987).

Alcoholism

The literature reports that Jews have had a low incidence of alcoholism in the past (Mourant, Kopec, & Domaniewsks-Sobczak, 1978). This assumption is questionable, and the incidence of cross-addiction—to both alcohol and another substance—may be higher among Jews than among non-Jews (Steinhardt, 1988). Lieberman (1987) has noted that Jews do not acknowledge a problem with alcohol because of their perception of what an alcoholic is: many Jews view the alcoholic as a skid-row bum, not a person who gets drunk and acts silly at a wedding, or maybe drinks too much when celebrating a holiday or festival, even if this behavior occurs on a regular basis.

All the behaviors that characterize the alcoholic in general—denial, isolation, ignorance of the disease, and guilt—seem to be intensified in the Jewish alcoholic because of the myth of Jewish sobriety. Orthodox Jews seem to suffer the greatest from these symptoms (Steinhardt, 1988).

Studies done in the United States indicate that drinking disorders tend to increase in Jews as religious affiliation shifts from Orthodox, to Conservative, to Reform, to secular (Mourant, Kopec, & Domaniewsks-Sobczak, 1978). Some sociologists have suggested that alcoholism among Jews may increase as acculturation proceeds.

Of greatest concern to the Jewish community, and to health care workers, is the increasing alcohol and drug abuse among the Jewish youth. It is important to educate the Jewish community on the facts that alcoholics are not just skid-row, homeless people and that the ceremonial and social drinking of the Jewish community can increase the potential for alcoholism if it is not tempered.

Holocaust survivors

Although the Holocaust has had a large effect on Jewish feelings regarding "Jewishness" and persecution, the Holocaust survivors have had very little effect on the

Jewish culture in America as a whole. The reason for this is the relatively small number of Jewish Americans who fall into this category.

Many studies have been done on the effects of the Holocaust on survivors (Kren & Rappoport, 1980; Rose & Garske, 1987). These studies have helped the medical profession, especially the psychiatric medical profession, to determine the effects of war atrocities on people who have experienced them.

Many Jews have a difficult time discussing the effects of the Holocaust and its devastation to Jewish families and communities. Jewish individuals sometimes leave the room when the Holocaust is mentioned or joke to relieve their distress or feelings of anger and bewilderment at how this type of event could occur in modern times in a country that was supposed to be "civilized."

The effects of the Holocaust on the survivors and their children are still being studied. From the literature comes evidence of anger, depression, withdrawal, and anxiety in the survivors (Krystal & Niederland, 1971; Steinitz & Szonyi, 1979). The bearing of children was seen as a means for the survivors to replace their loved ones who were lost during "The War," and the children were seen as a source of new hope and meaning. Because of this transference, the children of the survivors were usually overprotected and placed in situations that created unrealistic expectations on the growing child (Nadler, Kav-Venaki, & Gleitman, 1985).

Numerous studies have been done on children of Holocaust survivors. The results of these studies indicate that, on the whole, this population is well adjusted, with few significant psychopathological problems (Nadler, Kav-Venaki, & Gleitman, 1985; Rose & Garske, 1987; Steinitz & Szonyi, 1979). The biggest problems for these children seem to be related to the pressures they feel to protect their parents from any further physical or psychological pain, and to the desire to fulfill their parents' unrealistic need to have the child compensate for what has been lost. These feelings lead to feelings of guilt when the children attempt to become emancipated from their parents.

Types of personality characteristics that most studies have discovered in Holocaust survivors are repressed anger, feelings of guilt, depression, feelings of being different, a strong feeling of Jewishness (even if they are nonpracticing Jews), a concern for Jewish survival (often more intense than in non–Holocaust survivors), and a desire to maintain Jewish tradition that may border on obsession (Nadler, Kav-Venaki, & Gleitman, 1985; Rose & Garske, 1987; Steinitz & Szonyi, 1979).

Some Jewish people believe that it is important that the memory of the Holocaust never die and that no event like this should ever happen again. These same people believe there should never be mass destruction of any people. Perhaps protecting the memory of the Holocaust is one plausible explanation for the vast amount of literature that has been published regarding the Holocaust and its effect on the survivors. Some Jewish people believe that the Holocaust was just one more act of persecution against a people who have endured thousands of years of being victims to ignorance and misunderstandings.

Implications for Nursing Care

The nurse caring for a Jewish American patient should get a careful history of the patient's eating habits. Many ethnic Jewish foods are high in animal and saturated fats. Since these are known to influence the amount of cholesterol in the body and since high cholesterol is known to be a factor in heart disease, dietary education is important with this cultural group. In addition, many prepared kosher foods are made with eggs, as well as palm or coconut oil. Jewish patients who maintain a kosher diet must be cautioned to read labels carefully on all prepared kosher foods.

Because of the use of dairy products by this cultural group, as well as the high incidence of Crohn's disease and ulcerative colitis, a history regarding bowel habits and abdominal problems should be carefully obtained. The nurse needs to remain alert for any symptoms that may indicate lactose intolerance. In addition, the nurse needs to remain alert for signs of drug or alcohol abuse. Since alcohol consumption is considered permissible at religious and secular functions, excessive drinking on a routine basis may not be viewed as a problem by the individual or the family. Cultural beliefs and taboos may make educating the patient about the potential for alcohol abuse difficult.

Assisting Orthodox Jewish patients in areas of psychological needs takes patience and understanding on the part of the nurse. Not only may patients have concerns about personal acceptance by peers, but they may also worry that knowledge of psychiatric problems in the family will lead to potential problems in finding a suitable mate for themselves or future children. Going to counseling is equated with being "crazy," and being "crazy" is seen as a hereditary problem. Further education on psychiatric and emotional problems is needed to change negative attitudes about treatment.

SUMMARY

It is crucial that the nurse remember that not all Jewish patients are alike. While some Jewish patients are Orthodox and follow the commandments strictly, other Jewish people, with each successive generation, have become more acculturated to the behavior of the people around them.

Caring for the Jewish American patient can be a challenge. Although nursing education traditionally has prepared nurses to view health from a singular professional perspective, health must also be understood from a cultural perspective when care is being provided to patients whose cultural background differs from that of the nurse (Leininger, 1985). A number of educational programs are seeking to address this issue by providing transcultural experiences for student nurses. Other health care facilities are offering educational programs to new nurses and nurses already in practice. One such experience related to the Jewish patient is at Baycrest Centre for Geriatric Care in Toronto, Canada (Gorrie, 1989; Gould-Stuart, 1986; Rose, 1981). This program provides a transcultural experience for nurses in orientation and for selected nurses on a continuing care unit of the hospital. During this experience, differences between the Jewish culture and the secular culture are examined. Such educational programs can assist nurses in developing increased understanding of the universality of various cultural attributes and the importance of culture to all individuals.

CASE
STUDY   Esther Rosenbloom is admitted to a nursing home following a fall that resulted in a fractured hip. Esther, age 87, immigrated from Russia with her family in 1910, at the age of 8. She is brought to the nursing home by her son-in-law, Nat, and her daughter, Bernice. Esther is

being admitted for physical therapy and is expecting to be discharged to her home after learning to walk with a walker. Her home is a block away from her daughter and son-in-law's.

Esther was raised in an Orthodox home in Brooklyn, New York, but joined the Conservative movement when she married at age 24. Bernice, age 61, informs the nurse that although Esther follows Conservative thought, she maintains a kosher diet. The nursing home she is admitted to has very few Jewish patients and is not familiar with kosher diets. Bernice also mentions that her mother has abdominal difficulties if she ingests too much cheese or milk.

Esther appears worried, is moaning, and is complaining of pain in her hip. Bernice's eyes appear red, as if she has been crying. Bernice is wringing her hands and mentions that her mother has been uncomfortable and that she hopes the nurses at the nursing home will be able to keep Esther comfortable.

When the nurse asks Esther how she is feeling, she states in a whining tone of voice, "My hip hurts, and I want to go home. How are you going to feed me here? What do you know from kosher foods?"

When moving Esther from wheelchair to bed, the nurse notes that Esther does not seem to want to assist, despite the fact that the transfer sheet notes that Esther can move from wheelchair to bed with minimal assistance. When asked why she did not help, Esther replies, "I'm just too tired."

Esther is usually self-sufficient and very busy with her volunteer activities, despite decreased visual acuity, for which she wears glasses. Although Bernice mentions that her mother always worries about her bowels, Ester does not have a history of constipation. She is continent of urine and stool.

CARE PLAN

Nursing Diagnosis Pain related to fractured hip and anxiety. Supportive data: complains of pain, appears upset and tense, has difficulty transferring from chair to bed.

Patient Outcome	***Nursing Interventions***
Pain will decrease.	1 Medicate as ordered.
	2 Use comfort measures (e.g., relaxation techniques, diversional activities) to promote relaxation.
	3 Assist patient to a comfortable position.
	4 Spend at least 10 minutes per shift, while patient is awake, to allow for expression of feelings.

Nursing Diagnosis Nutrition, altered: less than body requirements, related to religious and cultural dietary restrictions plus possible lactose intolerance.

Patient Outcome	***Nursing Interventions***
Patient will maintain weight within normal limits.	1 Determine patient's likes and dislikes in foods that the institution can provide that meet with patient's religious restrictions.
	2 Request that family bring ethnic foods from home that patient would enjoy.

3 Serve foods on paper plates with plastic utensils to avoid mixing permissible foods with nonkosher foods.

4 Offer cheese or milk products in small amounts until tolerance can be determined.

5 If milk products are ingested, assess for abdominal cramps and diarrhea.

Nursing Diagnosis   Anxiety related to situational crisis.

Patient Outcome	**Nursing Interventions**
Patient will adust to new living arrangements with minimal difficulty.	1 Spend time with patient to allow verbalization of fears, discomforts. 2 Find activities patient is interested in and attempt to have patient participate in facility activities. 3 Encourage independence. 4 Include patient in decisions related to her care whenever feasible. 5 Allow family to spend as much time as desired with patient. 6 Give patient clear, concise explanations of anything that is about to occur. 7 Introduce patient to other Jewish patients and encourage them to visit with each other. 8 Remain nonjudgmental toward family and patient. 9 Contact rabbi and ask him to visit if patient wishes.

Nursing Diagnosis   Anxiety related to maturational crisis.

Patient Outcome	**Nursing Interventions**
Patient will identify potential and actual sources of anxiety.	1 Encourage patient to identify stressful life events experienced within the last year. 2 Spend specific amount of uninterrupted time with patient to listen to her concerns. 3 Allow family to spend as much time with patient as they desire. 4 Involve family in patient's care if desired. 5 Assist patient in identifying sources of fear or tension. 6 Assist patient in identifying activities that help decrease anxiety and encourage the use of these activities.

Nursing Diagnosis Mobility, impaired physical, related to discomfort, fractured hip, and
possible fear.

Patient Outcome	*Nursing Interventions*
Patient will be able to transfer easily by self from bed to chair and ambulate with walker with minimal assistance.	1 Provide physical therapy daily. 2 Reinforce what patient is learning in physical therapy. 3 Observe patient's functional ability daily. 4 Encourage and compliment patient liberally. 5 Encourage verbalization of fears and feelings regarding altered state of mobility. 6 Remain nonjudgmental when patient is unwilling to perform to her ability. 7 Provide comfort measures, such as medication as ordered and padding of extremities that may be prone to skin breakdown. 8 Do range-of-motion (ROM) exercises to increase strength; instruct family in ROM exercises and encourage them to encourage patient. 9 Promote progressive ambulation. 10 Discuss use of distraction and other nonpharmacological pain relief. 11 Explain necessity of moving, even when in pain, to prevent arthritic conditions or contractions and increased stiffness.

Nursing Diagnosis Injury, potential for, related to impaired mobility, decreased visual acuity, and new environment.

Patient Outcome	*Nursing Interventions*
Patient will sustain no injury.	1 Encourage use of a walker, with assistance. 2 Assist patient when getting slow of breath (SOB), out of chair or walking. 3 Be sure floor is dry and furniture and litter are out of the way when patient is engaging in activities that may cause falls. 4 Instruct patient and family regarding safety practices when using walker or transferring. 5 Keep side rails up when patient is in bed. 6 Maintain bed in low position.

Nursing Diagnosis   Constipation related to decreased mobility.

Patient Outcome	*Nursing Interventions*
Patient will not develop constipation.	1 Monitor frequency and characteristics of stools, and record.
	2 Recognize that patient may have concerns about bowels because of age and culture.
	3 Ask patient if she has a specific routine at home, such as a normal time for defecation or use of prune juice (a favorite "remedy" for Eastern European Jews).
	4 Encourage fluid intake of 2000 ml per day.

Nursing Diagnosis   Spiritual distress (potential for) related to separation from religious and cultural ties.

Patient Outcome	*Nursing Interventions*
Patient will express feelings of spiritual distress.	1 Listen for cues that patient may be having spiritual distress (e.g., "Why did God do this to me?").
	2 Remain nonjudgmental.
	3 Acknowledge spiritual concerns and encourage expression of thoughts and feelings.
	4 Find ways to help patient maintain kosher diet.
	5 Encourage patient to continue her religious practices during hospitalization, and do whatever is necessary to help facilitate this.
	6 Ask patient if she desires rabbi to visit, and contact synagogue if necessary.
	7 Introduce patient to and help foster friendships with other Jewish patients.
	8 If patient can have pass, and family and patient desire it, make arrangements for patient to attend Friday night or Saturday services.

STUDY
QUESTIONS

1. List ways that a kosher diet can be maintained while a patient is in the hospital.
2. List religious needs a Jewish patient may have while being hospitalized that nursing staff can assist with.
3. Identify three communication barriers that a nurse may encounter when giving care to a Jewish American patient.
4. List biological variations a patient who is Jewish may have that will affect care given by a nurse.

5. Explain relationship characteristics that families of Jewish patients usually display toward a hospitalized relative.
6. Explain how Jewish people may react toward the impending death of a relative.

REFERENCES

Bash, D.M. (1980, Sept./Oct.). Jewish religious practices related to childbearing. *Journal of Nurse-Midwifery, 25,* 5.

Dempsey, D. (1975). *The way we die.* New York: MacMillan.

Edelheit, J. (1989, July/Aug.). The rabbi and the abyss of AIDS. *Tikkun, 4*(4), 67-69.

Feldman, D.M. (1986). *Health and medicine in the Jewish tradition.* New York: Crossroad.

Ganzfried, S. (1927). *Code of Jewish law: A compilation of Jewish laws and customs.* New York: Hebrew Publishing.

Glazer, N. (1957). *American Judaism.* Chicago: University of Chicago Press.

Gold, M. (1988). *And Hannah wept: Infertility, adoption and the Jewish couple.* Philadelphia: Jewish Publication Society.

Goodman, R. (1979). *Genetic disorders among the Jewish people.* Baltimore: Johns Hopkins University Press.

Gorrie, M. (1989). Reaching clients through cross cultural education. *Journal of Gerontological Nursing, 15*(10), 29-31.

Gould-Stuart, J. (1986). Bridging the cultural gap between residents and staff. *Geriatric Nursing, 7,* 319-321.

Heller, Z. (1975). The Jewish view of death: Guidelines for dying. In E. Kubler-Ross (Ed.), *Death: The final stage of growth.* Englewood Cliffs, N.J.: Prentice Hall.

Howe, I. (1976). *World of our fathers.* New York: Harcourt Brace Jovanovich.

Jakobovits, I. (1959). *Jewish medical ethics.* New York: Philosophical Library.

Janowsky, O. (1964). *The American Jew: A reappraisal.* Philadelphia: Jewish Publication Society.

Kaplan, R. (1970, May 26). *An experience with residual populations in Detroit.* Paper presented at the annual meeting of the National Conference of Jewish Communal Service, Boston.

Kertzer, M. (1978). *What is a Jew* (4th ed.). New York: World Publishing.

Kolatch, A.J. (1985). *The second Jewish book of why.* New York: Jonathan David.

Kren, G.M., & Rappoport, L. (1980). *The Holocaust and the crisis of human behavior.* New York: Holmes & Meier.

Krystal, H., & Niederland, W.G. (1971). *Psychic traumatization: After effects in individuals and communities.* Boston: Little, Brown.

Leininger, M. (1985). Transcultural nursing: An essential knowledge and practice field for today. *Canadian Nurse, 80*(11), 41-45.

Lieberman, L. (1987). Jewish alcoholics and the disease concept. *Journal of Psychology and Judaism, 13*(3), 165-179.

Lutwak, R., Ney, A.M., & White, J.E. (1988, Jan./Feb.). Maternity nursing and Jewish law. *Maternal and Child Health, 13,* 3.

Meer, J. (1987, April). An open door. *Psychology Today,* p. 17.

Mourant, A.E., Kopec, A.C., & Domaniewsks-Sobczak, K. (1978). *The genetics of the Jews.* New York: Oxford University Press.

Nadler, A., Kav-Venaki, S., & Gleitman, B. (1985). Transgenerational effects of the Holocaust: Externalization of aggression in second generation of Holocaust survivors. *Journal of Consulting and Clinical Psychology, 53*(3), 365-369.

Novak, W., & Waldoks, M. (1981). *The big book of Jewish humor.* Philadelphia: Harper & Row.

Patai, R., & Wing, J.P. (1975). *The myth of the Jewish race.* New York: Charles Scribner's Sons.

Popenoe, D. (1977). *Sociology* (3rd ed.). Englewood Cliffs, N.J.: Prentice Hall.

Rose, A. (1981). The Jewish elderly: Behind the myths. In M. Weinfield, W. Whaffer, & I. Cotler (Eds.), *The Canadian Jewish mosaic* (pp. 199-200). New York: John Wiley & Sons.

Rose, S.L., & Garske, J. (1987). Family environment, adjustment, and coping among children of Holocaust survivors: A comparative investigation. *American Journal of Orthopsychiatrics, 57*(3), 332-342.

Ross, H.M. (1981, Oct.). Cultural views regarding death and dying. *Topics in Clinical Nursing,* pp. 1-16.

Rosten, L. (1968). *The joys of Yiddish*. New York: Pocket Books.

Rothchild, H. (1981). *Biocultural aspects of disease*. New York: Academic Press.

Sachar, A.L. (1964). *A history of the Jews*. New York: Alfred A. Knopf.

Schlesinger, B. (1971). *The Jewish family: A survey and annotated bibliography*. Toronto: University of Toronto Press.

Schneider, S. (1985). *The non-Orthodox Jewish perspective of dying and death*. Thesis submitted to the University of Arizona, Tucson.

Schwartz, E. (1984). The non-Orthodox Jewish perspective on dying and death. Thesis, University of Arizona, Tucson.

Sowell, T. (1981). *Ethnic America*. New York: Basic Books.

Sperling, A. (1968). *Reasons for Jewish customs and traditions*. New York: Bloch.

Steinhardt, D. (1988, Feb.). Alcoholism: The myth of Jewish immunity. *Psychology Today,* p. 10.

Steinitz, L.Y., & Szonyi, D.M. (Eds.). (1979). *Living after the Holocaust: Reflections by children of survivors in America*. New York: Bloch.

Stevenson, J.C., Schanfield, M.S., & Sandler, S.G. (1985). Immunoglobulin allotypes in Jewish populations living in Israel and the United States. *Immunoglobin Allotypes,* pp. 176-208.

Thompson, J.M., McFarland, G.K., Hirsch, J.E., Tucker, S.M., & Bowers, A.C. (1989). *Mosby's manual of clinical nursing* (2nd ed.). St. Louis: C.V. Mosby.

Trepp, L. (1980). *The complete book of Jewish observances*. New York: Behrman House.

Wikler, M. (1986). Pathways to treatment: How Orthodox Jews enter therapy. *Social Casework: The Journal of Contemporary Social Work,* pp. 113-118.

Zborowski, M. (1969). *People in pain*. San Francisco: Jossey-Bass.

Index